T0324122

Practical Guide to Obesity Medicine

Practical Guide to Obesity Medicine

JOLANTA URSZULA WEAVER, MRCS, MRCP, FRCP, PHD, CTLHE

Senior Lecturer in Diabetes Medicine
Institute of Cellular Medicine
Newcastle University
Newcastle upon Tyne, United Kingdom
Honorary Consultant Endocrinologist,
Queen Elizabeth Hospital, Gateshead Health,
NHS Foundation Trust,
Gateshead, United Kingdom.

ELSEVIER

ELSEVIER

3251 Riverport Lane
St. Louis, Missouri 63043

PRACTICAL GUIDE TO OBESITY MEDICINE
ISBN: 978-0-323-48559-3

Copyright © 2018 by Elsevier, Inc. All rights reserved.

No part of this publication may be reproduced or transmitted in any form or by any means, electronic or mechanical, including photocopying, recording, or any information storage and retrieval system, without permission in writing from the publisher. Details on how to seek permission, further information about the Publisher's permissions policies and our arrangements with organizations such as the Copyright Clearance Center and the Copyright Licensing Agency, can be found at our website: www.elsevier.com/permissions.

This book and the individual contributions contained in it are protected under copyright by the Publisher (other than as may be noted herein).

Notices

Knowledge and best practice in this field are constantly changing. As new research and experience broaden our understanding, changes in research methods, professional practices, or medical treatment may become necessary.

Practitioners and researchers must always rely on their own experience and knowledge in evaluating and using any information, methods, compounds, or experiments described herein. In using such information or methods they should be mindful of their own safety and the safety of others, including parties for whom they have a professional responsibility.

With respect to any drug or pharmaceutical products identified, readers are advised to check the most current information provided (i) on procedures featured or (ii) by the manufacturer of each product to be administered, to verify the recommended dose or formula, the method and duration of administration, and contraindications. It is the responsibility of practitioners, relying on their own experience and knowledge of their patients, to make diagnoses, to determine dosages and the best treatment for each individual patient, and to take all appropriate safety precautions.

To the fullest extent of the law, neither the Publisher nor the authors, contributors, or editors, assume any liability for any injury and/or damage to persons or property as a matter of products liability, negligence or otherwise, or from any use or operation of any methods, products, instructions, or ideas contained in the material herein.

Content Strategist: Kayla Wolfe
Content Development Manager: Taylor Ball
Content Development Specialist: Meredith Madeira
Publishing Services Manager: Deepthi Unni
Project Manager: Janish Ashwin Paul
Designer: Gopalakrishnan Venkatraman

Printed in United States of America

Last digit is the print number: 9   8   7   6   5   4   3   2   1

Working together
to grow libraries in
developing countries

www.elsevier.com • www.bookaid.org

List of Contributors

Ian A. Aird, MBChB, DA, FRCOG
Consultant Obstetrician and Gynaecologist
Queen Elizabeth Hospital
Gateshead, United Kingdom, Visiting Professor,
    Faculty of Health Sciences and Wellbeing
University of Sunderland
United Kingdom

**Nimantha M.W. de Alwis, MBBS, MD,
FRCP, PhD**
Consultant in Diabetes & Endocrinology
Department of Diabetes, Endocrinology &
    Metabolic Medicine
Sunderland Royal Hospital
Sunderland, United Kingdom

**Ananthi Anandhakrishnan MBBS, iBSc
Neuroscience (Hons)**
Centre for Endocrinology
William Harvey Research Institute
Barts and the London School of Medicine and
    Dentistry
Queen Mary University of London
London, United Kingdom

Stephen L. Atkin, MBBS, FRCP, PhD
Weill Cornell Medicine Education City, Qatar
    Foundation
Doha, Qatar

Anindo Banerjee, PhD, FRCP, Dr.
Department of Respiratory Medicine
Southampton General Hospital
Southampton, United Kingdom

Philippe Bareille, MD
Discovery Medicine, GSK
Stevenage, United Kingdom

Jordan Barnard, BSc (Hons)
South Tees Hospitals NHS Foundation Trust
SWMS Office, Langbaurgh House
Guisborough, United Kingdom

Ayat Bashir, MBBS
Newcastle Hospitals Trust
Newcastle upon Tyne, United Kingdom

Frauke Becker, PhD
Health Economics Research Centre
Nuffield Department of Population Health
University of Oxford
Oxford, United Kingdom
Health Economics Group
Institute of Health & Society
Newcastle University
Newcastle, United Kingdom

Helene Brandon, MBChB, FRCOG
Queen Elizabeth Hospital Gateshead Health NHS
    Foundation Trust
Queen Elizabeth Hospital
Sheriff Hill, United Kingdom

**Matthew D. Campbell, PhD, ACSM CES,
Bsc (Hons.)**
Institute of Sport, Physical Activity and Leisure
AGADA Diabetes Education and Research Institute
Leeds Beckett University
Leeds, United Kingdom

K. Clément, MD, PhD
Institute of Cardiometabolism and Nutrition (ICAN)
Nutrition Department and French Reference Centre
    for Prader-Willi Syndrome
Pitié-Salpêtrière Hospital
Assistance Publique-Hôpitaux de Paris
INSERM, Nutriomics UMR_S U1166, University
    Pierre et Marie Curie-Paris 6, 47–83 Boulevard de
    l'hôpital
Paris, France

**Esther M. Cohen-Tovée, BA, MA, MPhil,
DClinPsy, AFBPsS**
Northumberland, Tyne & Wear NHS Foundation Trust
St Nicholas Hospital
Newcastle upon Tyne, United Kingdom

Piers L Cornelissen BA, MBBS, DPhil
Professor of Cognitive Neuroscience
Department of Psychology
Northumbria University
United Kingdom

Caroline Day, PhD, FRSB
Diabetes Group
School of Life and Health Sciences
Aston University
Birmingham, United Kingdom

B. Dubern, MD, PhD
Institute of Cardiometabolism and Nutrition (ICAN)
Department of Pediatric Nutrition and Gastroenterology
Armand-Trousseau Hospital
Assistance Publique-Hôpitaux de Paris
INSERM, Nutriomics UMR_S U1166
University Pierre et Marie Curie-Paris 6, 47–83
    Boulevard de l'hôpital
Paris, France

Pamela Dyson, PhD, RD
Research Dietitian
OCDEM, Churchill Hospital
Oxford, United Kingdom

Javier T. Gonzalez, PhD, MRes, BSc (Hons)
Department for Health
University of Bath
Bath, United Kingdom

Yitka Graham, PhD, BSc (Hons)
Senior Lecturer in Public Health, Faculty of Health
    Sciences and Wellbeing
University of Sunderland
Honorary Specialty Lead, Health Services Research
Department of General Surgery
City Hospitals Sunderland NHS Foundation Trust
Sunderland, United Kingdom

Emily Heiden, BM, MRCP
Southampton General Hospital
Southampton, United Kingdom

Nicola Heslehurst, BSc (Hons), MSc, PhD
Institute of Health & Society
Newcastle University
Newcastle upon Tyne, United Kingdom

Lucy Hewitson, BMedSci, MA, PGDip
South Tees Hospitals NHS Foundation Trust
Nutrition and Dietetic Department
The James Cook University Hospital
Middlesbrough, United Kingdom

Sarah Hill, BA, MSc
Health Economics Group, Institute of Health &
    Society
Newcastle University
Newcastle upon Tyne, United Kingdom

Charlotte Hilton, BSc, PhD
Faculty of Health and Life Sciences
School of Psychological, Social and Behavioural
    Sciences
Coventry University
Coventry, United Kingdom

Ann L. Hunter, BSc (Hons), MBChB (Hons), MRCP
MRC Clinical Research Fellow, Faculty of Biology,
    Medicine and Health
The University of Manchester
Manchester, United Kingdom

**Lynne Johnston, BA, MSc, PhD, CBTDip,
DClinPsych, AfBPsS**
City Hospitals Sunderland NHS Foundation Trust and
    Halley Johnston Associates LTD
Specialist Weight Management Services, Psychology
    Services
Sunderland Royal Hospital
Sunderland, United Kingdom

Susan E. Jones, MBChB, MD, FRCP
Consultant Physician in Diabetes, Endocrinology &
    Medical Education
University Hospital of North Tees
Honorary Senior Clinical Lecturer
University of Newcastle
United Kingdom

Marta Korbonits, MD, PhD
Professor of Endocrinology and Metabolism
Centre for Endocrinology
William Harvey Research Institute
Barts and the London School of Medicine and
    Dentistry
Queen Mary University of London
London, United Kingdom

Angelos Kyriacou, MBChB, MRCP, DipPGME
Consultant in Endocrinology & Diabetes
CEDM Centre of Endocrinology, Diabetes & Metabolism
Limassol, Cyprus
Clinical Consultant Fellow, Salford NHS Foundation
    Trust, Salford, Greater Manchester, United Kingdom

Claire Lane, BA, PhD, DipPsych, DClinPsych
Gloucestershire Hospitals NHS Foundation Trust
Specialist Weight Management Service, Health
    Psychology
Beacon House, Gloucestershire Royal Hospital,
    United Kingdom

Helen Long, BSc (Hons)
QE Gateshead, HCPC and British Dietetic Association
Nutrition and Dietetics Department
Queen Elizabeth Hospital
Gateshead, United Kingdom

Floriana S. Luppino, MD, PhD
Medical Doctor at Eurocross International Assistance
Independent Researcher
Leiden, The Netherlands

Cristina G. Matei, MD, MRCPCH, MSc
East and North Herts Institute of Diabetes and
    Endocrinology
Department of Paediatrics, Lister Hopsital
East and North Herts NHS Trust
Stevenage, United Kingdom

Ray Meleady, MD, FRCP
Consultant Cardiologist
Department of Cardiology
Queen Elizabeth Hospital Gateshead NHS
    Foundation Trust
Gateshead, United Kingdom

Yemi Oluboyede, BA, MSc, PhD
Health Economics Group
Institute of Health & Society
Newcastle University
Newcastle upon Tyne, United Kingdom

C. Poitou, MD, PhD
Institute of Cardiometabolism and Nutrition (ICAN)
Nutrition Department and French Reference Centre
    for Prader-Willi Syndrome
Pitié-Salpêtrière Hospital, Assistance Publique-
    Hôpitaux de Paris
INSERM, Nutriomics UMR_S U1166, University Pierre
    et Marie Curie-Paris 6, 47–83 Boulevard de l'hôpital
Paris, France

Unaiza Qamar, MBBS, FCPS, FRCPath
Department of Academic Endocrinology, Diabetes
    and Metabolism
University of Hull
Hull, United Kingdom

Zoe H. Rutherford, PhD, MSc, BSc (Hons)
Institute of Sport, Physical Activity and Leisure
Leeds Beckett University
Leeds, United Kingdom

Thozhukat Sathyapalan, MBBS, FRCP, MD
Department of Academic Endocrinology, Diabetes
    and Metabolism
University of Hull
Hull, United Kingdom

Emma Slack, BSc (Hons), MSc
Institute of Health & Society
Newcastle University
Newcastle upon Tyne, United Kingdom

Deborah Snowdon, BSc (Hons)
South Tees Hospitals NHS Foundation Trust
Nutrition and Dietetic Department
Langbaurgh House, Guisborough
United Kingdom

Sarah Steven, MBChB (Hons), MRCP, PhD
Consultant Diabetologist
Central Manchester University Hospitals NHS
    Foundation Trust
Manchester, United Kingdom

Grace Stonebanks, BSc (Hons)
QE Gateshead, HCPC and British Dietetic Association
Nutrition and Dietetics Department
Queen Elizabeth Hospital
Gateshead, United Kingdom

Akheel A. Syed, MBBS, MRCP, PhD, FRCP
Honorary Senior Lecturer, Faculty of Biology,
    Medicine and Health
The University of Manchester
Manchester, United Kingdom, Consultant
    Endocrinologist & Clinical Lead
Department of Endocrinology, Diabetes & Obesity
    Medicine
Salford Royal NHS Foundation Trust
Greater Manchester, United Kingdom

Martin J. Tovée, PhD
Professor of Psychology
School of Psychology
Lincoln University
United Kingdom

Arutchelvam Vijayaraman, FRCP, MD, MSc, PGDME
Consultant in Obesity, Diabetes and Endocrinology
    and Metabolism
Diabetes Care Centre
The James Cook University Hospital
Middlesbrough, United Kingdom

Jolanta U. Weaver, MRCS, FRCP, PhD, CTLHE
Senior Lecturer in Diabetes Medicine
Institute of Cellular Medicine
Newcastle University
Newcastle upon Tyne, United Kingdom

Manoj Wickramasinghe, MBBS
Foundation Year 2 doctor in Leeds Teaching Hospital
    Trust
Leeds, United Kingdom

Leonore M. de Wit, MSc, PhD
Faculty of Behavioral and Movement Sciences
VU University
Amsterdam, The Netherlands

Stephen Hyer, PhD, MD, FRCP
Epsom & St Helier University Hospitals NHS Trust

Preface: Does "Benign Obesity" Exist?

Global obesity is an overwhelming challenge to our modern life. The latest World Health Organization (WHO) fact sheet states: "Worldwide obesity has more than doubled since 1980. In 2014, more than 1.9 billion adults, 18 years and older, were overweight. Of these over 600 million were obese. 39% of adults aged 18 years and over were overweight in 2014, and 13% were obese. Most of the world's population live in countries where overweight or obesity kills more people than being underweight. 41 million children under the age of 5 were overweight or obese in 2014. Obesity is preventable".[1]

One wonders how we can rise to this challenge, what resources are required, and who do we need to be concerned about?

Evidence-based policies are the only solution to this tsunami of economic, societal, and health burden. How do we prioritize our effort in preventing or treating obesity?

The World Health Organization provides several body mass index (BMI) categories for application to research, guidelines, and clinical practice.[2] The BMI categories are defined as underweight ($<18.5\,kg/m^2$), recommended normal weight range ($18.5-24.9\,kg/m^2$), overweight ($25-29.9\,kg/m^2$), and obese ($\geq30\,kg/m^2$). The obesity category can also be further subdivided into class I ($30-34.9\,kg/m^2$), class II ($35-39.9\,kg/m^2$), and class III obesity ($\geq40\,kg/m^2$).

An increased BMI in the range defined as obesity with BMI $\geq30\,kg/m^2$ has been associated with increased mortality.[3-5] However, detailed data from a large metaanalysis found that while a BMI $\geq35\,kg/m^2$ (grade 2-3 obesity) was associated with a higher hazard ratio (HR): 1.29 (95% CI 1.18-1.41) for all-cause mortality, paradoxically overweight individuals (BMI: $25-30\,kg/m^2$) had lower HR: 0.94 (95% CI 0.91-0.96) for all-cause mortality than individuals with a normal weight BMI ($18.5-25\,kg/m^2$).[6]

It is well known that individuals in the same BMI category can have substantial heterogeneity of metabolic features such as fat distribution, central versus peripheral, lipid profile, blood pressure, and glucose tolerance. Individuals of normal weight can display adverse metabolic features while obese individuals with normal metabolic features have been described as "metabolically healthy obese" or suffering from "benign obesity."[7-9] The "myth" of "benign obesity" and the paradox of lower all-cause mortality associated with being overweight have, however, been dispelled by the data from 61,386 individuals in eight separate studies from the past decade in a large metaanalysis, which identified 1455 studies published between 1950 and June 2013.[10]

In summary, Kramer and coworkers identified that when compared with metabolically healthy normal weight individuals, metabolically healthy obese individuals were at increased risk for all-cause mortality and cardiovascular (CV) events if followed up for long enough. The data from follow-up studies in excess of 10 years were crucial in addressing this important question. This observation is not surprising because a lower–CV risk population requires longer studies to detect the difference in CV events, and only robust long-term follow-up of epidemiologic data are of any value in addressing the issue of increased CV risk. Of note is that the Kramer study cannot be generalized to an older population because BMI had a lesser effect on relative mortality risk.[11,12]

Furthermore, Kramer and coresearchers have shown that all individuals with unhealthy metabolic status presented with increased CV risk regardless of their body weight or BMI, suggesting that the underlying metabolic alterations are more important than weight itself in predicting CV risk. This observation also has an impact on the comparator group for CV outcome studies, confirming that caution should be taken in defining metabolic profile in normal weight individuals.

These researchers have also shown that BMI had a worsening effect on the adverse metabolic profile of an individual by increasing blood pressure, central obesity, and insulin resistance while reducing HDL cholesterol across metabolically healthy and unhealthy groups.[10]

Therefore the term "benign obesity" is a thing of the past because the key finding of the Kramer study was that in the absence metabolic alterations, an obese person whose BMI is 30 or greater may be at 24% additional risk for a cardiovascular event or premature death compared with a person of normal weight. Consequently, an increasing BMI is harmful even when the metabolic profile is still normal and subclinical vascular disease is not apparent.[13] The rate of progression of metabolically healthy obesity to metabolically unhealthy obesity has been reported to be approximately 50% within 10 years.[14] Thus a high BMI and gaining weight should be avoided at all costs. By ignoring raised BMI in 200 million individuals with "metabolically healthy obesity," we are ignoring the potential of 1.4 million premature deaths or CV events worldwide.[10] Let us not ignore it.

This book aims to address some aspects of the up-to-date management of weight problems and provides relevant information for the professional advising individuals with an increased BMI.

Jolanta U. Weaver, MRCS, MRCP, FRCP, PhD, CTLHE

REFERENCES

1. WHO. Obesity and Overweight Fact Sheet Accessed at: www.who.int/mediacentre/fcs311/en/.
2. Obesity: preventing and managing the global epidemic. Report of a WHO consultation. *World Health Organ Tech Rep Ser.* 2000;894:i–xii. 1–253.
3. Adams KF, Schatzkin A, Harris TB, et al. Overweight, obesity, and mortality in a large prospective cohort of persons 50 to 71 years old. *N Engl J Med.* 2006;355(8):763–778.
4. Berrington de Gonzalez A, Hartge P, Cerhan JR, et al. Body-mass index and mortality among 1.46 million white adults. *N Engl J Med.* 2010;363(23):2211–2219.
5. Prospective Studies Collabration, Whitlock G, Lewington S, et al. Body-mass index and cause-specific mortality in 900 000 adults: collaborative analyses of 57 prospective studies. *Lancet.* 2009;373(9669):1083–1096.
6. Flegal KM, Kit BK, Orpana H, Graubard BI. Association of all-cause mortality with overweight and obesity using standard body mass index categories: a systematic review and meta-analysis. *JAMA.* 2013;309(1):71–82.
7. Karelis AD. Metabolically healthy but obese individuals. *Lancet.* 2008;372(9646):1281–1283.
8. Ruderman N, Chisholm D, Pi-Sunyer X, Schneider S. The metabolically obese, normal-weight individual revisited. *Diabetes.* 1998;47(5):699–713.
9. Wildman RP, Muntner P, Reynolds K, et al. The obese without cardiometabolic risk factor clustering and the normal weight with cardiometabolic risk factor clustering: prevalence and correlates of 2 phenotypes among the US population (NHANES 1999–2004). *Arch Intern Med.* 2008;168(15):1617–1624.
10. Kramer CK, Zinman B, Retnakaran R. Are metabolically healthy overweight and obesity benign conditions? A systematic review and meta-analysis. *Ann Intern Med.* 2013;159(11):758–769.
11. Heiat A, Vaccarino V, Krumholz HM. An evidence-based assessment of federal guidelines for overweight and obesity as they apply to elderly persons. *Arch Intern Med.* 2001;161(9):1194–1203.
12. Kvamme JM, Holmen J, Wilsgaard T, Florholmen J, Midthjell K, Jacobsen BK. Body mass index and mortality in elderly men and women: the Tromso and HUNT studies. *J Epidemiol Commun Health.* 2012;66(7):611–617.
13. Khan UI, Wang D, Thurston RC, et al. Burden of subclinical cardiovascular disease in "metabolically benign" and "at-risk" overweight and obese women: the Study of Women's Health across the Nation (SWAN). *Atherosclerosis.* 2011;217(1):179–186.
14. Munoz-Garach A, Cornejo-Pareja I, Tinahones FJ. Does metabolically healthy obesity exist? *Nutrients.* 2016;(6):8.

Contents

CHAPTER 1

The Global Problem of Obesity

DR. SUSAN E. JONES, MB, CHB, MD, FRCP

INTRODUCTION

Obesity increases the risk of a wide range of medical conditions including type 2 diabetes, cardiovascular disease, and all cancers, with the exception of pancreatic, prostate, and esophageal cancers (females).[1] Obesity costs the UK's National Health Service in excess of £5.1 billion per annum, and this figure is set to rise because the prevalence of the condition increases year on year.[2] The prevalence of obesity in the United Kingdom has nearly doubled between the years 1993 and 2011. Obesity rates in males rose from 13% to 24% and in females from 16% to 26%.[3] Total societal and economic burden of obesity and overweight in the United Kingdom was estimated at £16 billion per annum in 2007 (1% of GDP) and this is predicted to rise to £50 billion by 2050 if the prevalence of obesity continues to increase at the same rate.[3] Prevalence and economic data from the United Kingdom provide a "snapshot" of trends within Western healthcare systems but cannot be extrapolated widely because of a number of factors. Obesity is not just a "Western problem," and there are many confounding variables that need to be addressed. "Developed" nations invariably have a very robust dataset for their healthcare, and obesity rates in the West are relatively easy to find; therefore data can be correlated to look at the effect of obesity on chronic health conditions.

Worldwide, the data collection methods are less robust, but this chapter aims to give an overview of how obesity is a truly global problem that is increasing year on year. The World Health Organization (WHO) and United Nations (UN) data are a major source of information on a wide range of noncommunicable diseases (NCDs) and also provide data on obesity. Closer analysis of these data shows a wide range of methodologies over the years, but data from India provide a modern perspective on the current state of obesity, which can be extrapolated more easily to less well developed countries, and are used throughout this chapter.

DEFINITION OF OBESITY

WHO has classified obesity by body mass index (BMI),[4,5] but this classification is controversial. BMI is calculated by an individual's weight in kilograms divided by their height in meter squared and expressed as kg/m^2. The original calculation was devised by a Belgian statistician, Adolphe Quetelet, in 1832. His remit was to study growth of "normal" men and to produce an index of relative weight to predict growth, which became known as the "Quetelet index." From the outset he did not want to study obesity, but WHO adopted the index in 1995 to do just that[4] and renamed it BMI. BMI was ever validated only in Caucasian males and not immediately transferrable to females or non-Caucasians.

BMI takes no account of the distribution of body fat[6] and is a "blunt instrument" to identify individuals at risk of morbidity due to their weight. Waist circumference measurement can be used as a screening tool to identify individuals at risk of increased visceral fat deposition, which is an independent risk factor for cardiovascular disease and type 2 diabetes.[7-9] To identify "pathologic obesity," one, therefore, needs both waist circumference and BMI, but these data are not always available together; therefore BMI continues to be used as the main indicator of obesity.

Both BMI and waist circumference have been validated in Caucasian populations, but it is widely recognized that Southeast Asian (SE Asian) populations are different. SE Asians have higher rates of metabolic syndrome and type 2 diabetes than their age, BMI, and waist circumference matched Caucasian counterparts in the same environment.[10] This observation has been previously noted and led to redefinition of obesity among SE Asian population.[11-13] Table 1.1 shows classification of obesity between Caucasian and SE Asians and emphasizes how obesity rates can be underestimated among SE Asians if BMI standards for Caucasians are applied to them.

OBESITY RATES WORLDWIDE

WHO produces regular reports on a wide range of health issues among which are the NCDs that include, among others, diabetes and cardiovascular disease. The Global Health Observatory (GHO) data on NCD include rates of overweight and obesity based on BMI,

TABLE 1.1
Body Mass Index (BMI) Classification for Caucasians and Southeast (SE) Asians

	BMI KG/M^2	
	Caucasian	**SE Asian**
Underweight	<18.5	<18.5
Normal	18.5–24.9	18.5–22.9
Overweight	25.0–29.9	23.0–24.9
Obese I	30.0–34.9	25.0–29.9
Obese II	35.0–39.9	≥30.0
Obese III	≥40.0	

Data from WHO. Obesity: preventing and managing the global epidemic. Report of a WHO Expert Consultation. *WHO Technical Report Series 89*, Geneva: World Health Organisation; 2000, WHO/IASO/IOTF. *The Asia-Pacific Perspective: Redefining Obesity and Its Treatment*. Melbourne: Health Communications Australia; 2000, and WHO Expert Consultation. Appropriate body-mass index for Asian populations and its implications for policy and intervention strategies. *Lancet*. 2004:157–163.

but waist circumference data are not available. In 2014 GHO estimated that 39% adults aged 18 years and above were overweight and 13% were obese, and the mean BMI of the world's population was 24 kg/m^2.[14] It must be appreciated that these data are only estimates and as such can map trends in obesity by geographic region but cannot provide true prevalence data. Countries around the world report voluntarily to WHO on their NCD prevalence and WHO used a "standard year" of 2010 to provide baseline data. The figures produced are based on published and unpublished literature with a variety of statistical tests, including regression analysis, to produce the final data.[15] The data for countries with "developed" healthcare systems who publish epidemiologic and other research are likely to be very robust and the estimated rates are fairly accurate. In contrast, "developing" nations in whom NCD research and healthcare systems are not yet at the same level as Western nations will, by definition, have underestimation of obesity rates.

To produce its reports WHO divides the world into regions that have vastly different healthcare resources and a wide variation in NCD. In 2014 the global rate of obesity was determined to be 11.5% with higher rates in women (13.7%) than in men (9.3%).[14] All countries and regions show that women have higher obesity rates than men; therefore the discussion below is based on total obesity rates. These data seem to suggest a low obesity rate worldwide, but analysis of prevalence

within WHO region and by country within the regions tells a very different story.

For administrative and analysis purposes WHO has designated the world into regions for which they produce reports that can be subanalyzed by country. These regions are defined as Africa, Americas (Canada, the United States, Mexico, Central and South America), SE Asia, Europe (including Turkey and the former USSR), Eastern Mediterranean (includes all the Arab states, Egypt, Pakistan, and other countries such as Afghanistan, Somalia, and Yemen), and Western Pacific (including highly developed countries such as China, Japan, Malaysia, Singapore, Australia, and New Zealand plus 31 other smaller nations).

Fig. 1.1 shows the obesity rates by WHO region. The data from Africa and SE Asia illustrate the problems with defining obesity rates within countries and across the world.

Africa is defined as all the sub-Saharan African countries, which show huge heterogeneity of healthcare systems, NCD rates, and wide variation in wealth. This can be illustrated by the difference in obesity rates between Sierra Leone (7.6%), Zambia (8.9%), Nigeria (11%), and South Africa (26.8%). Some of this variation is due to the variables outlined above, but lack of robust data and low research activity will lead to underestimation of obesity rates for the region as a whole.

Waist measurement is not used by WHO to estimate obesity rates because of the paucity of these data; therefore BMI 30 kg/m^2 or higher is used instead. As discussed above, this will lead to underestimation of the problem in SE Asians where lower BMI cutoff should be used to define obesity.

The SE Asian cutoff BMI for obesity is ≥25.0 kg/m^2 with a BMI of 23–24.9 kg/m^2 being defined as overweight.[11–13] It is, therefore, inappropriate to compare BMI ≥ 30.0 kg/m^2 between SE Asia and the other WHO regions to define obesity. It is more accurate to compare WHO data for "overweight" for SE Asian with those of "obese" for the rest of the world. Fig. 1.1 shows this comparison, and the adjusted obesity rates for SE Asia are 22.2%, which places them as the third highest region for obesity in the world.

THE OBESITY EPIDEMIC AND URBANIZATION

Asian countries have traditionally seen the majority of their population living in rural rather than urban areas. The shift from rural to urban life is known as urbanization, and the United Nations Department of Economic and Social Affairs (UNESA) has collected data

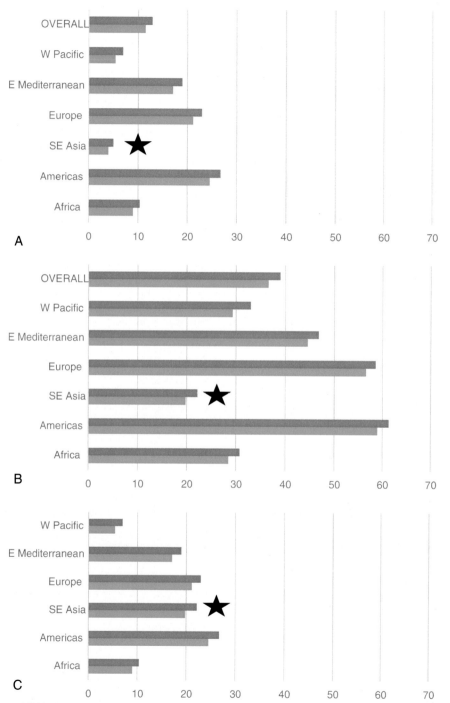

FIG. 1.1 WHO data for percentage obesity and overweight 2010 (*lower bars*) versus 2014 (*upper bars*) by region. **(A)** Obesity body mass index (BMI) > 30 kg/m². **(B)** Overweight BMI > 25 kg/m². **(C)** Obesity corrected for the fact that Southeast (SE) Asian obesity is defined as BMI > 25 kg/m² and the data for rates of "overweight" in SE Asia are plotted with "obesity" rates in all other regions. (Data from WHO. *Global Health Observatory (GHO) data overweight and obesity.* http://www.who.int/gho/ncd/risk_factors/overweight/en/; 2014.)

on urbanization rates since the 1950s.[16] UNESA classifies the countries of the world into different regions to those used by WHO. This difference can make extrapolation of data to examine the effect of urbanization on obesity difficult without careful analysis. UNESA divides Asia into subdivisions of Eastern Asia (includes China, Korea, and Japan plus other areas), Central Asia (includes former USSR countries), Southern Asia (includes India, Pakistan, Sri Lanka, and others), SE Asia (includes Cambodia, Malaysia, and Singapore plus others), and Western Asia (the WHO Eastern Mediterranean area plus Turkey).

In 2014 China's urban population of 758 billion represented 20% of the global total of urban dwellers followed by India with 410 billion urban dwellers and the United States with 263 billion.[16] India is predicted to double the size of its urban population between 2014 and 2050, which would place it first in the "world rankings" for urbanization.[16] Urbanization brings benefits of better access to healthcare, sanitation, and improved nutrition because of better availability of a wider range of food. The latter paves the way for increased obesity and by default increased risk of type 2 diabetes, cardiovascular disease, and hypertension. This effect is most pronounced in less developed countries.[17]

India's rapid increase in urbanization since the 1950s has produced a huge burden of NCD and obesity rates are rising exponentially. The Indian Council of Medical Research—India Diabetes (ICMR-INDIAB) Collaborative Study Group[18] has an ongoing cross-sectional national epidemiologic study to examine the prevalence type 2 diabetes, obesity, and hypertension. This is the largest study of its kind undertaken in India, and the ICMR-INDIAB aims at expanding its research to sample all 29 states, 2 union territories, and the national capital territory of Delhi.

Phase I of the ICMR-INDIAB study used robust sampling methodology of four areas of India representing both rural and urban populations. They collected data on weight, BMI, and waist circumference from a total of 4063 urban dwellers and 9737 rural dwellers.[19] The group used the WHO Asia Pacific guidelines[11-13] to classify individuals as overweight (BMI 23–24.9 kg/m^2), generalized obesity (GO, BMI ≥ 25 kg/m^2), and abdominal obesity (AO, waist circumference ≥90 cm males and ≥80 cm females). Combined obesity (CO) was defined as individuals with both GO and AO and nonobese was defined as individuals without either GO or AO. This study also ascertained diabetes and hypertension rates between rural and urban dwellers. Overall, women had higher mean BMI than men, but mean waist circumference was higher in men than in women. Urban dwellers had significantly higher mean BMI and mean waist circumference than rural dwellers. Urban dwellers also had significantly higher rates of GO, AO, and CO compared with rural dwellers. Of the four Indian states studied in Phase I, the states with highest income per capita had the highest rates of obesity (see Table 1.2).

The WHO data for the prevalence of overweight in India (BMI ≥ 25.0 kg/m^2)[14] are equivalent to the GO within the study. The WHO reports GO rates of 22.0%

TABLE 1.2
Obesity Rates (Percentage) in Urban Versus Rural India in Four Areas Studied in Phase I of the ICMR-INDIAB Study

	Combined Obesity (CO) Individuals With Both GO and AO		Generalized Obesity (GO) BMI ≥ 25 kg/m2		Abdominal Obesity (AO) Waist Circumference: Males ≥ 90 cm Females ≥ 80 cm	
	Urban	**Rural**	**Urban**	**Rural**	**Urban**	**Rural**
Chandigarh	34.0	24.0	40.3	27.9	46.6	32.1
Tamil Nadu	28.8	15.3	35.7	20.0	37.4	22.1
Jharkhand	26.3	3.1	30.4	4.3	37.2	8.7
Maharashtra	20.2	9.7	26.1	12.2	26.7	15.0
WHO (2014)			22.0			

Chandigarh has the highest income per capita. The WHO data are the estimated rate of BMI ≥ 25 kg/m^2 for the whole of India in 2014.
Data from Pradeepa R, Anjan RM, Joshi SR, et al. Prevalence of generalized and abdominal obesity in urban and rural India – the ICMR-INDIAB Study (Phase-1) [ICMR-INDIAB-3]. *Indian J Med Res*. 2015;142(2):139–150 and WHO. *Global Health Observatory (GHO) data overweight and obesity*. http://www.who.int/gho/ncd/risk_factors/overweight/en/; 2014.

for India in 2014, but this study reports rates from 26.1% to 40.3% in urban dwellers and 4.3% to 27.9% in rural dwellers. This illustrates how the current WHO obesity rates for India, and other developing nations, are an underestimation and fail to truly represent the real problem of obesity worldwide.

CHILDHOOD OBESITY

In 2014 WHO estimated that 41 million children aged <5 years of age were overweight or obese and 50% of them were residents of Asian countries and 25% are residents of African countries.[20] As detailed above, obesity rates in adults in Asian countries are rising and the rise in childhood obesity will further add to the burden of NCD in the future. African countries have seen a rise in childhood obesity from 5.4 to 10.3 million for 1990–2014.[20] Childhood overweight and obesity are defined as weight-for-height z-score values more than 2 standard deviations (SDs) and 3 SDs, respectively, from the WHO growth standard median for age <5 years.[21] In children aged 5 to <19 years overweight and obesity are defined as BMI-for-age more than 1 SD and 2 SDs above the WHO growth reference median, respectively.[22,23] More overweight and obese children live in low- and middle-income countries compared with high-income countries.[22,23] Childhood obesity is a strong predictor of adult obesity and is associated with increased risk of metabolic syndrome and cardiovascular disease in adulthood.[24,25]

There are many factors that influence infant and childhood obesity, and in some nations the rates are plateauing. Absolute numbers of overweight and obese children vary according to the income status of their country of residence. The numbers are highest in low- and middle-income countries compared with high-income countries.[22]

Thanks to immunization programs, improved sanitation, improved maternal healthcare, increasing urbanization, and other factors, there has been a reduction in infant (aged <12 months) and childhood (aged <5 years) mortality in the majority of countries of the world. Worldwide infant mortality rates per live births have reduced from 63 deaths per 1000 to 32 deaths per 1000 in 2015.[26] This reduced mortality, combined with increased obesity, will inevitably lead to increased adulthood obesity unless programs to address childhood obesity are initiated. WHO has established a commission to implement measures to reduce childhood obesity because previous measures to tackle the problem have been patchy and inconsistent.[20] The program outlined by WHO to tackle childhood obesity will take time to implement and the current cohort of obese children are highly likely to become obese adults.

THE BARKER HYPOTHESIS AND OBESITY

Intrauterine malnutrition or prematurity (birth before 37 weeks gestation) leads to low birth weight (LBW), which is defined as a weight at birth <2500 g,[27] and this is linked to chronic diseases such as hypertension, cardiovascular disease, and type 2 diabetes in adulthood. This phenomenon is known as the Barker hypothesis,[28] and there have been numerous papers showing the link between LBW and chronic disease in adulthood, the effect of which is magnified if LBW infants become obese adults.

Data for LBW by country are patchy as the data are not robustly collected in many developing countries where access to maternal healthcare is not always highly structured. In 2011 worldwide LBW rates were estimated to be 15% (more than 20 million infants). India alone accounted for one-third of these births, and one in four newborns in South Asia are of LBW.[29] For the purposes of the UNICEF report[29] South Asia was defined as Afghanistan, Bangladesh, Bhutan, India, Maldives, Nepal, Pakistan, and Sri Lanka. UNICEF states that 69% of infants born in South Asia are not weighed at birth, which means that LBW rates are an underestimate.[29]

Within the UNICEF-defined South Asian regions, data collection and healthcare systems are highly developed in India. In 2005 the Indian state of Maharashtra (one of the four regions subsequently studied in Phase I of INCR-INDIAB study[18]) established an "Independent State Nutrition Mission" (ISNM), which focused on infants and children <2 years of age and was sponsored by UNICEF.[30] In contrast to figures for the South Asian region,[29] 92.9% of children in Maharashtra (91.0% rural and 95.0% urban) were weighed at birth. In 2012, the incidence of LBW was 19.9% in Maharashtra with similar rates in both rural and urban communities (19.8% and 20.0%, respectively). A retrospective study of birth weight data in the Nasik district of Maharashtra (1989–2007) showed an LBW rate of 24.2% (17.5–34.3).[31] These two publications imply that LBW rates have changed little over the last three decades in Maharashtra. Changes in birth weight take time, but Maharashtra has been cited in the UNICEF report as an area of good practice having reduced the rates of many key indicators of childhood malnutrition since the inception of the ISMN.[29,30] Ultimately, this will have a positive effect on health, but the impact of LBW combined with improved nutrition may lead to adulthood obesity, which will increase the risk of NCD such as type 2 diabetes mellitus, cardiovascular disease, and hypertension. The better nourished cohort of Maharashtra will hopefully produce less LBW infants in the future, and this may slow the rate of rise in NCD, but obesity rates will continue to rise. Maharashtra had the lowest obesity rates in Phase I of the ICMR-INDIAB study[18] (see Table 1.2), and approximately a quarter of the population were LBW. With the recent improvement in childhood nutrition it will be interesting to look at obesity and other NCD rates in the next few decades to see if the "Barker hypothesis" is proven as children in Maharashtra born in the early 21st century reach adulthood.

LEAST DEVELOPED COUNTRIES AND OBESITY

The UN has defined countries into "development groups" according to a variety of parameters including income, healthcare, infant mortality, and education and classified them as more developed, less developed, and least developed.[16] A total of 48 countries are categorized the "least developed countries" of the world and 71% of these are in sub-Saharan Africa. The rate of urbanization is rapidly increasing in the less and least developed countries (see Fig. 1.2), which will ultimately lead to more people being exposed to the "obesogenic environment" of urban life.[32] An obesogenic environment is one that promotes high energy intake and sedentary behavior. The availability of affordable accessible food that is freely advertised is the norm in urban areas and this plus mechanized transportation with a more sedentary lifestyle promotes obesity.

Based on previous urbanization and current urbanization rates, the least developed countries are predicted to have a 3% increase year on year from 2014 to 30.[16]

CONCLUSION

Current UN and WHO data underestimate the true global problem of obesity. Analysis of trends in urbanization combined with modern epidemiologic studies, in countries such as India, gives a much more accurate representation of the scale of the problem. Urgent action is required to reduce obesity rates, but whether this is achievable is debatable. Individuals aspire to achieve their goals of achieving the "Western dream" of affluence and by doing so increase their exposure to obesogenic environments and further fuel the worldwide obesity epidemic.

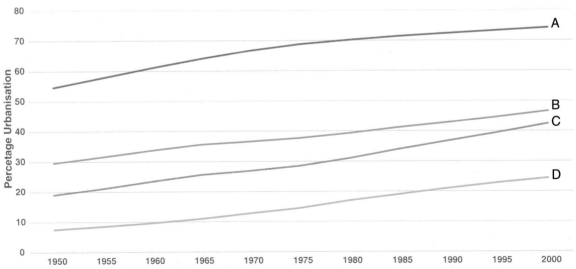

FIG. 1.2 United Nations Department of Economic and Social Affairs data for percentage urbanization from 1950 to 2000. "More developed" countries **(A)** show a plateauing of urbanization rates compared with the "less developed" countries **(C)**, which have increased urbanization rates from 19% to 42.4% over the same period and are the major contributor to the increase in worldwide urbanization **(B)**. The "least developed" countries **(D)** are predicted to show an annual 3% rise in urbanization between 2014 and 2030. (Data from United Nations, Department of Economic and Social Affairs, Population Division. *World Urbanization Prospects: The 2014 Revision*, (ST/ESA/SER.A/366); 2015.)

REFERENCES

1. Guh DP, Zhang W, Bansback N, et al. The incidence of co-morbidities related to obesity and overweight: a systematic review and meta-analysis. *BMC Public Health.* 2009;9:88 (Online Publication).
2. Scarborough P, Bhatnagar P, Wickramasinghe KK, et al. The economic burden of ill health due to diet, physical inactivity, smoking, alcohol and obesity in the UK: an update 2006 – 07 NHS costs. *J Public Health.* 2001;33: 527–535.
3. National Institute for Health and Care Excellence (NICE). *Obesity: Identification, Assessment and Management CG 189;* November 27, 2014:5.
4. WHO. Physical status; the use and interpretation of anthropometry. Report of a WHO Expert Committee. In: *WHO Technical Report Series 854.* Geneva World Health Organisation; 1995.
5. WHO. Obesity: preventing and managing the global epidemic. Report of a WHO Expert Consultation. In: *WHO Technical Report Series 89.* Geneva: World Health Organisation; 2000.
6. Chan DC, Watts GF, Barrett PHR, et al. Waist circumference, waist-to hip ratio and body mass as predictors of adipose tissue compartments in men. *Q Med.* 2003;96: 441–447.
7. Despres J-P, Lemieux I, Prud'homme D. Treatment of obesity: need to focus on high risk abdominally obese patients. *BMJ.* 2001;322:716–720.
8. Pischon T, Boeing H, Hoffman K, et al. General and abdominal adiposity and risk of death in Europe. *N Eng J Med.* 2008;359:2105–2120.
9. St-Pierre J, Lemieux I, Perron P, et al. Hyper-triglyceridaemic waist and 7.5 year prospective risk of cardiovascular disease in asymptomatic middle aged men. *Int J Obes.* 2007;31:791–796.
10. Wulan SN, Westerterp KR, Plasqui G. Ethnic differences in body composition and the associated metabolic profile: a comparative study between Asians and Caucasians. *Maturitas.* 2010;65(4):315–319.
11. WHO/IASO/IOTF. *The Asia-Pacific Perspective: Redefining Obesity and Its Treatment.* Melbourne: Health Communications Australia; 2000.
12. James WPT, Chen C, Inoue S. Appropriate Asian body mass indices? *Obes Rev.* 2002;3:139.
13. WHO Expert Consultation. Appropriate body-mass index for Asian populations and its implications for policy and intervention strategies. *Lancet.* 2004:157–163.
14. WHO. *Global Health Observatory (GHO) Data Overweight and Obesity;* 2014. http://www.who.int/gho/ncd/risk_factors/overweight/en/.
15. WHO. *Global Observatory (GHO) Data Information on Estimation Methods;* 2014. http://www.who.int/gho/ncd/methods/en/.
16. United Nations, Department of Economic and Social Affairs, Population Division. *World Urbanization Prospects: The 2014 Revision* (ST/ESA/SER.A/366); 2015.
17. Godfrey R, Julien M. Urbanisation and health. *Clin Med.* 2005;5(2):137–141.
18. Anjan RM, Pradeepa R, Deepa M, et al. The Indian Council of Medical Research – India Diabetes (ICMR-INDIAB) study: methodological details. *J Diabetes Sci Technol.* 2011;5:906–914.
19. Pradeepa R, Anjan RM, Joshi SR, et al. Prevalence of generalized and abdominal obesity in urban and rural India – the ICMR-INDIAB Study (Phase-1) [ICMR-INDIAB-3]. *Indian J Med Res.* 2015;142(2):139–150.
20. WHO. *Report of the Commission on Ending Childhood Obesity;* 2016.
21. WHO Multi-centre Growth Reference Study Group. WHO child growth standards based on length/height weight and age. *Acta Paediatr Suppl.* 2006;450:76–85.
22. Ng M, Fleming T, Robinson M, et al. Global, regional and national prevalence of overweight and obesity in children and adults during 1980–2013: a systematic analysis for the Global Burden of Disease Study 2013. *Lancet.* 2014;384:766–781.
23. Roberto CA, Swinburne B, Hawkes C, et al. Patchy progress on obesity prevention: emerging examples, entrenched barriers, and new thinking. *Lancet.* 2015;385:2400–2409.
24. Miller AL, Lee HJ, Lumeng JC. Obesity-associated biomarkers and executive function in children. *Pediatr Res.* 2015;77:143–147.
25. Litwin SE. Childhood obesity and adulthood cardiovascular disease: quantifying the lifetime cumulative burden of cardiovascular burden of cardiovascular risk factors. *J Am Coll Cardiol.* 2014;64:1588–1590.
26. Global Health Observatory (GHO) Data. *Infant Mortality Situations and Trends.* WHO; 2015. www.who.int/gho/child_health/mortality/neonatal_infant_text/en/.
27. World Health Organisation (WHO). *International Statistical Classification of Diseases and Related Health Problems.* Geneva: World Health Organisation; 1992.
28. Barker DJP, ed. *Fetal and Infant Origins of Adult Disease.* London: BMJ Books; 1992.
29. United Nations Children Fund (UNICEF). *Improving Child Nutrition. The Achievable Imperative for Global Progress.* New York: UNICEF; 2013.
30. *Comprehensive Nutrition Survey in Maharashtra* Mumbai; 2012.
31. Ashtekar SV, Kulkarni MB, Sadvarte VS, et al. Analysis of birth weights of a rural hospital. *Indian J Community Med.* 2010;35(2):252–255.
32. Lake A, Townshed T. Obesogenic environments: exploring the built and food environments. *J R Soc Promot Health.* 2006;126:262–267.

CHAPTER 2

Health Economics of Obesity

SARAH HILL, BA, MSc • YEMI OLUBOYEDE, BA, MSc, PHD •
FRAUKE BECKER, DIPL OEC, PHD

BACKGROUND

Obesity is considered one of the most important medical and public health problems of our time.[1] Excess body fat has been identified as a major risk factor for several common disorders, including diabetes and cardiovascular diseases,[2] and the associated consequences for healthcare systems, as well as health policy implications, have been well documented.[3,4]

While obesity-related diseases are the main cause of increased morbidity and mortality within populations, obesity itself is considered a preventable condition.[1] Defining excessive weight gain as the consequence of a continuous positive energy balance (where the calorie intake exceeds energy expenditure) describes obesity as the result of individual behaviors associated with specific food patterns, dietary compositions, and calorie expenditure.[5-9] However, the system of factors affecting individual choices and weight-related behaviors is complex and multifaceted. The UK Government's Foresight Programme[a] used a strategic approach to describe influences on and implications of obesity. It developed an obesity map describing the obesogenic environment as a system of intercorrelated influences of weight gain, integrating evidence from various fields of relevant research without identifying a single dominating factor[10] (see Fig. 2.1).

Although the influences of body weight have been identified, the pathways leading to obesity are not entirely clear. This lack of evidence combined with ever-increasing overweight and obesity rates suggests that to develop effective interventions promoting a healthy body weight, a better understanding is required of:

- which factors influence individual weight-related choices the most and
- how a combination of behaviors and interaction of factors might moderate their separate effects.

In addition to influences on individual quality of life and self-esteem, as well as the clinical implications of obesity and the associated costs to healthcare

systems, economic frameworks can be used to analyze obesity from a behavioral point of view. Once the obesogenic environment has been defined, economic frameworks allow to model and predict long-term behaviors and their effect on body weight as well as cost implications. Thus, the effectiveness of treatments can be estimated, which may help to derive implications for interventions and policy recommendations.

INDIVIDUAL CHOICES AND BEHAVIOR

Explaining human behavior and its underlying motivations is a complex process (see, e.g., Ref. 12). Determinants of weight-related behaviors are characterized by a complex relationship between biologic and lifestyle factors and various influences from the physical, social, and economic environment.[13] The interactions within this system of influences characterize pathways to a healthy body weight while capturing indirect effects of the socioeconomic environment on weight-related choices at the same time.

From an economic point of view, individuals engage in a behavior because it delivers an immediate reward (i.e., *utility*).[12,14] Therefore, uptake of certain dietary and activity behaviors may be explained primarily by the immediate satisfaction they provide rather than the behaviors' impact on body weight. Accounting for effects on weight would require individuals to consider long-term consequences, including general health, which may only be indirectly affected by current behaviors.

According to behavioral economics, individuals make rational choices to maximize their own overall utility. A healthy body weight should be one of the overall rationales of a healthy lifestyle, which is associated with a lower risk of morbidity and mortality in the long run. "Healthy time" can be spent on any type of activity from which the individual would generate satisfaction, utility, or income. However, to understand the observable trend of increased obesity prevalence in both developed and developing countries and given the negative implications of excessive body weight on

---

[a] https://www.gov.uk/government/publications/reducing-obesity-future-choices.

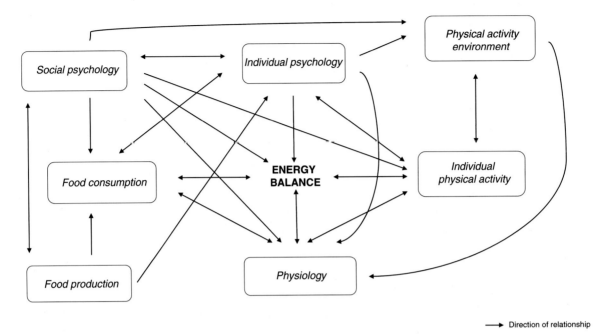

FIG. 2.1 Key determinants of the individual energy balance. (Adapted from Butland B, Jebb S, Kopelman P, et al. *Foresight Tackling Obesities: Future Choices – Project Report*; 2007, with permission.)

health, other approaches are required to explain supposedly irrational weight-related behaviors. From the individual perspective, a weight-related behavior may be rational within a specific context, e.g., for reasons of convenience when considering time constraints. However, maximizing individual utility may be counterproductive for society's overall welfare. This issue arises especially in healthcare systems that are mainly publicly funded such as the National Health Service (NHS) in the United Kingdom or that are set up as pooled private health insurances, e.g., in the United States where some employers provide health insurance coverage for their employees. In contrast, individual private health insurance premiums may account for the individual risk of disease more directly, therefore forcing individuals to take on more responsibility for their health-related behaviors (see for more details, e.g., Ref. 15). To tackle the obesity problem and develop effective targeted policy recommendations and interventions, the pathways leading to obesity must be clearly defined and related behaviors be identified. Preventative measures aimed at maintaining healthy weight would need to consider various weight-related choices individuals make over time, how the accumulation of their effects may impact on an individual's body weight, and, finally, determining which behavior, situation, or population group to target for effective interventions. Understanding triggers

of individual choices would need to account for external influences, as well as forming of habits and routines (especially during childhood) or even addictive behaviors that could pose substantial barriers to a more healthy lifestyle, and would need to be addressed when aiming at changing behaviors on population level. Although the treatment of obesity follows a similar pattern, especially when behavioral interventions are involved, it may constitute a more individual approach, where a required change in weight-related behaviors or even in medical procedures is considered based on the individual situation and personal requirements.

The more individualized the approach to tackle obesity, the more costly it is for both the individual and society in terms of time and financial resources required. Prevention of obesity may seem to be the favorable approach because it is potentially more cost-effective than obesity treatment.[16] However, the increasing obesity prevalence and large proportions of populations being overweight and obese require a dual approach to reduce excess body weight within the population to improve the general health of the population and reduce future cost implications.

COSTS OF OBESITY

While the effects of excess body weight on an individual's self-esteem and health-related quality of life may

TABLE 2.1
Types of Costs

Type of Cost	Examples
Individual	• Lower wages • Increased risks of mortality and morbidity
Societal	• Productivity losses through absenteeism, presenteeism, disability, and premature death • Increased welfare payments for those unable to work because of obesity-related disability • Opportunity cost of obesity-related treatment or prevention
Healthcare	• Costs of treatment for obesity directly (e.g., bariatric surgery or counseling) • Costs of treatment for obesity-related comorbidities such as type 2 diabetes

require specifically tailored instruments to measure the impact for adults and children separately (see US Food and Drug Administration report on the development of robust Patient-Reported Outcome Measures[17]), the associated costs can be more easily quantified. Direct (e.g., medical costs) and indirect costs (e.g., productivity losses) can be divided into three main areas: individual-level costs (i.e., those that fall on the obese individual themselves), costs to society, and costs to the healthcare system (see Table 2.1).

The described types of costs are not necessarily financial, but may be adverse effects of being overweight or obese; in economic terms such negative effects can be considered a cost to whoever experiences them. While there is undoubtedly overlap between the three areas, certain costs will affect specific recipients to a greater extent than others. Each of the aforementioned types of costs will be outlined in detail below.

Individual Level

In terms of physical health, a wide range of health risks are associated with increased body weight, such as type 2 diabetes, hypertension, coronary heart disease and stroke, cancers, osteoarthritis, cancers, and gall bladder disease. The risk of developing each of the above conditions was found to be positively correlated with higher body mass index (BMI).[18]

Compared with those of normal weight, obese individuals have higher risks of mortality and morbidity[19,20]

alongside the potential for a lower quality of life from both physical and mental health problems. Mental health and well-being can also be negatively affected by excess body fat, which is particularly notable in children and adolescents. Studies have suggested links between obesity and reduced mental well-being in the form of depression and/or low self-esteem (see review by Caird et al.[21]). Discrimination and stigma toward those who are overweight and obese can also contribute toward reductions in mental well-being.[21] The media plays a part in stigmatizing those who are overweight and obese from "fat-shaming" headlines to the often negative portrayal of overweight characters in television and films, who are usually depicted as unfriendly, undesirable, or lazy.[22] Discrimination in the workplace can also be a contributing factor to mental ill-health. A study conducted in a Finnish population[23] found that several measures of obesity (BMI, fat mass, and waist circumference) are associated with lower labor force participation for women while higher fat mass predicted lower probability of employment in men. While causality cannot be confirmed in this study, the use of more "visible" obesity indicators (such as waist circumference and fat mass) suggests that discrimination by employers could be a contributing factor to lower employment probabilities for obese individuals.

Additionally, several studies[24-26] have documented the negative effects of obesity on employment and wages. Therefore, regardless of causality it has been shown that individuals who are obese may face costs in terms of lower financial compensation for work compared with their normal weight colleagues.

Societal Level

The costs of obesity to society refer to those that fall on all individuals in a population. In other words, societal costs affect both the obese population causing the costs and normal weight individuals who do not contribute to the obesity problem. The effects of obesity on society include productivity losses, increased welfare costs, and the opportunity cost of expenditures for obesity reduction.

Lost workforce productivity can arise in a number of ways. Firstly, foregone productivity can occur when individuals of working-age who would otherwise be employed are unable to work for obesity-related health reasons such as sick leave, disability, or premature death.[27] Secondly, rates of absenteeism (i.e., being absent from work) and presenteeism (i.e., being present at work but working at a lower rate of productivity than in perfect health) have been positively associated with a higher BMI.[28-30] It can be difficult to quantify productivity losses due to the data available and the confounding effects of alternative factors other than obesity. However, a number of attempts have been made to place a value on lost productivity from obesity in various countries. Estimates for Europe range from over EUR2000 per year difference in presenteeism and absenteeism costs between the most obese workers (BMI ≥ 40 kg/m²) and their normal weight coworkers[29] to a lifetime difference in productivity losses of EUR60,000 for obese Swedish workers compared with normal weight workers.[27]

Individuals who are unable to work because of health conditions related to obesity also incur additional costs on society from increased welfare payments. Many countries, such as the United Kingdom and the United States, provide disability benefit payments to those who are unable to work due to ill-health. A number of studies have examined the association between obesity and an increased receipt of disability payments,[31,32] which imposes an avoidable burden on social welfare. The increasing prevalence of obesity in children is particularly concerning for the future workforce. The effect of long-term habit-forming in childhood has implications for obese children who are likely to retain unhealthy behaviors into adulthood, putting them at greater risk of remaining obese and developing a range of chronic diseases.[33] This trend of youth obesity could have economic repercussions because more individuals may be prevented from entering the workforce when working-age is reached due to obesity-related chronic disease.

Finally, society faces the opportunity cost of spending on treatment for obesity and related diseases. An opportunity cost refers to the cost of foregone spending because resources have been deployed elsewhere. In other words, when resources available are limited or fixed and a proportion of those resources are spent on one good (A), those same resources cannot be used to purchase a different good (B). The opportunity cost of spending the resources on good A is what you could have received had you used them to buy good B instead. Therefore, by spending limited healthcare resources on treating obesity and related diseases, society faces the opportunity cost of not being able to use those resources to treat other conditions. How great the opportunity costs are will depend on the weight that society places on treating all other health conditions compared with obesity-related ones.

Healthcare System

The healthcare costs of obesity are the costs associated with either treating obesity itself (e.g., bariatric surgery or counseling) or treating diseases related to obesity,

such as type 2 diabetes where 90% of type 2 diabetics have a BMI > 23 kg/m².[18] The cost burden of obesity will vary by country depending on its prevalence and medical costs. For instance in the United Kingdom, in 2006–07 the NHS spent over £5 billion GBP (Great British Pound; more than 10% of the total NHS budget) on ill-health related to overweight and obesity.[34] By 2050, if current obesity trends continue, this has been predicted[11] to double to £10 billion per year.[b] In the United Kingdom diabetes care alone costs the NHS around 14 billion GBP per year.[35] Similar trends can be observed on an international level. In the United States it has been estimated[36] that, on average, obesity increases the average individual annual medical costs by almost USD3,000.[c]

PREDICTIONS AND MODELING

To reduce the economic burden related to increasing obesity rates, models of potential obesity interventions can predict future consequences and may therefore help in guiding health policy. Especially regarding scarce health resources, economic evaluations can be used to model the long-term costs and health-related outcomes as well as the relative cost-effectiveness of interventions and treatments compared with alternative measures.[37,38] While the direct treatment costs of obesity fall within the responsibility of the NHS (United Kingdom) (or the specific healthcare provider in other countries), interventions aimed at preventing and/or reducing levels of obesity can be categorized primarily as public health interventions which, in the United Kingdom, are the responsibility of local authorities (following the Health and Social Care Act 2012 in the United Kingdom[d]). Evidence on the cost-effectiveness and therefore the economic case for investment in specific interventions is increasingly required to justify the use of public resources.

A major challenge for the modeling of obesity and its implications is described by the complex system of the obesogenic environment. Influences may vary during the lifetime and different modeling approaches may be required for adults and children. Although it is desirable to develop models that capture the individual's or a cohort's pathways over the predefined time horizon as realisticly as possible, it might not be feasible or even possible to do so. For any type of weight

---

[b] In 2007 GBP.
[c] In 2005 USD.
[d] https://www.gov.uk/government/publications/health-and-social-care-act-2012-fact-sheets.

model, this would imply considering the increasing obesity prevalence on population level, combining it with individual characteristics and the probabilities of engaging in certain behaviors and capture how these potentially changed behaviors relate to the onset of weight-related diseases and associated treatment costs. Epidemiologic models can be useful for predicting the pathway between specific health issues and estimating the probabilities of future health problems as well as treatment outcomes. However, the long-term modeling of weight is more complex than the usual disease model. The complexity is due to various influences of obesity and weight-related behaviors as well as the absence of evidence around the effectiveness and cost-effectiveness of interventions (including the lack of robust longitudinal data), uncertainty around the duration of specific behaviors, and the combined effect of weight-related behaviors that needs to be considered in addition to the unique effect of each behavior.

In the United Kingdom, the National Institute for Health and Care Excellence (NICE) has specified the gaps in evidence in several of its recent obesity-related guidelines (Preventing excess weight gain [NG7],[e] Obesity prevention [CG43],[f] Exercise referral schemes to promote physical activity [PH54],[g] Behavior change: individual approaches [PH49][h]). They all highlight the lack of evidence around evaluations of effectiveness and cost-effectiveness of interventions. From current evidence, it is not possible to determine the most effective and cost-effective intervention targeted at a specific behavior or population group, which makes the modeling of economic benefits of potential interventions and healthcare expenditures for the treatment of obese patients even more challenging.

Following the Health and Social Care Act 2012, Public Health England was established as a new executive agency of the Department of Health. They have developed a tool for the economic assessment of weight management interventions in adults[39] to help estimate costs and potential cost savings of weight management interventions and to provide an economic model for (or against) investing in those interventions.

POLICY IMPLICATIONS

In the United Kingdom, institutions such as NICE and the government publish guidelines and policies related to obesity, the purpose of which is to improve the effectiveness of interventions and treatments that reduce the burden of obesity and improve patient care for those at risk. NICE offers a number of different approaches to tackling the obesity problem through its clinical guidelines, public health guidelines, and quality standards. The most recently published guidance on the topic of obesity covers obesity identification, assessment, and management (CG189)[i]; preventing excess weight gain (NG7); lifestyle services for overweight or obese adults (PH53)[j] and children (PH47)[k]; and obesity prevention and lifestyle weight management programs (QS111).[l] The clinical guidelines, which are aimed at health professionals specifically, emphasize the role of general practitioners in providing information to patients on how to lose weight and maintain a healthy lifestyle. A major focus of these guidelines is the education of individuals to promote behavior change as either prevention or intervention. On the other hand, the public health guidelines, which are directed toward local authorities and community services in addition to clinical practitioners, encourage practices such as the development of healthy environments (via targets such as providing healthy eating choices in workplaces, cycle routes, and safe play areas) and specialist training for professionals in lifestyle weight management.

While being a useful resource for those in contact with obese or at risk individuals, the NICE guidance does not discuss in detail specific policies or interventions that could help address the obesity problem in the United Kingdom. With the exception of brief advice interventions on effective ways to lose weight and maintain a healthy lifestyle, a lack of evidence on the most (cost-) effective policies to reduce obesity could explain this omission as discussed earlier. There are, however, several other policies and interventions with potential to reduce the current obesity burden.

Ensuring a healthy environment is a point raised by NICE in its public health guidelines that could also be particularly relevant for tackling childhood obesity because young people generally have less influence on their surroundings than adults. The idea of creating an environment to foster healthy eating behaviors is highlighted in the recent publication by the government on childhood obesity.[40] Plans to challenge industry to reduce the sugar content of food and drink and making school food healthier demonstrate attempts to shape

---

[e] http://www.nice.org.uk/guidance/ng7.

[f] https://www.nice.org.uk/guidance/cg43.

[g] https://www.nice.org.uk/guidance/ph54.

[h] https://www.nice.org.uk/guidance/ph49.

[i] https://www.nice.org.uk/guidance/cg189.

[j] https://www.nice.org.uk/guidance/ph53.

[k] https://www.nice.org.uk/guidance/ph47.

[l] https://www.nice.org.uk/guidance/qs111.

the food environment such that improvements can be made to eating habits without relying on individual behavior change.

Providing incentives to incite behavior change is a commonly used economic tool in many sectors, not just health. While the use of financial incentives to adapt the behavior of specific groups or individuals can be controversial, those which are nonexclusive are better accepted.[41] The ultimate success of financial incentives, such as those to promote engagement in physical activity, relies on whether longitudinal behavior change can be achieved through the formation of new habits because often financial rewards will only be available for a determined period. Without alternative incentives, such as enjoyment, to continue with the desired activity once financial incentives are removed, a risk is run that individuals will cease to engage in the healthy behavior and return to their previous practices.[42]

Indirect incentives, such as taxation and minimum pricing, which can reduce consumption of goods by raising prices for consumers, can also be used to alter the behavior of individuals and nudge them toward making healthier purchases (of goods not subject to increased taxes). An added bonus of such schemes is that additional tax revenue can be directed toward subsidizing healthier goods or funding alternative interventions, as with the case of the soft drinks levy proposed by the UK government.[40] The success of such schemes will, however, depend on how much of a tax is passed onto consumers through increased prices and the flexibility of consumers to adapt their behavior.

Health insurance can also be utilized to encourage healthy behavior if premiums are suitably related to the risk of obesity. By attaching a premium to obesity, the costs of the risky behavior can be transferred from society to the individual thus at worst reducing some of the financial burden on society and at best incentivizing obese individuals to lose weight.[43] This option is less useful in the United Kingdom where the health system is publicly funded, wherein countries such as the United States it could be more viable although potentially controversial.

Prevention Versus Treatment

Public health policies to prevent obesity have great potential to be cost-effective due to their relatively low cost and potential for long-run benefits. Despite this, a lack of evidence on cost-effectiveness and future funding cuts to local authorities in England jeopardizes the implementation of many preventive policies.[44] However, continual focus on treating obesity at the expense of prevention is likely to result in a burgeoning burden of disease and spiraling health costs in the future, especially given the rate of increase in obesity in younger generations. While the current prevalence of obesity warrants action in the form of treatment for obese individuals, a dual approach incorporating appropriate preventive efforts is necessary to stem the rising trend before the demand on healthcare as a result of obesity becomes unmanageable.

CONCLUSIONS

Obesity rates have been increasing over recent decades, causing significant concern among policy makers. Excess body fat is considered a major risk factor for several common disorders, placing a substantial burden on healthcare systems. In order (1) to prevent obesity and guide effective public health policies and (2) to identify effective treatments in a clinical context, we need to understand the complex system of factors affecting individual choices and weight-related behaviors.

Economic evaluations can help in modeling long-term costs and health-related consequences as well as the relative cost-effectiveness of interventions and treatments compared with alternative measures. These models allow for consideration of varying environmental factors as well as individual characteristics and can help in predicting outcomes on individual and societal levels. Results can be used to identify the best-targeted approaches and the most effective and cost-effective interventions when tackling the obesity problem.

REFERENCES

1. World Health Organization. *Obesity and Overweight Fact Sheet*; 2016. http://www.who.int/mediacentre/factsheets/fs311/en/.
2. Guh DP, Zhang W, Bansback N, Amarsi Z, Birmingham CL, Anis AH. The incidence of co-morbidities related to obesity and overweight: a systematic review and meta-analysis. *BMC Public Health*. 2009;9(1):88.
3. Popkin BM. Using research on the obesity pandemic as a guide to a unified vision of nutrition. *Public Health Nutr*. September 1, 2005;8(6A):724–729.
4. World Health Organisation. *Global Action Plan for the Prevention and Control of NCDs 2013-2020*; 2013.
5. Paineau DL, Beaufils F, Boulier A, et al. Family dietary coaching to improve nutritional intakes and body weight control: a randomized controlled trial. *Arch Pediatr Adolesc Med*. 2008;162(1):34–43.
6. Malik VS, Hu FB. Popular weight-loss diets: from evidence to practice. *Nat Clin Pract Cardiovasc Med*. January 2007;4(1):34–41.

7. Blundell JE, Stubbs J. Diet composition and the control of food intake in humans. In: Bray GA, Bouchard C, eds. *Handbook of Obesity*. CRC Press; 2003:427–460.

8. Wilkinson W, Blair S. Physical activity, obesity and health outcomes. In: Bray GA, Bouchard C, eds. *Handbook of Obesity*. CRC Press; 2003:983–1004.

9. Mutikainen S, Perhonen M, Alén M, et al. Effects of long-term physical activity on cardiac structure and function: a twin study. *J Sports Sci Med*. 2009;8(4):533–542.

10. Vandenbroeck I, Goossens J, Clemens M. *Tackling Obesities: Future Choices – Building the Obesity System Map*; 2007.

11. Butland B, Jebb S, Kopelman P, et al. *Foresight Tackling Obesities: Future Choices – Project Report*; 2007.

12. Ajzen I. The theory of planned behavior. *Organ Behav Hum Decis Process*. December 1, 1991;50(2):179–211.

13. Birch S, Jerrett M, Eyles J. Heterogeneity in the determinants of health and illness: the example of socioeconomic status and smoking. *Soc Sci Med*. July 16, 2000;51(2):307–317.

14. Hill JO, Wyatt HR, Reed GW, Peters JC. Obesity and the environment: where do we go from here? *Science*. 2003;299(5608):853–855.

15. Bhattacharya J, Sood N. Who pays for obesity? *J Econ Perspect*. Winter 2011;25(1):139–158.

16. van Baal PHM, Polder JJ, de Wit GA, et al. Lifetime medical costs of obesity: prevention no cure for increasing health expenditure. *PLoS Med*. 2008;5(2):e29.

17. Food and Drug Administration. Guidance for industry, patient-reported outcome measures: use in medical product development to support labeling claims. In: *U.S. Department of Health and Human Services*. ; 2009.

18. Kopelman P. Health risks associated with overweight and obesity. *Obes Rev*. 2007;8:13–17.

19. Olshansky SJ, Passaro DJ, Hershow RC, et al. A potential decline in life expectancy in the United States in the 21st century. *New Engl J Med*. March 17, 2005;352(11):1138–1145.

20. Sturm R. The effects of obesity, smoking, and drinking on medical problems and costs. *Health Aff*. March 1, 2002;21(2):245–253.

21. Caird J, Kavanagh J, Oliver K, et al. *Childhood Obesity and Educational Attainment: A Systematic Review*. EPPI-Centre, Social Science Research Unit, Institute of Education, University of London; 2011.

22. Puhl RM, Heuer CA. The stigma of obesity: a review and update. *Obesity*. 2009;17(5):941–964.

23. Johansson E, Böckerman P, Kiiskinen U, Heliövaara M. Obesity and labour market success in Finland: the difference between having a high BMI and being fat. *Econ Hum Biol*. March 2009;7(1):36–45.

24. Baum CL, Ford WF. The wage effects of obesity: a longitudinal study. *Health Econ*. 2004;13(9):885–899.

25. Han E, Norton EC, Stearns SC. Weight and wages: fat versus lean paychecks. *Health Econ*. 2009;18(5):535–548.

26. Cawley J. The impact of obesity on wages. *J Hum Resour*. 2004;39(2):451–474.

27. Neovius K, Rehnberg C, Rasmussen F, Neovius M. Lifetime productivity losses associated with obesity status in early adulthood: a population-based study of Swedish men. *Appl Health Econ Health Policy*. September 1, 2012;10(5):309–317.

28. Goetzel RZ, Gibson TB, Short ME, et al. A multi-worksite analysis of the relationships among body mass index, medical utilization, and worker productivity. *J Occup Environ Med*. January 2010;52(suppl 1):S52–S58.

29. Gupta S, Richard L, Forsythe A. The humanistic and economic burden associated with increasing body mass index in the EU5. *Diabetes Metab Syndr Obesity*. 2015;8:327–338.

30. Wang YC, McPherson K, Marsh T, Gortmaker SL, Brown M. Health and economic burden of the projected obesity trends in the USA and the UK. *Lancet*. August–September 2011;378(9793):815–825.

31. Narbro K, Jonsson E, Larsson B, Waaler H, Wedel H, Sjostrom L. Economic consequences of sick-leave and early retirement in obese Swedish women. *Int J Obes Relat Metab Disord*. October 1996;20(10):895–903.

32. Burkhauser RV, Cawley J. *Obesity, Disability and Movement onto the Disability Insurance Rolls*; 2004.

33. Wang Y, Lim H. The global childhood obesity epidemic and the association between socio-economic status and childhood obesity. *Int Rev Psychiatry*. June 1, 2012;24(3):176–188.

34. Scarborough P, Bhatnagar P, Wickramasinghe KK, Allender S, Foster C, Rayner M. The economic burden of ill health due to diet, physical inactivity, smoking, alcohol and obesity in the UK: an update to 2006–07 NHS costs. *J Public Health*. December 1, 2011;33(4):527–535.

35. Gulliford MC, Charlton J, Booth HP, et al. Costs and outcomes of increasing access to bariatric surgery for obesity: cohort study and cost-effectiveness analysis using electronic health records. *Health Serv Deliv Res*. 2016;4(17).

36. Cawley J, Meyerhoefer C. The medical care costs of obesity: an instrumental variables approach. *J Health Econ*. January 2012;31(1):219–230.

37. Briggs AH, Claxton K, Sculpher MJ. *Decision Modelling for Health Economic Evaluation*. Oxford University Press; 2006.

38. Gray AM, Clarke PM, Wolstenholme JL. *Applied Methods of Cost-Effectiveness Analysis in Healthcare*. Oxford: OUP; 2011.

39. Copely V. *User Guide: Weight Management Economic Assessment Tool Version 2*. Oxford: Public Health England; 2016. Obesity Risk Factors Intelligence.

40. HM Government. Childhood obesity. A plan for action. In: *Health Do*. ; 2016.

41. Giles EL, Sniehotta FF, McColl E, Adams J. Acceptability of financial incentives for health behaviour change to public health policymakers: a qualitative study. *BMC Public Health*. September 15, 2016;16.

42. Gneezy U, Meier S, Rey-Biel P. When and why incentives (don't) work to modify behavior. *J Econ Perspect*. Fall 2011;25(4):191–209.

43. Bhattacharya J, Sood N. Health insurance and the obesity externality. In: *The Economics of Obesity*. ; 2006:279–318.

44. Taylor-Robinson DC, Lloyd-Williams F, Orton L, Moonan M, O'Flaherty M, Capewell S. Barriers to partnership working in public health: a qualitative study. *PLoS One*. 2012;7(1).

CHAPTER 3

Glucagon-Like Peptide 1 and Human Obesity

ANANTHI ANANDHAKRISHNAN (MBBS, IBSC, BMEDSCI) •
MÁRTA KORBONITS MD, PHD

INTRODUCTION

The ideal management of any illness involves an understanding of its underlying pathophysiology: greater understanding facilitates the development of targeted pharmacotherapies to either replete physiologic factors pathologically depleted or antagonize pathologic processes. The pathophysiology of obesity, however, remains poorly understood and may explain the currently suboptimal medical management of obesity[1]; the transient weight loss effects of some agents[2]; and potentially fatal adverse effects of others, meaning that until very recently the pancreatic lipase inhibitor orlistat was the only licensed antiobesity agent in the United Kingdom. Although lifestyle intervention is currently the first-line treatment for obesity,[1] weight loss effects are poorly sustained[3–5]; and the only proven treatment to achieve and maintain weight loss in obesity is bariatric surgery.[6–8] Excess surgical[9] and anesthetic[10] risks of obesity, together with treatment-related costs, see such invasive procedures reserved as a last resort.[1] The minimally invasive and efficacious management of obesity, therefore, remains an unmet clinical need.

Among its pleiotropic central and peripheral effects, the enteroendocrine hormone glucagon-like peptide 1 (GLP-1) acts as a potent incretin first clinically used in the medical management of overweight or obese individuals with type 2 diabetes (T2DM) (reviewed in Ref. 11). The repeatedly demonstrated ability of GLP-1 analogues to induce weight loss in this cohort[12,13] has prompted phase III trials studying the weight loss efficacy of the GLP-1 analogue liraglutide (3 mg) versus placebo[14] and the pancreatic lipase inhibitor orlistat[15,16] in nondiabetic overweight and obese adults. The greater weight loss efficacy achieved and maintained by GLP-1 agonism has prompted the Food and Drug Administration (FDA) in 2014 and

the European Medical Association (EMA) in 2015[17] to approve 3 mg liraglutide as the first GLP-1 analogue for use as a weight loss aid in obese adults and overweight adults with at least one weight-related comorbidity.[18] Although the current postmarketing surveillance suggests a low risk-benefit to treatment, launched in April 2015 in the United States at a cost of over $1000 per patient a month,[19] cost-benefit is of greater issue in nations such as the United Kingdom where healthcare is primarily socially funded. Clinical evidence, however, implicates a role for functional impairments in GLP-1 signaling in the pathophysiology of obesity, suggesting that GLP-1 agonists may be the first targeted therapeutic agents for use in the medical management of obesity and possibly explaining the superior weight loss efficacy of such agents. With greater sustained weight loss having the potential to reduce direct and indirect long-term financial burdens of obesity, cost-benefit may be swayed to favor the use of GLP-1 agonists as first-line agents in the medical management of obesity.[19]

GLUCAGON-LIKE PEPTIDE 1 PHYSIOLOGY
Synthesis Secretion and Degradation
GLP-1 is a 31 amino acid polypeptide derived from posttranslational processing of the native 160 amino acid peptide proglucagon by the enzyme prohormone convertase 1 (PC1/3) peripherally expressed in enteroendocrine L-cells and pancreatic α-cells and centrally in brainstem regions such as the nucleus of the solitary tract.[20–22] Tissue-specific posttranslational processing liberates different proglucagon-derived peptides,[23] depending on the subtype of prohormone convertase (PC) enzyme present (Fig. 3.1).

GLP-1 is primarily synthesized by PC1/3 activity in the intestinal L-cells,[29] most densely located in the

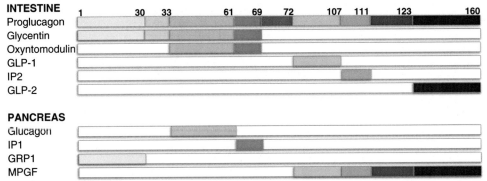

FIG. 3.1 Tissue-dependent proglucagon processing.[24–26] The 160 amino acid proglucagon gene (GCG), encoded on chromosome 2, undergoes tissue-specific posttranslational cleavage by prohormone convertase (PC) 1/3 and PC2 in central and peripheral sites (*numbers* indicate the amino acids bordering the cleavage products or at which the PC enzymes act). In the pancreas, PC2 dominates and liberates glucagon. In the intestine PC1/3 activity dominates and produces glucagon-like peptide 1 (GLP-1); of note, other products of proglucagon cleavage by PC1/3 are produced in a 1:1 ratio with GLP-1.[27,28] The PC responsible for cleaving GCG in the central nervous system is not well established; both PC1/3 and PC 2 may play a role. *GRP*, gastrin-releasing peptide; *IP*, intervening peptide; *MPGF*, major proglucagon fragment.

ileum[30,31] and colon.[32] L-cell GLP-1 secretion is biphasic: an initial rapid rise occurring within 10–15 min postprandial, attributed to neural signals from the parasympathetic vagal nerve and neurotransmitters such as gastrin-releasing peptide and acetylcholine, followed by a second longer phase peaking at 30–60 min most likely mediated via direct nutrient sensing. Fig. 3.2 details intestinal L-cell GLP-1 secretagogues, of which glucose has been implicated as the most potent in both healthy and type 2 diabetic humans.[33] Secreted GLP-1 is rapidly degraded by the ubiquitously expressed enzyme dipeptidyl peptidase IV,[34] most abundantly expressed in the hepatic portal system,[35] resulting in a short half-life of approximately 2 min. As such, only about 10%–15% of GLP-1 secreted from intestinal L-cells reaches peripheral downstream targets. The amount of GLP-1 reaching potential central targets is unknown. As parenteral administration of GLP-1 avoids this physiologic first-pass effect, the supraphysiologic plasma concentrations achieved by subcutaneous (SC) administration may explain the powerful weight loss effect of these agents.

Role in Energy Balance

Physiologically, energy balance is a closely regulated system involving peripheral signals to central controllers that act to modulate energy expenditure and food intake to maintain body weight (Fig. 3.3). Overall, energy status is signaled to central controllers of energy balance by long- or short-acting peripheral signals. Long-acting signals include the white adipocyte

hormone leptin[38] and pancreatic hormone insulin and provide information about available energy stores in response to which the brain makes corrective adjustments to food intake and energy expenditure to maintain body weight (reviewed in Ref. 39). In the short term, food intake and energy expenditure are governed by interactions between situational and meal-related factors that act to signal acute energy status. Information conveyed by gastric chemo- and mecho-receptors and gut-derived hormones such as GLP-1 play a key role in the short-term regulation of energy balance.

The hypothalamic arcuate nucleus (ARC) is believed to play a crucial role in the homeostatic control of energy balance, with distinct populations of orexigenic (appetite-stimulating)[40,41] and anorexigenic (appetite-suppressing) neurons[42,43] projecting to effectors in intrahypothalamic and extrahypothalamic sites. Despite a robust homeostatic system governing energy balance, feeding and meal termination are also influenced by hedonic, reward-related factors such as palatability; the drive to pursue such pleasurable experiences is largely mediated by the mesolimbic rewards system originating from dopaminergic neurons in ventral tegmental area (VTA) that terminate on neurons in the nucleus accumbens. Interestingly, where the homeostatic control of energy balance modulates food intake to regulate the amount of body fat an individual maintains,[54] despite an overall positive energy balance, hyperphagia is the norm and suggests a skew toward hedonic drivers to food intake in obesity. Where previously the neurocircuits mediating the homeostatic and hedonistic control

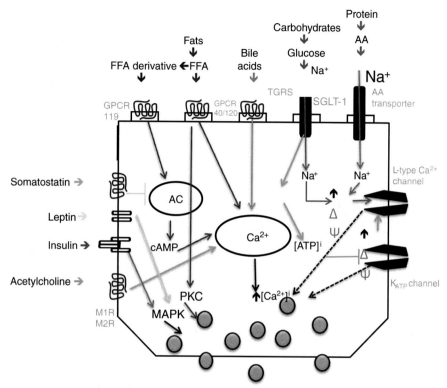

FIG. 3.2 Nutrient and neural glucagon-like peptide 1 (GLP-1) secretagogues in L-cell (reviewed in Refs. 24, 25, 36, and 37). Nutrients: Glucose derived from carbohydrate metabolism is the most potent stimuli for GLP-1 secretion and stimulates GLP-1 release via membrane depolarization ($\Delta\Psi$) secondary to sodium (Na) influx with glucose via sodium-glucose cotransporter 1 (SGLT-1), increasing intracellular Ca levels ([Ca^{2+}]i) by opening L-type Ca channels and causing subsequent GLP-1 release (*red arrows*). Glucose metabolism generates adenosine triphosphate (ATP) and increased intracellular ATP concentrations [ATP]i close KATP channels causing $\Delta\Psi$ increasing intracellular Ca levels ([Ca^{2+}]i) by opening L-type Ca channels and causing subsequent GLP-1 release. Fats are also potent stimuli for GLP-1 secretion. Free fatty acids (FFAs) (*blue arrows*) interact with G protein–coupled receptors (GPCRs) that trigger Ca^{2+} release from internal stores and also activate protein kinase C (PKC). FFA derivates (*purple arrows*) interact with GPCRs that activate second messenger systems involving adenylate cyclase (AC) and cyclic AMP (cAMP), which increases [Ca^{2+}]i. Bile acids (*orange arrows*) and short-chained fatty acids (not shown) also increase [Ca^{2+}]I by GPCR interactions. Protein is a weak stimulator of GLP-1 release. Amino acids (AAs) derived from protein breakdown are transported intracellularly with Na+ via Na+-dependent AA transporters. Na+ influx causes membrane depolarization and elevated [Ca^{2+}]i with resultant GLP-1 exocytosis (*pink arrows*). Somatostatin inhibits GLP-1 release by blocking AC activation (*light blue arrows*). The peripheral adiposity signals leptin (*yellow arrows*) and insulin (*brown arrows*) are thought to stimulate GLP-1 release via activation of mitogen-activated protein kinase (MAPK) signaling pathway. Neural signals: Acetylcholine binding to muscarinic receptors (M1R, M2R) elevates [Ca^{2+}]I stimulating GLP-1 release (*gray arrows*). Gastrin-releasing peptide is thought to stimulate GLP-1 release in association with the activation of mitogen-activated protein kinase kinase (MAPKK) and subsequent phosphorylation and activation of MAPK (not shown). (Figure modified from Anandhakrishnan, A. & Korbonits, M. (2016) Glucagon-like peptide 1 in the pathophysiology and pharmacotherapy of clinical obesity. *World Journal of Diabetes* **7**, 572-598.)

of energy balance were considered distinct entities, it has now emerged that considerable cross talk exists with central GLP-1 signaling implicated as a mediator (detailed in a number of excellent reviews[51–53]); GLP-1 receptors (GLP-1Rs) have localized preclinically in the ARC[47] and paraventricular nucleus[48] of the hypothalamus, with stimulation of these receptors reducing the food intake to induce weight loss in rodents, and in the dopaminergic neurons of the VTA[55] where activation inhibits neural firing, potentially reducing hedonic

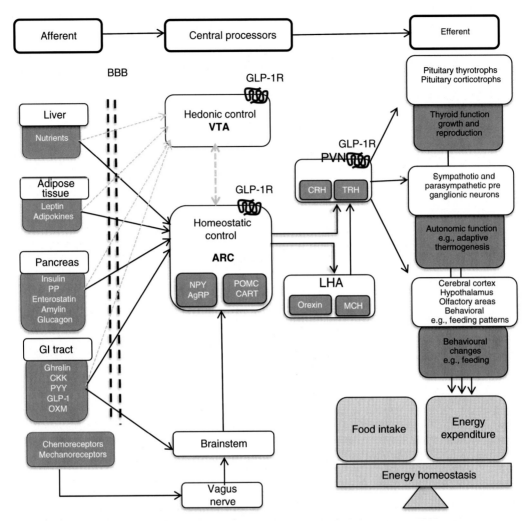

FIG. 3.3 The energy balance equation. (1) Afferent peripheral signals from the liver, adipose tissue, pancreas, and gastrointestinal tract (GI-tract) cross the blood-brain barrier (BBB) to signal directly to the central controllers of energy balance. Peripheral afferents can also indirectly activate central controllers via the vagus nerve and brainstem. (2) Central controllers: The hypothalamic arcuate nucleus (ARC) is believed to play a crucial role in the homeostatic control of energy balance containing two distinct neural populations exerting antagonistic effects on food intake: a medially located orexigenic population coexpressing Agouti-related peptide (AgRP) and neuropeptide Y (NPY)[40,41] and a laterally located anorexigenic population coexpressing proopiomelanocortin (POMC) and cocaine and amphetamine related transcript (CART).[42,43] Both neural subsets project to melanocortin 4 receptor (MC4R), where POMC is cleaved to produce α-MSH, an agonist of MC4R,[44] and AgRP acts an inverse agonist.[45,46] MC4R are located in intrahypothalamic (paraventricular nucleus [PVN] and lateral hypothalamic area [LHA]) and extrahypothalamic sites. GLP-1Rs have been localized preclinically in the ARC[47] and PVN.[48] Hedonic control of energy balance is mediated in then ventral tegmental area (VTA). GLP-1Rs have been localized preclinically in the VTA.[49] Cross-interactions exist between central homeostatic and hedonic control centers[50] potentially mediated by central GLP-1 signaling (reviewed in Refs. 51–53) (3) Efferent pathways: Overall energy balance can be modulated by altering food intake and energy expenditure; to date evidence hedonic controls of energy balance are thought to exert their effects mainly by modulating food intake. Downstream effectors of homeostatic controllers of energy balance involve the activation of thyrotropin releasing hormone (TRH) and corticotropin releasing hormone (CRH) expressing neurons and preganglionic sympathetic and parasympathetic neurons that may modulate energy balance by energy expenditure as well as food intake. CKK, cholecystokinin; OXM, oxyntomodulin; PP, pancreatic polypeptide; PYY, polypeptide-YY. (Figure modified from Anandhakrishnan, A. & Korbonits, M. (2016) Glucagon-like peptide 1 in the pathophysiology and pharmacotherapy of clinical obesity. World Journal of Diabetes 7, 572-598.)

drives toward food consumption. With evidence existing to suggest that clinical obesity is associated with functional deficits in GLP-1, perhaps this deficit contributes toward the hedonic hyperphagia, promoting weight gain despite an overall positive energy balance.

GLUCAGON-LIKE PEPTIDE 1 AND THE REGULATION OF ENERGY BALANCE IN MAN

Several clinical studies report the relationship of acute physiologic[56] and supraphysiologic[57] administration of GLP-1 to mimic that of postprandial release with measures of food intake and levels of hunger and satiety in lean[57] and obese adults with[58] and without T2DM.[59] With results from individual studies summarized in Fig. 3.4, a metaanalysis reports a mean 11.7% decrease in food intake following acute GLP-1 infusion when compared with saline control.[60] The long-acting GLP-1 analogue liraglutide administered at supraphysiologic doses (3 mg) has shown a superior weight loss efficacy in nondiabetic obese subjects when compared with currently licensed antiobesity agents and saline control; to date, however, clinical studies assessing the comparative efficacy of acute versus continuous GLP-1 administration on energy balance remain scarce. One study[61] compared the effects on food intake and weight loss after four doses of acute GLP-1 infused 30 min before meals with those of an equivalent dose of continuous SC GLP-1 infusion and reported a greater weight loss compared with placebo following acute administration. Data are limited, however, by potential biases

introduced by the significantly greater peak plasma GLP-1 concentrations observed following acute dosing. In view of the lack of data to suggest significant differences in efficacy, and bearing in mind the negative impacts on adherence posed by multidose regimes, once-daily bolus administration, at present, seems to be the most clinically efficacious means of therapeutic GLP-1 analogue delivery. Although evidence suggests that acute postprandial GLP-1 secretion contributes to negative energy balance by decreasing the food intake, its effects on energy expenditure are less clear; some studies reported reduced energy expenditure following physiologic infusions of GLP-1 in lean[62] and nondiabetic obese patients,[59] whereas others observed increases in energy expenditure in response to supraphysiologic dosing.[63]

Mediators of Glucagon-Like Peptide 1–Induced Negative Energy Balance in Man

GLP-1 exerts its effects by intracellular signaling pathways activated after binding to the G protein–coupled receptor (GPCR) GLP-1R.[68] The extensive central and peripheral expression of the GLP-R[24] reflecting the pleiotropic physiologic roles of GLP-1 is summarized in Fig. 3.5 and extensively reviewed elsewhere.[36] Together, evidence from clinical interventional studies suggests that acute postmeal rises in GLP-1 contribute to negative energy balance primarily through an anorexigenic effect, potentially mediated by GLP-1 interactions with peripheral afferents and central controllers of the hedonic and homeostatic energy balance equation.

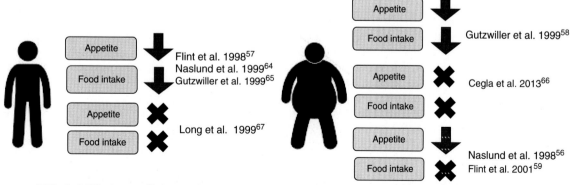

FIG. 3.4 Effects on self-assessed appetite scores and ad libitum food intake in lean and obese subjects following physiologic[56,59,64–66] and supraphysiologic[57,58,65,67] infusions of glucagon-like peptide 1 (GLP-1). Although individual studies report conflicting data, a metaanalysis of clinical studies evaluating the acute effects of GLP-1 infusion on food intake reports a mean 11.7% decrease when compared with saline control.[60] (Figure modified from Anandhakrishnan, A. & Korbonits, M. (2016) Glucagon-like peptide 1 in the pathophysiology and pharmacotherapy of clinical obesity. *World Journal of Diabetes* **7**, 572-598.)

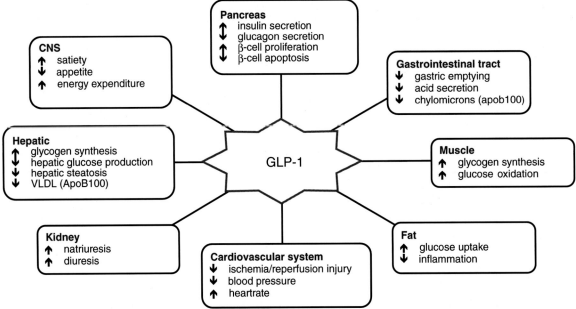

FIG. 3.5 Peripheral effects of glucagon-like peptide 1 (GLP-1). The peripheral effects of GLP-1 may be classed broadly as pancreatic or extrapancreatic. Pancreatic effects of GLP-1 act to promote insulin secretion (incretin effect). Extrapancreatic effects of GLP-1 include (1) regulation of energy metabolism and nutrient storage (the liver, muscle, and fat), (2) efficient nutrient handling (the stomach and gastrointestinal tract), and (3) others: cardiovascular repair, blood pressure control, diuresis (reviewed in Ref. 36). Interactions with peripheral afferents of the energy balance equation. *VLDL*, very low-density lipoproteins. (Figure modified from Anandhakrishnan, A. & Korbonits, M. (2016) Glucagon-like peptide 1 in the pathophysiology and pharmacotherapy of clinical obesity. *World Journal of Diabetes* **7**, 572-598.)

Gastric mechanoreceptors

Gastric mechanoreceptors are activated by gastric distension following acute nutrient intake and act as meal-to-meal satiety signals to ARC and the VTA (reviewed in Ref. 69; see Role in energy balance and Figure 3.3 Delayed gastric emptying is associated with increased mechanoreceptor firing and is also positively associated with increased satiety and fullness in both healthy and obese patients.[70-74] GLP-1 has been found to delay gastric emptying in healthy lean,[75-77] obese,[56] and type 2 diabetic[78] subjects, and histologic studies in man have shown that GLP-1Rs are expressed in gastric mucosa.[79] Postprandial GLP-1 secretion may therefore exert its anorectic effect through activating GLP-1Rs in gastric mucosa.

Incretin effect

The most extensively studied physiologic role of GLP-1 is as a positive modulator of insulin secretion from pancreatic β-cells (reviewed in Ref. 80). Insulin has been traditionally viewed as a long-acting anorectic signal in the energy balance equation (reviewed in Refs. 39 and 51). Insulin, however, displays both basal and acute meal-related secretion,[81] and acute insulin administration has been associated with reduced food intake in lean individuals,[82] suggesting a role as a short-term satiety signal. Insulin receptors are widely expressed in the ARC[83,84] and VTA[85]; thus GLP-1–induced insulin secretion and secondary signaling to homeostatic and hedonic appetite controllers may be the means by which GLP-1 achieves its anorectic effects.

Ghrelin

Ghrelin is the only orexigenic peripheral afferent in the energy balance equation released preprandially by the G-cells of the stomach to promote feeding, with postmeal ghrelin suppression contributing to meal termination. Ghrelin receptors have been identified preclinically in ARC[86] and VTA[87] neurons; receptor stimulation is positively associated with food consumption. GLP-1 infusion in lean humans has been associated with significant suppression of postprandial rises in ghrelin,[88] the decline in orexigenic signaling a potential mediator of GLP-1's anorectic effect.

Interactions with central controllers of the energy balance equation

Functional neuroimaging in man has provided in vivo evidence to suggest GLP-1 may mediate its anorectic effect through direct signaling to central hedonic and homeostatic appetite controllers. PET studies have demonstrated that GLP-1 infusion in lean individuals reduces glucose metabolism in the hypothalamus and brainstem,[89] with correlations between hypothalamic blood flow and physiologic postprandial rises in serum GLP-1 observed elsewhere.[90] Although findings may represent altered neural activity in brain regions associated with homeostatic energy balance secondary to central GLP-1 signaling, the effects of this altered neural activity on food intake and appetite have not been explored. Elsewhere, fMRI[91] has demonstrated that GLP-1 infusion in lean individuals attenuates neuronal activity in brain regions involved in rewards processing accompanied with reductions in food intake. Findings suggest that postprandial GLP-1 may induce its anorectic effect by direct signaling to hedonic appetite control centers to suppress pleasurable drives to food consumption, allowing physiologic anorectic signals to initiate meal termination.

GLUCAGON-LIKE PEPTIDE 1 IN THE PATHOPHYSIOLOGY OF CLINICAL OBESITY

Functional Glucagon-Like Peptide 1 Deficits as a Risk Factor Toward the Obesity Phenotype

Genetic analyses in human monogenic and polygenic obesity suggest that a lack of functional GLP-1 signaling may act as a risk factor toward the development of the obesity phenotype.

Monogenic obesity

Accounting for less than 1% of total cases of obesity worldwide, monogenic human obesity is a rare form of clinical obesity that shows Mendelian patterns of inheritance.[92] Six studies to date document the relationship between autosomal recessive, compound heterozygous[93–95] or homozygous[96] mutations in PCSK1 encoding the enzyme PC1/3 in 21 probands, all of whom presented with an early onset hyperphagic obesity with varying endocrine phenotypes. Although the cause of obesity and endocrine phenotypes associated with PCSK1 mutation are unknown,

they may well be attributed to impaired intestinal PC1/3 prohormone processing of proglucagon,[96] and indeed enteroendocrine expression of GLP-1 is significantly reduced compared with control in children with PCSK1 monogenic obesity.[96] Disappointingly, only two of six studies detailing the phenotypes PCSK1-mutant probands assess postprandial GLP-1 secretory responses and reports are conflicting; while an oral glucose load (oral glucose tolerance test, OGTT) yields significantly reduced GLP-1 response in three child probands compared with age-matched controls,[96] postprandial responses in a 40-year-old proband match those of healthy age-matched controls.[93] Interestingly, GLP-1 secretion following OGTT in the three paediatric probands suggested an inverse relationship between GLP-1 secretory impairment and age. This may represent another manifestation of the age-dependent impairments in endocrine function seen in PCSK1 mutant probands.[97] Comparing the enteroendocrine expression of GLP-1 in adult PCSK1-mutant probands against the documented reduced expression documented in children[96] may allow such a relationship to be quantified.

Polygenic obesity

Instead of being attributed to the phenotypic result of single gene defects, the pathogenesis behind the current clinical obesity epidemic is complex and poorly understood. Defined by some as the interaction between the "obesogenic environment" (reviewed in Refs. 98,99) and a genetic predisposition (reviewed in Refs. 100–102), genomewide association studies have identified 119 independent gene loci implicated as risk factors toward "common" or polygenic obesity.[103,104] One such gene is *PCSK1*: single-nucleotide polymorphisms at three independent *PCSK1* consistently linked to an increased risk of obesity.[105–109] Although it is unclear how these minor alleles predispose to obesity, in vitro studies suggest that the encoded PC1/3 variants may not be as enzymatically active or physiologically available as the common form, potentially resulting in a partial GLP-1 deficiency that may confer an increased risk toward obesity.

Obesity as a Risk Factor Toward Functional Glucagon-Like Peptide 1 Deficits

Although genetic studies implicate a role for primary alterations in GLP-1 signaling as a risk factor toward obesity, clinical studies assessing physiologic GLP-1 responses in normal-weight and obese subjects suggest that weight gain may induce functional deficits in GLP-1 that may maintain and propagate weight gain.

Post–oral glucose tolerance test glucagon-like peptide 1 secretory responses

A number of clinical studies have assessed the effect of GLP-1 secretion in obese and lean subjects following an oral 75 g glucose load (OGTT)[110–113] or postprandial following a balanced meal. Studies consistently demonstrate a reduced GLP-1 secretion post-OGTT in obese subjects compared with lean control; however, postprandial GLP-1 responses are conflicting: some observing significant reductions[114–116] and others with no change[117–120] (Fig. 3.6).

In vivo neuroimaging and self-assessments of appetite

Functional GLP-1 signaling in hedonic brain regions is associated with reduced food consumption.[121] fMRI studies have provided evidence in vivo to suggest that hedonic brain regions show altered patterns of functioning in obese subjects: reduced brain activity in response to the consumption of, and increased activity in response to the anticipation of palatable food consistently observed when compared with lean control.[121–123] Interestingly, GLP-1 agonism reverses these functional changes to match those of lean control with associated reductions in food intake,[121] an effect prevented by pretreatment with a GLP-1 antagonist.[124] Subjectively assessed, emotional eating scores have been defined as hedonic markers of appetite[125] that display strong positive associations with the degree of human obesity[126] and, in obese subjects, are inversely correlated with GLP-1R signaling in brain regions involved in rewards processing.[127]

Although GLP-1 secretory response and results from fMRI and appetite scores support a role for

obesity-induced GLP-1 functional impairments in human obesity, observing demonstrable deficits in GLP-1 secretion following weight gain in a normal-weight individual would provide greater support to such a claim.

Potential Mechanisms of Obesity-Induced Functional Deficits in Glucagon-Like Peptide 1

L-cell glucose sensing deficits

Clinical studies consistently demonstrate a decreased GLP-1 secretory response following an OGTT in obese subjects. With glucose being the most potent GLP-1 secretagogue, such responses may be secondary to obesity-induced reductions in L-cell glucose sensing capacity. Support for such a postulate comes from findings by Ranganath et al.[116] who demonstrate that while GLP-1 secretion to an oral fat load remains intact, GLP-1 secretion in response to an oral carbohydrate load is decreased in obesity.

Target organ hyposensitivity

Although supraphysiologic doses of GLP-1 reduces appetite and food intake in both lean[57,65] and obese subjects,[58] physiologic GLP-1 doses achieve a similar effect in only lean subjects,[64,65] suggesting resistance to physiologic GLP-1 signaling and obesity.

Interactions with peripheral efferents of the energy balance equation

Although the mechanisms of reduced functional postprandial GLP-1 signaling in obesity remain to be defined, clinical evidence implicates a role for interactions between GLP-1 and other short- and long-term peripheral effectors of energy balance.

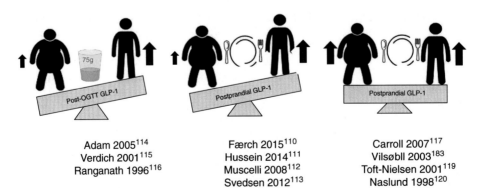

Adam 2005[114]
Verdich 2001[115]
Ranganath 1996[116]

Færch 2015[110]
Hussein 2014[111]
Muscelli 2008[112]
Svedsen 2012[113]

Carroll 2007[117]
Vilsøbll 2003[183]
Toft-Nielsen 2001[119]
Naslund 1998[120]

FIG. 3.6 Effects of obesity on glucagon-like peptide 1 (GLP-1) responses post-OGTT and postprandial. Obese subjects consistently demonstrate reduced GLP-1 secretory responses following a 75 g oral glucose load (OGTT, oral glucose tolerance test)[110–113] compared with lean controls. Postprandial GLP-1 secretory responses in obese subjects are conflicting, with some studies observing significant reductions[114–116] and others observing no change[117–120] when compared with lean controls. (Figure modified from Anandhakrishnan, A. & Korbonits, M. (2016) Glucagon-like peptide 1 in the pathophysiology and pharmacotherapy of clinical obesity. *World Journal of Diabetes* 7, 572-598.)

Insulin. The most extensively studied of physiologic role of GLP-1 is as an insulin secretagogue (reviewed in Ref. 80). Hyperinsulinemia is positively associated with increased BMI in individuals with normal glucose tolerance,[117,128] and increased BMI and increasing glucose intolerance have been shown to independently and additively impair GLP-1 secretion.[110] The chronic hyperinsulinemia is positively associated with increasing levels of obesity; therefore, it may act as a negative feedback signal to downregulate physiologic postprandial GLP-1 release in obese subjects.

Leptin. Leptin acts as a satiety signal governing long-term energy balance. Increased BMI has been shown to be positively correlated with fasted leptin[129]; however, obese subjects are thought to be resistant to leptin's effects (reviewed in Ref. 130). In vitro studies of human intestinal L-cells have shown that leptin acts a GLP-1 secretagogue[131]; thus perhaps the leptin resistance associated with obesity may account for the decreased postprandial GLP-1 secretion observed.[114]

Ghrelin. Released preprandially, the orexigenic hormone ghrelin promotes meal initiation and increases food intake. It has also been shown to enhance postprandial GLP-1 release in pre-clinical studies.[132] Clinical obesity has been associated with reductions in both fasting ghrelin levels and postprandial GLP-1.[114] Whilst reductions in baseline ghrelin levels may facilitate the lowered postprandial GLP-1 levels seen in clinical obesity, suppression of late postprandial rises in ghrelin has been shown clinically to be one mechanism by which GLP-1 exerts its anorectic effect,[88] an action that is impaired in obese individuals.[133,134] Derangements in both orexigneic and anorexigenic enteroendocrine signaling associated with clinical obesity create a feed-forward cycle facilitating hyperphagia despite an overall energy balance.

Interactions with the central controllers of energy balance
Where the homeostatic control of energy balance modulates food intake to regulate the amount of body fat an individual maintains,[54] in obesity, despite an overall positive energy balance, hyperphagia is the norm. Excessive consumption of palatable food can trigger neuroadaptive responses in brain reward circuits similar to that of alcohol and drugs of abuse (reviewed in Ref. 135), and clinical studies provide evidence to suggest that human obesity is associated with altered rewards processing that may render the hyperphagia of obesity the manifestation of a "food addiction"; fMRI studies provide evidence in vivo to suggest that hedonic

brain regions show GLP-1-dependant altered patterns of functioning in obese subjects.[121,124]; where GLP-1 infusions induce similar reducations in appetite reductions in obese subjects to their lean peers[59], unlike their lean peers this reduction in appetite is not translated to reduced food consumption. Such findings perhaps the result of an end-organ hyposensitivity to GLP-1 in obesity. Irrespective of the cause, GLP-1-associated altered signaling to central controllers of appetite in obesity potentially reinforces hedonic feeding despite a reduced physiologic drive to food intake, resulting in continued weight gain.

GLUCAGON-LIKE PEPTIDE 1 IN THE PHARMACOTHERAPY OF CLINICAL OBESITY
Restoration of Functional Glucagon-Like Peptide 1 Signaling as a Weight Loss Agent in Obesity
Roux-en-y gastric bypass
Bariatric surgery remains the most effective treatment modality for morbid obesity, with a metaanalysis reporting the Roux-en-y gastric bypass (RYGB) to produce a greater and more sustained weight loss than currently available pharmacotherapy, lifestyle interventions, or other bariatric options.[136] Prospective studies assessing the effects of RYGB on postprandial GLP-1 responses in nondiabetic obese patients consistently report statistically significant increases in postprandial GLP-1 when compared with the preoperative state,[137–143] following equivalent weight losses with gastric banding,[138,139,141,143] and when compared with healthy lean control[141] (Fig. 3.7). This postoperative supraphysiologic GLP-1 secretory response perhaps explains the greater short- and long-term weight loss efficacy achieved with this treatment modality.

Glucagon-like peptide 1 agonists
A phase II (NCT00422058)[16] and a number of phase III multinational double-blinded randomized control trials conducted in nondiabetic obese adults (NCT00480909),[15] overweight adults with at least one weight-related comorbidity (SCALE Obesity and Prediabetes and SCALE Maintenance[144,145]), nondiabetic obese adults with obstructive sleep apnea (SCALE OSA[14]), and obese adults with T2DM (SCALE Diabetes[146]) have established the efficacy of once-daily 3 mg SC GLP-1 analogue liraglutide as an adjunct to lifestyle interventions for weight management in morbidly obese or comorbidly obese individuals. Results from the first study, a 20-week phase II trial in nondiabetic obese subjects, showed that weight loss with liraglutide is dose-dependent up to

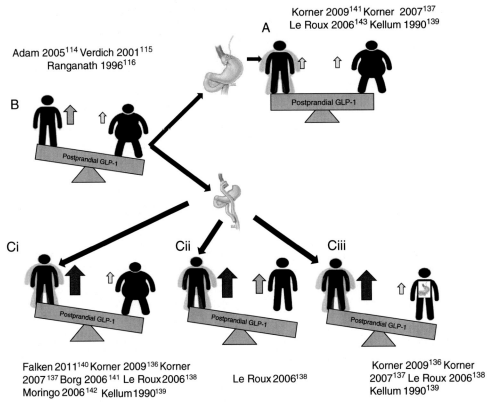

FIG. 3.7 Effects of weight loss induced by gastric banding and Roux-en-Y gastric bypass (RYGB) on postprandial glucagon-like peptide 1 (GLP-1) secretion. Weight loss following gastric banding **(A)** induces no changes in postprandial GLP-1 levels from preoperative levels **(B)**. All seven studies assessing the effects of postprandial GLP-1 secretion following weight loss with RYGB show significantly increased responses compared with presurgery responses and healthy obese controls **(Ci)**, healthy lean controls **(Cii)**, and following weight losses following gastric banding **(Ciii)**. (Figure modified from Anandhakrishnan, A. & Korbonits, M. (2016) Glucagon-like peptide 1 in the pathophysiology and pharmacotherapy of clinical obesity. *World Journal of Diabetes* **7**, 572-598.)

3.0 mg once daily,[15,145] with significantly more liraglutide 3 mg/day recipients than placebo or orlistat recipients achieving a 5% or 10% reduction in body weight at 20 weeks. In a 2-year phase III extension of the same study,[15] double-blind treatment (liraglutide 1.2–3 mg/day) was continued until week 52, after which all liraglutide (<2.4 mg/day) and placebo recipients were switched to liraglutide 2.4 mg, then to 3.0 mg (week 70–96) based on 20-week and 1-year results, respectively, which indicated that this was the optimal dosage. At 2 years, mean body weight reductions in those randomized to liraglutide were significantly greater than pancreatic lipase inhibitor orlistat, the only alternative licensed weight loss agent in the United Kingdom. A similarly significant reduction in body weight and increased 5% and 10% responder rates were observed in subjects randomized to 3 mg liraglutide when compared with placebo in all

four subsequent phase III trials,[14,144–146] depicted in Fig. 3.8. With even modest losses of 5%–10% of total body weight associated with reduced risk of comorbidities in obese individuals,[147–149] findings provide rationale for the use of 3 mg liraglutide as an adjunct to lifestyle alteration and as the first-line antiobesity pharmaceutical agent for weight management in obese and comorbidly overweight adults.

Potential Mechanisms of Weight Loss Induced by Supraphysiologic Glucagon-Like Peptide 1 Levels

Weight losses following bariatric surgery, pharmacotherapy or diet, and lifestyle modification are all associated with decreases in circulating leptin and improved insulin sensitivity. The resultant reductions in anorexigenic signaling of these long-term afferents of the

Labels within figure:
Korner 2009[141] Korner 2007[137] Le Roux 2006[143] Kellum 1990[139] A
Adam 2005[114] Verdich 2001[115] Ranganath 1996[116] B
Postprandial GLP-1
Ci Cii Ciii
Falken 2011[140] Korner 2009[136] Korner 2007[137] Borg 2006[141] Le Roux 2006[138] Moringo 2006[142] Kellum 1990[139]
Le Roux 2006[138]
Korner 2009[136] Korner 2007[137] Le Roux 2006[138] Kellum 1990[139]

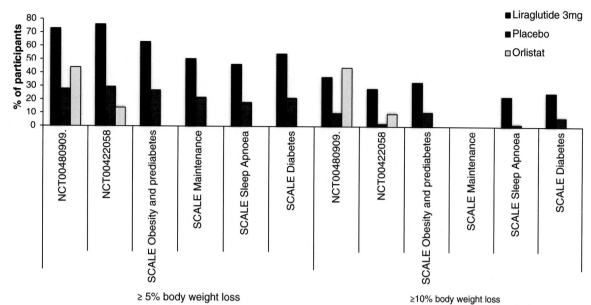

FIG. 3.8 5% and 10% weight loss achieved following 3 mg subcutaneous (SC) liraglutide compared with placebo and orlistat. Liraglutide 3 mg is consistently associated with higher 5% and 10% responder rates in nondiabetic obese subjects when compared with orlistat and placebo at 1 and 2 years (NCT00480909 and NCT00422058).[15] Liraglutide was superior in nondiabetic obese subjects in the Sleep Apnoea trial,[14] SCALE Maintenance,[145] and SCALE Obesity and Prediabetes[144] trials when compared with placebo alone, and also in obese diabetic in the SCALE Diabetes trial.[146] (Figure modified from Anandhakrishnan, A. & Korbonits, M. (2016) Glucagon-like peptide 1 in the pathophysiology and pharmacotherapy of clinical obesity. *World Journal of Diabetes* **7**, 572-598.)

energy balance equation potentially facilitate weight gain and may explain the difficulty obese subjects have in attaining and maintaining weight loss. Supraphysiologic GLP-1 levels achieved following RYGB and treatment with high-dose GLP-1 analogues may antagonize the orexigenic drives associated with weight loss, explaining the weight loss efficacy of RYGB and 3 mg liraglutide.

Roux-en-y gastric bypass

Postprandial GLP-1 responses following RYGB are significantly greater than those following gastric banding (that show no change from preoperative levels[137,138,140]) and when compared with responses observed in lean controls. GLP-1 responses post-RYGB are also positively associated with the amount of weight lost. Deranged L-cell carbohydrate sensing has been implicated in the pathophysiology of human obesity, and 1 year post-RYGB a significantly greater achieved and maintained weight loss was associated with significantly increased GLP-1 responses to a carbohydrate meal.[143] Perhaps therefore the feedforward effect of weight loss on GLP-1 signaling and the resultant supraphysiologic GLP-1 signaling allows for a resensitzation

of end organs to GLP-1, allowing long-term weight loss maintenance in the face of increased orexigenic drives.

Liraglutide 3 mg

Excessive consumption of palatable food can trigger neuroadaptive responses in brain reward circuits similar to that of alcohol and drugs of abuse (reviewed in Ref. 135), and clinical studies provide evidence to suggest that human obesity is associated with altered rewards processing mediated in part by altered GLP-1 function that may render the hyperphagia of obesity the manifestation of a "food addiction." As such, perhaps GLP-1 agonism may produce its weight loss effects by attenuating the negative reinforcement to hyperphagia in obesity. Although 3 mg liraglutide has been shown to induce weight loss in man by reducing appetite,[150] preclinically, liraglutide has been shown to attenuate the reinforcing properties of alcohol.[151] Interestingly, although all aforementioned trials[15] advise the participants to restrict food consumption throughout treatment, adherence rates are not reported. If GLP-1 agonism induced its weight loss effects, at least in part, by modulating food-related rewards, an increased adherence to caloric restriction would be expected. It would be interesting to see if this were the case.

Glucagon-Like Peptide 1 Agonism in the Clinic

Greater understanding of the underlying disease pathophysiology facilitates the development of targeted therapeutics with the potential for greater efficacy in managing medical illness, whereas the poorly understood pathophysiology of clinical obesity perhaps explains the scarcity of clinically efficacious pharmacotherapeutics to date. Several lines of clinical evidence, however, implicate a role for altered GLP-1 function in the pathophysiology of human obesity, and a number of recent clinical trials have validated the efficacy of once-daily SC 3 mg liraglutide as an antiobesity agent in obese and overweight individuals with at least one weight-related comorbidity. Balancing drug efficacy against tolerability and cost, however, ultimately determines the selection of a pharmacologic agent for widespread clinical use.

Cost-benefit of 3 mg liraglutide as an antiobesity agent

Treatment period. Follow-up period (FUP) assessments in the SCALE Maintenance[144,145] and SCALE Diabetes[146] trials suggest that weight loss with 3 mg liraglutide is treatment dependent; weight gains in excess to those seen in placebo control and subjects rerandomized to treatment were observed in liraglutide-treated participants on treatment cessation (Fig. 3.9A). Reducing

the prevalance of obesity and overweight has been shown to significantly improve health outcomes and reduce healthcare costs long term.[152] However, in spite of their proven clinical efficacy, the cost (over $1000 per patient a month) associated with the use of GLP-1 agonists as weight loss agents in countries, such as the United Kingdom, where healthcare is primarily socially funded, seems unsustainable. A potential solution comes from longitudinal observations from demonstrating that subjects randomized to liraglutide 3 mg achieve maximal rates of weight loss in the initial 0- to 20-week treatment period, with a tendency toward weight gain beyond 36 weeks.[16] Findings suggest that although initially treatment with a GLP-1 analogue may compensate for functional deficits in obesity, prolonged treatment may be associated with the development of treatment resistance (Fig. 3.9B). Based on this, perhaps treatment with liraglutide 3 mg should be prescribed for 20 to a maximum of 36 weeks alongside behavioral therapies promoting lifestyle changes to combat the addiction-driven hyperphagia implicated in obesity pathophysiology. This approach, integrating the psychosocial empowerment associated with patient self-management of chronic illness, alongside cost-benefits associated with limited in-treatment period, seems to be an attractive one, especially if sustainable long-term weight losses with resultant reductions in the socioeconomic impacts of weight-related comorbidities can be achieved.

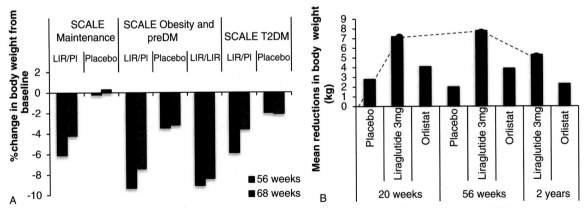

FIG. 3.9 Body weight changes associated with treatment with 3 mg liraglutide. **(A)** Follow-up period (FUP) analyses: following the 56-week treatment period a 12 week FUP was conducted in SCALE Maintenance, SCALE Obesity and Prediabetes, and SCALE Diabetes trials. 12 week FUP was an off-treatment period in SCALE Maintenance and SCALE Diabetes. In SCALE Obesity and Prediabetes FUP period involved a rerandomization to either 3 mg liraglutide (LIR/LIR) or placebo (LIR/Pl) and although weight gain occurred in all three groups weight gain was significantly higher following cessation of liraglutide. **(B)** In-treatment analyses: 3 mg liraglutide shows greater, dose-dependent reductions in body weight compared with placebo and orlistat with maximal effect between 0 and 20 weeks of treatment reducing from 20 to 36 with a tendency toward weight gain from 36 weeks and beyond; *red line dotted trace* shows patters of weight loss from baseline in those subjects treated with 3 mg liraglutide. (Figure modified from Anandhakrishnan, A. & Korbonits, M. (2016) Glucagon-like peptide 1 in the pathophysiology and pharmacotherapy of clinical obesity. *World Journal of Diabetes* **7**, 572-598.)

Reducing indirect healthcare costs of obesity and overweight. Being overweight or obese is the main modifiable risk factor for T2DM.[155] T2DM is one of the major indirect financial burdens of obesity and overweight. Increased BMI and impaired glucose tolerance have been shown to independently and additively impair post-OGTT GLP-1 responses,[110] and treatment with the first-line anti-diabetic agent metformin upregulates GLP-1 secretory response following an OGTT[153] perhaps explaining its weight loss[154] properties. Such observations suggest that functional deficits of GLP-1 may underpin a common pathophysiology to obesity and T2DM. Although costly, in addition to a superior weight loss efficacy, treatment with 3 mg liraglutide[15,145] is associated with a greater reversion to normal glycemic control and reduced T2DM incidence[144] in nondiabetic obese subjects. Findings suggests that treatment with GLP-1 analogues may be associated with reductions in both direct and indirect costs of obesity and overweight. However, weight loss in itself is associated with improvements in glycemic control, and true cost-benefit of funding liraglutide 3 mg on the rationale of T2DM prevention may exist only if the improved glucose tolerance achieved following a quantified weight loss with liraglutide 3 mg exceeds that attained following an equivalent weight loss achieved by using other, arguably cheaper treatment modalities. Statistically comparing the correlations between percentage weight lost with changes in glucose tolerance in nondiabetic obese subjects randomized to liraglutide 3 mg compared with those administered orlistat[15,145] or placebo[16] in aforementioned phase III trials may be one way this could be assessed (modeled in Fig. 3.10). If indeed pharmacologic GLP-1 agonism improves glucose tolerance in excess to that achieved with equivalent weight loss induced by other treatment modalities, then the potential of GLP-1 agonists to curb the prevalence and resultant socioeconomic burden of T2DM provides further rationale for the use of liraglutide 3 mg as the first-line antiobesity agent for weight management in obese and comorbidly overweight individuals.

Adverse drug events
In-treatment period. The safety and efficacy of liraglutide 3 mg has been evaluated in five phase III double-blind placebo-controlled trials[15] comprising 3384 overweight or obese subjects receiving liraglutide 3 mg and 1941 placebo controls for treatment periods of 32,[14] 52,[15] and 56[144,145] weeks. In a pooled analysis of the five aforementioned trials, liraglutide 3 mg in obese and overweight subjects was generally well tolerated, with most adverse drug events being gastrointestinal in nature, transient, and of mild to moderate intensity.[15,16,144–146] However, 9.8% of liraglutide and 4.3% of placebo recipients discontinued treatment because of an adverse event.[156] Of interest, 0.6% of subjects receiving liraglutide 3 mg experienced increases in mean heart rate (an average baseline increase of 2.5 beats/min) compared with 0.1% of placebo recipients.[157]

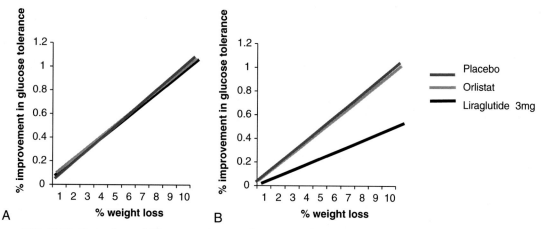

FIG. 3.10 Theoretic model to assess glucose tolerance as a factor of weight. **(A)** If the greater glucose sensitivity seen following treatment with liraglutide 3 mg is secondary to the greater weight loss achieved, the relationship between a given weight reduction and the percentage improvement in glucose tolerance should be the same in all treatment groups. **(B)** If, however, the relationship between a given weight loss and change in glucose tolerance is less strong following treatment with liraglutide, findings would suggest that mechanisms beyond weight loss contribute to the greater improvements of glucose tolerance seen following glucagon-like peptide 1 (GLP-1) agonism, perhaps an effect mediated by supraphysiologic GLP-1 counteracting the end-organ GLP-1 hyposensitivity associated with obesity.

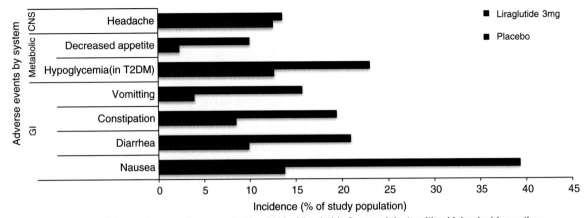

FIG. 3.11 Adverse drug reactions reported in ≥10% of liraglutide 3 mg recipients with a higher incidence than placebo stratified by system. CNS: Dizziness, malaise, and fatigue were also more prevalent in liraglutide-treated participants but occurred with incidence ≤10%, not shown. Metabolic: Liraglutide reduces blood glucose and thus, there is a potential for hypoglycemia to occur. In the SCALE Diabetes trial severe hypoglycemia occurred in 3 (0.7%) of 422 liraglutide-treated patients and in none of the 212 placebo-treated patients. In clinical trials involving patients without type 2 diabetes (T2DM)[15,16,144,145] no systematic reporting of hypoglycaemia occurred but spontaneously reported symptomatic episodes potentially hypoglycemic in cause were reported by 1.6% (46/2962) of liraglutide 3 mg and 1.1% of (19/1729) placebo-treated nondiabetic patients. GI: Dyspepsia, abdominal pain, dry mouth, gastritis, gastroesophageal reflux disease, flatulence, eructation, and abdominal distension were also more prevalent in liraglutide-treated participants but occurred with incidence ≤10%, not shown. 6.2% with liraglutide versus 0.8% with placebo discontinued treatment as a result of gastrointestinal adverse reactions. (Figure modified from Anandhakrishnan, A. & Korbonits, M. (2016) Glucagon-like peptide 1 in the pathophysiology and pharmacotherapy of clinical obesity. *World Journal of Diabetes* **7**, 572-598.)

This increased heart rate is perhaps a manifestation of GLP-1-induced increase in sympathetic nervous system activity (NEW REFERENCE Exenatide acutely increases heart rate in parallel with augmentedsympathetic nervous system activation in healthy overweight males. Br J Clin Pharmacol. 2016 Apr;81(4):613-20. doi: 10.1111/bcp.12843. Epub 2016 Jan 25.Smits MM1, Muskiet MH1, Tonneijck L1, Hoekstra T2,3, Kramer MH1, Diamant M1, van Raalte DH1.) contributing to the weight loss effect of GLP-1 through increased energy expenditure. In other studies, however, the tachycardia associated with 3 mg liraglutide treatment in non-diabetic obese subjects yielded no such increases in energy expenditure.[150] Thus, while the clinical significance of this finding remains to be determined, observations may warrant more intense monitoring in patients with preexisting cardiovascular disease. Fig. 3.11 details adverse reactions occurring with a higher incidence to placebo with an incidence of ≥10% in liraglutide 3 mg recipients, stratified by system.

Follow-up period assessment and postmarketing surveillance. Although generally well tolerated in the acute setting, safety concerns have been raised regarding the long-term use of GLP-1 analogues,[158,159]

and confirmed cases of acute pancreatitis and papillary thyroid carcinoma were reported in 0.3% of liraglutide 3 mg–treated participants compared with 0.2% of those placebo treated. Fig. 3.12 details other potentially serious medical conditions observed during in-treatment and FUP assessments.[15,16,144–146] The relative rarity of events, however, means that the relationship between treatment and disease incidence and severity remains to be defined. Ongoing clinical experience and thorough postmarketing surveillance should help clarify any such associations and also identify other potential adverse drug events. To this end, episodes of acute renal failure and medullary thyroid carcinoma (not observed during in-treatment and FUP assessments[15,16,144–146]) have been reported in the postmarketing period, although again, insufficient data exist to establish or exclude a causal relationship.

CONCLUSIONS AND FUTURE PERSPECTIVE

The current medical management of obesity is suboptimal, with the only treatment modality with proven long-term efficacy being bariatric surgery; treatment-related risk and cost, however, limits its use for the

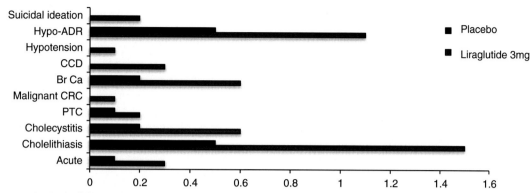

FIG. 3.12 Adverse drug reactions. Reported incidences of serious medical conditions from pooled analyses of five double-blinded placebo-controlled trials studying the safety and efficacy of 3 mg liraglutide in 3384 overweight or obese subjects receiving liraglutide and 1941 placebo controls; hypotension associated adverse reactions (Hypo-ADR) refer to hypotension, orthostatic hypotension, circulatory collapse, and decreased blood pressure. One of the six (0.2%) liraglutide-treated subjects reporting suicidal ideations attempted suicide. (Figure modified from Anandhakrishnan, A. & Korbonits, M. (2016) Glucagon-like peptide 1 in the pathophysiology and pharmacotherapy of clinical obesity. *World Journal of Diabetes* 7, 572-598.)

widespread management of obesity. The ideal medical management of any illness uses a targeted pharmacotherapy that restores physiologic factors pathologically depleted or antagonizes pathologic processes; the development of such an agent requires an understanding of the pathophysiology underpinning a disease; the poorly understood pathology of clinical obesity perhaps explains the limited success of pharmacologic disease management to date. Although undoubtedly multifactorial, recent clinical evidence has come to light implicating a role for functional impairments of the acute anorectic peptide GLP-1 in human obesity pathology. Where genetic studies suggest that primary alterations to GLP-1 signaling may confer an increased susceptibility to obesity, physiologic GLP-1 responses in normal-weight and obese subjects suggest that weight gain may induce functional deficits in GLP-1. Independent of this relationship, either cause or effect, reductions in functional GLP-1 seem to play a role in clinical obesity; pharmacologically replenishing this deficit therefore is a viable target for a novel antiobesity agent. Indeed, the GLP-1 analogue liraglutide 3 mg has shown promising results in achieving and maintaining greater weight loss in obese individuals when compared with control or currently licensed antiobesity medication. Although generally well tolerated, extended phase III and phase IV studies have reported associations with potentially fatal adverse drug events. The rarity of events, however, limits interpretations into the relationship with drug treatment, seeing potential risks outweighed by proven superior efficacy of liraglutide

3 mg as an antiobesity agent. Cost-benefit, however, may pose a barrier toward viable funding, although this may be overcome by strategic treatment delivery, combining short-term in-treatment period with behavioral therapies targeted toward promoting lifestyle change. With drug-induced weight loss potentially reinforcing adherence to long-term lifestyle changes, if successful, shortened in-treatment period, alongside decreases in direct and indirect socioeconomic burdens of obesity and overweight associated with the superior short- and long-term weight loss efficacy of 3 mg liraglutide, confers a long-term cost-benefit to treatment. Together, clinical studies suggest that liraglutide 3 mg may be the first targeted pharmacotherapeutic agent in the medical management of obesity with risk and cost-benefit analyses supporting its use as the first-line antiobesity agent, when lifestyle management alone has failed to achieve and sustain significant weight loss in comorbidly overweight or obese adults.

REFERENCES

1. [Internet]. *Obesity: Identification, Assessment and Management of Overweight and Obesity in Children, Young People and Adults*; 2014. Available from: http://www.nice.org.uk/guidance/cg189/chapter/1-recommendations#footnote_12.
2. Yanovski SZ, Yanovski JA. Obesity. *N Engl J Med.* 2002;346(8):591–602.
3. Holzapfel C, Hauner H. Weight maintenance after weight loss – how the body defends its weight. *Dtsch Med Wochenschr.* 2011;136(3):89–94.

4. Loveman E, Frampton GK, Shepherd J, et al. The clinical effectiveness and cost-effectiveness of long-term weight management schemes for adults: a systematic review. *Health Technol Assess.* 2011;15(2):1–182.

5. Greenway FL. Physiological adaptations to weight loss and factors favouring weight regain. *Int J Obes.* 2015;39(8):1188–1196.

6. Golomb I, Ben David M, Glass A, Kolitz T, Keidar A. Long-term metabolic effects of laparoscopic sleeve gastrectomy. *JAMA Surg.* 2015;150(11).

7. Hirth DA, Jones EL, Rothchild KB, Mitchell BC, Schoen JA. Laparoscopic sleeve gastrectomy: long-term weight loss outcomes. *Surg Obes Relat Dis.* 2015;11(5).

8. Costa RC, Yamaguchi N, Santo MA, Riccioppo D, Pinto-Junior PE. Outcomes on quality of life, weight loss, and comorbidities after Roux-en-Y gastric bypass. *Arq Gastroenterol.* 2014;51(3):165–170.

9. Pasulka PS, Bistrian BR, Benotti PN, Blackburn GL. The risks of surgery in obese patients. *Ann Intern Med.* 1986;104(4):540–546.

10. Dority J, Hassan ZU, Chau D. Anesthetic implications of obesity in the surgical patient. *Clin Colon Rectal Surg.* 2011;24(4):222–228.

11. Prasad-Reddy L, Isaacs D. A clinical review of GLP-1 receptor agonists: efficacy and safety in diabetes and beyond. *Drugs Context.* 2015;4:212283.

12. Monami M, Dicembrini I, Marchionni N, Rotella CM, Mannucci E. effects of glucagon-like peptide-1 receptor agonists on body weight: a meta-analysis. *Exp Diabetes Res.* 2012;2012:672658.

13. Vilsbøll T, Christensen M, Junker AE, Knop FK, Gluud LL. Effects of glucagon-like peptide-1 receptor agonists on weight loss: systematic review and meta-analyses of randomised controlled trials. *BMJ.* 2012;344:d7771.

14. Collier A, Blackman A, Foster G, et al. Liraglutide 3.0 mg reduces severity of obstructive sleep apnea and body weight in obese individuals with moderate or severe disease: scale sleep apnea trial. *Thorax.* 2014;69:A16–A17.

15. Astrup A, Carraro R, Finer N, et al. Safety, tolerability and sustained weight loss over 2 years with the once-daily human GLP-1 analog, liraglutide. *Int J Obes.* 2012;36(6):843–854.

16. Astrup A, Rössner S, Van Gaal L, et al. Effects of liraglutide in the treatment of obesity: a randomised, double-blind, placebo-controlled study. *Lancet.* 2009;374(9701):1606–1616.

17. *Saxenda® Approved in Europe for the Treatment of Obesity;* 2015. [Press Release].

18. Briefing Document [Internet]. *Liraglutide 3.0 mg for Weight Management;* 2014. Available from: http://www.fda.gov/downloads/advisorycommittees/committeesmeetingmaterials/drugs/endocrinologicandmetabolicdrugsadvisorycommittee/ucm413318.pdf.

19. New Drugs Online: Liraglutide [Internet]. *UK Medicines Information;* 2015. Available from: http://www.ukmi.nhs.uk/applications/ndo/record_view_open.asp?newDrugID=4884.

20. Drucker DJ, Asa S. Glucagon gene expression in vertebrate brain. *J Biol Chem.* 1988;263(27):13475–13478.

21. Lee YC, Brubaker PL, Drucker DJ. Developmental and tissue-specific regulation of proglucagon gene expression. *Endocrinology.* 1990;127(5):2217–2222.

22. Merchenthaler I, Lane M, Shughrue P. Distribution of pre-pro-glucagon and glucagon-like peptide-1 receptor messenger RNAs in the rat central nervous system. *J Comp Neurol.* 1999;403(2):261–280.

23. Mojsov S, Heinrich G, Wilson IB, Ravazzola M, Orci L, Habener JF. Preproglucagon gene expression in pancreas and intestine diversifies at the level of post-translational processing. *J Biol Chem.* 1986;261(25):11880–11889.

24. Baggio LL, Drucker DJ. Biology of incretins: GLP-1 and GIP. *Gastroenterology.* 2007;132(6):2131–2157.

25. Holst JJ. The physiology of glucagon-like peptide 1. *Physiol Rev.* 2007;87(4):1409–1439.

26. Pocai A. Unraveling oxyntomodulin, GLP1's enigmatic brother. *J Endocrinol.* 2012;215(3):335–346.

27. Orskov C, Holst JJ, Knuhtsen S, Baldissera FG, Poulsen SS, Nielsen OV. Glucagon-like peptides GLP-1 and GLP-2, predicted products of the glucagon gene, are secreted separately from pig small intestine but not pancreas. *Endocrinology.* 1986;119(4):1467–1475.

28. Rocca AS, Brubaker PL. Role of the vagus nerve in mediating proximal nutrient-induced glucagon-like peptide-1 secretion. *Endocrinology.* 1999;140(4):1687–1694.

29. Tucker JD, Dhanvantari S, Brubaker PL. Proglucagon processing in islet and intestinal cell lines. *Regul Pept.* 1996;62(1):29–35.

30. Bryant MG, Bloom SR, Polak JM, et al. Measurement of gut hormonal peptides in biopsies from human stomach and proximal small intestine. *Gut.* 1983;24(2):114–119.

31. Eissele R, Göke R, Willemer S, et al. Glucagon-like peptide-1 cells in the gastrointestinal tract and pancreas of rat, pig and man. *Eur J Clin Invest.* 1992;22(4):283–291.

32. Knudsen JB, Holst JJ, Asnaes S, Johansen A. Identification of cells with pancreatic-type and gut-type glucagon immunoreactivity in the human colon. *Acta Pathol Microbiol Scand A.* 1975;83(6):741–743.

33. O'Donovan DG, Doran S, Feinle-Bisset C, et al. Effect of variations in small intestinal glucose delivery on plasma glucose, insulin, and incretin hormones in healthy subjects and type 2 diabetes. *J Clin Endocrinol Metab.* 2004;89(7):3431–3435.

34. Kieffer TJ, McIntosh CH, Pederson RA. Degradation of glucose-dependent insulinotropic polypeptide and truncated glucagon-like peptide 1 in vitro and in vivo by dipeptidyl peptidase IV. *Endocrinology.* 1995;136(8):3585–3596.

35. Deacon CF, Pridal L, Klarskov L, Olesen M, Holst JJ. Glucagon-like peptide 1 undergoes differential tissue-specific metabolism in the anesthetized pig. *Am J Physiol.* 1996;271(3 Pt 1):E458–E464.

36. Cho YM, Fujita Y, Kieffer TJ. Glucagon-like peptide-1: glucose homeostasis and beyond. *Annu Rev Physiol.* 2014;76:535–559.

37. Lim GE, Brubaker PL. Glucagon-like peptide 1 secretion by the L-cell; the view from within. *Diabetes.* 2006;55(suppl 2).

38. Zhang Y, Proenca R, Maffei M, Barone M, Leopold L, Friedman JM. Positional cloning of the mouse obese gene and its human homologue. *Nature.* 1994;372(6505):425–432.

39. Gao Q, Horvath TL. Neurobiology of feeding and energy expenditure. *Annu Rev Neurosci.* 2007;30:367–398.

40. Broberger C, Johansen J, Johansson C, Schalling M, Hökfelt T. The neuropeptide Y/agouti gene-related protein (AGRP) brain circuitry in normal, anorectic, and monosodium glutamate-treated mice. *Proc Natl Acad Sci USA.* 1998;95(25):15043–15048.

41. Hahn TM, Breininger JF, Baskin DG, Schwartz MW. Co-expression of Agrp and NPY in fasting-activated hypothalamic neurons. *Nat Neurosci.* 1998;1(4):271–272.

42. Millington GW. The role of proopiomelanocortin (POMC) neurones in feeding behaviour. *Nutr Metab.* 2007;4:18.

43. Dhillo WS, Small CJ, Stanley SA, et al. Hypothalamic interactions between neuropeptide Y, agouti-related protein, cocaine- and amphetamine-regulated transcript and alpha-melanocyte-stimulating hormone in vitro in male rats. *J Neuroendocrinol.* 2002;14(9):725–730.

44. Haskell-Luevano C, Hendrata S, North C, et al. Discovery of prototype peptidomimetic agonists at the human melanocortin receptors MC1R and MC4R. *J Med Chem.* 1997;40(14):2133–2139.

45. Nijenhuis WA, Oosterom J, Adan RA. AgRP(83-132) acts as an inverse agonist on the human-melanocortin-4 receptor. *Mol Endocrinol.* 2001;15(1):164–171.

46. Haskell-Luevano C, Monck EK. Agouti-related protein functions as an inverse agonist at a constitutively active brain melanocortin-4 receptor. *Regul Pept.* 2001;99(1):1–7.

47. Secher A, Jelsing J, Baquero AF, et al. The arcuate nucleus mediates GLP-1 receptor agonist liraglutide-dependent weight loss. *J Clin Invest.* 2014;124(10):4473–4488.

48. Katsurada K, Maejima Y, Nakata M, et al. Endogenous GLP-1 acts on paraventricular nucleus to suppress feeding: projection from nucleus tractus solitarius and activation of corticotropin-releasing hormone, nesfatin-1 and oxytocin neurons. *Biochem Biophys Res Commun.* 2014;451(2):276–281.

49. Koob GF, Volkow ND. Neurocircuitry of addiction. *Neuropsychopharmacology.* 2010;35(1):217–238.

50. Figlewicz DP. Adiposity signals and food reward: expanding the CNS roles of insulin and leptin. *Am J Physiol Regul Integr Comp Physiol.* 2003;284(4):R882–R892.

51. Ulrich-Lai YM, Ryan KK. Neuroendocrine circuits governing energy balance and stress regulation: functional overlap and therapeutic implications. *Cell Metab.* 2014;19(6):910–925.

52. Williams DL. Neural integration of satiation and food reward: role of GLP-1 and orexin pathways. *Physiol Behav.* 2014;136:194–199.

53. Skibicka KP. The central GLP-1: implications for food and drug reward. *Front Neurosci.* 2013;7:181.

54. Kennedy GC. The role of depot fat in the hypothalamic control of food intake in the rat. *Proc R Soc Lond B Biol Sci.* 1953;140(901):578–596.

55. Richard JE, Anderberg RH, Göteson A, Gribble FM, Reimann F, Skibicka KP. Activation of the GLP-1 receptors in the nucleus of the solitary tract reduces food reward behavior and targets the mesolimbic system. *PLoS One.* 2015;10(3):e0119034.

56. Näslund E, Gutniak M, Skogar S, Rössner S, Hellström PM. Glucagon-like peptide 1 increases the period of postprandial satiety and slows gastric emptying in obese men. *Am J Clin Nutr.* 1998;68(3):525–530.

57. Flint A, Raben A, Astrup A, Holst JJ. Glucagon-like peptide 1 promotes satiety and suppresses energy intake in humans. *J Clin Invest.* 1998;101(3):515–520.

58. Gutzwiller JP, Drewe J, Göke B, et al. Glucagon-like peptide-1 promotes satiety and reduces food intake in patients with diabetes mellitus type 2. *Am J Physiol.* 1999;276(5 Pt 2):R1541–R1544.

59. Flint A, Raben A, Ersbøll AK, Holst JJ, Astrup A. The effect of physiological levels of glucagon-like peptide-1 on appetite, gastric emptying, energy and substrate metabolism in obesity. *Int J Obes Relat Metab Disord.* 2001;25(6):781–792.

60. Verdich C, Flint A, Gutzwiller JP, et al. A meta-analysis of the effect of glucagon-like peptide-1 (7-36) amide on ad libitum energy intake in humans. *J Clin Endocrinol Metab.* 2001;86(9):4382–4389.

61. Näslund E, King N, Mansten S, et al. Prandial subcutaneous injections of glucagon-like peptide-1 cause weight loss in obese human subjects. *Br J Nutr.* 2004;91(3):439–446.

62. Flint A, Raben A, Rehfeld JF, Holst JJ, Astrup A. The effect of glucagon-like peptide-1 on energy expenditure and substrate metabolism in humans. *Int J Obes Relat Metab Disord.* 2000;24(3):288–298.

63. Shalev A, Holst JJ, Keller U. Effects of glucagon-like peptide 1 (7-36 amide) on whole-body protein metabolism in healthy man. *Eur J Clin Invest.* 1997;27(1):10–16.

64. Näslund E, Barkeling B, King N, et al. Energy intake and appetite are suppressed by glucagon-like peptide-1 (GLP-1) in obese men. *Int J Obes Relat Metab Disord.* 1999;23(3):304–311.

65. Gutzwiller JP, Göke B, Drewe J, et al. Glucagon-like peptide-1: a potent regulator of food intake in humans. *Gut.* 1999;44(1):81–86.

66. Cegla J, Troke RC, Jones B, et al. Coinfusion of low-dose GLP-1 and glucagon in man results in a reduction in food intake. *Diabetes.* 2014;63(11):3711–3720.

67. Long SJ, Sutton JA, Amaee WB, et al. No effect of glucagon-like peptide-1 on short-term satiety and energy intake in man. *Br J Nutr.* 1999;81(4):273–279.

68. Donnelly D. The structure and function of the glucagon-like peptide-1 receptor and its ligands. *Br J Pharmacol.* 2012;166(1):27–41.

69. Travagli RA, Hermann GE, Browning KN, Rogers RC. Brainstem circuits regulating gastric function. *Annu Rev Physiol.* 2006;68:279–305.

70. Hunt JN. A possible relation between the regulation of gastric emptying and food intake. *Am J Physiol.* 1980;239(1):G1–G4.

71. Di Lorenzo C, Williams CM, Hajnal F, Valenzuela JE. Pectin delays gastric emptying and increases satiety in obese subjects. *Gastroenterology.* 1988;95(5):1211–1215.

72. Clegg ME, Ranawana V, Shafat A, Henry CJ. Soups increase satiety through delayed gastric emptying yet increased glycaemic response. *Eur J Clin Nutr.* 2013;67(1):8–11.

73. Hlebowicz J, Darwiche G, Björgell O, Almér LO. Effect of cinnamon on postprandial blood glucose, gastric emptying, and satiety in healthy subjects. *Am J Clin Nutr.* 2007;85(6):1552–1556.

74. Hlebowicz J, Hlebowicz A, Lindstedt S, et al. Effects of 1 and 3 g cinnamon on gastric emptying, satiety, and postprandial blood glucose, insulin, glucose-dependent insulinotropic polypeptide, glucagon-like peptide 1, and ghrelin concentrations in healthy subjects. *Am J Clin Nutr.* 2009;89(3):815–821.

75. Nauck MA, Niedereichholz U, Ettler R, et al. Glucagon-like peptide 1 inhibition of gastric emptying outweighs its insulinotropic effects in healthy humans. *Am J Physiol.* 1997;273(5 Pt 1):E981–E988.

76. Schirra J, Wank U, Arnold R, Göke B, Katschinski M. Effects of glucagon-like peptide-1(7-36)amide on motility and sensation of the proximal stomach in humans. *Gut.* 2002;50(3):341–348.

77. Little TJ, Pilichiewicz AN, Russo A, et al. Effects of intravenous glucagon-like peptide-1 on gastric emptying and intragastric distribution in healthy subjects: relationships with postprandial glycemic and insulinemic responses. *J Clin Endocrinol Metab.* 2006;91(5):1916–1923.

78. Meier JJ, Gallwitz B, Salmen S, et al. Normalization of glucose concentrations and deceleration of gastric emptying after solid meals during intravenous glucagon-like peptide 1 in patients with type 2 diabetes. *J Clin Endocrinol Metab.* 2003;88(6):2719–2725.

79. Broide E, Bloch O, Ben-Yehudah G, Cantrell D, Shirin H, Rapoport MJ. GLP-1 receptor is expressed in human stomach mucosa: analysis of its cellular association and distribution within gastric glands. *J Histochem Cytochem.* 2013;61(9):649–658.

80. Meloni AR, DeYoung MB, Lowe C, Parkes DG. GLP-1 receptor activated insulin secretion from pancreatic β-cells: mechanism and glucose dependence. *Diabetes Obes Metab.* 2013;15(1):15–27.

81. Polonsky KS, Given BD, Hirsch L, et al. Quantitative study of insulin secretion and clearance in normal and obese subjects. *J Clin Invest.* 1988;81(2):435–441.

82. Benedict C, Kern W, Schultes B, Born J, Hallschmid M. Differential sensitivity of men and women to anorexigenic and memory-improving effects of intranasal insulin. *J Clin Endocrinol Metab.* 2008;93(4):1339–1344.

83. Niswender KD, Morrison CD, Clegg DJ, et al. Insulin activation of phosphatidylinositol 3-kinase in the hypothalamic arcuate nucleus: a key mediator of insulin-induced anorexia. *Diabetes.* 2003;52(2):227–231.

84. Watanabe M, Hayasaki H, Tamayama T, Shimada M. Histologic distribution of insulin and glucagon receptors. *Braz J Med Biol Res.* 1998;31(2):243–256.

85. Iñiguez SD, Warren BL, Neve RL, Nestler EJ, Russo SJ, Bolaños-Guzmán CA. Insulin receptor substrate-2 in the ventral tegmental area regulates behavioral responses to cocaine. *Behav Neurosci.* 2008;122(5):1172–1177.

86. Wang Q, Liu C, Uchida A, et al. Arcuate AgRP neurons mediate orexigenic and glucoregulatory actions of ghrelin. *Mol Metab.* 2014;3(1):64–72.

87. Skibicka KP, Hansson C, Alvarez-Crespo M, Friberg PA, Dickson SL. Ghrelin directly targets the ventral tegmental area to increase food motivation. *Neuroscience.* 2011;180:129–137.

88. Hagemann D, Holst JJ, Gethmann A, Banasch M, Schmidt WE, Meier JJ. Glucagon-like peptide 1 (GLP-1) suppresses ghrelin levels in humans via increased insulin secretion. *Regul Pept.* 2007;143(1–3):64–68.

89. Alvarez E, Martínez MD, Roncero I, et al. The expression of GLP-1 receptor mRNA and protein allows the effect of GLP-1 on glucose metabolism in the human hypothalamus and brainstem. *J Neurochem.* 2005;92(4):798–806.

90. Pannacciulli N, Le DS, Salbe AD, et al. Postprandial glucagon-like peptide-1 (GLP-1) response is positively associated with changes in neuronal activity of brain areas implicated in satiety and food intake regulation in humans. *Neuroimage.* 2007;35(2):511–517.

91. De Silva A, Salem V, Long CJ, et al. The gut hormones PYY 3-36 and GLP-1 7-36 amide reduce food intake and modulate brain activity in appetite centers in humans. *Cell Metab.* 2011;14(5):700–706.

92. Huvenne H, Dubern B. Monogenic forms of obesity. In: Nóbrega C, Rodriguez-López R, eds. *Molecular Mechanisms Underpinning the Development of Obesity.* Switzerland: Springer International Publishing; 2014:9–21.

93. Jackson RS, Creemers JW, Farooqi IS, et al. Small-intestinal dysfunction accompanies the complex endocrinopathy of human proprotein convertase 1 deficiency. *J Clin Invest.* 2003;112(10):1550–1560.

94. Jackson RS, Creemers JW, Ohagi S, et al. Obesity and impaired prohormone processing associated with mutations in the human prohormone convertase 1 gene. *Nat Genet.* 1997;16(3):303–306.

95. Frank GR, Fox J, Candela N, et al. Severe obesity and diabetes insipidus in a patient with PCSK1 deficiency. *Mol Genet Metab.* 2013;110(1–2):191–194.

96. Bandsma RH, Sokollik C, Chami R, et al. From diarrhea to obesity in prohormone convertase 1/3 deficiency: age-dependent clinical, pathologic, and enteroendocrine characteristics. *J Clin Gastroenterol.* 2013;47(10):834–843.

97. Parker JA, McCullough KA, Field BC, et al. Glucagon and GLP-1 inhibit food intake and increase c-fos expression in similar appetite regulating centres in the brainstem and amygdala. *Int J Obes.* 2013;37(10):1391–1398.

98. Lake A, Townshend T. Obesogenic environments: exploring the built and food environments. *J R Soc Promot Health*. 2006;126(6):262–267.

99. Mackenbach JD, Rutter H, Compernolle S, et al. Obesogenic environments: a systematic review of the association between the physical environment and adult weight status, the SPOTLIGHT project. *BMC Public Health*. 2014;14:233.

100. O'Rahilly S, Farooqi IS. Human obesity as a heritable disorder of the central control of energy balance. *Int J Obes*. 2008;32(suppl 7):S55–S61.

101. O'Rahilly S, Farooqi IS. Human obesity: a heritable neurobehavioral disorder that is highly sensitive to environmental conditions. *Diabetes*. 2008;57(11):2905–2910.

102. Hebebrand J, Hinney A. Environmental and genetic risk factors in obesity. *Child Adolesc Psychiatr Clin N Am*. 2009;18(1):83–94.

103. Locke AE, Kahali B, Berndt SI, et al. Genetic studies of body mass index yield new insights for obesity biology. *Nature*. 2015;518(7538):197–206.

104. Choquet H, Meyre D. Genetics of obesity: what have we learned? *Curr Genomics*. 2011;12(3):169–179.

105. Benzinou M, Creemers JW, Choquet H, et al. Common nonsynonymous variants in PCSK1 confer risk of obesity. *Nat Genet*. 2008;40(8):943–945.

106. Choquet H, Kasberger J, Hamidovic A, Jorgenson E. Contribution of common PCSK1 genetic variants to obesity in 8,359 subjects from multi-ethnic American population. *PLoS One*. 2013;8(2):e57857.

107. Kilpeläinen TO, Bingham SA, Khaw KT, Wareham NJ, Loos RJ. Association of variants in the PCSK1 gene with obesity in the EPIC-Norfolk study. *Hum Mol Genet*. 2009;18(18):3496–3501.

108. Qi Q, Li H, Loos RJ, et al. Association of PCSK1 rs6234 with obesity and related traits in a Chinese Han population. *PLoS One*. 2010;5(5):e10590.

109. Chang YC, Chiu YF, Shih KC, et al. Common PCSK1 haplotypes are associated with obesity in the Chinese population. *Obesity*. 2010;18(7):1404–1409.

110. Færch K, Torekov SS, Vistisen D, et al. GLP-1 response to oral glucose is reduced in prediabetes, screen-detected type 2 diabetes, and obesity and influenced by sex: the addition-pro study. *Diabetes*. 2015;64(7):2513–2525.

111. Hussein MS, Abushady MM, Refaat S, Ibrahim R. Plasma level of glucagon-like peptide 1 in obese Egyptians with normal and impaired glucose tolerance. *Arch Med Res*. 2014;45(1):58–62.

112. Muscelli E, Mari A, Casolaro A, et al. Separate impact of obesity and glucose tolerance on the incretin effect in normal subjects and type 2 diabetic patients. *Diabetes*. 2008;57(5):1340–1348.

113. Svendsen PF, Jensen FK, Holst JJ, Haugaard SB, Nilas L, Madsbad S. The effect of a very low calorie diet on insulin sensitivity, beta cell function, insulin clearance, incretin hormone secretion, androgen levels and body composition in obese young women. *Scand J Clin Lab Invest*. 2012;72(5):410–419.

114. Adam TC, Westerterp-Plantenga MS. Glucagon-like peptide-1 release and satiety after a nutrient challenge in normal-weight and obese subjects. *Br J Nutr*. 2005;93(6):845–851.

115. Verdich C, Toubro S, Buemann B, Lysgård Madsen J, Juul Holst J, Astrup A. The role of postprandial releases of insulin and incretin hormones in meal-induced satiety-effect of obesity and weight reduction. *Int J Obes Relat Metab Disord*. 2001;25(8):1206–1214.

116. Ranganath LR, Beety JM, Morgan LM, Wright JW, Howland R, Marks V. Attenuated GLP-1 secretion in obesity: cause or consequence? *Gut*. 1996;38(6):916–919.

117. Carroll JF, Kaiser KA, Franks SF, Deere C, Caffrey JL. Influence of BMI and gender on postprandial hormone responses. *Obesity*. 2007;15(12):2974–2983.

118. Vilsbøll T, Krarup T, Sonne J, et al. Incretin secretion in relation to meal size and body weight in healthy subjects and people with type 1 and type 2 diabetes mellitus. *J Clin Endocrinol Metab*. 2003;88(6):2706–2713.

119. Toft-Nielsen MB, Damholt MB, Madsbad S, et al. Determinants of the impaired secretion of glucagon-like peptide-1 in type 2 diabetic patients. *J Clin Endocrinol Metab*. 2001;86(8):3717–3723.

120. Näslund E, Grybäck P, Backman L, et al. Distal small bowel hormones: correlation with fasting antroduodenal motility and gastric emptying. *Dig Dis Sci*. 1998;43(5):945–952.

121. van Bloemendaal L, Veltman DJ, Ten Kulve JS, et al. Brain reward-system activation in response to anticipation and consumption of palatable food is altered by glucagon-like peptide-1 receptor activation in humans. *Diabetes Obes Metab*. 2015;17(9):878–886.

122. Stice E, Spoor S, Bohon C, Small DM. Relation between obesity and blunted striatal response to food is moderated by TaqIA A1 allele. *Science*. 2008;322(5900):449–452.

123. Stice E, Spoor S, Bohon C, Veldhuizen MG, Small DM. Relation of reward from food intake and anticipated food intake to obesity: a functional magnetic resonance imaging study. *J Abnorm Psychol*. 2008;117(4):924–935.

124. van Bloemendaal L, IJzerman RG, Ten Kulve JS, et al. GLP-1 receptor activation modulates appetite- and reward-related brain areas in humans. *Diabetes*. 2014;63(12):4186–4196.

125. Witt AA, Raggio GA, Butryn ML, Lowe MR. Do hunger and exposure to food affect scores on a measure of hedonic hunger? An experimental study. *Appetite*. 2014;74:1–5.

126. Singh M. Mood, food, and obesity. *Front Psychol*. 2014;5:925.

127. van Bloemendaal L, Veltman DJ, Ten Kulve JS, et al. Emotional eating is associated with increased brain responses to food-cues and reduced sensitivity to GLP-1 receptor activation. *Obesity*. 2015;23(10):2075–2082.

128. McKeigue PM, Pierpoint T, Ferrie JE, Marmot MG. Relationship of glucose intolerance and hyperinsulinaemia to body fat pattern in south Asians and Europeans. *Diabetologia*. 1992;35(8):785–791.

129. Mannucci E, Ognibene A, Cremasco F, et al. Glucagon-like peptide (GLP)-1 and leptin concentrations in obese patients with type 2 diabetes mellitus. *Diabet Med.* 2000;17(10):713–719.

130. Zhang Y, Scarpace PJ. The role of leptin in leptin resistance and obesity. *Physiol Behav.* 2006;88(3):249–256.

131. Anini Y, Brubaker PL. Role of leptin in the regulation of glucagon-like peptide-1 secretion. *Diabetes.* 2003;52(2):252–259.

132. Gagnon J, Baggio LL, Drucker DJ, Brubaker PL. Ghrelin is a novel regulator of GLP-1 secretion. *Diabetes.* 2015;64(5):1513–1521.

133. Daghestani MH. A preprandial and postprandial plasma levels of ghrelin hormone in lean, overweight and obese Saudi females. *J King Saud Univ Sci.* 2009;21(2):119–124.

134. English PJ, Ghatei MA, Malik IA, Bloom SR, Wilding JP. Food fails to suppress ghrelin levels in obese humans. *J Clin Endocrinol Metab.* 2002;87(6):2984.

135. Kenny PJ. Reward mechanisms in obesity: new insights and future directions. *Neuron.* 2011;69(4):664–679.

136. Maggard MA, Shugarman LR, Suttorp M, et al. Meta-analysis: surgical treatment of obesity. *Ann Intern Med.* 2005;142(7):547–559.

137. Falkén Y, Hellström PM, Holst JJ, Näslund E. Changes in glucose homeostasis after Roux-en-Y gastric bypass surgery for obesity at day three, two months, and one year after surgery: role of gut peptides. *J Clin Endocrinol Metab.* 2011;96(7):2227–2235.

138. Korner J, Inabnet W, Febres G, et al. Prospective study of gut hormone and metabolic changes after adjustable gastric banding and Roux-en-Y gastric bypass. *Int J Obes.* 2009;33(7):786–795.

139. Korner J, Bessler M, Inabnet W, Taveras C, Holst JJ. Exaggerated glucagon-like peptide-1 and blunted glucose-dependent insulinotropic peptide secretion are associated with Roux-en-Y gastric bypass but not adjustable gastric banding. *Surg Obes Relat Dis.* 2007;3(6):597–601.

140. Borg CM, le Roux CW, Ghatei MA, Bloom SR, Patel AG, Aylwin SJ. Progressive rise in gut hormone levels after Roux-en-Y gastric bypass suggests gut adaptation and explains altered satiety. *Br J Surg.* 2006;93(2):210–215.

141. le Roux CW, Aylwin SJ, Batterham RL, et al. Gut hormone profiles following bariatric surgery favor an anorectic state, facilitate weight loss, and improve metabolic parameters. *Ann Surg.* 2006;243(1):108–114.

142. Morínigo R, Moizé V, Musri M, et al. Glucagon-like peptide-1, peptide YY, hunger, and satiety after gastric bypass surgery in morbidly obese subjects. *J Clin Endocrinol Metab.* 2006;91(5):1735–1740.

143. Kellum JM, Kuemmerle JF, O'Dorisio TM, et al. Gastrointestinal hormone responses to meals before and after gastric bypass and vertical banded gastroplasty. *Ann Surg.* 1990;211(6):763–770. Discussion 70–71.

144. Pi-Sunyer X, Astrup A, Fujioka K, et al. A randomized, controlled trial of 3.0 mg of liraglutide in weight management. *N Engl J Med.* 2015;373(1):11–22.

145. Wadden TA, Hollander P, Klein S, et al. Weight maintenance and additional weight loss with liraglutide after low-calorie-diet-induced weight loss: the SCALE maintenance randomized study. *Int J Obes.* 2013;37(11):1443–1451.

146. Davies MJ, Bergenstal R, Bode B, et al. Efficacy of liraglutide for weight loss among patients with type 2 diabetes: the SCALE diabetes randomized clinical trial. *JAMA.* 2015;314(7):687–699.

147. Vidal J. Updated review on the benefits of weight loss. *Int J Obes Relat Metab Disord.* 2002;26(suppl 4):S25–S28.

148. Goldstein DJ. Beneficial health effects of modest weight loss. *Int J Obes Relat Metab Disord.* 1992;16(6):397–415.

149. Blackburn G. Effect of degree of weight loss on health benefits. *Obes Res.* 1995;3(suppl 2):S211–S216.

150. van Can J, Sloth B, Jensen CB, Flint A, Blaak EE, Saris WH. Effects of the once-daily GLP-1 analog liraglutide on gastric emptying, glycemic parameters, appetite and energy metabolism in obese, non-diabetic adults. *Int J Obes.* 2014;38(6):784–793.

151. Vallöf D, Maccioni P, Colombo G, et al. The glucagon-like peptide 1 receptor agonist liraglutide attenuates the reinforcing properties of alcohol in rodents. *Addict Biol.* 2015;21(2).

152. Bray GA. Why do we need drugs to treat the patient with obesity? *Obesity.* 2013;21(5):893–899.

153. Mannucci E, Ognibene A, Cremasco F, et al. Effect of metformin on glucagon-like peptide 1 (GLP-1) and leptin levels in obese nondiabetic subjects. *Diabetes Care.* 2001;24(3):489–494.

154. Campbell IW, Howlett HC. Worldwide experience of metformin as an effective glucose-lowering agent: a meta-analysis. *Diabetes Metab Rev.* 1995;11(suppl 1):S57–S62.

155. [Internet]. *Adult Obesity and Type 2 Diabetes*; 2014. Available from: https://www.gov.uk/government/uploads/system/uploads/attachment_data/file/338934/Adult_obesity_and_type_2_diabetes_.pdf.

156. Drugs Information Leaflet ONLINE [Internet]. *Saxenda; Injectable Liraglutide for Obesity*; 2015. Available from: http://www.novo-pi.com/saxenda.pdf.

157. [Internet]. *Assessment Report: Saxenda*; 2015. Available from: http://www.ema.europa.eu/docs/en_GB/document_library/EPAR_-_Public_assessment_report/human/003780/WC500185788.pdf.

158. Haluzík M, Mráz M, Svačina Š. Balancing benefits and risks in patients receiving incretin-based therapies: focus on cardiovascular and pancreatic side effects. *Drug Saf.* 2014;37(12):1003–1010.

159. Nauck MA, Friedrich N. Do GLP-1-based therapies increase cancer risk? *Diabetes Care.* 2013;36(suppl 2):S245–S252.

CHAPTER 4

Obesity, Cortisol Excess, and the Hypothalamic–Pituitary–Adrenal Axis

ANN L. HUNTER, BSC (HONS), MBCHB (HONS), MRCP (UK) •
AKHEEL A. SYED, MBBS, MRCP (UK), PHD, FRCP (EDIN)

INTRODUCTION

Glucocorticoid hormones, chiefly cortisol in man, are critical regulators of metabolism and essential for life. They are secreted by the adrenal glands under the control of the pituitary gland, which in turn is regulated by the hypothalamus. Primary pathologies of the hypothalamic–pituitary–adrenal (HPA) axis (e.g., Cushing's syndrome), on the one hand, are associated with obesity and other metabolic derangements such as hyperglycemia and hypertriglyceridemia. Idiopathic obesity, on the other hand, can be associated with subtle perturbations of HPA axis function.

In this chapter, we firstly examine what is known about the role of glucocorticoids in the regulation of adipose tissue biology and distribution. We, secondly, discuss the abnormalities of HPA function observed in obese individuals in the laboratory and in the clinical setting. We consider how glucocorticoid excess, both pathophysiologic and iatrogenic, affects adipose tissue and body weight. We then explore the important question of circadian disruption and its implications for our metabolic health. Finally, we discuss how this current understanding might be applied for therapeutic benefit, and what questions should be the focus of future research.

GLUCOCORTICOIDS—STEROID HORMONES ESSENTIAL FOR LIFE

Glucocorticoids or corticosteroids are four-ring steroid hormones produced by the zona fasciculata of the adrenal cortex. In man, the major glucocorticoid is cortisol; in most rodents used in laboratory studies, it is corticosterone. Glucocorticoid production is stimulated by adrenocorticotrophic hormone (ACTH), in health produced by the anterior pituitary. This in turn is positively regulated by hypothalamic corticotrophin-releasing hormone/factor (CRH/CRF). Glucocorticoid feedback at the level of the pituitary and hypothalamus serves to negatively regulate glucocorticoid production (Fig. 4.1).

The HPA axis plays a key role in the organism's response to stress. Thus, the prime metabolic action of glucocorticoids is to mobilize energy substrates, chiefly glucose and fatty acids. Glucocorticoid deficiency manifests classically as Addison's disease (primary adrenal failure) in man, is incompatible with life, and is rapidly fatal if left untreated.

Glucocorticoid actions are mediated by the glucocorticoid receptor (GR); the predominant human isoform, GRα, is a 777 amino acid protein. Unliganded GR largely resides in the cytoplasm, complexed with chaperone proteins. Ligand binding induces conformational change and nuclear translocation. GR then regulates gene transcription by direct DNA-binding, or by "tethering" other transcription factors.[1] GR is also found at the cell membrane,[2] but it is currently unclear how important this is to the metabolic actions of glucocorticoids.

Circulating glucocorticoid levels demonstrate diurnal variation; the importance of this circadian rhythm is explored in more detail later in this chapter. The local availability of glucocorticoids is regulated by the 11β-hydroxysteroid dehydrogenase (11β-HSD) enzymes. The 11β-HSD1 isoform is bidirectional and can interconvert active cortisol and inactive cortisone, whereas the 11β-HSD2 isoform is unidirectional and inactivates cortisol to cortisone.[3] Availability of the active hormone can therefore vary between tissues, because of differential expression of the 11β-HSD isoforms. Historically, this has been considered important in tissues such as the kidney, where the mineralocorticoid receptor (MR)—which has far higher affinity for glucocorticoids than GR—is "protected" from physiologic levels of circulating cortisol by 11β-HSD2, the action of which results in a lower cortisol:cortisone ratio in the kidney than in the systemic circulation. More recently, 11β-HSD1 has become a potential therapeutic target to attenuate the metabolic effects of glucocorticoids on adipose tissue and the liver.[4]

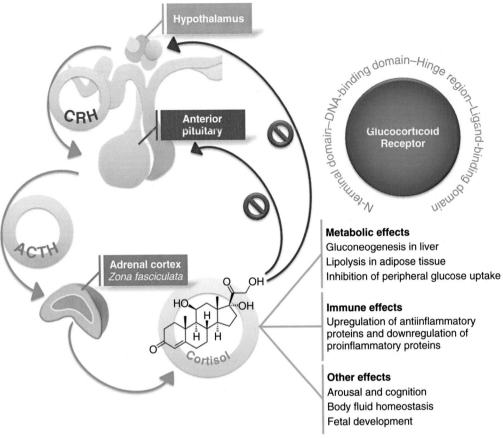

FIG. 4.1 The hypothalamic–pituitary–adrenal axis. The hypothalamic nuclei secrete corticotrophin-releasing hormone (CRH), which stimulates the anterior pituitary to release adrenocorticotrophic hormone (ACTH), which in turn stimulates the zona fasciculata in the adrenal cortex to produce glucocorticoids, chiefly cortisol in man. The concentration of cortisol in the circulation is finely regulated by negative feedback inhibition of ACTH and CRH. Cortisol exerts its peripheral actions by activation of the glucocorticoid receptor, which comprises an N-terminal domain, a DNA-binding domain, a hinge region, and a ligand-binding domain.

In clinical practice, exogenous glucocorticoids are potent antiinflammatory therapy and are employed in oral, parenteral, topical, inhaled, and intraarticular preparations to treat a wide range of inflammatory and neoplastic disorders. Their use is ubiquitous; in England, for instance, 28 million prescriptions were issued for oral and inhaled glucocorticoid preparations in 2014–15.[5] Oral preparations are also used as glucocorticoid replacement in patients with adrenal or pituitary insufficiency. However, when used for their antiinflammatory activity, glucocorticoids are often used at supraphysiologic doses. This leads to a great exaggeration of their metabolic effects, as will be discussed below, in addition to other important adverse outcomes such as osteoporosis, skin changes, myopathy, and dysphoria.

Minimizing these unwanted effects, while preserving the desirable antiinflammatory action, is a significant challenge facing the field of glucocorticoid research.

GLUCOCORTICOID REGULATION OF ADIPOSE TISSUE FUNCTION AND DISTRIBUTION

The metabolic effects of glucocorticoids are numerous and complex.[6] In the liver, glucocorticoids induce gluconeogenesis and hepatosteatosis. They reduce glucose uptake and utilization in skeletal muscle and inhibit β-cell function in the pancreas.

Here, we explore the effects of glucocorticoids on adipose tissue. Far from being an inert depot, adipose tissue should be regarded as both a metabolically and hormonally active organ.

Glucocorticoids and White Adipose Tissue

The adipocytes of white adipose tissue (WAT) store energy as triglyceride (triacylglycerol) and release fatty acids in times of starvation. Triglyceride is usually stored as a single large intracellular lipid droplet. The majority of the triglyceride store is synthesized from free fatty acids taken up from circulating lipoproteins; de novo lipogenesis also contributes. In starvation, triglyceride is broken down into glycerol and free fatty acids, which can then serve as an energy substrate.

As would be expected from their role in the stress response, glucocorticoids upregulate the lipase enzymes responsible for triglyceride breakdown and thus enhance lipolysis and free fatty acid mobilization.[7,8] However, in the clinical state of glucocorticoid excess (Cushing's syndrome), central obesity is seen. Indeed, glucocorticoids have also been shown to promote adipogenesis (see below) and lipogenesis,[9] and their direction of action may be context-dependent, depending on the endocrine milieu, for example. In a human adipocyte cell line, a low dose of the synthetic glucocorticoid, dexamethasone, has a synergistic effect with insulin in increasing lipogenesis yet decreases lipogenesis in the absence of insulin[10] (see Table 4.1). This suggests that the effects of glucocorticoids may vary between the fed and fasted state.

Glucocorticoids and Brown Adipose Tissue

Brown adipose tissue (BAT) has been demonstrated in adult humans and is chiefly an organ of thermogenesis. BAT possesses uncoupling protein 1 (UCP1) in the inner membrane of its mitochondria, generating heat from mitochondrial oxidation, thus causing energy expenditure and conferring metabolic benefit.[11] White and brown adipocytes can be found within the same adipose depot, with one more preponderant than the other. Cold temperature, or β-adrenergic stimulation, promotes "browning" of adipose tissue; "browning" currently attracts much interest as a potential therapeutic option in obesity.[12]

Similar to WAT, experimental evidence as to the effects of glucocorticoids on BAT suggests context-specificity. A study in cultured adipocytes from human brown adipose biopsy demonstrates that, in the absence of dexamethasone, noradrenergic stimulation increases the expression of UCP1, with opposite effects in the presence of dexamethasone.[13] This is supported by work in a brown adipocyte cell line[14] (Table 4.1).

Glucocorticoid Regulation of Adipose Tissue Mass and Distribution

Glucocorticoids are critical for the accumulation of fat mass; the absence of glucocorticoid or the GR prevents adipogenesis and the development of obesity.[9] It should also be noted that the MR is proposed to play a key role in facilitating adipocyte maturation.[15] In vitro, glucocorticoids promote adipocyte differentiation and maturation.[16,17] They can also promote adipocyte hypertrophy.[7] Therefore, increased adipose tissue mass in the presence of glucocorticoids may reflect increased adipocyte cell number, increased cell size, or both.

That glucocorticoids influence adipose distribution has been inferred from clinical observations of central obesity and peripheral wasting in Cushing's syndrome and from animal studies. For example, accumulation of visceral rather than subcutaneous adiposity is seen in a mouse model of glucocorticoid excess (corticosteroid binding globulin [CBG] deficiency),[18] supporting the notion that glucocorticoids regulate lipid partitioning.

It has been shown that dexamethasone may lead to lipolysis and the development of insulin resistance in mature adipocytes,[19] as would be found in preexisting adipose depots. It is also known that the distribution of adipose tissue is important in determining its biology. In humans, visceral adipose—intraabdominal adipose tissue deposited around the viscera—is distinguished from peripheral subcutaneous depots and is thought to contribute to insulin resistance and the metabolic syndrome. It is also differentially responsive to glucocorticoids; there are differences in both gene expression and tissue function between subcutaneous and visceral adipose deposits (Table 4.1).[9,20,21]

Therefore, we can hypothesize that glucocorticoid effects on adipose are context- and tissue-specific, varying between visceral and subcutaneous depots. Lipolysis in one depot may be simultaneous with adipogenesis in another. This may go some way toward explaining the dyslipidemia and abnormal adipose distribution seen in Cushing's syndrome, but highlights the complexity that any therapeutics must address as well.

HYPOTHALAMIC–PITUITARY–ADRENAL AXIS FUNCTION IN THE OBESE

Obesity causes abnormalities in HPA axis function, and therefore abnormalities of glucocorticoid levels and availability. Here, we compare what is seen in animal models with what is observed in human studies.

TABLE 4.1
Laboratory Observations of Glucocorticoid Effects on White and Brown Adipose Tissue

Treatment	Human Adipocyte Cell Line (Chub-S7)[10]	Primary Rat Stromal-Vascular Cells[17]	3T3-F442A CELL LINE (WHITE ADIPOCYTE MODEL)[19]		Primary Human White Adipocytes[20]	Primary Human White Adipose Tissue Culture[21]	Primary Human Brown Adipocytes[13]	Brown Adipocyte Cell Line (HIB-1B)[14]
			Proliferating	Terminally Differentiated (Mature)				
+dexamethasone −insulin	↓ lipogenesis	No significant change in differentiation to preadipocytes				Greater increase in lipoprotein lipase activity in visceral adipose than subcutaneous adipose		
+dexamethasone +insulin	↑ lipogenesis	Significant ↑ in differentiation to preadipocytes			In visceral adipose, greater induction of DEX-responsive genes involved in carbohydrate and lipid metabolism, compared with subcutaneous adipose	Lipoprotein lipase activity increased in both visceral and subcutaneous adipose		
+dexamethasone (in nonadipogenic media)			↑ recruitment of progenitors toward adipogenesis	↑ lipolysis ↓ glucose uptake				
+dexamethasone +noradrenergic stimulation							Dexamethasone inhibits isoprenaline-incuced increase in UCP1 expression	Dexamethasone inhibits norepinephrine-induced increase in UCP1 expression. Effect reversed by RU486

UCP1, uncoupling protein 1.

Experimental Models of Obesity

Obesity has been modeled in laboratory animals for many years, and there are both polygenic and monogenic models that are well-established.[22] Polygenic models usually use an environmental change; the diet-induced obesity rat and the high-fat diet (HFD) model are two of the most common. The most popular monogenic models are those where animals have mutations affecting leptin function. Leptin is produced by adipocytes and promotes satiety; hence leptin deficiency or resistance is associated with obesity, and obese individuals generally display higher leptin levels.[23] The ob/ob mouse has a mutation in the leptin gene and is deficient in leptin, whereas the db/db mouse has a mutation in the leptin receptor gene and is leptin-resistant.[24] Abnormalities of brain leptin signaling characterize another group of monogenic obesity models, namely, the POMC knockout mouse and the MCR4 knockout.[22]

Data from animal studies suggest hyperactivity of the HPA axis in these models of obesity. In the HFD model, obese male rats have been found to have higher basal levels of corticosterone and elevated plasma ACTH.[25] In 1975, Edwardson & Hough reported that adult ob/ob mice had higher pituitary levels of ACTH than lean controls, with corticosterone levels in plasma and the adrenal being similarly higher.[26] This difference was found to persist over the life span of the animals, in the later study of Garthwaite et al.[27] In obese Zucker rats with leptin resistance, levels of corticosterone in both plasma and urine are higher than in lean controls,[28] interestingly with lower activity of 11β-HSD1 in the liver.

Clinical Studies

In human obesity, the studies characterizing HPA axis function have recently been systematically reviewed.[29] As might be expected, there is much variation in the quality and design of studies. In the 34 papers meeting their inclusion criteria, the authors report a trend toward greater abdominal fat being associated with greater HPA axis reactivity. Some studies, however, for example that of Abraham et al.,[30] did not find any correlation between measures of HPA function (urinary free cortisol and salivary cortisol in this study) and weight in 369 participants, albeit in a secondary analysis.

In obese women undergoing insulin tolerance testing, greater obesity has been found to correlate with greater ACTH response.[31] Obese women with their body fat distributed around their abdomen have also been found to have higher morning salivary cortisol levels, compared with obese women with their fat distributed peripherally.[32] It is proposed that this might reflect altered HPA feedback sensitivity in these women, in addition to providing further support to the hypothesis that glucocorticoids influence fat distribution.[33] Indeed, greater glucocorticoid sensitivity has been demonstrated in a proportion of obese people of Cushingoid appearance (a clinical picture, which includes central obesity, usually indicative of glucocorticoid excess; see Obesity in Glucocorticoid Excess: Cushing's Syndrome section).[34]

There have also been efforts to study 11β-HSD1 activity in obese humans (11β-HSD1 predominantly converts inactive cortisone to active cortisol and thus has been proposed as a local enhancer of glucocorticoid action), and indeed, elevated 11β-HSD1 has been demonstrated ex vivo in subcutaneous adipose tissue of men with obesity,[35] which the authors suggest might serve to enhance local cortisol levels. However, this has not been seen in a polygenic mouse model,[36] and 11β-HSD1 knockout mice on the ALIOS diet (American lifestyle-induced obesity syndrome diet—high in fat and sugar) do not appear to be protected from the metabolic syndrome.[37]

In terms of the effectors of glucocorticoid action, a polymorphism in the GRβ isoform of the GR is associated with lesser central obesity in European women, but not in South Asian women, or in men.[38] A polymorphism in intron 2 of the GR gene has been linked with insulin resistance in Caucasian men.[39] Expression (mRNA levels) of GRα has been shown to be lower in the subcutaneous adipose of black South African women compared with white South African women, with lower levels associated with greater abdominal subcutaneous adipose tissue.[40]

The effect on the HPA axis of rapid weight loss (induced by a very-low-calorie diet) has been studied by Yanovski et al.[41] While they observed a 19% weight loss in their participants and a concomitant fall in AUC (area under the curve) for plasma cortisol levels with CRH testing, the authors concluded that effects on HPA function were not significant, because of observed cortisol changes likely caused by the fall in CBG levels with weight loss.

OBESITY IN GLUCOCORTICOID EXCESS

Primary HPA perturbation similarly has an important effect on body weight. Glucocorticoid deficiency is associated with weight loss, whereas glucocorticoid excess is associated with weight gain. We focus here on the latter.

Obesity in Glucocorticoid Excess: Pathophysiology

Glucocorticoids have complex actions on adipose tissue and in excess lead to altered adipocyte function and distribution. Glucocorticoid excess also affects energy balance by influencing energy intake. For example, chronic hydrocortisone administration to mice increases appetite, body weight, and fat pad weight, in addition to increasing hypothalamic glucocorticoid levels, which may influence control of energy balance beyond simply appetite control.[42] The picture is less clear in humans, with a systematic review of therapeutic glucocorticoid use reporting equivocal findings regarding altered energy intake.[43] Choice of food is thought to be different in people with Cushing's syndrome, however.[44] With myopathy and changes in body shape, it is also feasible that glucocorticoid excess reduces activity levels, and this has indeed been demonstrated in the mouse chronic hydrocortisone model.[45]

Here, we discuss obesity in association with frank glucocorticoid excess, namely Cushing's syndrome and iatrogenic steroid administration. It should be noted that the hyperactivity of the HPA axis seen in chronic stress, and the subsequent adverse effect on metabolism also attracts considerable research interest. Peters and McEwen[46] put forward the argument that the ability to cope with, or habituate to, chronic stress may influence body habitus, with high levels of visceral fat despite a lean body shape, representing "nonhabituation" and carrying increased mortality risk. Interestingly, the mesenteric fat depot is the most susceptible to the effects of chronic stress in a rat model.[47] This may well have relevance to the excess morbidity and mortality seen with socioeconomic deprivation but has yet to achieve clear clinical translation.

Obesity in Glucocorticoid Excess: Cushing's Syndrome

Cushing's syndrome due to endogenous glucocorticoid excess may be ACTH-dependent, being caused by either pituitary ACTH excess (Cushing's disease) or ectopic ACTH production, or is less commonly ACTH-independent (e.g., excess adrenal steroid secretion) (Fig. 4.2). Obesity is seen in 95% of affected individuals with Cushing's syndrome,[48] with mean body mass index (BMI) reported as 31 kg/m^2 by the European Registry on Cushing's Syndrome (ERCUSYN) and weight gain a reported symptom in 81% (more commonly so in women than in men).[49] The syndrome also comprises other significant metabolic abnormalities such as glucose intolerance and dyslipidemia (reviewed by Ferrau & Korbonits[50]). Cushing's syndrome may initially

be treated medically, with agents such as metyrapone and ketoconazole used with the aim of blocking steroid synthesis, but this is not curative. Surgical intervention to reduce glucocorticoid secretion is usually the goal, by removing either the culprit tumor, or—if it cannot be found—the adrenal glands.

Mortality is increased two- to four-fold with Cushing's syndrome[51] and does not normalize with remission. Similarly, it would appear that there is marked persistence of obesity, although waist–hip ratio does improve with treatment.[52] In an older study, despite treatment leading to clinical response, obesity persisted in 55% of patients during follow-up lasting up to 30 years.[53] More recent studies also report greater abdominal obesity in Cushing's patients, compared with controls, 5 years after cure.[54,55]

The recognition and diagnosis of Cushing's syndrome remains difficult, and obesity may be the presenting symptom. Javorsky et al.[56] report a series of Cushing's patients (15 with Cushing's disease and 1 with an adrenal adenoma) who underwent weight-loss surgery; in 12 of these, the diagnosis of Cushing's was not made until after bariatric surgery. Clinicians must therefore be alert to other symptoms and signs of Cushing's (or indeed any other endocrinopathy) in their assessment of the obese patient. Similarly, we must hope that the drive to improve diagnosis and management of Cushing's syndrome[57] is able to reduce the burden of the associated obesity. While bariatric surgery is not a primary treatment for Cushing's syndrome, BMI has been demonstrated to fall with obesity surgery in Cushing's patients.[56]

Obesity in Glucocorticoid Excess: Iatrogenic Steroid Excess

Glucocorticoid prescription, as discussed earlier, is widespread and is not without significant morbidity. Recent studies using the Clinical Practice Research Datalink have found that, in patients with rheumatoid arthritis, glucocorticoid prescription is a risk factor for the development of diabetes mellitus[58] and is associated with a hazard ratio of 1.97 for all-cause mortality.[59] Importantly, they do report a dose-dependent effect, with doses equivalent to 5 mg prednisolone daily or lower not conferring increased mortality risk.[59]

Berthon et al.[43] have recently systematically reviewed risk of weight gain with oral glucocorticoid use and conclude that chronic use may indeed lead to weight gain. However, they were not able to describe a dose-response relationship. The same group has since studied the effects of a short course (10 days) of oral prednisolone 50 mg daily in asthmatic adults and did not observe an increase in body weight or body fat.[60] Although weight

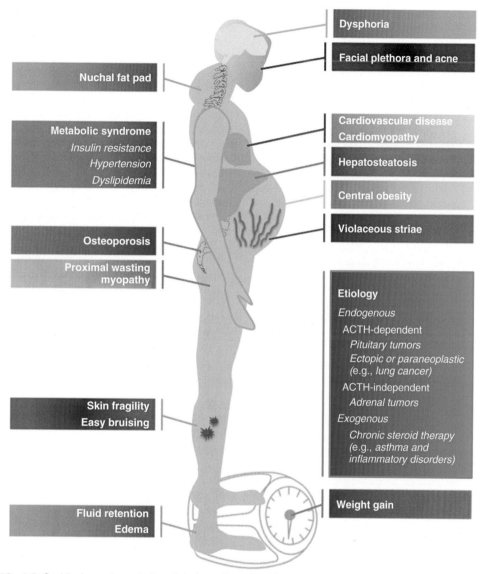

FIG. 4.2 Cushing's syndrome is the clinical manifestation of chronic hypercortisolism and can result from endogenous or iatrogenic glucocorticoid excess. It may comprise some or all of the clinical features indicated here.

gain is listed as an adverse effect of corticosteroid preparations in the British National Formulary, it is unclear how rigorously patients are counseled about the risks of weight gain and about what they can do to try and prevent excessive weight gain while on steroid therapy.

Pseudo Cushing's Syndrome

It is worth noting that obesity may also be a feature of pseudo Cushing's syndrome. Pseudo Cushing's syndrome is a clinical state thought to reflect physiologic hypercortisolism.[61] It is associated with alcohol excess and mental illness such as depression, and it is also reported in people taking antiretroviral therapy.[62,63] In states of alcohol excess, the proposed mechanisms include elevated CRH production and greater levels of free cortisol (due to reduced CBG production in end-stage liver failure).[64] However, while obesity can be a feature of both pseudo Cushing's syndrome and Cushing's syndrome, the presence of clinical features such as skin fragility, myopathy, and bruising is thought to be more indicative of Cushing's.[63] Both the dexamethasone–CRH test and serum or salivary midnight cortisol have recently been demonstrated as reliable biochemical means of distinguishing between the two conditions.[61]

CIRCADIAN DISRUPTION AND OBESITY

Circulating glucocorticoid levels peak at the start of the active phase (dawn in humans, dusk in nocturnal animals) and reach a nadir during the middle of the rest phase (typically around midnight in humans). Superimposed on this circadian rhythm is an ultradian rhythm of approximately hourly pulses of secretion. The circadian rhythm of glucocorticoid secretion and action is governed by the circadian clock.

The Clock

The circadian clock (or body clock) is the internal timing mechanism of an organism, which anticipates rhythmic changes in the environment and thus promotes homeostasis. External cues or "zeitgebers"—chiefly light, but also temperature, nutrient intake, and social interaction—serve to set or synchronize the clock. The hypothalamic master clock is found in the suprachiasmatic nucleus and receives signals from the retinohypothalamic tract, but peripheral organs, including the liver and the pancreas, also demonstrate rhythms of function and gene expression. At a molecular level, the circadian clock is driven by transcription–translation feedback loops between the core clock proteins, with these cycles having a periodicity close to 24 h. The activating limb of the clock comprises the proteins CLOCK (Circadian Locomotor Output Cycles Kaput) and BMAL1 (brain muscle ARNT-like 1), which together drive the transcription of their repressors, the Period, Cryptochrome, and REV-ERB proteins.[65] Rhythmic programs of clock-controlled genes serve to regulate the metabolism (for example) of an organism, so that it is appropriate to its rhythms of activity, feeding behavior, and nutrient intake. Dyssynchrony between these rhythms, such as might occur in shift workers or with travel across time zones, is emerging as a significant factor in the development of metabolic disease.[66]

Circadian Disruption and Obesity

The internal body clock plays a key role in maintaining homeostasis in the face of oscillating environmental signals (light, temperature, availability of nutrition, for example). Growing evidence (recently summarized by West and Bechtold[67]) suggests that circadian dyssynchrony, promoted by modern 24-h lifestyles, shift work, and travel across time zones, can lead to obesity and the metabolic syndrome. Indeed, the phenomenon of "social jetlag," when sleep and activity patterns vary between work and leisure periods, seems to confer increased risk of obesity and metabolic syndrome, as demonstrated in the large Dunedin-based study of 815 participants.[68] Exposure to light at night, a risk factor for sleep disruption, significantly increased the risk of obesity in a questionnaire-based study of over 100,000 women.[69]

As discussed above, physiologic glucocorticoid secretion by the HPA axis follows a circadian rhythm. In the systematic review by Incollingo Rodriguez et al.,[29] five studies reported a "flatter" diurnal slope in cortisol levels with greater BMI or waist–hip ratio. However, it is not yet understood whether this finding is simply a consequence of obesity, reflects circadian disruption, or is contributing to the phenotype. There is undoubtedly great need for further study of the HPA axis and obesity in those exposed to shift work and social jetlag, and it will be especially interesting to see whether the growing efforts to improve shift work result in improvements in metabolic parameters.

OPPORTUNITIES FOR THERAPEUTIC INTERVENTION AND QUESTIONS FOR FUTURE RESEARCH

Greater understanding of the role of glucocorticoids in obesity has two important translational applications. Firstly, it is highly desirable that we mitigate the adverse metabolic effects of glucocorticoid therapy. Secondly, targeting the mechanisms involved may be of potential value in the treatment of obesity and obesity-related metabolic disorders.

Can We Employ Glucocorticoids More Smartly?

Given their potency, availability, ease of administration, and relatively low cost, glucocorticoids are unlikely to lose their popularity for treating inflammatory disorders. The challenge for the field is to exploit growing understanding of glucocorticoid biology to preserve their antiinflammatory effects while reducing or eliminating their undesirable effects. As the unwanted actions of glucocorticoids are largely thought to be mediated by GR transactivation of target genes, whilst antiinflammatory actions are mediated by both transactivation and transrepression, alternative GR ligands—termed Selective Glucocorticoid Receptor

Agonists and Modulators (SEGRAMs)—have been the focus of much work (reviewed in Refs. 70,71). Some of these agents have reached Phase II trials; none have yet to enter clinical practice.

Whereas adverse effects are common, less commonly patients may fail to experience the full intended therapeutic benefits of steroid treatment. Examples include steroid-resistant asthma, nephrotic syndrome, and inflammatory bowel disease. That there is interindividual variability in glucocorticoid sensitivity[34] raises the possibility of tailoring glucocorticoid treatments to likely responders versus nonresponders. It is becoming more evident than ever, however, that the actions of glucocorticoids are context- and tissue-specific. It has been demonstrated in vitro that the cistrome of the GR changes markedly in the inflammatory state.[72] Therefore, the effects and mechanisms of action of glucocorticoids observed in the healthy experimental participant may be different from what occurs in an individual with an inflammatory disorder. This unfortunately limits the extrapolation of some of the animal and human research that has been done into glucocorticoid side effects. There is therefore an urgent need for further studies in either patients (with obvious ethical considerations) or in experimental models of inflammation.

Can We Exploit Understanding of Glucocorticoid Biology to Treat Obesity and the Metabolic Syndrome?

Glucocorticoid availability, at the level of the tissue, is regulated by the 11β-HSD enzymes, and inhibition of 11β-HSD1, with the aim of reducing local concentrations of active cortisol, continues to receive considerable interest as a potential treatment for the metabolic syndrome. Studies in humans (reviewed by Gathercole et al.[73]) have demonstrated modest but significant improvements in body weight, but with effects on other metabolic parameters, such as glucose handling and lipid profile, varying between compounds.

The understanding that the MR and GR play a role in adipogenesis and adipocyte maturation has triggered Mammi et al.[74] to study the effects of combined MR and GR antagonism on the weight gain and development of fat mass normally induced by an HFD. They report that their compound, CORT118335, did indeed have significant beneficial effects in their mouse model, with reduction in overall weight gain, prevention of fat mass gain, and improvement of glucose tolerance, compared with vehicle treatment.

SUMMARY

Glucocorticoids are enormously useful antiinflammatory agents, used to treat large numbers of people with inflammatory disorders. In contrast, endogenous glucocorticoid excess is a rare condition. However, both these situations are associated with considerable morbidity related to the weight gain and adverse metabolic effects caused by glucocorticoids.

Similarly, as human societies move toward cultures of work and behavior that promote disharmony between our circadian rhythms of activity, feeding, and circulating glucocorticoid, there is greater impetus to address the obesity and metabolic dysfunction associated with this.

There is therefore scope for research and therapeutic intervention at all levels, from molecular to cultural, within this field, to improve health and treat disease. However, as we hope this chapter highlights, glucocorticoid actions are complex, and it may be some time before a fuller understanding is translated into human benefit.

REFERENCES

1. Caratti G, Matthews L, Poolman T, Kershaw S, Baxter M, Ray D. Glucocorticoid receptor function in health and disease. *Clin Endocrinol.* 2015;83:441–448.
2. Arango-Lievano M, Lambert WM, Jeanneteau F. Molecular biology of glucocorticoid signaling. *Adv Exp Med Biol.* 2015;872:33–57.
3. Draper N, Stewart PM. 11beta-hydroxysteroid dehydrogenase and the pre-receptor regulation of corticosteroid hormone action. *J Endocrinol.* 2005;186:251–271.
4. Morgan SA, McCabe EL, Gathercole LL, et al. 11beta-HSD1 is the major regulator of the tissue-specific effects of circulating glucocorticoid excess. *Proc Natl Acad Sci USA.* 2014;111:E2482–E2491.
5. Health, Social Care Information Centre. *Clinical Commissioning Group Prescribing Data (Quarters 1-4, 2014-15);* June 18, 2015. Ref Type: Online Source.
6. Magomedova L, Cummins CL. Glucocorticoids and metabolic control. *Handb Exp Pharmacol.* 2016;233:73–93.
7. de Guia RM, Herzig S. How do glucocorticoids regulate lipid metabolism? *Adv Exp Med Biol.* 2015;872: 127–144.
8. Peckett AJ, Wright DC, Riddell MC. The effects of glucocorticoids on adipose tissue lipid metabolism. *Metabolism.* 2011;60:1500–1510.
9. Lee MJ, Pramyothin P, Karastergiou K, Fried SK. Deconstructing the roles of glucocorticoids in adipose tissue biology and the development of central obesity. *Biochim Biophys Acta.* 2014;1842:473–481.
10. Gathercole LL, Morgan SA, Bujalska IJ, Hauton D, Stewart PM, Tomlinson JW. Regulation of lipogenesis by glucocorticoids and insulin in human adipose tissue. *PLoS One.* 2011;6:e26223.

11. Thuzar M, Ho KK. Mechanisms in endocrinology: brown adipose tissue in humans: regulation and metabolic significance. *Eur J Endocrinol.* 2016;175:R11–R25.

12. Giordano A, Frontini A, Cinti S. Convertible visceral fat as a therapeutic target to curb obesity. *Nat Rev Drug Discov.* 2016;15:405–424.

13. Barclay JL, Agada H, Jang C, Ward M, Wetzig N, Ho KK. Effects of glucocorticoids on human brown adipocytes. *J Endocrinol.* 2015;224:139–147.

14. Soumano K, Desbiens S, Rabelo R, Bakopanos E, Camirand A, Silva JE. Glucocorticoids inhibit the transcriptional response of the uncoupling protein-1 gene to adrenergic stimulation in a brown adipose cell line. *Mol Cell Endocrinol.* 2000;165:7–15.

15. Caprio M, Feve B, Claes A, Viengchareun S, Lombes M, Zennaro MC. Pivotal role of the mineralocorticoid receptor in corticosteroid-induced adipogenesis. *FASEB J.* 2007;21:2185–2194.

16. Hausman DB, DiGirolamo M, Bartness TJ, Hausman GJ, Martin RJ. The biology of white adipocyte proliferation. *Obes Rev.* 2001;2:239–254.

17. Kras KM, Hausman DB, Hausman GJ, Martin RJ. Adipocyte development is dependent upon stem cell recruitment and proliferation of preadipocytes. *Obes Res.* 1999;7:491–497.

18. Gulfo J, Ledda A, Serra E, Cabot C, Esteve M, Grasa M. Altered lipid partitioning and glucocorticoid availability in CBG-deficient male mice with diet-induced obesity. *Obesity (Silver Spring).* 2016;24:1677–1686.

19. Ayala-Sumuano JT, Velez-delValle C, Beltran-Langarica A, Marsch-Moreno M, Hernandez-Mosqueira C, Kuri-Harcuch W. Glucocorticoid paradoxically recruits adipose progenitors and impairs lipid homeostasis and glucose transport in mature adipocytes. *Sci Rep.* 2013;3:2573.

20. Lee MJ, Gong DW, Burkey BF, Fried SK. Pathways regulated by glucocorticoids in omental and subcutaneous human adipose tissues: a microarray study. *Am J Physiol Endocrinol Metab.* 2011;300:E571–E580.

21. Fried SK, Russell CD, Grauso NL, Brolin RE. Lipoprotein lipase regulation by insulin and glucocorticoid in subcutaneous and omental adipose tissues of obese women and men. *J Clin Invest.* 1993;92:2191–2198.

22. Lutz TA, Woods SC. Overview of animal models of obesity. *Curr Protoc Pharmacol.* 2012. http://dx.doi.org/10.1002/0471141755.ph0561s58. Chapter 5.

23. Lean ME, Malkova D. Altered gut and adipose tissue hormones in overweight and obese individuals: cause or consequence? *Int J Obes.* 2016;40:622–632.

24. Wong SK, Chin K-Y, Suhaimi FH, Fairus A, Ima-Nirwana S. Animal models of metabolic syndrome: a review. *Nutr Metab.* 2016;13.

25. Tannenbaum BM, Brindley DN, Tannenbaum GS, Dallman MF, McArthur MD, Meaney MJ. High-fat feeding alters both basal and stress-induced hypothalamic-pituitary-adrenal activity in the rat. *Am J Physiol.* 1997;273:E1168–E1177.

26. Edwardson JA, Hough CA. The pituitary-adrenal system of the genetically obese (ob/ob) mouse. *J Endocrinol.* 1975;65:99–107.

27. Garthwaite TL, Martinson DR, Tseng LF, Hagen TC, Menahan LA. A longitudinal hormonal profile of the genetically obese mouse. *Endocrinology.* 1980;107:671–676.

28. Livingstone DE, Jones GC, Smith K, et al. Understanding the role of glucocorticoids in obesity: tissue-specific alterations of corticosterone metabolism in obese Zucker rats. *Endocrinology.* 2000;141:560–563.

29. Incollingo Rodriguez AC, Epel ES, White ML, Standen EC, Seckl JR, Tomiyama AJ. Hypothalamic-pituitary-adrenal axis dysregulation and cortisol activity in obesity: a systematic review. *Psychoneuroendocrinology.* 2015;62:301–318.

30. Abraham SB, Rubino D, Sinaii N, Ramsey S, Nieman LK. Cortisol, obesity, and the metabolic syndrome: a cross-sectional study of obese subjects and review of the literature. *Obesity (Silver Spring).* 2013;21:E105–E117.

31. Weaver JU, Kopelman PG, McLoughlin L, Forsling ML, Grossman A. Hyperactivity of the hypothalamo-pituitary-adrenal axis in obesity: a study of ACTH, AVP, beta-lipotrophin and cortisol responses to insulin-induced hypoglycaemia. *Clin Endocrinol.* 1993;39:345–350.

32. Duclos M, Marquez PP, Barat P, Gatta B, Roger P. Increased cortisol bioavailability, abdominal obesity, and the metabolic syndrome in obese women. *Obes Res.* 2005;13:1157–1166.

33. Syed AA, Weaver JU. Glucocorticoid sensitivity: the hypothalamic-pituitary-adrenal-tissue axis. *Obes Res.* 2005;13:1131–1133.

34. Syed AA, Redfern CP, Weaver JU. In vivo and in vitro glucocorticoid sensitivity in obese people with cushingoid appearance. *Obesity (Silver Spring).* 2008;16:2374–2378.

35. Rask E, Olsson T, Söderberg S, et al. Tissue-specific dysregulation of cortisol metabolism in human obesity. *J Clin Endocrinol Metab.* 2001;86:1418–1421.

36. Morton NM, Densmore V, Wamil M, et al. A polygenic model of the metabolic syndrome with reduced circulating and intra-adipose glucocorticoid action. *Diabetes.* 2005;54:3371–3378.

37. Larner DP, Morgan SA, Gathercole LL, et al. Male 11β-HSD1 knockout mice fed trans-fats and fructose are not protected from metabolic syndrome or nonalcoholic fatty liver disease. *Endocrinology.* 2016;157:3493–3504.

38. Syed AA, Irving JA, Redfern CP, et al. Association of glucocorticoid receptor polymorphism A3669G in exon 9beta with reduced central adiposity in women. *Obesity (Silver Spring).* 2006;14:759–764.

39. Syed AA, Halpin CG, Irving JA, et al. A common intron 2 polymorphism of the glucocorticoid receptor gene is associated with insulin resistance in men. *Clin Endocrinol.* 2008;68:879–884.

40. Goedecke JH, Chorell E, Livingstone DE, et al. Glucocorticoid receptor gene expression in adipose tissue and associated metabolic risk in black and white South African women. *Int J Obes.* 2015;39:303–311.

41. Yanovski JA, Yanovski SZ, Gold PW, Chrousos GP. Differences in corticotropin-releasing hormone-stimulated adrenocorticotropin and cortisol before and after weight loss. *J Clin Endocrinol Metab.* 1997;82:1874–1878.

42. Sefton C, Harno E, Davies A, et al. Elevated hypothalamic glucocorticoid levels are associated with obesity and hyperphagia in male mice. *Endocrinology.* 2016;157:4257–4265.

43. Berthon BS, MacDonald-Wicks LK, Wood LG. A systematic review of the effect of oral glucocorticoids on energy intake, appetite, and body weight in humans. *Nutr Res.* 2014;24:179–190.

44. Moeller SJ, Couto L, Cohen V, et al. Glucocorticoid regulation of food-choice behavior in humans: evidence from Cushing's syndrome. *Front Neurosci.* 2016;10.

45. Karatsoreos IN, Bhagat SM, Bowles NP, Weil ZM, Pfaff DW, McEwen BS. Endocrine and physiological changes in response to chronic corticosterone: a potential model of the metabolic syndrome in mouse. *Endocrinology.* 2010;151:2117–2127.

46. Peters A, McEwen BS. Stress habituation, body shape and cardiovascular mortality. *Neurosci Biobehav Rev.* 2015;56:139–150.

47. Rebuffé-Scrive M, Walsh UA, McEwen BS, Rodin J. Effect of chronic stress and exogenous glucocorticoids on regional fat distribution and metabolism. *Physiol Behav.* 1992;52:583–590.

48. Newell-Price J, Bertagna X, Grossman A, Nieman LK. Cushing's syndrome. *Lancet.* 2006;367:1605–1617.

49. Valassi E, Santos A, Yaneva M, et al. The European registry on Cushing's syndrome: 2-year experience. Baseline demographic and clinical characteristics. *Eur J Endocrinol.* 2011;165:383–392.

50. Ferrau F, Korbonits M. Metabolic comorbidities in Cushing's syndrome. *Eur J Endocrinol.* 2015;173:M133–M157.

51. Lacroix A, Feelders RA, Stratakis CA, Nieman LK. Cushing's syndrome. *Lancet.* 2015;386:913–927.

52. Faggiano A, Pivonello R, Spiezia S, et al. Cardiovascular risk factors and common carotid artery caliber and stiffness in patients with Cushing's disease during active disease and 1 year after disease remission. *J Clin Endocrinol Metab.* 2003;88:2527–2533.

53. Ross EJ, Linch DC. The clinical response to treatment in adult Cushing's syndrome following remission of hypercortisolaemia. *Postgrad Med J.* 1985;61:205–211.

54. Colao A, Pivonello R, Spiezia S, et al. Persistence of increased cardiovascular risk in patients with Cushing's disease after five years of successful cure. *J Clin Endocrinol Metab.* 1999;84:2664–2672.

55. Wagenmakers M, Roerink S, Gil L, et al. Persistent centripetal fat distribution and metabolic abnormalities in patients in long-term remission of Cushing's syndrome. *Clin Endocrinol.* 2015;82:180–187.

56. Javorsky BR, Carroll TB, Tritos NA, et al. Discovery of Cushing's syndrome after bariatric surgery: multicenter series of 16 patients. *Obes Surg.* 2015;25:2306–2313.

57. Reincke M. Improving outcome in Cushing's syndrome. *Eur J Endocrinol.* 2015;173:E3–E5.

58. Movahedi M, Beauchamp ME, Abrahamowicz M, et al. Risk of incident diabetes mellitus associated with the dosage and duration of oral glucocorticoid therapy in patients with rheumatoid arthritis. *Arthritis Rheumatol.* 2016;68:1089–1098.

59. Movahedi M, Costello R, Lunt M, Pye SR, Sergeant JC, Dixon WG. Oral glucocorticoid therapy and all-cause and cause-specific mortality in patients with rheumatoid arthritis: a retrospective cohort study. *Eur J Epidemiol.* 2016;31:1045–1055.

60. Berthon BS, Gibson PG, McElduff P, MacDonald-Wicks LK, Wood LG. Effects of short-term oral corticosteroid intake on dietary intake, body weight and body composition in adults with asthma – a randomized controlled trial. *Clin Exp Allergy.* 2015;45:908–919.

61. Alwani RA, Schmit Jongbloed LW, de Jong FH, van der Lely AJ, de Herder WW, Feelders RA. Differentiating between Cushing's disease and pseudo-Cushing's syndrome: comparison of four tests. *Eur J Endocrinol.* 2014;170:477–486.

62. Miller KK, Daly PA, Sentochnik D, et al. Pseudo-Cushing's syndrome in human immunodeficiency virus-infected patients. *Clin Infect Dis.* 1998;27:68–72.

63. Newell-Price J, Trainer P, Besser M, Grossman A. The diagnosis and differential diagnosis of Cushing's syndrome and pseudo-Cushing's states. *Endocr Rev.* 1998;19:647–672.

64. Groote VR, Meinders AE. On the mechanism of alcohol-induced pseudo-Cushing's syndrome. *Endocr Rev.* 1996;17:262–268.

65. Gustafson CL, Partch CL. Emerging models for the molecular basis of mammalian circadian timing. *Biochemistry.* 2015;54:134–149.

66. Bechtold DA, Gibbs JE, Loudon AS. Circadian dysfunction in disease. *Trends Pharmacol Sci.* 2010;31:191–198.

67. West AC, Bechtold DA. The cost of circadian desynchrony: evidence, insights and open questions. *Bioessays.* 2015;37:777–788.

68. Parsons MJ, Moffitt TE, Gregory AM, et al. Social jetlag, obesity and metabolic disorder: investigation in a cohort study. *Int J Obes.* 2015;39:842–848.

69. McFadden E, Jones ME, Schoemaker MJ, Ashworth A, Swerdlow AJ. The relationship between obesity and exposure to light at night: cross-sectional analyses of over 100,000 women in the Breakthrough Generations Study. *Am J Epidemiol.* 2014;180:245–250.

70. McMaster A, Ray DW. Drug insight: selective agonists and antagonists of the glucocorticoid receptor. *Nat Clin Pract Endocrinol Metab.* 2008;4:91–101.

71. Sundahl N, Bridelance J, Liebert C, De Bosscher K, Beck IM. Selective glucocorticoid receptor modulation: new directions with non-steroidal scaffolds. *Pharmacol Ther.* 2015;152:28–41.

72. Uhlenhaut NH, Barish GD, Yu RT, et al. Insights into negative regulation by the glucocorticoid receptor from genome-wide profiling of inflammatory cistromes. *Mol Cell.* 2013;49:158–171.

73. Gathercole LL, Lavery GG, Morgan SA, et al. 11β-Hydroxysteroid dehydrogenase 1: translational and therapeutic aspects. *Endocr Rev.* 2013;34:525–555.

74. Mammi C, Marzolla V, Armani A, et al. A novel combined glucocorticoid-mineralocorticoid receptor selective modulator markedly prevents weight gain and fat mass expansion in mice fed a high-fat diet. *Int J Obes.* 2016;40:964–972.

CHAPTER 5

Thyroid and Weight

ANGELOS KYRIACOU, MBCHB, MRCP

INTRODUCTION

Both obesity and thyroid dysfunction are common in modern society. Weight-related complaints are very common among patients with thyroid dysfunction. Obese patients are more likely to suffer from thyroid dysfunction as well, with one study reporting that 20% of morbidly obese patients had either subclinical or overt hypothyroidism.[1] The thyroid gland produces thyroid hormones (THs) that are essential for the various metabolic processes in our body and our resting energy expenditure (REE), which forms approximately 60% of the total energy expenditure in adults. It is common for patients, and indeed the general public, to complain of unexplained weight gain or difficulty in losing weight while dieting and attribute this to "thyroid dysfunction." In fact, in daily clinical practice this is likely to be the most common presenting complaint, and this was confirmed in a study where weight-related complaints formed the presenting complaint of 50%–60% of the overall, normal body mass index (BMI) and euthyroid populations attending a general endocrine clinic.[2]

PATHOPHYSIOLOGY

TH physiology is discussed in Fig. 5.1.

HYPOTHYROIDISM AND WEIGHT

Hypothyroidism decreases REE and thermogenesis and clinically causes a decrease in mental and physical functioning. Hence, it is common for patients with overt hypothyroidism to complain of weight gain. Treatment with levothyroxine (L-t4) reduces weight in about half of the hypothyroid patients. It is worth remembering that hypothyroidism is intrinsically associated with cardiovascular (CVS) risk factors, such as hyperlipidemia, hypertension, and nonalcoholic fatty liver disease, and the association between hypothyroidism and either preexistent or evolving obesity can exacerbate such an adverse CVS profile. It is therefore imperative to exclude hypothyroidism as a potential cause of obesity and the accompanied metabolic syndrome, because prompt therapy with thyroxine will not only reduce weight but also improve the various metabolic parameters and ultimately reduce CVS risk. Similarly, it is our practice to encourage such patients with newly diagnosed hypothyroidism and the metabolic-syndrome profile to avoid complacency and not only be commenced on L-t4 therapy, but also to pay attention to lifestyle factors to maximize weight loss.

Subclinical Hypothyroidism

Regarding subclinical hypothyroidism (SCH) the picture is less clear-cut with many, but not all, studies linking it with weight gain, as well as dyslipidemia and CVS disease and even mortality. Data from a longitudinal study with individuals above the age of 65 years showed that increased baseline TSH by 1 mIU/L was associated with a 0.5 kg increase in weight; both associations were seen only in females.[5] Adjusted analysis of longitudinal weight changes again revealed a modest weight increase of 0.3 and 0.2 kg in females and males, respectively, with a 1 mIU/L increase in TSH.[5] In another study, obese individuals with SCH were compared with age-, gender- and BMI-matched obese patients with normal TSH.[6] SCH has not been identified to alter body composition as measured by bioelectrical impedance[6] or dual energy X-ray absorptiometry (DXA).[5] A prospective population-based observational study with about 600 patients investigated the effect that SCH has on elderly patients at 85 years of age and followed up these patients for 4 years.[7] A gradual increase in weight was observed in this study with a transition from hyperthyroidism to euthyroidism and then to hypothyroidism; for example, the SCH group was on average a modest 0.6 kg heavier than the euthyroid group.[7] Another cross-sectional study of elderly patients (>65 years) found a similar association between SCH and increased BMI in women, but the opposite effect in men.[8] Three other longitudinal studies have also reported an association between change in TSH and change in BMI.[9–11]

In conclusion, although many studies report an association between SCH and increased weight, it is unclear what is the cause and what is the effect on this relationship. Moreover, even with studies indicating a positive correlation, the effect is very modest and of debatable clinical significance.

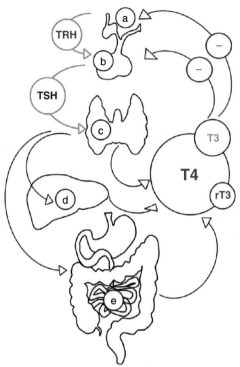

FIG. 5.1 Thyroid physiology. *Central regulation*: Thyrotropin-releasing hormone (TRH) is produced by the hypothalamus **(A)** and stimulates production and release of thyroid-stimulating hormone (TSH) from the anterior pituitary **(B)**. TSH stimulates secretion of the thyroid hormones (THs), tetraiodothyronine (T4), and triiodothyronine (T3) produced by follicular cells in the thyroid gland **(C)**. Iodine is a mineral that is essential for TH production. *TH transport in plasma and action at a cellular level*: THs are poorly soluble in water and hence bind reversibly to plasma proteins all of which are synthesized in the liver **(D)**. The free hormones are the ones available at the tissue level for intracellular transport and feedback regulation and control of the various metabolic processes. THs bind to thyroid receptors intracellularly and form a heterodimer with retinoid X receptor; this whole complex binds to the TH response element in DNA to increase (or decrease) transcription and translation. *Peripheral TH metabolism*: For every 100 mcg of T4 produced by the thyroid gland, approximately 6 mcg of T3 is produced.[4] T4 undergoes peripheral conversion to the more active molecule T3. Given that some of the peripherally produced T3 escapes back to the circulation, the ratio between serum T4 to T3 is 80%:20%. Both T4 and T3 are inactivated by inner ring deiodination. The deiodinase enzymes occur in three isoforms. *Deiodinases*: D1 is a plasma membrane protein mainly present in the liver **(D)**, kidney, and thyroid **(C)** and is involved not only in T4 to T3 activation, but also in the degradation of the inactive TH, reverse triiodothyronine (rT3). D2 is an intracellular protein found mainly in the central nervous system, pituitary **(A)**, and brown adipose tissue; it induces T4 to T3 activation intracellularly and is a source of plasma T3. D3 is a plasma membrane protein found in the central nervous system, placenta, and liver **(D)** and is involved in TH inactivation, e.g., conversion of T4 to rT3. All three isoforms contain the rare amino acid, selenocysteine, in the active catalytic center, of which selenium is an essential component. *TH excretion*: T4 and T3 breakdown involves the conjugation of the phenolic hydroxyl group with glucuronic acid or sulfate. Glucuronidated T4 and T3 are excreted in the bile but may be partially reabsorbed after deglucuronidation in the intestine **(E)**. (From Kyriacou A, McLaughlin J, Syed AA. Thyroid disorders and gastrointestinal and liver dysfunction: a state of the art review. *Eur J Intern Med*. 2015;26(8):563–571, with permission.)

Management of Hypothyroidism and Weight Changes

Although the benefits of treatment with L-t4 are undeniable in cases of overt hypothyroidism, there is ongoing debate if and when SCH should be treated, with guidelines recommending L-t4 for persistent SCH if the TSH is above 10 mIU/L and a trial of L-t4 therapy for symptomatic patients who have a TSH above the normal range and below 10 mIU/L; for the more elderly patients (e.g., above the age of 70 years) the threshold for treatment is higher, with L-t4 not recommended for TSH below 10 mIU/L.[12] However, a common clinical scenario is of overweight or obese asymptomatic patients with a mildly raised TSH (but below 10 mIU/L), and the question arises whether such patients are likely to benefit from treatment. In the majority of such patients L-t4 is not indicated given that it is unlikely to exert any significant beneficial effect, but an individualized approach to treatment is required. Once L-t4 is commenced, the conventional treatment goal is to achieve a TSH in the lower half of the normal range. The rationale for this is that only a small fragment (2.5%–9%) of the general population has a TSH that is higher than 2.5 mIU/L.[13,14] However, this has been challenged because achieving a TSH in the lower half of the normal range did not have a significant impact on the BMI or body composition[15] and small changes in L-t4 dose did not seem to alter the weight, symptomatology, or the quality of life in patients with hypothyroidism.[16]

Levothyroxine versus combination therapies

Many patients who are well controlled on L-t4, as judged by a TSH well into the normal range, do still complain of "hypothyroid-related symptomatology" including weight gain and difficulty with weight loss. There is a debate regarding the effectiveness of a combination of L-t4 and liothyronine (L-t3) versus L-t4 alone or even L-t4 versus L-t3 in the treatment of hypothyroidism. The use of L-t3 has been associated with better weight loss of about 2 kg in two small randomized controlled trials (RCTs).[17,18] A metaanalysis concluded a statistically, but not clinically, significant weight drop at 100 g with combination therapy versus L-t4 monotherapy.[19] Not only does the utilization of T3 in these studies provided only a modest clinical benefit, but also other studies did not find any added benefit to standard L-t4 therapy, and there are difficulties with current T3 preparations including their nonphysiologic profiles with short-term peaks and short duration of action, unclear long-term safety profile, and need to rely on TSH alone for dosing. Therefore most endocrinologists and relevant guidelines discourage the use of T3 in

hypothyroidism, but a window for its use, in combination with L-t4, on selected, refractory cases, and on a trial basis, has been opened by the European Thyroid Association guidelines.[20]

Treatment with levothyroxine and body composition

Body composition studies indicate that the main compartment affected by the treatment of hypothyroidism is that of lean body mass. This is defined as the total body weight after the subtraction of total body fat. In a Danish study that included 12 patients with overt hypothyroidism (mean TSH = 102 mIU/L), the mean weight loss achieved with L-t4 therapy for a year and the establishment of euthyroidism (mean TSH = 2 mIU/L) was about 4 kg; the corresponding BMI reduction was at 2 kg/m^2 and both were statistically significant.[21] Body composition analysis before and after L-t4 therapy showed that most of the weight loss was due to reduction in lean body mass, itself likely to indicate a total body fluid reduction.[21] Various theories may explain the observed weight loss with treatment of hypothyroidism: (1) reversal of the reduced free-water excretion by the kidneys, (2) reversal of the increased vasopressin release, and (3) reversal of the increased amount of glycosaminoglycans (which can retain water), all three of which are hypothyroidism-induced phenomena. Similarly, lean body mass has been proven to be the main factor determining the dose of L-t4 in hypothyroid patients (see Fig. 5.2).

HYPERTHYROIDISM AND WEIGHT

Hyperthyroidism causes the inverse phenomenon to what you get with hypothyroidism with increased REE and thermogenesis and a more catabolic picture. The appetite increases, but the energy expenditure increase is usually more prominent, hence the weight decreases in about 90% of such patients. In the remaining patients, the appetite effect and increased energy intake are more significant to the extent that they gain weight. Weight reduction with hyperthyroidism is estimated to be at around 16% or on average about 7 kg compared with 1 year before presentation.[23] It is of course very difficult to measure the premorbid weight for the great majority of the patients, and hence one has to rely more on self-reported weight alterations, which are subjected to recall bias.

Treatment of Hyperthyroidism

Numerous, but not all, studies report overshoot of weight regain following treatment of hyperthyroidism

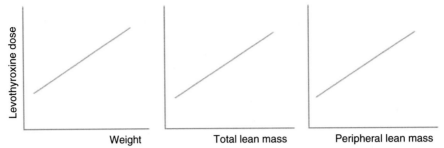

FIG. 5.2 Levothyroxine dosing in relation to body weight and body composition analysis by dual energy X-ray absorptiometry scan. (Adapted from Santini F, Pinchera A, Marsili A, et al. Lean body mass is a major determinant of levothyroxine dosage in the treatment of thyroid diseases. *J Clin Endocrinol Metab.* 2005;90(1):124–127, with permission.)

in a range from 1 to 16 kg[23–25]; this is something that concerns the majority of such patients with 69% identified to have more weight gain than previous weight loss.[26] The reason why there is such weight gain may relate to a reduced REE that is comparatively more than the fall of the reduced appetite, which occurs with thyrotoxicosis treatment, or alternatively a leftover deregulation of appetite from the hyperthyroid phase. One of the limitations of research on this field is that the weight gain posttreatment has been traditionally compared with the presentation weight, but ideally the comparison should be with the premorbid weight. Furthermore, many studies used the thyroid cancer cohort to study the effects of thyroidectomy on weight, given that such patients have all received total thyroidectomy; however, one needs to bear in mind that the effect of thyroidectomy on weight may be different when the procedure is done for thyroid cancer treatment and, of course, that with this pathology invariably there is no weight loss preoperatively. Furthermore, thyroid cancer patients are often given L-t4 to such doses so as to keep the TSH suppressed, which may in itself be causing some weight loss (albeit not proven so).

Body composition analysis in hyperthyroidism and with its treatment

In terms of which body compartment is affected by hyperthyroidism, it seems that mainly lean body mass is reduced with the disease state per se whether this was estimated from percutaneous biopsies[27] or DXA scan.[28] In terms of the effect of treatment, a study assessed body composition using both DXA and computed tomography (CT) scan protocols on presentation and after treatment for hyperthyroidism, with a variety of treatment modalities, in nine patients.[23] Firstly, this study showed that at 1 year the regained weight

exceeded the premorbid, self-reported, weight by over 1 kg.[23] Secondly, they showed that in the first instance at 3 months the lean body mass (namely skeletal tissue) and intraperitoneal adipose tissue increased, whereas at a later point at 12 months posttreatment the retroperitoneal and subcutaneous adipose tissue increased; the 8.7 kg gained by the end of the study was the aggregate of about 5 kg of fat and 3.5 kg of fat-free mass.[23] Studies also exist that report a more synchronous rise in total lean and fat mass (as measured by DXA scan) within the first year of treatment with thionamides.[28]

Management of hyperthyroidism and weight changes

A study has indicated that significantly more weight gain occurs when hyperthyroid patients are operated on. In particular, in this study they had 136 subjects who underwent treatment for hyperthyroidism and were followed for up to 10 years.[29] The mean weight gain observed at 2 years was 5.4 kg; both thionamides and radioactive iodine therapy caused on average a weight gain of about 5 kg, whereas the corresponding weight gain with thyroidectomy was significantly higher at 10 kg.[29] Independent risk factors for weight gain included (1) a history of weight loss before presentation with hyperthyroidism, (2) preexisting obesity, (3) a diagnosis of Graves' disease, (4) development of iatrogenic hypothyroidism requiring L-t4 therapy, and (5) increasing follow-up time.[29] Limitations of this study include its retrospective design and the lack of a euthyroid or other control group. Another retrospective study documented that the development of hypothyroidism postthyroidectomy or postradioidine therapy (for Graves' disease) was associated with significantly higher weight gain compared with patients who were rendered euthyroid with thionamides or hemithyroidectomy; all these patients experienced more weight gain compared with patients with thyroid cancer who were subjected to total thyroidectomy (mean weight gain of about 10 kg vs. 4 kg vs. 0.6 kg, respectively).[30] Therefore, on balance, there seems to be a significant amount of weight gain following the diagnosis and treatment of hyperthyroidism. Such weight gain is due to a regain of the lost weight that occurred before the illness was treated and to some extent due to iatrogenic hypothyroidism. Although a few studies indicate that the weight regain is more than the premorbid weight loss, further prospective studies would be beneficial to confirm this observation.

Radioiodine therapy is associated with significant weight gain in most studies. A prospective study included 75 patients with hyperthyroidism who received radioactive iodine and showed a mean weight gain at approximately 5 kg in 5 years; such weight rise was attained early within 6 months.[31] The average BMI increase was 2.3 kg/m^2 versus a recorded average BMI increase of 1.2 kg/m^2 in the general population in the surrounding region.[31] Nevertheless, no matched-control group was used and the weight comparison was done against the weight at presentation. DXA studies before and after radioactive iodine therapy revealed that most of the weight increase was due to increases in lean body mass, which demonstrated a statistically significant 20% rise at 1 year.[31]

Induction of Iatrogenic Thyrotoxicosis for Weight Loss Purposes

Going back to the original realization that most of our patients with hyperthyroidism will lose weight because of it, the following question transpires: Why not use TH replacement to tackle the modern obesity epidemic? There are two reasons why we should resist this temptation. Firstly, L-t4 or L-t3 does not seem to be particularly effective in bringing about weight loss. Short-term intervention studies did not find any significant reduction in BMI with L-t4 use in mild hypothyroidism. Similarly, postthyroid cancer iatrogenic thyrotoxicosis does not seem to reduce weight.[25] More evidence on the lack of efficacy of TH therapy for weight loss purposes in euthyroid obese populations on existing caloric restriction comes from a systematic review that included only RCTs or prospective observational studies.[32] The included studies were characterized by marked heterogeneity, poor quality, small study samples, and variable TH dosages and duration of use. Nevertheless, some deductions can be drawn: (1) overall, there seems to be no significant benefit in weight reduction when THs are added in euthyroid obese individuals, and (2) mild or full thyrotoxicosis is a concern

with TH use and TSH reduction is possible even with "physiologic" doses of THs.[32] The second reason why we should avoid inducing iatrogenic thyrotoxicosis for weight loss purposes rests on the fact that such hormone therapy can potentially cause adverse effects and complications such as osteoporosis, osteoporotic fractures, arrhythmias and CVS diseases, and mortality. It is plausible that if we could selectively target certain tissues (e.g., adipose tissue) with TH therapy that would benefit the weight, lipogenesis, and other parameters of the metabolic syndrome and avoid targeting tissues and organs (e.g., myocardium and bone) that can produce complications, then higher doses could be used that may cause weight loss. A synthetic TH analogue called GC-1 exists, which is selective for the β-isoform of TH receptor and which in animal studies seems promising with reduced fat mass, triglycerides, and α-lipoprotein without the adverse effect of T3 on the heart, muscle, or bone.[33,34]

EUTHYROIDISM AND WEIGHT

Results from a population study in Denmark suggest that even small differences in thyroid function may be important for the BMI level and the prevalence of obesity in a population.[35] In this study about 4000 people were included without any overt thyroid dysfunction and they observed that there was an independent, positive linear relationship between the TSH and BMI; therefore, for example, females with a TSH at the upper side of the normal range (3.6 mIU/L) were on average 5.5 kg heavier compared with females with TSH at the lower side of normal (0.4 mIU/L).[35] Significant positive associations were also noticed between TSH and self-reported weight changes in the past 5 years, but not with free T4 (fT4), free T3 (fT3), and thyroid peroxidase (TPO) antibodies (see Fig. 5.3).[35] A Norwegian population–based 10.5 years longitudinal study of about 15,000 euthyroid individuals revealed a weight increase by approximately 2 kg in the study period with no corresponding rise in the median TSH; the change in TSH over the follow-up period was positively associated with a change in body weight, BMI, and waist circumference.[11] A cross-sectional substudy of NHANES found that as BMI increased TSH also increased; fT3 and fT4 were found to be positively and negatively correlated with obesity, respectively.[36] The relationship between thyroid function and weight seems to be independent of the thyroid autoimmunity status.[37]

A study that assessed in 275 healthy volunteers (but with a median BMI of 26 kg/m^2) used abdominal

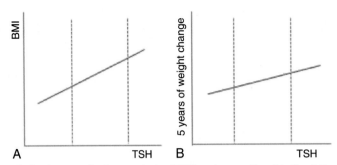

FIG. 5.3 The association between body mass index (BMI) and serum thyroid-stimulating hormone (TSH) **(A)** and 5 years of change in weight and serum TSH **(B)** in mostly euthyroid individuals or individuals with mild thyroid dysfunction. The *vertical interrupted lines* represent the normal reference range. (Adapted from Knudsen N, Laurberg P, Rasmussen LB, et al. Small differences in thyroid function may be important for body mass index and the occurrence of obesity in the population. *J Clin Endocrinol Metab.* 2005;90(7):4019–4024, with permission.)

ultrasonography.[38] It showed that fT4 was modestly, independently, and inversely associated with subcutaneous fat.[38] Another study assessed 201 euthyroid females with a BMI ≥ 25 kg/m² and found that both TSH and fT3, but not fT4, were independently associated with waist circumference; fT3 was also correlated with BMI.[39]

However, the association between increasing BMI, obesity, and increased TSH is not consistent between all studies. A retrospective review included about 400 euthyroid patients presenting with thyroid nodules; no significant correlation was identified between TSH or fT4 and BMI.[37] Another retrospective review of over 1200 obese euthyroid patients has found that those with BMI of 30–35 kg/m² had similar TSH to patients with BMI ≥ 40 kg/m².[40] Interestingly, in this same study fT3 and T4 were both significantly elevated in the morbidly obese and were positively associated with BMI,[40] whereas the obese population in another study had significantly lower fT3 and fT4.[41]

A single systematic review study has been performed examining the connection between TSH and weight indices; a total of 29 studies were included with about 56,000 participants.[42] Of 17 clinical studies, 11 showed a positive correlation between TSH and measures of adiposity; overall, this correlation was more pronounced in the obese and female cohorts.[42] Of 12 population-based studies, 7 showed a positive correlation between TSH and measures of adiposity; 2 of these studies were longitudinal and both confirmed the same positive relationship.[42] This study may be critiqued in that it did not include fT3, fT4, or TPO antibody data; that it did not attempt to merge and analyze data (which would admittedly be very difficult given the heterogeneity

of these studies); and finally that it used a composite "measure of adiposity" and that it did not specifically study body composition as measured by DXA scan. Nevertheless, the question arises as to why there is such a difference between these studies considering that 11 of the 29 studies did not show a link between TSH and measures of adiposity? The following explanations may apply: (1) different baseline weights were used between the studies, (2) different TSH normal reference ranges (and assays) were used between studies, (3) a lack of adjustment for confounders in about half of these studies was found, (4) different populations in terms of ethnic background and/or iodine sufficiency status prevailed, (5) only two of these studies were longitudinal and therefore causality cannot be claimed, (6) a difference between community[35] versus hospital-based studies was found,[37] and (7) other methodological factors may be at play.

OBESITY AND IMPACT ON THYROID FUNCTION

As already discussed most studies concur that obesity is associated with higher TSH and fT3 and a variable fT4 level. Significantly increased levels of hypothyroidism have been reported in obese individuals.[41] Raised TSH and fT3, but with raised fT4 as well, have been observed in obese children, 12% of which had a TSH above the normal reference level.[43] For balance, we ought to mention that there are a lesser amount of studies that did not identify any relationship between obesity and thyroid dysfunction.[37] Various theories have been put forward to explain the relationship between thyroid function and weight. Overall, there seems to be an activation of the hypothalamic–pituitary–thyroid axis in human obesity.[44] Leptin may be the mediator to the relationship,[44] but cause-and-effect is difficult to differentiate. The opposite effect may be true in that primary TSH hypersecretion may induce proadipocyte differentiation and proliferation. Other changes seen in obesity that may explain or contribute to the altered TFTs observed include (1) TH resistance, (2) central T3 receptor resistance in the hypothalamus, and (3) increased peripheral activity of deiodinases, which may explain the commonly observed increased fT3 and T3:T4 ratio and reduced fT4.[40]

WEIGHT LOSS AND THYROID FUNCTION

Non-surgically accomplished weight loss generally leads to reversal of the thyroid changes that are usually observed with obesity (high fT3 and high TSH), with consequent reductions in fT3, fT4, and total T3, where reverse T3 (rT3) seems to increase, changes not dissimilar to what is observed with nonthyroidal illness, which in turn may at least to some extent reflect starvation-related changes occurring with an acute illness.

Weight loss surgery is also accompanied by many hormonal changes, including alterations in thyroid function, and a catabolic state observed in the postoperative period must be contributing. As a general principle, different types of surgery appear to influence thyroid function differently:

- Roux-en-Y gastric bypass (RYGB), overall, appears to reduce fT3, TSH, or T3 without the expected rise in TSH[45–48]; it also seems to reverse SCH in many patients not on L-t4, whereas in patients taking L-t4 for hypothyroidism-spectrum disease it allows for a drop, or even, discontinuation of L-t4 in up to half of such patients.[47,48]
- Sleeve gastrectomy: although the evidence base is smaller regarding sleeve gastrectomy, its impact on the thyroid function seems similar to that of RYGB with a decrease in TSH.[49]
- Laparoscopic adjustable gastric banding effect on thyroid function is inconsistent between studies with some showing a lack of any impact while others demonstrate a reduction in TSH with/without a concomitant reduction in fT3.[3,45,46]
- Severely malabsorptive procedures can impair bioavailability of THs, which can presumably impair L-t4 absorption.[3]

CONCLUSIONS

In summary, hypothyroidism usually causes weight gain and treatment with L-t4 causes weight loss, which is mostly due to lean body mass reduction. Hyperthyroidism per se usually, but not always, causes weight loss. Its therapy is associated with weight gain; lean body mass seems to be increasing first followed by adipose tissue buildup. Weight gain with the therapy given for hyperthyroidism often exceeds premorbid levels. Patients should be warned about the possibility of excessive weight gain with such therapies, and those at high risk (e.g., overweight) should be preemptively encouraged to commit to lifestyle changes for weight loss and be referred to a dietitian. Overall, there is a bidirectional relationship between TSH and BMI. Most studies show that as TSH increases the weight increases, even within the normal reference range. Conversely, obese individuals seem to have higher TSH. We recommend against using TH replacement for treating obesity. Synthetic TH analogues that can act on specific TH receptor isoforms may prove promising in the future for treating obesity. In the meantime, for the majority of patients who complain of unexplained weight gain or difficulty with weight loss, there is no thyroid-related explanation for it and no thyroid-related intervention that can help. Hence, we encourage lifestyle interventions, medication manipulation whenever possible, and bariatric surgery in a carefully selected subgroup of patients, instead of trialing L-t4.

ACKNOWLEDGMENTS

I would like to thank Dr. Akheel Syed (Consultant in Endocrinology and Diabetes) and Alexis Kyriacou (Clinical Dietitian and Nutritionist) for providing feedback for this work.

REFERENCES

1. Michalaki MA, Vagenakis AG, Leonardou AS, et al. Thyroid function in humans with morbid obesity. *Thyroid*. 2006; 16(1):73–78. http://dx.doi.org/10.1089/thy.2006.16.73.
2. Kyriacou A, Kyriacou A, Economides N. Weight-related concerns in endocrine outpatients and its relationship to thyroid function. *Endocr Abstr*. October 2016. http://dx.doi.org/10.1530/endoabs.44.P252.
3. Kyriacou A, McLaughlin J, Syed AA. Thyroid disorders and gastrointestinal and liver dysfunction: a state of the art review. *Eur J Intern Med*. 2015;26(8):563–571. http://dx.doi.org/10.1016/j.ejim.2015.07.017.
4. Santoro N, Braunstein GD, Butts CL, Martin KA, McDermott M, Pinkerton JV. Compounded bioidentical hormones in endocrinology practice: an endocrine society scientific statement. *J Clin Endocrinol Metab*. 2016;101(4):1318–1343. http://dx.doi.org/10.1210/jc.2016-1271.

5. Garin MC, Arnold AM, Lee JS, Tracy RP, Cappola AR. Subclinical hypothyroidism, weight change, and body composition in the elderly: the cardiovascular health study. *J Clin Endocrinol Metab*. 2014;99(4):1220–1226. http://dx.doi.org/10.1210/jc.2013-3591.

6. Tagliaferri M, Berselli ME, Calò G, et al. Subclinical hypothyroidism in obese patients: relation to resting energy expenditure, serum leptin, body composition, and lipid profile. *Obes Res*. 2001;9(3):196–201. http://dx.doi.org/10.1038/oby.2001.21.

7. Gussekloo J, van Exel E, de Craen AJM, Meinders AE, Frölich M, Westendorp RGJ. Thyroid status, disability and cognitive function, and survival in old age. *JAMA*. 2004;292(21):2591. http://dx.doi.org/10.1001/jama.292.21.2591.

8. Lindeman RD, Romero LJ, Schade DS, Wayne S, Baumgartner RN, Garry PJ. Impact of subclinical hypothyroidism on serum total homocysteine concentrations, the prevalence of coronary heart disease (CHD), and CHD risk factors in the New Mexico elder health survey. *Thyroid*. 2003;13(6):595–600. http://dx.doi.org/10.1089/105072503322238863.

9. Nyrnes A, Jorde R, Sundsfjord J. Serum TSH is positively associated with BMI. *Int J Obes*. 2006;30(1):100–105. http://dx.doi.org/10.1038/sj.ijo.0803112.

10. Fox CS, Pencina MJ, D'Agostino RB, et al. Relations of thyroid function to body weight: cross-sectional and longitudinal observations in a community-based sample. *Arch Intern Med*. 2008;168(6):587. http://dx.doi.org/10.1001/archinte.168.6.587.

11. Svare A, Nilsen TI, Bjoro T, Asvold BO, Langhammer A. Serum TSH related to measures of body mass: longitudinal data from the HUNT Study, Norway. *Clin Endocrinol*. 2011;74(6):769–775. http://dx.doi.org/10.1111/j.1365-2265.2011.04009.x.

12. Pearce SHS, Brabant G, Duntas LH, et al. 2013 ETA guideline: management of subclinical hypothyroidism. *Eur Thyroid J*. 2013;2(4):215–228. http://dx.doi.org/10.1159/000356507.

13. Hollowell JG, Staehling NW, Flanders WD, et al. Serum TSH, T$_4$, and thyroid antibodies in the United States population (1988 to 1994): National Health and Nutrition Examination Survey (NHANES III). *J Clin Endocrinol Metab*. 2002;87(2):489–499. http://dx.doi.org/10.1210/jcem.87.2.8182.

14. Baloch Z, Carayon P, Conte-Devolx B, et al. Laboratory support for the diagnosis and monitoring of thyroid disease. *Thyroid*. 2003;13(1):3. http://dx.doi.org/10.1089/105072503321086962.

15. Boeving A, Paz-Filho G, Radominski RB, Graf H, de Carvalho GA. Low-normal or high-normal thyrotropin target levels during treatment of hypothyroidism: a prospective, comparative study. *Thyroid*. 2011;21(4):355–360. http://dx.doi.org/10.1089/thy.2010.0315.

16. Walsh JP, Ward LC, Burke V, et al. Small changes in thyroxine dosage do not produce measurable changes in hypothyroid symptoms, well-being, or quality of life: results of a double-blind, randomized clinical trial. *J Clin Endocrinol Metab*. 2006;91(7):2624–2630. http://dx.doi.org/10.1210/jc.2006-0099.

17. Celi FS, Zemskova M, Linderman JD, et al. Metabolic effects of liothyronine therapy in hypothyroidism: a randomized, double-blind, crossover trial of liothyronine versus levothyroxine. *J Clin Endocrinol Metab*. 2011;96(11):3466–3474. http://dx.doi.org/10.1210/jc.2011-1329.

18. Appelhof BC, Fliers E, Wekking EM, et al. Combined therapy with levothyroxine and liothyronine in two ratios, compared with levothyroxine monotherapy in primary hypothyroidism: a double-blind, randomized, controlled clinical trial. *J Clin Endocrinol Metab*. 2005;90(5):2666–2674. http://dx.doi.org/10.1210/jc.2004-2111.

19. Grozinsky-Glasberg S, Fraser A, Nahshoni E, Weizman A, Leibovici L. Thyroxine-triiodothyronine combination therapy versus thyroxine monotherapy for clinical hypothyroidism: meta-analysis of randomized controlled trials. *J Clin Endocrinol Metab*. 2006;91(7):2592–2599. http://dx.doi.org/10.1210/jc.2006-0448.

20. Wiersinga WM, Duntas L, Fadeyev V, Nygaard B, Vanderpump MPJ. 2012 ETA guidelines: the use of L-T4 + L-T3 in the treatment of hypothyroidism. *Eur Thyroid J*. 2012;1(2):55–71. http://dx.doi.org/10.1159/000339444.

21. Karmisholt J, Andersen S, Laurberg P. Weight loss after therapy of hypothyroidism is mainly caused by excretion of excess body water associated with myxoedema. *J Clin Endocrinol Metab*. 2011;96(1):E99–E103. http://dx.doi.org/10.1210/jc.2010-1521.

22. Santini F, Pinchera A, Marsili A, et al. Lean body mass is a major determinant of levothyroxine dosage in the treatment of thyroid diseases. *J Clin Endocrinol Metab*. 2005;90(1):124–127. http://dx.doi.org/10.1210/jc.2004-1306.

23. Lönn L, Stenlöf K, Ottosson M, Lindroos A-K, Nyström E, Sjöström L. Body weight and body composition changes after treatment of hyperthyroidism. *J Clin Endocrinol Metab*. 1998;83(12):4269–4273. http://dx.doi.org/10.1210/jcem.83.12.5338.

24. Pears J, Jung RT, Gunn A. Long-term weight changes in treated hyperthyroid and hypothyroid patients. *Scott Med J*. 1990;35(6):180–182. http://www.ncbi.nlm.nih.gov/pubmed/2077652.

25. Weinreb JT, Yang Y, Braunstein GD. Do patients gain weight after thyroidectomy for thyroid cancer? *Thyroid*. 2011;21(12):1339–1342. http://dx.doi.org/10.1089/thy.2010.0393.

26. O'Malley B, Hickey J, Nevens E. Thyroid dysfunction – weight problems and the psyche: the patients' perspective. *J Hum Nutr Diet*. 2000;13(4):243–248. http://dx.doi.org/10.1046/j.1365-277x.2000.00238.x.

27. Martin WH, Spina RJ, Korte E, et al. Mechanisms of impaired exercise capacity in short duration experimental hyperthyroidism. *J Clin Invest*. 1991;88(6):2047–2053. http://dx.doi.org/10.1172/JCI115533.

28. Zimmermann-Belsing T, Dreyer M, Holst JJ, Feldt-Rasmussen U. The relationship between the serum leptin concentrations of thyrotoxic patients during treatment and their total fat mass is different from that of normal subjects. *Clin Endocrinol*. 1998;49(5):589–595. http://www.ncbi.nlm.nih.gov/pubmed/10197073.

29. Dale J, Daykin J, Holder R, Sheppard MC, Franklyn JA. Weight gain following treatment of hyperthyroidism. *Clin Endocrinol*. 2001;55(2):233–239. http://dx.doi.org/10.1046/j.1365-2265.2001.01329.x.

30. Tigas S, Idiculla J, Beckett G, Toft A. Is excessive weight gain after ablative treatment of hyperthyroidism due to inadequate thyroid hormone therapy? *Thyroid*. 2000;10(12):1107–1111. http://dx.doi.org/10.1089/thy.2000.10.1107.

31. de la Rosa RE, Hennessey JV, Tucci JR. A longitudinal study of changes in body mass index and total body composition after radioiodine treatment for thyrotoxicosis. *Thyroid*. 1997; 7(3):401–405. http://dx.doi.org/10.1089/thy.1997.7.401.

32. Kaptein EM, Beale E, Chan LS. Thyroid hormone therapy for obesity and nonthyroidal illnesses: a systematic review. *J Clin Endocrinol Metab*. 2009;94(10):3663–3675. http://dx.doi.org/10.1210/jc.2009-0899.

33. Baxter JD, Webb P, Grover G, Scanlan TS. Selective activation of thyroid hormone signaling pathways by GC-1: a new approach to controlling cholesterol and body weight. *Trends Endocrinol Metab*. 2004;15(4):154–157. http://dx.doi.org/10.1016/j.tem.2004.03.008.

34. Villicev CM, Freitas FRS, Aoki MS, et al. Thyroid hormone receptor – specific agonist GC-1 increases energy expenditure and prevents fat-mass accumulation in rats. *J Endocrinol*. 2007;193(1):21–29. http://dx.doi.org/10.1677/joe.1.07066.

35. Knudsen N, Laurberg P, Rasmussen LB, et al. Small differences in thyroid function may be important for body mass index and the occurrence of obesity in the population. *J Clin Endocrinol Metab*. 2005;90(7):4019–4024. http://dx.doi.org/10.1210/jc.2004-2225.

36. Kitahara CM, Platz EA, Ladenson PW, et al. Body fatness and markers of thyroid function among U.S. men and women. *PLoS One*. 2012;7(4):e34979. http://dx.doi.org/10.1371/journal.pone.0034979.

37. Manji N, Boelaert K, Sheppard MC, Holder RL, Gough SC, Franklyn JA. Lack of association between serum TSH or free T4 and body mass index in euthyroid subjects. *Clin Endocrinol*. 2006;64(2):125–128. http://dx.doi.org/10.1111/j.1365-2265.2006.02433.x.

38. Alevizaki M, Saltiki K, Voidonikola P, Mantzou E, Papamichael C, Stamatelopoulos K. Free thyroxine is an independent predictor of subcutaneous fat in euthyroid individuals. *Eur J Endocrinol*. 2009;161(3):459–465. http://dx.doi.org/10.1530/EJE-09-0441.

39. De Pergola G, Ciampolillo A, Paolotti S, Trerotoli P, Giorgino R. Free triiodothyronine and thyroid stimulating hormone are directly associated with waist circumference, independently of insulin resistance, metabolic parameters and blood pressure in overweight and obese women. *Clin Endocrinol*. 2007;67(2):265–269. http://dx.doi.org/10.1111/j.1365-2265.2007.02874.x.

40. Temizkan S, Balaforlou B, Ozderya A, et al. Effects of thyrotrophin, thyroid hormones and thyroid antibodies on metabolic parameters in a euthyroid population with obesity. *Clin Endocrinol*. 2016;85(4):616–623. http://dx.doi.org/10.1111/cen.13095.

41. Marzullo P, Minocci A, Tagliaferri MA, et al. Investigations of thyroid hormones and antibodies in obesity: leptin levels are associated with thyroid autoimmunity independent of bioanthropometric, hormonal, and weight-related determinants. *J Clin Endocrinol Metab*. 2010;95(8): 3965–3972. http://dx.doi.org/10.1210/jc.2009-2798.

42. de Moura Souza A, Sichieri R. Association between serum TSH concentration within the normal range and adiposity. *Eur J Endocrinol*. 2011;165(1):11–15. http://dx.doi.org/10.1530/EJE-11-0261.

43. Reinehr T, Andler W. Thyroid hormones before and after weight loss in obesity. *Arch Dis Child*. 2002;87(4):320–323. http://www.ncbi.nlm.nih.gov/pubmed/12244007.

44. Laurberg P, Knudsen N, Andersen S, Carlé A, Pedersen IB, Karmisholt J. Thyroid function and obesity. *Eur Thyroid J*. 2012;1(3):159–167. http://dx.doi.org/10.1159/000342994.

45. Chikunguwo S, Brethauer S, Nirujogi V, et al. Influence of obesity and surgical weight loss on thyroid hormone levels. *Surg Obes Relat Dis*. 2007;3(6):631–636. http://dx.doi.org/10.1016/j.soard.2007.07.011. pii:S1550-7289(07)00576-X.

46. Korner J, Inabnet W, Febres G, et al. Prospective study of gut hormone and metabolic changes after adjustable gastric banding and Roux-en-Y gastric bypass. *Int J Obes*. 2009;33(7):786–795. http://dx.doi.org/10.1038/ijo.2009.79.

47. Raftopoulos Y, Gagné DJ, Papasavas P, et al. Improvement of hypothyroidism after laparoscopic Roux-en-Y gastric bypass for morbid obesity. *Obes Surg*. 2004;14(4):509–513. http://dx.doi.org/10.1381/096089204323013514.

48. Moulin de Moraes CM, Mancini MC, de Melo ME, et al. Prevalence of subclinical hypothyroidism in a morbidly obese population and improvement after weight loss induced by Roux-en-Y gastric bypass. *Obes Surg*. 2005;15(9):1287–1291. http://dx.doi.org/10.1381/096089205774512537.

49. Abu-Ghanem Y, Inbar R, Tyomkin V, et al. Effect of sleeve gastrectomy on thyroid hormone levels. *Obes Surg*. 2014. http://dx.doi.org/10.1007/s11695-014-1415-7.

CHAPTER 6

Obesity and Polycystic Ovary Syndrome

UNAIZA QAMAR, MBBS, FCPS, FRCPATH • STEPHEN L. ATKIN, MBBS, FRCP, PHD • THOZHUKAT SATHYAPALAN, MBBS, FRCP, MD

INTRODUCTION

Overweight and obesity are defined as an abnormal or excessive fat accumulation[1] based on body mass index (BMI), which is defined as a person's weight in kilograms divided by the square of his height in meters (kg/m^2). A BMI of 25.0 to <30 kg/m^2 is classified as overweight, >30 kg/m^2 is defined as obesity, and >40 kg/m^2 is defined as morbid obesity.[2,3] Obesity is now considered a global epidemic with the percentage of women with a BMI of 25 kg/m^2 or greater having increased from 29.8% to 38.0%, from 1980 to 2013. In 2010, obesity caused 3.4 million deaths, 3.9% of years of life lost, and 3.8% of disability-adjusted life-years worldwide. This increase in obesity has called for a need for monitoring the prevalence of overweight and obesity in all populations to combat its deleterious effects.

Polycystic ovary syndrome (PCOS) is a disorder of chronically abnormal ovarian function and hyperandrogenism (elevated androgen levels). It affects 3%–20% of women of reproductive age depending on the diagnostic criteria used.[4] PCOS is a diagnosis of exclusion (congenital adrenal hyperplasia, androgen-secreting tumors, Cushing's syndrome, hyperprolactinemia, hypothalamic anovulation)[5] followed by the application of specific criteria. There is broad agreement among specialty guidelines[6–8] that PCOS diagnosis must be based on the presence of two of the following three findings—hyperandrogenism (increased free androgen index), ovulatory dysfunction (presenting as irregularity of menstrual cycle), and polycystic ovaries (on ultrasound). Elevated androgens disrupt the normal menstrual cycle leading to infertility, acne, and abnormal hair growth, such as excess facial hair or male pattern baldness. Women with PCOS are at significantly higher risk for high blood pressure, diabetes, heart disease, and cancer of the uterus (endometrial cancer).[9]

It has been suggested that the hormonal abnormalities of PCOS begin soon after menarche. PCOS is associated with insulin resistance[10]; however, insulin resistance is also related to obesity.[11] Therefore, the question arises: Do all obese women have PCOS? In the United States 80% of the women with PCOS are obese although in Spain, a study reported 28% of overweight and obese women had PCOS, giving a strong association.[12,13] The importance of the role of obesity in PCOS is also reflected in the data showing that treating obesity addresses many of the problems associated with PCOS. Most of the treatments meant for obesity have helped in only achieving modest reductions in weight and improvements in PCOS symptoms. Bariatric surgery, on the other hand, is a treatment modality that leads to dramatic change in altering PCOS phenotype (discussed below). Despite that, weight loss by lifestyle changes remains the foremost option; further studies are, however, needed to determine the role of lifestyle changes.[14] Considering the risk of obesity-related morbidities, interventions to combat obesity in these patients is needed for the prevention of the development of metabolic syndrome (MBS).[15]

Obesity and PCOS both run in a vicious circle.[16] During the last 20 years, the rate of obesity has increased more than threefold.[17] A parallel increase in obesity and diabetes has been witnessed, but this is not known for PCOS. One study has shown that weight gain is reported by the patients before the development of PCOS,[18] further supporting the obesity as a contributory cause in the development of PCOS.

There are two theories in support of a contributory effect of obesity on the development of PCOS. One suggests that the adipose tissue behaves like a gland that secretes several hormones known collectively as adipokines. It is the aberrant adipokine secretion that may cause the development of PCOS.[19] Another theory is that when adipose tissue mass increases, there comes a stage when it can no longer store more fat subcutaneously, and it causes a state of lipotoxicity. The fat then accumulates around tissues and it starts to deposit in other tissues such as the liver, muscles, and pancreas, i.e., ectopic fat deposition. This state of lipotoxicity causes insulin resistance and subsequently hyperandrogenism commonly seen in PCOS women.[20] Obesity aggravates hyperandrogenism and menstrual disturbances in PCOS[21] and also contributes to the psychologic comorbidities in women with PCOS, such as anxiety and depression.[22]

A metaanalysis comparing the Caucasian versus Asian women showed that Caucasian women with PCOS have a higher prevalence of obesity[23] that was in accord with a study comparing Eastern Asian women with PCOS with American and European patients.[24]

Central Obesity/Fat Distribution in Polycystic Ovary Syndrome

Central or visceral obesity has been associated with PCOS.[25,26] Various large population studies have revealed that central obesity causes more insulin resistance and thus carries increased risk for developing cardiovascular disease (CVD), anovulation, type 2 diabetes mellitus (T2DM), and dyslipidemia as compared with BMI-matched controls.[27] Conversely, high insulin levels due to insulin resistance in PCOS and androgens may cause central body fat distribution that could sustain the centrally obese condition of women with PCOS.[28–30] The studies conducted on fat distribution even in lean PCOS women have shown that they also have increased visceral fat deposition, whereas healthy controls have gynoid fat distribution.[31] However, there remains some controversy on the association of central obesity with PCOS within the few studies performed.[32]

Morbidities Aggravated by Obesity in Polycystic Ovary Syndrome
Cardiovascular disease risk

Obesity contributes to around 43% prevalence of the MBS in women with PCOS.[33] This can be attributed to insulin resistance, which is the central connection in both obesity and PCOS.[34,35] The traditional CVD risk factor assessment tools such as the Framingham risk score are based on low-density lipoprotein (LDL) cholesterol, low-density lipoprotein (HDL) cholesterol, hypertension, age, and smoking status do not provide a true picture of CVD risk in women with PCOS.[36] According to the Androgen Excess-PCOS Society, the risk factors for CVD in women with PCOS include most of the factors that are commonly associated with PCOS including central obesity, impaired glucose tolerance (IGT), and subclinical vascular disease, and those with MBS and T2DM further increase that

risk particularly with increasing age. Other risk factors include cigarette smoking, dyslipidemia, and hypertension.[7,36,37] Dyslipidemia is considered the most common metabolic abnormality in PCOS. Increased systolic blood pressure is reported in these individuals even after adjustment for body fat and insulin resistance. They have increased levels of circulating inflammatory markers such as PAI-1, endothelin-1, and C-reactive protein concentrations. Flow-mediated dilatation studies have demonstrated impaired endothelial function. These factors put these patients at a heightened risk for MBS in terms of developing diabetes, CVD, and mortality.[38] Vascular pathology assessed by endothelial function, carotid-intima media thickening, and coronary artery calcification have been found to be increased in patients with PCOS than controls.[39,40] In a metaanalysis of cardiovascular risk for T2DM and CVD in PCOS including 2256 PCOS women and 4130 controls, the odds ratio of developing CVD in women with PCOS was 2.2 when compared with BMI-matched controls, suggesting the potential benefit from aggressive lifestyle intervention.[41] Therefore, BMI, waist circumference, serum lipid, OGTT, and blood pressure measurements are recommended for all women with PCOS.[42,43]

Infertility

Women with PCOS show an increased prevalence of anovulation and infertility (50% primary infertility, 25% secondary infertility, and 70%–90% of ovulatory disorders).[44] Nonetheless, fertility is also affected by obesity. There is an association of menstrual irregularities, infertility, increased risk of miscarriages, and poor outcome of assisted reproductive technologies and pregnancy with the BMI exceeding 30 kg/m[2].[45] The spontaneous abortion rate in women with PCOS is 20%–40% higher than the baseline in the general obstetric population.[46]

The effect of obesity on the metabolic and reproductive symptoms in PCOS is likely to be mediated by insulin resistance, and for any given BMI women with PCOS are more insulin resistant as compared with BMI-matched controls.[30,47]

Gestational diabetes

The prevalence of gestational diabetes is 6%–16% depending on ethnicity, and up to 66% of the patients who develop gestational diabetes have underlying PCOS. Gestational diabetes puts these patients at further risk for premature delivery, preeclampsia, and shoulder dystocia. The metabolic profile of women with gestational diabetes is exacerbated by obesity[48];

therefore it is recommended to assess BMI, blood pressure, and oral glucose tolerance in such patients before conception.[49,50] However, there are no trials in PCOS to show that a preconception intervention to lose weight would improve maternal or neonatal outcomes.[51]

Endometrial cancer

Chronic unopposed estrogen exposure and reduction in ovulatory events leading to deficient progesterone secretion for differentiation of endometrium in PCOS is thought to increase the risk of endometrial hyperplasia and endometrial carcinoma by three times.[52] Obesity, hyperinsulinemia, diabetes, and abnormal uterine bleeding have been considered to contribute to the development of endometrial cancer, which are commonly seen in PCOS patients also. While these women are therefore at an increased risk of endometrial cancer, the routine use of ultrasound has not been recommended for screening.[53]

Type 2 diabetes mellitus

These patients by virtue of insulin resistance are prone to develop IGT and there is a two- to threefold increased risk of developing T2DM. Presence of obesity further aggravate the insulin-resistant state and is most common if BMI is more than 30 with central obesity. An OGTT (consisting of a fasting and 2-h glucose level using a 75-g oral glucose load) is recommended for IGT and T2DM screening in adolescents and adult women with PCOS.[54] Screening is done on a 3- to 5-yearly basis according to the guidelines of Endocrine Society of the United States.[53]

Obstructive sleep apnea

Obesity is a major risk factor for the development and exacerbation of obstructive sleep apnea (OSA),[55] which in itself is an important determinant of insulin resistance, glucose intolerance, and type 2 diabetes. Likewise, OSA is common in obese women with PCOS.[56–58] However, in one study it was found that the risk of OSA in PCOS parallels the high prevalence of obesity in these patients.[59] In one study, treatment with continuous positive airway pressure (CPAP) improved insulin sensitivity and reduced diastolic blood pressure in women with PCOS. The guidelines suggest to screen patients with PCOS for OSA.[14]

Cutaneous findings

Patients with PCOS are known to have hyperandrogenemia. The clinical cutaneous manifestations of hyperandrogenism are hirsutism, acne, seborrhea, alopecia,

acanthosis nigricans, and skin tags.[60] Obese patients with PCOS show an exaggeration of cutaneous manifestations mentioned above when compared with lean patients with PCOS, because obesity itself aggravates hyperandrogenism.[14,53]

Nonalcoholic fatty liver disease

Obesity is a great risk factor for the development of nonalcoholic fatty liver disease (NAFLD). When the uptake of fatty acids by the liver from plasma is more as compared with its metabolism in the liver and its export as a very-low-density lipoprotein (VLDL) triglyceride, there is an excessive deposition of intrahepatic triglycerides that results in complicated metabolic events. This results in aberrations of glucose, fatty acid, and lipoprotein metabolism, which initiate a constant environment of low-grade inflammation that results in the development of insulin resistance, dyslipidemia, and other cardiometabolic risk factors.[61]

The prevalence of NAFLD, including nonalcoholic steatohepatitis (NASH), may be increased in women with PCOS.[62] The prevalence of NAFLD in one study was found to be 39% in lean women with PCOS, suggesting that the risk is independent of obesity. However, screening for NAFLD is not routinely recommended in United States.[63]

OBESITY, HYPERANDROGENISM, HYPERINSULINEMIA, AND POLYCYSTIC OVARY SYNDROME—PATHOPHYSIOLOGY

It can be inferred from the above discussion that obesity and PCOS are interrelated in terms of their clinical manifestations, but what happens at the biochemical and molecular level shows how both these phenomena are intertwined.

Obesity Causes Insulin Resistance and Hyperinsulinemia

Insulin resistance is the most common and significant finding in the obese and in hyperandrogenic women with PCOS.[64] Insulin resistance is present in 20%–43% of the women with PCOS; it can be attributed to intrinsic defects in insulin signaling and receptor activity and a decrease in insulin clearance due to the inhibitory effect of high testosterone levels, free fatty acids (FFAs), and cytokine production such as tumor necrosis factor α (TNF-α) and interleukin 6.[26]

The mechanisms involved in insulin resistance in PCOS show some differences from insulin-resistant

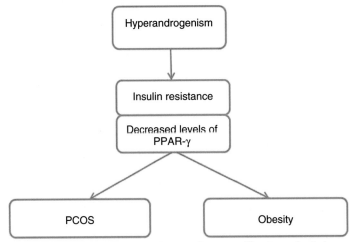

FIG. 6.1 Relationship between hyperandrogenism, peroxisome proliferator-activated receptor gamma (PPAR-γ), obesity, and polycystic ovary syndrome (PCOS).

states such as obesity and T2DM, given the fact that hepatic insulin resistance is present only in obese women with PCOS, on top of decreased glucose entry into the muscles. It is crucial that this category of PCOS patients are optimally managed taking into account their increased propensity to develop metabolic problems.[65] Several underlying mechanisms for insulin resistance in PCOS have been suggested:

- Adipose tissue expansion increases the availability of several metabolic products (i.e., FFAs, lactate, etc.), which interfere with the functions of insulin by decreasing the tissue sensitivity for insulin.[66]
- Adipose tissue also releases also TNF-α,[67] which interferes with the actions of insulin-like growth factor (IGF), which is produced by the liver in response to growth hormone and plays a crucial role in growth and differentiation.[68]
- TNF-α also mediates serine phosphorylation of IRS-1 (which is a key mediator in insulin functions and is located downstream of the insulin receptor), thus inhibiting insulin signaling leading to insulin resistance that would result in hyperinsulinemia.
- At the molecular level TNF-α as well as hyperandrogenism inhibit signaling through peroxisome proliferator-activated receptor gamma (PPAR-γ) (which under normal conditions increases fatty acid oxidation and glucose metabolism), thus causing a state of insulin resistance and excess FFA.[69]
- Also the mutations in PPAR-γ, which is a nuclear receptor as described above, lead to obesity and/or PCOS, making a genetic link between obesity and PCOS[70] (see Fig. 6.1).

Hyperinsulinemia Leading to Ovarian Follicular Arrest

A further adverse effect of hyperinsulinemia on the ovary in women with PCOS includes the arrest at 5–10 mm of ovarian follicle development due to aberrant intraovarian signaling. Higher insulin levels, secondary to insulin resistance, cause premature luteinization of oocytes by increasing the luteinizing hormone (LH) receptors on them and alter the oocyte quality, leading to impaired blastocyst development. It has been found that oocytes contain a functional insulin-signaling pathway, and hyperinsulinemia can lead to chromatin remodeling and embryonic developmental aberrations.[10,71,72]

Obesity and Hyperinsulinemia Leading to Hyperandrogenism

Hyperinsulinemia mediates the following effects (see Fig. 6.2):

- Hyperinsulinemia may also exert undesirable effects in women with PCOS through its action at nonovarian sites. These include the pituitary causing a greater pituitary LH pulse amplitude by increasing the sensitivity to gonadotropin-releasing hormone,[73] and on the adrenal through stimulation of P450c17α activity, the same enzyme that is present in theca cells of the ovaries mentioned above, thereby further increasing adrenal androgen production.[74]
- The increased levels of both insulin and LH present within the theca cells of ovaries cause activation of the enzyme, P450c17α, which is the main enzyme in the cascade of ovarian androgen production, resulting in hyperandrogenism.[74]

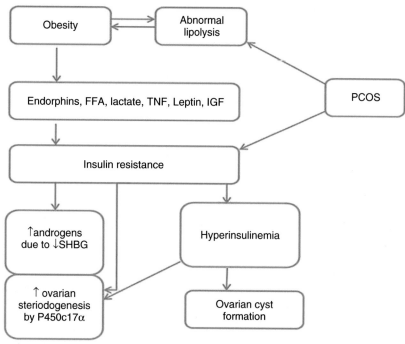

FIG. 6.2 Flow chart illustrating pathophysiology of polycystic ovary syndrome (PCOS) and obesity. *FFA*, free fatty acid; *IGF*, insulin-like growth factor; *P450c17α*, cytochrome P450 17 α-hydroxylase; *SHBG*, sex hormone–binding globulin; *TNF*, tumor necrosis factor; *↑*, increased; *↓*, decreased.

- Sex hormone–binding globulin (SHBG) is negatively correlated with hyperinsulinemia. By acting on the liver, the insulin causes suppression of SHBG (thereby increasing the circulating free androgen).[75] At the same time, abdominal obesity seems to be associated with slight Hypocortisolemia and increased sensitivity to exogenous adrenocorticotropic stimulation, which may contribute to the hyperinsulinemia by causing aberrant release of FFA from adipose tissue and the related metabolic changes including decreased SHBG levels—functional hyperandrogenism.[76,77]

Various studies evaluated the impact of obesity on the hyperandrogenic state in women with PCOS; it has been repeatedly described that a higher proportion of obese PCOS women complained of hirsutism and menstrual disturbances than normal-weight PCOS women did.[78] Therefore, there is consistent evidence that the increase in body weight may favor a worsened hyperandrogenic state in women with PCOS.[79] Although PCOS may be associated with alterations of both lipid and lipoprotein metabolism, the presence of obesity usually leads to a more atherogenic lipoprotein pattern because they tend to have an increase in VLDL particle number, LDL particle number, and a decrease in HDL size.[80,81] A greater reduction in HDLs together with a higher increase in both triglycerides and total cholesterol levels was, in fact, observed in obese women with respect to the normal-weight PCOS women.[82] From the above facts, it can be clearly inferred that reversal of insulin resistance by various mechanisms can lead to reversal of the majority of the morbidities associated with it.[83]

Dietary habits: a link between obesity and polycystic ovary syndrome

There is also evidence suggesting that PCOS contributes to obesity. Women with high androgen levels independent of PCOS status were found to have greater cravings for high-fat foods and carbohydrate-rich foods[84] and possibly a greater intake of these foods.[85] Dietary habits have a strong association with obesity. In fact very high lipid intake has been found to decrease SHBG blood levels and increase free androgen index.[86] In some reports, PCOS women were found to have a higher intake of saturated lipids and a lower intake of fibers when compared with control groups.[87]

Genetic Link Between Obesity and Polycystic Ovary Syndrome

PPAR-γ is a nuclear receptor that regulates downstream transcription of many genes. Studies on women with mutations in *PPARγ* reveal that, in addition to severe insulin resistance, hyperinsulinemia, partial lipodystrophy, and features of the MBS, they also present with features of PCOS including oligomenorrhea and hirsutism.[88]

Also the serine phosphorylation of both the ovarian P450c17 enzymatic system (associated with androgen production) and the insulin receptor substrate may be a genetic link that may explain the association between hyperandrogenism and insulin resistance in PCOS women.[89] Women with PCOS have been found to have increased 5α-reductase activity in the adipocyte, skin, and other organs,[89] which could therefore be one mechanism by which obese women with PCOS display increased androgenicity. The cause of the increased 5α-reductase activity remains unknown.[90,91]

Chronic Low-Grade Inflammation and Insulin Resistance

Low-grade inflammation is another potential factor leading to PCOS. The study conducted by Kelly et al.[92] showed that CRP concentrations are increased in women with PCOS relative to those in healthy subjects after adjusting them for BMI. At the same time an expanding fat mass releases increasing amounts of inflammatory compounds, such as FFA, angiotensin 2, resistin, TNF-α, interleukin 6, and interleukin 1-β.[93] One hypothesis of obesity-associated insulin resistance suggests that during the development of obesity, inflammation in fat tissue causes insulin resistance throughout the body.[94] Hence chronic low-grade inflammation although an independent risk factor of PCOS is further aggravated by obesity.[95]

TREATMENT OF POLYCYSTIC OVARY SYNDROME—AIMING TO TREAT OBESITY AND INSULIN RESISTANCE

Even modest weight loss of less than 10% of initial body weight has been shown to increase the frequency of ovulation, improve conception, and reduce testosterone, free androgen index, hyperlipidemia, hyperglycemia, and insulin resistance in women with PCOS.[96] Weight loss improves chances of ovulation and pregnancy and normalization of the menstrual cycles with weight loss of as little as 5%. It can also decrease the androgen and glucose levels in obese women with PCOS; however, weight loss is beneficial only for overweight women with a BMI > 25–27 kg/m². The treatment of obesity includes modifications in lifestyle (diet and exercise) and medical and surgical treatment. All these treatments must be performed before and not with reproduction therapies.[83]

Treating Obesity—Lifestyle Modifications

Taking into account the high risk of overweight, obesity, and central obesity in PCOS, obesity management should precede all other interventions for the treatment of PCOS. In addition, awareness regarding the risk of central obesity should be created among these patients because it can affect these patients even with normal BMI. Overweight and obese adolescents with PCOS should always be advised to lose weight. This, on one hand, helps to relieve the immediate morbidities related to obesity such as cutaneous manifestations and infertility and, on the other, would also relieve long-term sequel of MBS. The trend of weight gain among PCOS women should be discouraged and ideally prevented from the beginning.[97] Benefits of weight loss in PCOS have the following effects:

- It has been shown to improve hyperandrogenism, hirsutism, body weight, waist circumference, and insulin resistance in women with PCOS.[98]
- Exercise and weight loss also improves insulin resistance calculated using the homeostasis model of assessment for insulin resistance (HOMA-IR) method. 44%–57% of PCOS women had improvement in either menstrual cycle or ovulation after lifestyle changes and subsequent weight loss. A knowledge gap exists regarding the optimal type, duration, and frequency of exercise.[83] Exercise can also improve the phenotypic features of PCOS. But maintaining weight loss and exercise programs have faced the challenge of low participants' compliance rate over time.[99] Therefore, pharmaceutical intervention is an additional essential therapeutic tool to lifestyle changes in many patients (discussed in the next section).[100,101]
- Various trials have been conducted where different diet types have been tried in the PCOS women that revealed weight loss, independent of the type of diet, has always helped patients in alleviating PCOS morbidities, especially in the reduction in fasting blood glucose and insulin; in fact the effect might be equivalent to that of metformin.[100] Goss and Gower[102] studied the effects of various types of diets (low carbohydrate with 41%:19%:40% energy from CHO: protein: fat, and standard diets 55%:18%:27%) and observed that the low-carbohydrate diet led to a

decrease in intraabdominal adipose tissue, subcutaneous abdominal adipose tissue, and thigh intermuscular adipose tissue, whereas a high-carbohydrate diet would lead to redistribution of lean mass to fat mass.[103]

Treating Obesity—Medical Therapy

Pharmacologic therapy has proved to be disappointing in treating obesity and only orlistat is currently available. Orlistat is a lipase inhibitor that decreases fat absorption from the intestine by approximately 30%. The results of a metaanalysis estimated that orlistat treatment led to an average placebo-subtracted weight loss of 2.7 kg at 1 year[104] and a 3.6-kg weight loss compared with 1.4 kg for placebo at 4 years in another trial.[105]

In women with PCOS, orlistat reduced both total testosterone levels and insulin resistance (quantified by HOMA-IR) by around 20% and a weight loss of 4.69%[106,107]; however, the use of orlistat is limited by its gastrointestinal side effects such as oily stools, spotting, and fecal incontinence, especially at the start of treatment. Despite these adverse effects, it is still useful in the management of weight loss in obese patients.[105]

Treating Insulin Resistance in Polycystic Ovary Syndrome—Medical Therapy
Metformin

Metformin is a biguanide used in the treatment of T2DM. It mainly reduces gluconeogenesis in liver but also acts on the extrahepatic sites such as skeletal muscles, adipose tissue, endothelium, and the ovary. The use of metformin in PCOS is justified by improvement in insulin resistance that further leads to improvements in SHBG levels, hyperandrogenemia, and ovulation.[108] However, metformin's effect on weight loss remains controversial. Metformin has been found to be more useful at higher doses in obese women.[42,109] In the United States the use of metformin is recommended as a first-line therapy in women who have type 2 diabetes, whereas in IGT lifestyle modifications show promising results.[110]

A report suggested that metformin when given to obese PCOS women who had lost weight earlier with rimonabant, an endocannabinoid receptor blocker removed from the market because of adverse effect profile, helped in maintaining the weight loss, decrease in waist circumference, testosterone levels, and insulin resistance determined by HOMA-IR. It is possible that the insulin sensitization action of metformin was complementary to the weight loss caused by rimonabant.[111]

The side effects of metformin include nausea, anorexia, vomiting, abdominal discomfort, and diarrhea and occur in up to one-fifth of patients. In 3%–5% cases, patients have to discontinue metformin because of severe intolerance.

Glucagon-like peptide-1 receptor agonist therapy

Glucagon-like peptide (GLP) is secreted by intestinal cells; causes insulin release; inhibits glucagon secretion, appetite, and energy intake; and delays gastric emptying because GLP receptors are located on the gut, pancreas, brainstem, hypothalamus, and vagal-afferent nerves.[112]

In a 12-week randomized controlled trial in women with PCOS, a combination treatment with liraglutide (GLP-1 mimetic) and metformin was found to be superior to liraglutide or metformin monotherapy in reducing weight and improving menstrual cycles, ovulation rate, free androgen index, and insulin sensitivity evaluated by euglycemic-hyperinsulinemic clamp[113] and has better side effect profile compared with orlistat.[114,115]

Most commonly reported side effects of GLP-1 analogues are nausea, vomiting, and an increased risk of pancreatitis. Once-daily 3 mg of subcutaneous liraglutide has been shown to cause weight loss when combined with low-calorie diet and increased physical activity.[116,117]

Bariatric Surgery

Lifestyle changes remain the first-line treatment for weight loss; however, for morbid obesity, bariatric surgery has proven to be more effective, and hence this is the case for obese patients with PCOS.[118] In one study,[119] 17 PCOS patients underwent bariatric surgery indicated for morbid obesity; the mean weight loss in them after surgery was calculated to be 41 ± 9 kg (95% confidence interval, 36–47 kg; $P < .001$) after 12 ± 5 months and was accompanied by resolution of features of hyperandrogenism and biochemical and hormonal profile. Patients had more regular menstrual cycles and ovulation. On reevaluation after the weight loss, patients did not fit into PCOS diagnostic criteria anymore, and the metabolic abnormalities of prediabetes, hypertension, and dyslipidemia resolved completely. However, it is clear that the underlying pathophysiology of PCOS did not reverse completely and the bariatric surgery by helping lose weight allays severity of clinical manifestations of PCOS. Another study conducted by Eid et al.[120] showed similar results in that the MBS associated with PCOS improved by gastric bypass surgery independent of weight loss achieved. Another study[121] showed that such improvement is similar for both PCOS and non-PCOS patients with obesity. Both Roux-en-Y gastric bypass and laparoscopic adjustable gastric banding are FDA approved in young patients. One of the aspects these young patients might consider by having surgical weight loss is improving the chances of pregnancy. As in one study 30% of these patients admitted to have undergone this surgery to improve their chances of getting pregnant,[122] although it is advised to wait for 12 months at least postsurgery to get pregnant to allow for rapid metabolic, nutritional, and weight loss changes to subside.[123] The bariatric surgery is still a weight loss measure rather than treatment for PCOS.

TREATING MORBIDITIES AGGRAVATED BY OBESITY IN POLYCYSTIC OVARY SYNDROME

Infertility

Lifestyle modifications to encourage weight loss serve as the first-line treatment for infertility in PCOS. Not only does it decrease the chances of infertility, but also it would reduce the maternal and neonatal morbidities.[124] Obesity is the major predictor of reduced response to in vitro fertilization (IVF) therapy and studies show restoration of fertility or response to IVF therapy with weight loss. Therefore fertility treatment given to anyone with BMI > 35 kg/m² has not shown promising results.[125]

The second-line treatment is ovulation induction by clomiphene citrate. Metformin as a single agent has not proved to be beneficial in terms of fertility and pregnancy outcomes; however, its concomitant use with clomiphene citrate doubled the chances of pregnancy.[126]

IVF remains the third-line treatment modality; however, these have promising results with weight loss. Obesity decreases the chances of success with these modalities.[127]

Cutaneous Manifestations

Weight loss is the most effective and convenient approach, without adverse reactions. As little as 2%–7% of weight loss improves most of the cutaneous manifestations of PCOS such as acne and hirsutism by reducing androgen levels and improvement in insulin resistance.[60] According to the UK Endocrine Society Practice Guidelines, oral contraceptive pills (OCPs) or direct hair removal should be used initially. If hirsutism does not decrease after 6 months of OCP therapy, 50–200 mg antiandrogens may be added daily for another 6 months. OCPs and antiandrogens have proven to be useful in the management of acne and alopecia as well.[83]

Obstructive Sleep Apnea

Obese women with PCOS frequently complain of sleep apnea. Again lifestyle approach remains the first-line nonsurgical and nonpharmacologic treatment for patients with OSA.[128] Treatment with CPAP can improve blood pressure, improve insulin levels, and reduce the risk for diabetes and MBS in 13% of the patients.[129,130]

Cardiovascular Risks

CVD is responsible for the increased mortality and morbidity not only in the general population but also in patients with PCOS. The Endocrine Society Clinical Practice Guideline stated to take into account early detection of the MBS to prevent serious outcomes. It recommends screening for IGT, diabetes, dyslipidemia, and hypertension in PCOS patients.[38,53]

CONCLUSION

It is clear that obesity may exaggerate all the manifestations of the PCOS phenotype. PCOS patients have higher insulin resistance at a given BMI, and many of the features seen in PCOS are exacerbated by obesity. Treating obesity by weight loss, pharmacologically, especially by bariatric surgery, has shown that many of the features of PCOS can be reversed. While the cause and the etiology of PCOS remain elusive, pragmatically the support of patients to lose weight through lifestyle changes in the first instance will help their response to the treatment strategies available.

REFERENCES

1. Haslam DW, James WP. Obesity. *Lancet.* 2005;366(9492): 1197–1209.
2. Bray GA. Medical consequences of obesity. *J Clin Endocrinol Metab.* 2004;89(6):2583–2589.
3. Striegel-Moore RH, Rosselli F, Perrin N, et al. Gender difference in the prevalence of eating disorder symptoms. *Int J Eat Disord.* 2009;42(5):471–474.
4. Sirmans SM, Pate KA. Epidemiology, diagnosis, and management of polycystic ovary syndrome. *Clin Epidemiol.* 2013;6:1–13.
5. Trivax B, Azziz R. Diagnosis of polycystic ovary syndrome. *Clin Obstet Gynecol.* 2007;50(1):168–177.
6. Rotterdam EA-SPCWG. Revised 2003 consensus on diagnostic criteria and long-term health risks related to polycystic ovary syndrome. *Fertil Steril.* 2004;81(1):19–25.
7. Azziz R, Carmina E, Dewailly D, et al. The androgen excess and PCOS society criteria for the polycystic ovary syndrome: the complete task force report. *Fertil Steril.* 2009;91(2):456–488.

8. Carmina E. Diagnosis of polycystic ovary syndrome: from NIH criteria to ESHRE-ASRM guidelines. *Minerva Ginecol.* 2004;56(1):1–6.

9. Karaer A, Cavkaytar S, Mert I, Buyukkagnici U, Batioglu S. Cardiovascular risk factors in polycystic ovary syndrome. *J Obstet Gynaecol.* 2010;30(4):387–392.

10. Poretsky L, Cataldo NA, Rosenwaks Z, Giudice LC. The insulin-related ovarian regulatory system in health and disease. *Endocr Rev.* 1999;20(4):535–582.

11. Goossens GH, Bizzarri A, Venteclef N, et al. Increased adipose tissue oxygen tension in obese compared with lean men is accompanied by insulin resistance, impaired adipose tissue capillarization, and inflammation. *Circulation.* 2011;124(1):67–76.

12. Motta AB. The role of obesity in the development of polycystic ovary syndrome. *Curr Pharm Des.* 2012;18(17): 2482–2491.

13. Alvarez-Blasco F, Botella-Carretero JI, San Millan JL, Escobar-Morreale HF. Prevalence and characteristics of the polycystic ovary syndrome in overweight and obese women. *Arch Intern Med.* 2006;166(19):2081–2086.

14. Legro RS. Obesity and PCOS: implications for diagnosis and treatment. *Semin Reprod Med.* 2012;30(6):496–506.

15. Buggs C, Rosenfield RL. Polycystic ovary syndrome in adolescence. *Endocrinol Metab Clin North Am.* 2005;34(3): 677–705.

16. Vrbikova J, Hainer V. Obesity and polycystic ovary syndrome. *Obes Facts.* 2009;2(1):26–35.

17. Rubenstein AH. Obesity: a modern epidemic. *Trans Am Clin Climatol Assoc.* 2005;116:103–111. Discussion 112–103.

18. Laitinen J, Taponen S, Martikainen H, et al. Body size from birth to adulthood as a predictor of self-reported polycystic ovary syndrome symptoms. *Int J Obes Relat Metab Disord.* 2003;27(6):710–715.

19. Rabe K, Lehrke M, Parhofer KG, Broedl UC. Adipokines and insulin resistance. *Mol Med.* 2008;14(11–12): 741–751.

20. Slawik M, Vidal-Puig AJ. Adipose tissue expandability and the metabolic syndrome. *Genes Nutr.* 2007;2(1):41–45.

21. Ahmadi A, Akbarzadeh M, Mohammadi F, Akbari M, Jafari B, Tolide-Ie HR. Anthropometric characteristics and dietary pattern of women with polycystic ovary syndrome. *Indian J Endocrinol Metab.* 2013;17(4):672–676.

22. Conte F, Banting L, Teede HJ, Stepto NK. Mental health and physical activity in women with polycystic ovary syndrome: a brief review. *Sports Med.* 2015;45(4): 497–504.

23. Lo JC, Feigenbaum SL, Yang J, Pressman AR, Selby JV, Go AS. Epidemiology and adverse cardiovascular risk profile of diagnosed polycystic ovary syndrome. *J Clin Endocrinol Metab.* 2006;91(4):1357–1363.

24. Swinburn BA, Sacks G, Hall KD, et al. The global obesity pandemic: shaped by global drivers and local environments. *Lancet.* 2011;378(9793):804–814.

25. Cosar E, Ucok K, Akgun L, et al. Body fat composition and distribution in women with polycystic ovary syndrome. *Gynecol Endocrinol.* 2008;24(8):428–432.

26. Lim SS, Norman RJ, Davies MJ, Moran LJ. The effect of obesity on polycystic ovary syndrome: a systematic review and meta-analysis. *Obes Rev.* 2013;14(2): 95–109.

27. Kalra P, Bansal B, Nag P, et al. Abdominal fat distribution and insulin resistance in Indian women with polycystic ovarian syndrome. *Fertil Steril.* 2009;91(4 suppl): 1437–1440.

28. Arpaci D, Gurkan Tocoglu A, Yilmaz S, et al. The relationship between epicardial fat tissue thickness and visceral adipose tissue in lean patients with polycystic ovary syndrome. *J Ovarian Res.* 2015;8:71.

29. Millar SR, Perry IJ, Van den Broeck J, Phillips CM. Optimal central obesity measurement site for assessing cardiometabolic and type 2 diabetes risk in middle-aged adults. *PLoS One.* 2015;10(6):e0129088.

30. Sam S. Obesity and polycystic ovary syndrome. *Obes Manag.* 2007;3(2):69–73.

31. Kirchengast S, Huber J. Body composition characteristics and body fat distribution in lean women with polycystic ovary syndrome. *Hum Reprod.* 2001;16(6):1255–1260.

32. Faloia E, Canibus P, Gatti C, et al. Body composition, fat distribution and metabolic characteristics in lean and obese women with polycystic ovary syndrome. *J Endocrinol Invest.* 2004;27(5):424–429.

33. Mandrelle K, Kamath MS, Bondu DJ, Chandy A, Aleyamma T, George K. Prevalence of metabolic syndrome in women with polycystic ovary syndrome attending an infertility clinic in a tertiary care hospital in south India. *J Hum Reprod Sci.* 2012;5(1):26–31.

34. Dunaif A. Insulin resistance and the polycystic ovary syndrome: mechanism and implications for pathogenesis. *Endocr Rev.* 1997;18(6):774–800.

35. Ibricevic D, Asimi ZV. Frequency of prediabetes in women with polycystic ovary syndrome. *Med Arch.* 2013;67(4): 282–285.

36. Lloyd-Jones DM, Wilson PW, Larson MG, et al. Framingham risk score and prediction of lifetime risk for coronary heart disease. *Am J Cardiol.* 2004;94(1): 20–24.

37. Ramezani Tehrani F, Montazeri SA, Hosseinpanah F, et al. Trend of cardio-metabolic risk factors in polycystic ovary syndrome: a population-based prospective cohort study. *PLoS One.* 2015;10(9):e0137609.

38. Sharma ST, Nestler JE. Prevention of diabetes and cardiovascular disease in women with PCOS: treatment with insulin sensitizers. *Best Pract Res Clin Endocrinol Metab.* 2006;20(2):245–260.

39. Meyer ML, Malek AM, Wild RA, Korytkowski MT, Talbott EO. Carotid artery intima-media thickness in polycystic ovary syndrome: a systematic review and meta-analysis. *Hum Reprod Update.* 2012;18(2):112–126.

40. Talbott EO, Zborowski J, Rager J, Stragand JR. Is there an independent effect of polycystic ovary syndrome (PCOS) and menopause on the prevalence of subclinical atherosclerosis in middle aged women? *Vasc Health Risk Manag.* 2008;4(2):453–462.

41. Yusuf S, Hawken S, Ounpuu S, et al. Effect of potentially modifiable risk factors associated with myocardial infarction in 52 countries (the INTERHEART study): case-control study. *Lancet*. 2004;364(9438):937–952.

42. Sheehan MT. Polycystic ovarian syndrome: diagnosis and management. *Clin Med Res*. 2004;2(1):13–27.

43. Sardinha LB, Santos DA, Silva AM, Grontved A, Andersen LB, Ekelund U. A comparison between BMI, waist circumference, and waist-to-height ratio for identifying cardio-metabolic risk in children and adolescents. *PLoS One*. 2016;11(2):e0149351.

44. Homburg R. The management of infertility associated with polycystic ovary syndrome. *Reprod Biol Endocrinol*. 2003;1:109.

45. Pasquali R, Patton L, Gambineri A. Obesity and infertility. *Curr Opin Endocrinol Diabetes Obes*. 2007;14(6):482–487.

46. Glueck CJ, Wang P, Goldenberg N, Sieve-Smith L. Pregnancy outcomes among women with polycystic ovary syndrome treated with metformin. *Hum Reprod*. 2002;17(11):2858–2864.

47. Diamanti-Kandarakis E. Role of obesity and adiposity in polycystic ovary syndrome. *Int J Obes*. 2007;31(suppl 2):S8–S13. Discussion S31–12.

48. Ramirez VI, Miller E, Meireles CL, Gelfond J, Krummel DA, Powell TL. Adiponectin and IGFBP-1 in the development of gestational diabetes in obese mothers. *BMJ Open Diabetes Res Care*. 2014;2(1):e000010.

49. Katulski K, Czyzyk A, Podfigurna-Stopa A, Genazzani AR, Meczekalski B. Pregnancy complications in polycystic ovary syndrome patients. *Gynecol Endocrinol*. 2015;31(2):87–91.

50. Kim LH, Taylor AE, Barbieri RL. Insulin sensitizers and polycystic ovary syndrome: can a diabetes medication treat infertility? *Fertil Steril*. 2000;73(6):1097–1098.

51. Kamalanathan S, Sahoo JP, Sathyapalan T. Pregnancy in polycystic ovary syndrome. *Indian J Endocrinol Metab*. 2013;17(1):37–43.

52. Haoula Z, Salman M, Atiomo W. Evaluating the association between endometrial cancer and polycystic ovary syndrome. *Hum Reprod*. 2012;27(5):1327–1331.

53. Legro RS, Arslanian SA, Ehrmann DA, et al. Diagnosis and treatment of polycystic ovary syndrome: an Endocrine Society clinical practice guideline. *J Clin Endocrinol Metab*. 2013;98(12):4565–4592.

54. De Leo V, Musacchio MC, Morgante G, La Marca A, Petraglia F. Polycystic ovary syndrome and type 2 diabetes mellitus. *Minerva Ginecol*. 2004;56(1):53–62.

55. Romero-Corral A, Caples SM, Lopez-Jimenez F, Somers VK. Interactions between obesity and obstructive sleep apnea: implications for treatment. *Chest*. 2010;137(3):711–719.

56. Vgontzas AN, Legro RS, Bixler EO, Grayev A, Kales A, Chrousos GP. Polycystic ovary syndrome is associated with obstructive sleep apnea and daytime sleepiness: role of insulin resistance. *J Clin Endocrinol Metab*. 2001;86(2):517–520.

57. Tasali E, Van Cauter E, Ehrmann DA. Relationships between sleep disordered breathing and glucose metabolism in polycystic ovary syndrome. *J Clin Endocrinol Metab*. 2006;91(1):36–42.

58. Fogel RB, Malhotra A, Pillar G, Pittman SD, Dunaif A, White DP. Increased prevalence of obstructive sleep apnea syndrome in obese women with polycystic ovary syndrome. *J Clin Endocrinol Metab*. 2001;86(3):1175–1180.

59. Mokhlesi B, Scoccia B, Mazzone T, Sam S. Risk of obstructive sleep apnea in obese and nonobese women with polycystic ovary syndrome and healthy reproductively normal women. *Fertil Steril*. 2012;97(3):786–791.

60. Moura HH, Costa DL, Bagatin E, Sodre CT, Manela-Azulay M. Polycystic ovary syndrome: a dermatologic approach. *An Bras Dermatol*. 2011;86(1):111–119.

61. Kelley CE, Brown AJ, Diehl AM, Setji TL. Review of nonalcoholic fatty liver disease in women with polycystic ovary syndrome. *World J Gastroenterol*. 2014;20(39):14172–14184.

62. Vassilatou E. Nonalcoholic fatty liver disease and polycystic ovary syndrome. *World J Gastroenterol*. 2014;20(26):8351–8363.

63. Gambarin-Gelwan M, Kinkhabwala SV, Schiano TD, Bodian C, Yeh HC, Futterweit W. Prevalence of nonalcoholic fatty liver disease in women with polycystic ovary syndrome. *Clin Gastroenterol Hepatol*. 2007;5(4):496–501.

64. Carmina E. Metabolic syndrome in polycystic ovary syndrome. *Minerva Ginecol*. 2006;58(2):109–114.

65. Wajchenberg BL. Subcutaneous and visceral adipose tissue: their relation to the metabolic syndrome. *Endocr Rev*. 2000;21(6):697–738.

66. Boden G. Obesity and free fatty acids. *Endocrinol Metab Clin North Am*. 2008;37(3):635–646. viii-ix.

67. Tzanavari T, Giannogonas P, Karalis KP. TNF-alpha and obesity. *Curr Dir Autoimmun*. 2010;11:145–156.

68. Samy N, Hashim M, Sayed M, Said M. Clinical significance of inflammatory markers in polycystic ovary syndrome: their relationship to insulin resistance and body mass index. *Dis Markers*. 2009;26(4):163–170.

69. Kajita K, Mune T, Kanoh Y, et al. TNFalpha reduces the expression of peroxisome proliferator-activated receptor gamma (PPARgamma) via the production of ceramide and activation of atypical PKC. *Diabetes Res Clin Pract*. 2004;66(suppl 1):S79–S83.

70. Sikaris KA. The clinical biochemistry of obesity. *Clin Biochem Rev*. 2004;25(3):165–181.

71. Acevedo N, Ding J, Smith GD. Insulin signaling in mouse oocytes. *Biol Reprod*. 2007;77(5):872–879.

72. Dumesic DA, Richards JS. Ontogeny of the ovary in polycystic ovary syndrome. *Fertil Steril*. 2013;100(1):23–38.

73. Adashi EY, Hsueh AJ, Yen SS. Insulin enhancement of luteinizing hormone and follicle-stimulating hormone release by cultured pituitary cells. *Endocrinology*. 1981;108(4):1441–1449.

74. Katakam PV, Hoenig M, Ujhelyi MR, Miller AW. Cytochrome P450 activity and endothelial dysfunction in insulin resistance. *J Vasc Res*. 2000;37(5):426–434.

75. Ding EL, Song Y, Manson JE, et al. Sex hormone-binding globulin and risk of type 2 diabetes in women and men. *N Engl J Med.* 2009;361(12):1152–1163.

76. Hautanen A. Synthesis and regulation of sex hormone-binding globulin in obesity. *Int J Obes Relat Metab Disord.* 2000;24(suppl 2):S64–S70.

77. Wang M. The role of glucocorticoid action in the pathophysiology of the metabolic syndrome. *Nutr Metab.* 2005;2(1):3.

78. Kopera D, Wehr E, Obermayer-Pietsch B. Endocrinology of hirsutism. *Int J Trichology.* 2010;2(1):30–35.

79. Mueller A, Dittrich R, Binder H, Hoffmann I, Beckmann MW, Cupisti S. Endocrinological markers for assessing hyperandrogenemia in women classified as having polycystic ovary syndrome (PCOS) according to the revised 2003 diagnostic criteria. *Eur J Med Res.* 2006;11(12):540–544.

80. Teede H, Deeks A, Moran L. Polycystic ovary syndrome: a complex condition with psychological, reproductive and metabolic manifestations that impacts on health across the lifespan. *BMC Med.* 2010;8:41.

81. Sidhwani S, Scoccia B, Sunghay S, Stephens-Archer CN, Mazzone T, Sam S. Polycystic ovary syndrome is associated with atherogenic changes in lipoprotein particle number and size independent of body weight. *Clin Endocrinol.* 2011;75(1):76–82.

82. Rajkhowa M, Neary RH, Kumpatla P, et al. Altered composition of high density lipoproteins in women with the polycystic ovary syndrome. *J Clin Endocrinol Metab.* 1997;82(10):3389–3394.

83. Badawy A, Elnashar A. Treatment options for polycystic ovary syndrome. *Int J Womens Health.* 2011;3:25–35.

84. Lim SS, Davies MJ, Norman RJ, Moran LJ. Overweight, obesity and central obesity in women with polycystic ovary syndrome: a systematic review and meta-analysis. *Hum Reprod Update.* 2012;18(6):618–637.

85. Bajramovic JJ, Volmer R, Syan S, Pochet S, Gonzalez-Dunia D. 2′-fluoro-2′-deoxycytidine inhibits Borna disease virus replication and spread. *Antimicrob Agents Chemother.* 2004;48(4):1422–1425.

86. Fontana R, Della Torre S. The deep correlation between energy metabolism and reproduction: a view on the effects of nutrition for women fertility. *Nutrients.* 2016;8(2):87.

87. Pasquali R, Gambineri A. Role of changes in dietary habits in polycystic ovary syndrome. *Reprod Biomed Online.* 2004;8(4):431–439.

88. Meirhaeghe A, Cottel D, Amouyel P, Dallongeville J. Association between peroxisome proliferator-activated receptor gamma haplotypes and the metabolic syndrome in French men and women. *Diabetes.* 2005;54(10):3043–3048.

89. Baptiste CG, Battista MC, Trottier A, Baillargeon JP. Insulin and hyperandrogenism in women with polycystic ovary syndrome. *J Steroid Biochem Mol Biol.* 2010;122(1–3):42–52.

90. McAllister JM, Legro RS, Modi BP, Strauss 3rd JF. Functional genomics of PCOS: from GWAS to molecular mechanisms. *Trends Endocrinol Metab.* 2015;26(3):118–124.

91. Vassiliadi DA, Barber TM, Hughes BA, et al. Increased 5 alpha-reductase activity and adrenocortical drive in women with polycystic ovary syndrome. *J Clin Endocrinol Metab.* 2009;94(9):3558–3566.

92. Kelly CC, Lyall H, Petrie JR, Gould GW, Connell JM, Sattar N. Low grade chronic inflammation in women with polycystic ovarian syndrome. *J Clin Endocrinol Metab.* 2001;86(6):2453–2455.

93. Duleba AJ, Dokras A. Is PCOS an inflammatory process? *Fertil Steril.* 2012;97(1):7–12.

94. Heilbronn LK, Campbell LV. Adipose tissue macrophages, low grade inflammation and insulin resistance in human obesity. *Curr Pharm Des.* 2008;14(12):1225–1230.

95. Puder JJ, Varga S, Kraenzlin M, De Geyter C, Keller U, Muller B. Central fat excess in polycystic ovary syndrome: relation to low-grade inflammation and insulin resistance. *J Clin Endocrinol Metab.* 2005;90(11):6014–6021.

96. Moran LJ, Misso ML, Wild RA, Norman RJ. Impaired glucose tolerance, type 2 diabetes and metabolic syndrome in polycystic ovary syndrome: a systematic review and meta-analysis. *Hum Reprod Update.* 2010;16(4):347–363.

97. Teede HJ, Joham AE, Paul E, et al. Longitudinal weight gain in women identified with polycystic ovary syndrome: results of an observational study in young women. *Obesity (Silver Spring).* 2013;21(8):1526–1532.

98. Moran LJ, Ranasinha S, Zoungas S, McNaughton SA, Brown WJ, Teede HJ. The contribution of diet, physical activity and sedentary behaviour to body mass index in women with and without polycystic ovary syndrome. *Hum Reprod.* 2013;28(8):2276–2283.

99. Moran LJ, Brinkworth G, Noakes M, Norman RJ. Effects of lifestyle modification in polycystic ovarian syndrome. *Reprod Biomed Online.* 2006;12(5):569–578.

100. Douglas CC, Gower BA, Darnell BE, Ovalle F, Oster RA, Azziz R. Role of diet in the treatment of polycystic ovary syndrome. *Fertil Steril.* 2006;85(3):679–688.

101. Haqq L, McFarlane J, Dieberg G, Smart N. Effect of lifestyle intervention on the reproductive endocrine profile in women with polycystic ovarian syndrome: a systematic review and meta-analysis. *Endocr Connect.* 2014;3(1):36–46.

102. Goss AM, Chandler-Laney PC, Ovalle F, et al. Effects of a eucaloric reduced-carbohydrate diet on body composition and fat distribution in women with PCOS. *Metabolism.* 2014;63(10):1257–1264.

103. de Souza RJ, Bray GA, Carey VJ, et al. Effects of 4 weight-loss diets differing in fat, protein, and carbohydrate on fat mass, lean mass, visceral adipose tissue, and hepatic fat: results from the POUNDS LOST trial. *Am J Clin Nutr.* 2012;95(3):614–625.

104. Sjostrom L, Rissanen A, Andersen T, et al. Randomised placebo-controlled trial of orlistat for weight loss and prevention of weight regain in obese patients. European Multicentre Orlistat Study Group. *Lancet.* 1998;352(9123):167–172.

105. Drew BS, Dixon AF, Dixon JB. Obesity management: update on orlistat. *Vasc Health Risk Manag*. 2007;3(6): 817–821.

106. Diamanti-Kandarakis E, Katsikis I, Piperi C, Alexandraki K, Panidis D. Effect of long-term orlistat treatment on serum levels of advanced glycation end-products in women with polycystic ovary syndrome. *Clin Endocrinol*. 2007;66(1):103–109.

107. Jayagopal V, Kilpatrick ES, Holding S, Jennings PE, Atkin SL. Orlistat is as beneficial as metformin in the treatment of polycystic ovarian syndrome. *J Clin Endocrinol Metab*. 2005;90(2):729–733.

108. Johnson NP. Metformin use in women with polycystic ovary syndrome. *Ann Transl Med*. 2014;2(6):56.

109. Fulghesu AM, Romualdi D, Di Florio C, et al. Is there a dose-response relationship of metformin treatment in patients with polycystic ovary syndrome? Results from a multicentric study. *Hum Reprod*. 2012;27(10):3057–3066.

110. Lashen H. Role of metformin in the management of polycystic ovary syndrome. *Ther Adv Endocrinol Metab*. 2010;1(3):117–128.

111. Sathyapalan T, Cho LW, Kilpatrick ES, Coady AM, Atkin SL. Metformin maintains the weight loss and metabolic benefits following rimonabant treatment in obese women with polycystic ovary syndrome (PCOS). *Clin Endocrinol*. 2009;70(1):124–128.

112. MacDonald PE, El-Kholy W, Riedel MJ, Salapatek AM, Light PE, Wheeler MB. The multiple actions of GLP-1 on the process of glucose-stimulated insulin secretion. *Diabetes*. 2002;51(suppl 3):S434–S442.

113. Jensterle M, Goricar K, Janez A. Metformin as an initial adjunct to low-dose liraglutide enhances the weight-decreasing potential of liraglutide in obese polycystic ovary syndrome: randomized control study. *Exp Ther Med*. 2016;11(4):1194–1200.

114. Kang JG, Park CY. Anti-obesity drugs: a review about their effects and safety. *Diabetes Metab J*. 2012;36(1):13–25.

115. Niswender K, Pi-Sunyer X, Buse J, et al. Weight change with liraglutide and comparator therapies: an analysis of seven phase 3 trials from the liraglutide diabetes development programme. *Diabetes Obes Metab*. 2013;15(1):42–54.

116. Garber AJ. Long-acting glucagon-like peptide 1 receptor agonists: a review of their efficacy and tolerability. *Diabetes Care*. 2011;34(suppl 2):S279–S284.

117. Pi-Sunyer X, Astrup A, Fujioka K, et al. A randomized, controlled trial of 3.0 mg of liraglutide in weight management. *N Engl J Med*. 2015;373(1):11–22.

118. Skubleny D, Switzer NJ, Gill RS, et al. The impact of bariatric surgery on polycystic ovary syndrome: a systematic review and meta-analysis. *Obes Surg*. 2016;26(1):169–176.

119. Escobar-Morreale HF, Botella-Carretero JI, Alvarez-Blasco F, Sancho J, San Millan JL. The polycystic ovary syndrome associated with morbid obesity may resolve after weight loss induced by bariatric surgery. *J Clin Endocrinol Metab*. 2005;90(12):6364–6369.

120. Eid GM, McCloskey C, Titchner R, et al. Changes in hormones and biomarkers in polycystic ovarian syndrome treated with gastric bypass. *Surg Obes Relat Dis*. 2014;10(5):787–791.

121. Kyriacou A, Hunter AL, Tolofari S, Syed AA. Gastric bypass surgery in women with or without polycystic ovary syndrome–a comparative observational cohort analysis. *Eur J Intern Med*. 2014;25(2):e23–e34.

122. Gosman GG, King WC, Schrope B, et al. Reproductive health of women electing bariatric surgery. *Fertil Steril*. 2010;94(4):1426–1431.

123. American College of Obstetricians, Gynecologists. ACOG practice bulletin no. 105: bariatric surgery and pregnancy. *Obstet Gynecol*. 2009;113(6):1405–1413.

124. Palomba S, Santagni S, Falbo A, La Sala GB. Complications and challenges associated with polycystic ovary syndrome: current perspectives. *Int J Womens Health*. 2015;7:745–763.

125. Pandey S, Pandey S, Maheshwari A, Bhattacharya S. The impact of female obesity on the outcome of fertility treatment. *J Hum Reprod Sci*. 2010;3(2):62–67.

126. Palomba S, Falbo A, La Sala GB. Metformin and gonadotropins for ovulation induction in patients with polycystic ovary syndrome: a systematic review with meta-analysis of randomized controlled trials. *Reprod Biol Endocrinol*. 2014;12:3.

127. Melo AS, Ferriani RA, Navarro PA. Treatment of infertility in women with polycystic ovary syndrome: approach to clinical practice. *Clinics*. 2015;70(11):765–769.

128. Kline CE, Crowley EP, Ewing GB, et al. The effect of exercise training on obstructive sleep apnea and sleep quality: a randomized controlled trial. *Sleep*. 2011;34(12):1631–1640.

129. Pepin JL, Tamisier R, Levy P. Obstructive sleep apnoea and metabolic syndrome: put CPAP efficacy in a more realistic perspective. *Thorax*. 2012;67(12):1025–1027.

130. Tasali E, Chapotot F, Leproult R, Whitmore H, Ehrmann DA. Treatment of obstructive sleep apnea improves cardiometabolic function in young obese women with polycystic ovary syndrome. *J Clin Endocrinol Metab*. 2011;96(2):365–374.

CHAPTER 7

The Role of Human Gut Microbiota in Obesity

STEPHEN HYER, PHD, MA, MD, FRCP

INTRODUCTION

In recent years, there has been increasing interest in the microbial populations that reside in the human gut. It is estimated that these comprise at least 10^{12} bacteria and 10^{15} viruses, which collectively constitute the *gut microbiota*, whereas their genes comprise the *gut microbiome*.[1] Numbers of microorganisms differ at different sites within the gastrointestinal tract, reflecting their physiological roles.[2] These roles, until recently, have been found to help in the digestion of food, production of vitamins such as vitamin K, and providing protection from pathogens.

Evidence is accumulating that the gut microbiota interact with the host in far more complex ways, contributing in important ways to overall energy homeostasis. Alterations in the composition of gut microbiota are associated with several clinical disorders.[3] This review will consider their putative role in the development of obesity and obesity-related metabolic disorders collectively described as the metabolic syndrome. This syndrome includes visceral adiposity, impaired glucose tolerance, fatty liver, and high plasma triglycerides and is strongly associated with insulin resistance.[4]

There are several ways in which the gut microbiota could influence host metabolism and fat deposition, and these will be briefly reviewed. In the healthy gut, a thick mucosal layer separates the intestinal epithelium from the lumen acting as a protective barrier that prevents the absorption of lipopolysaccharides (LPSs) and other harmful bacterial products. Significantly, the mucosal layer contains many of the populations of intestinal bacteria and viruses.[5]

Changes in the composition and numbers of gut microbiota, as occurs in obesity, are associated with increased intestinal permeability of this layer.[6] The effect is to increase the absorption of bacterial endotoxins and circulating LPS. This, in turn, stimulates an immune response of low-grade inflammation, increases

fatty acid metabolism and storage of fat in the liver, and increases insulin resistance. The ensuing phenotype, at least in animal models, has many of the features of the metabolic syndrome.[7] The situation in human obesity, as will be reviewed here, is less certain because many of the studies demonstrate associations rather than providing clear evidence of cause and effect.

EXPERIMENTAL MODELS OF OBESITY

When the gut microbiota of lean wild-type mice are compared with those of genetically obese mice (*ob/ob* mice), consistent differences are found with higher numbers of *Firmicutes* and fewer *Bacteroidetes* in the obese mice despite similar diet and activity.[8] Similar changes in gut microbiota are reported when comparing diet-induced obese and lean mice.[9] This alteration in the relative proportions of these populations of bacteria results in an increased capacity of the microbiota to harvest energy and hence makes the animal prone to obesity. For example, a 20% increase in *Firmicutes* with a 20% decrease in *Bacteroidetes* is estimated to provide an additional 150 kcal of energy per day.[10]

However, the observation that the gut microbiome is altered in obese animals (and, as we shall see, in humans) does not prove a causal relationship. More convincing are experimental data in which gut microbial material is transferred from obese animals into lean controls under carefully controlled conditions of diet and physical activity (Table 7.1).

More than a decade ago, Fredrik Bäckhed and colleagues at Washington University reported that transfer of microbiota from conventionally raised mice into germfree lean mice resulted in a 60% increase in body fat and insulin resistance despite a 29% reduction in chow consumption and 27% increased activity compared with control germfree mice.[11] Furthermore, the

TABLE 7.1
Mouse Transfer Experiments

Investigators	Experiment	Result
Backhed et al.[11]	Transfer of microbes from cecum of conventionally raised mice into lean germfree mice	60% increase in body fat and insulin resistance despite reduction in chow intake and increased activity
Turnbaugh et al.[9]	Microbiota harvested from the cecum of obese (*ob/ob*) mice into lean germfree mice	Obesity phenotype transferred
	Microbiota from lean donors into lean germfree mice	Decreased body fat
Ridaura et al.[21]	Transfer of microbiota from human female donor from twin pairs into adult germfree mice	Higher adiposity if microbiota from obese donor Lower adiposity if microbiota from lean donor

Adapted from Jayasinghe TN, Chiavaroli V, Holland DJ, Cutfield WS, O'Sullivan JM. The new era of treatment for obesity and metabolic disorders: evidence and expectations for gut microbiome transplantation. *Front Cell Infect Microbiol*. 2016;6:15 with permission.

obese phenotype of genetically obese (*ob/ob*) mice was shown to be transmitted to lean germfree mice by simply taking microbiota harvested from the gut of the genetically obese mice.[12] Intestinal microbiota were shown to interact with the host by suppressing the expression of an inhibitor (fasting-induced adipose factor, FIAF) of lipoprotein lipase (LPL), leading to increased LPL activity and hence enhanced lipogenesis and fat storage.[13]

Of note, when *ob/ob* mice are fed a high-fat diet, the *Firmicutes:Bacteroidetes* ratio (F/B ratio) increases compared with those that are fed a low-fat diet, implying that the profile of gut microbiota seen in these mice are related to their diet as much as their genetic makeup.[14] A similar finding is observed when a high-fat diet is fed to germfree lean mice.[15] Nevertheless, the role of the gut microbiome in obesity is likely to be far more complex than simply an imbalance in the proportion of these major classes of bacteria.

The importance of bacterial LPS in the pathogenesis of obesity and the metabolic syndrome was demonstrated in experiments in which 4 weeks of high-fat feeding to lean mice resulted in the expected changes in gut microbiota and a two- to threefold increase in circulating LPS levels.[7] Furthermore, continuous subcutaneous infusion of LPS resulted in excessive weight gain

and insulin resistance. The same group showed that LPS receptor knockout mice are hypersensitive to insulin and resistant to inflammation when fed a high-fat diet.[16]

Observations in obese mice have demonstrated that gut microbiota increase gut permeability, which enhances plasma LPS levels and exacerbates gut barrier disruption. They do so by activating the endocannabinoid (eCB) system.[17]

The increased eCB tone is associated with increased fat mass, insulin resistance, and fatty liver. A vicious cycle arises because the increased bacterial LPS will further activate the eCB system.[17]

Another approach to understanding the role of gut microbiota in obesity is examination of the effect of weight loss interventions and changes in microbial populations. Long-term calorie restriction, for example, results in a reduction in the F/B ratio in mice, particularly in those that are fed a low-fat diet.[18] A fall in LPS-binding protein is also observed, suggesting less metabolic endotoxaemia and inflammation. When bariatric surgery is performed on mice and compared with sham-operated controls, changes can be detected in the gut microbial ecology within 2 weeks with a relative abundance of *Verrucomicrobia* (genus *Akkermansia*) and *Gammaproteobacteria* (genus *Escherichia*).[19]

Interestingly, germfree mice inoculated with cecal material from the operated animals lost significantly more weight than controls receiving fecal material from sham-operated animals, implying that decreased adiposity is also transmissible through the gut microbiota.

Investigators have also examined whether *human* gut microbiota can induce obesity in lean mice. Germfree mice colonized with microbiota from high fat–fed mice that had previously received human microbiota ("humanized mice") gained more adiposity than mouse recipients from low fat–fed humanized mice reared under similar conditions.[20] The same researchers went on to show that when mice received human microbiota from obese patients, they gained more adiposity and hence more weight, as well as increased metabolic disturbances.[21]

More evidence for a role of microbiota in obesity comes from a study in which fecal material from morbidly obese patients, who had undergone bariatric surgery before 9 years, was transferred into germfree mice and the composition of gut microbiota compared.[22] Roux-en-Y gastric bypass surgery or vertical banded gastroplasty induced similar long-term changes on the gut microbiome. Germfree mice colonized with stools from these patients promoted reduced fat deposition in recipient mice, and the mice receiving the gastric bypass microbiota gained the least fat mass. The evidence provided by these studies suggests a role of the gut microbiota in the reduction of adiposity after bariatric surgery.

HUMAN STUDIES

Similar to animal models, differences have been reported in the gut microbiota of lean and obese human subjects with most studies showing greater proportions of the group *Firmicutes* in relation to *Bacteroidetes* in obese humans expressed as an increased F/B ratio.[24,25] However, this is not a consistent finding and a recent metaanalysis indicated no significant differences.[26] A possible explanation for the inconsistencies derives from studies comparing obese subjects with and without features of the metabolic syndrome. Investigators from Finland demonstrated a relative abundance of *Firmicutes* bacteria (*Eubacterium rectale*/*Clostridium coccoides*) and an increased F/B ratio only in the group with metabolic abnormalities and also reported significant associations between this ratio and body fat composition (percentage fat mass, visceral fat area) and lipid metabolism (high-density lipoprotein, triglycerides).[27] Hence, alterations of the gut microbiota may be more closely related to human obesity when metabolic abnormalities are also present.

Obesity and fat mass are associated with reduced bacterial diversity. In a MetaHit study of 169 obese versus 123 nonobese Danish individuals, those with low bacterial richness (23% of the population) had greater adiposity and features of the metabolic syndrome and also gained more weight over time.[28] Those individuals whose samples were most abundant in bacteria as assessed by gene diversity had an increased proportion of *anti*inflammatory species such as *Faecalibacterium prausnitzii* and *Akkermansia muciniphila*. Conversely, there was evidence of more *pro*inflammatory *Bacteroidetes* spp. and genes involved in oxidative stress in those with low gene counts. Importantly, gene count correlated with variables of the metabolic syndrome, such as insulin resistance. In another study, 6 weeks of calorie restriction followed by 8 weeks of weight maintenance significantly increased gene richness in subjects with low gene counts and partially improved the metabolic abnormalities but was less efficient in improving the low-grade inflammation.[29]

Increased microbial richness has also been reported 3 months after bariatric surgery remaining stable thereafter.[30,31] However, results need to be interpreted with caution because of dietary changes after surgery and the influence of medication. The presence of certain beneficial bacterial species could promote the growth of other species, leading to greater bacterial diversity.

In this regard, it has been postulated that the degradation of mucin by *A. muciniphila* to produce a supply of short-chain fatty acids could provide an energy source for other bacteria as well as for the host.[32] There is evidence that individuals with high gene richness and fecal abundance of *A. muciniphila* have the healthiest metabolic profile as reflected by fat distribution, plasma triglycerides, and fasting plasma glucose, but the precise role of this species in the human gut is still unclear.[33]

These observations have led investigators to assess the potential of *prebiotics* (nondigestible compounds that are metabolized by gut microorganisms, thereby modulating the composition or activity of the gut microbiota)[34] and *probiotics* (live microbial supplements, which beneficially affect the host by improving its intestinal microbial balance)[35] in the management of obesity. Manipulation of the gut microbiota in obese subjects could improve the metabolic abnormalities, reduce fat mass, and reduce gut-related inflammation.

Limited evidence exists in human studies.[36] A prebiotic approach offers the potential of encouraging the growth of a variety of beneficial microbiota, thereby improving microbial diversity. Of interest, supplementation of inulin-type fructans has been shown to

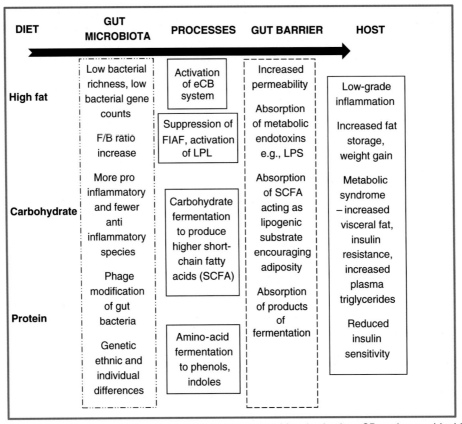

FIG. 7.1 Schematic representation of putative role of gut microbiota in obesity. *eCB*, endocannabinoid system; *F/B*, *Firmicutes:Bacteroidetes*; *FIAF*, fasting-induced adipose factor; *LPL*, lipoprotein lipase; *LPS*, lipopolysaccharide.

increase *bifidobacteria* and *F. prausnitzii*.[37] Probiotics, on the other hand, directly alter gut microbial composition by introducing bacteria such as *lactobacillus* and *bifidobacterium* shown experimentally to modulate inflammation or metabolic markers.[38] Although encouraging results have been reported in reducing fatty liver and nonalcoholic steatohepatitis, the impact of this therapeutic approach to reduce body weight or fat mass in human obesity has, to date, been limited.

Transplantation of fecal microbial material from lean individuals to recipients with metabolic syndrome has also been attempted in human studies.[39] An increase in gut bacterial diversity and specifically *Eubacterium hallii* was observed, which was associated with improvement in insulin sensitivity. However, body weight and adiposity did not change.

SUMMARY

Fig. 7.1 summarizes the putative role of the gut microbiota in obesity. The complex interactions between the host and the environment, especially diet and gut microbiota, are only just beginning to be unraveled. The interactions between the various microbes, including the effect of the phage component of the gut virome in modulating intestinal bacteria[40] and the metabolic consequences for the host, are currently under intense study. It is clear that gut microbiota are far more important in the metabolic health of the individual than was previously appreciated. Future research is aimed at a greater understanding of the role of intestinal microbiota in order that the adverse effects of obesity can, as far as possible, be mitigated.

REFERENCES

1. Clemente JC, Ursell LK, Parfrey LW, Knight R. The impact of the gut microbiota on human health: an integrative view. *Cell.* 2012;148:1258–1270.

2. Zhang Z, Geng J, Tang X, et al. Spatial heterogeneity and co-occurrence patterns of human mucosal-associated intestinal microbiota. *ISME J.* 2014;8:881–893.

3. Carding S, Verbeke K, Vipond DT, Corfe BM, Owen LJ. Dysbiosis of the gut microbiota in disease. *Microb Ecol Health Dis.* 2015;26. http://dx.doi.org/10.3402/mehd.v26.26191.

4. Alberti KG, Eckel RH, Grundy SM, et al. Harmonizing the metabolic syndrome: a joint interim statement of the International Diabetes Federation Task Force on Epidemiology and Prevention; National Heart, Lung, and Blood Institute; American Heart Association; World Heart Federation; International Atherosclerosis Society; and International Association for the Study of Obesity. *Circulation.* 2009;120:1640–1645.

5. Barr JJ, Auro R, Furlan M, et al. Bacteriophage adhering to mucus provides a non-host-derived immunity. *Proc Natl Acad Sci USA.* 2013;110:10771–10776.

6. Bischoff SC, Barbara G, Buurman W, et al. Intestinal permeability – a new target for disease prevention and therapy. *BMC Gastroenterol.* 2014;14:189.

7. Cani PD, Amar J, Iglesias MA, et al. Metabolic endotoxemia initiates obesity and insulin resistance. *Diabetes.* 2007;56:1761–1772.

8. Ley RE, Backhed F, Turnbaugh P, et al. Obesity alters gut microbial ecology. *Proc Natl Acad Sci USA.* 2005;102:11070–11075.

9. Turnbaugh PJ, Backhed F, Fulton L, et al. Diet-induced obesity is linked to marked but reversible alterations in the mouse distal gut microbiome. *Cell Host Microbe.* 2008;3:213–223.

10. Jumpertz R, Le DS, Turnbaugh PJ, et al. .Energy-balance studies reveal associations between gut microbes, caloric load, and nutrient absorption in humans. *Am J Clin Nutr.* 2011;94:58–65.

11. Backhed F, Ding H, Wang T, et al. The gut microbiota as an environmental factor that regulates fat storage. *Proc Natl Acad Sci USA.* 2004;101:15718–15723.

12. Turnbaugh PJ, Levy RE, Mahowald MA, et al. An obesity-associated gut microbiome with increased capacity for energy harvest. *Nature.* 2006;444:1027–1031.

13. Backhed F, Manchester JK, Semenkovich CF, et al. Mechanisms underlying the resistance to diet-induced obesity in germ-free mice. *Proc Natl Acad Sci USA.* 2007;104:979–984.

14. Murphy EF, Cotter PD, Healy S, et al. Composition and energy harvesting capacity of the gut microbiota: relationship to diet, obesity and time in mouse models. *Gut.* 2010;59:1635–1642.

15. Fleissner CK, Huebel N, Abd El-Bary MM, et al. Absence of intestinal microbiota does not protect mice from diet-induced obesity. *Br J Nutr.* 2010;104:919–929.

16. Cani PD, Bibiloni R, Knauf C, et al. Changes in gut microbiota control metabolic endotoxemia-induced inflammation in high-fat diet-induced obesity and diabetes in mice. *Diabetes.* 2008;57:1470–1481.

17. Muccioli GG, Naslain D, Bäckhed F, et al. The endocannabinoid system links gut microbiota to adipogenesis. *Mol Syst Biol.* 2010;6(1):392.

18. Zhang C, Li S, Yang L, et al. Structural modulation of gut microbiota in life-long calorie-restricted mice. *Nat Commun.* 2013;4.

19. Liou AP, Paziuk M, Luevano J-M, Machineni S, Turnbaugh PJ, Kaplan LM. Conserved shifts in the gut microbiota due to gastric bypass reduce host weight and adiposity. *Sci Transl Med.* 2013;5:178ra41.

20. Turnbaugh PJ, Ridaura VK, Faith JJ, Rey FE, Knight R, Gordon JI. The effect of diet on the human gut microbiome: a metagenomic analysis in humanized gnotobiotic mice. *Sci Transl Med.* 2009;1(6):6ra14.

21. Ridaura VK, Faith JJ, Rey FE, et al. Gut microbiota from twins discordant for obesity modulate metabolism in mice. *Science.* 2013;341:1241214. http://dx.doi.org/10.1126/science.1241214.

22. Tremaroli V, Karlsson F, Werling M, et al. Roux-en-Y gastric bypass and vertical banded gastroplasty induce long-term changes on the human gut microbiome contributing to fat mass regulation. *Cell Metab.* 2015;22:228–238.

23. Jayasinghe TN, Chiavaroli V, Holland DJ, Cutfield WS, O'Sullivan JM. The new era of treatment for obesity and metabolic disorders: evidence and expectations for gut microbiome transplantation. *Front Cell Infect Microbiol.* 2016;6:15.

24. Ley RE, Turnbaugh PJ, Klein S, Gordon JI. Microbial ecology: human gut microbes associated with obesity. *Nature.* 2006;444:1022–1023.

25. Turnbaugh PJ, Hamady M, Yatsunenko T, et al. A core gut microbiome in obese and lean twins. *Nature.* 2009;457:480–484.

26. Arumugam M, Raes J, Pelletier E, et al. MetaHIT Consortium. Enterotypes of the human gut microbiome. *Nature.* 2011;473:174–180.

27. Munukka E, Wiklund P, Pekkala S, et al. Women with and without metabolic disorder differ in their gut microbiota composition. *Obesity.* 2012;20:1082–1087.

28. Le Chatelier E, Nielsen T, Qin J, et al. Richness of human gut microbiome correlates with metabolic markers. *Nature.* 2013;500:541–546.

29. Cotillard A, Kennedy SP, Kong LC, et al. Dietary intervention impact on gut microbial gene richness. *Nature.* 2013;500:585–588.

30. Furet J-P, Kong L-C, Tap J, et al. Differential adaptation of human gut microbiota to bariatric surgery-induced weight loss: links with metabolic and low-grade inflammation markers. *Diabetes.* 2010;59:3049–3057.

31. Kong L-C, Tap J, Aron-Wisnewsky J, et al. Gut microbiota after gastric bypass in human obesity: increased richness and associations of bacterial genera with adipose tissue genes. *Am J Clin Nutr.* 2013;98:16–24.

32. Dao MC, Everard A, Aron-Wisnewsky J, et al. *Akkermansia muciniphila* and improved metabolic health during a dietary intervention in obesity: relationship with gut microbiome richness and ecology. *Gut.* 2016;65:426–436.

33. Khan MT, Nieuwdorp M, Bäckhed F. Microbial modulation of insulin sensitivity. *Cell Metab.* 2014;20:753–760.

34. Delzenne NM, Cani PD. Interaction between obesity and the gut microbiota: relevance in nutrition. *Annu Rev Nutr.* 2011;31:15–31.

35. Fuller R. Probiotics in man and animals. *J Appl Bacteriol.* 2004;66:365–378.

36. Dao MC, Clement K, Everard A, Cani PD. Losing weight for a better health: role for the gut microbiota. *Clin Nutr Exp.* 2016;6:39–58.

37. Ramirez-Farias C, Slezak K, Fuller Z, Duncan A, Holtrop G, Louis P. Effect of insulin on the human gut microbiota: stimulation of *Bifidobacterium adolescentis* and *Faecalibacterium prausnitzii*. *Br J Nutr.* 2009;101:541–550.

38. Kobyliak N, Conte C, Cammarota G, et al. Probiotics in prevention and treatment of obesity: a critical view. *Nutr Metab.* 2016;13:14.

39. Vrieze A, Van Nood E, Holleman F, et al. Transfer of intestinal microbiota from lean donors increases insulin sensitivity in individuals with metabolic syndrome. *Gastroenterology.* 2012;143(4):913–916.

40. Ogilvie LA, Jones BV. The human gut virome: a multifaceted majority. *Front Microbiol.* 2015;6:918.

CHAPTER 8

Obesity and Cardiovascular Disease Prevention

RAY MELEADY, MD, FRCP

DEFINITIONS AND ABBREVIATIONS

BMI Body mass index—the weight in kilograms divided by the height in meters squared

CAD Coronary artery disease

CHD Coronary heart disease

FDA Food and Drug Administration

HFpEF Heart failure preserved ejection fraction, equates to diastolic heart failure

HFrEF Heart failure reduced ejection fraction, equates to systolic heart failure

LDL Low-density lipoprotein

LVH Left ventricular hypertrophy

Metabolic syndrome Insulin resistance in association with clinical findings including abdominal obesity, raised systemic blood pressure, and an atherogenic lipid profile including low serum HDL cholesterol and raised serum triglycerides

NICE National Institute for Clinical Excellence

Obesity A body mass index of >30 kg/m²

Overweight A body mass index of 25–29.9 kg/m²

T2DM Type 2 diabetes mellitus

USPSTF U.S. Preventive Service Task Force

WC Waist circumference

WHR Waist-to-hip ratio

WHtR Waist-to-height ratio

INTRODUCTION

Prospective epidemiological studies have shown a consistent relationship between overweight or obesity and cardiovascular morbidity, mortality, and total mortality.[1-5] Obesity is strongly related to major cardiovascular risk factors, such as raised blood pressure, glucose intolerance, type 2 diabetes mellitus (T2DM), and dyslipidemia.[6-10] Given that the prevalence of obesity among children and adolescents is increasing,[11,12] there is growing concern for the cardiovascular future that lies in store for a generation of obese children who are likely to become obese adults and who already display an increased prevalence of T2DM.[13] Some have suggested that it is unrealistic to expect a continuation

of the improvement in life expectancy witnessed in the 20th century and indeed that there might even be a reversal owing to an array of factors, including obesity and T2DM.[14] Only with more detailed knowledge of such factors can we hope to find solutions to this burgeoning global phenomenon. Worldwide, noting that this epidemic affects both developed and developing economies,[15] the large scale of the problem involved means that treatment options need to be cost-effective, systemic, and take a societal and public health perspective. However, given that members of the public have more immediate contact with and look to clinicians rather than to public health foundations for advice on health, an opportunity presents itself for us as clinicians to act as opinion formers. This chapter, having considered theoretical aspects of the relationship between cardiovascular risk and obesity, sets out the background to such advice with the evidence cited for each treatment option.

PATHOPHYSIOLOGY OF CARDIOVASCULAR DISEASE IN OBESITY

Limitation of Using Body Mass Index as Predictor of Cardiovascular Risk

Definitions of obesity are weight based with the most prevalent measure being the body mass index (BMI) derived from the weight in kilograms divided by the height in meters squared. This is easy to measure, reproducible, and recommended by the World Health Organization because of its simplicity.[15] However, the BMI may fail to represent accurately the relative amounts of adipose tissue and lean body mass, especially in young children and adolescents, and may lead to misclassification. Furthermore, the point has been made that it does not constitute an index because an index ought to be dimensionless and it is further limited given that mass increases with the *cube* rather than the *square* of the height.[16] Body surface area was found to be a superior measure of prognosis in one study[16] and is commonly used by way of adjustment in measurements derived from echocardiography. Waist circumference (WC), waist-to-height ratio (WHtR), BMI, and waist-to-hip ratio (WHR) were compared as predictors of incident cardiovascular events and death in a European study of over 10,000 subjects. Of these, WHtR was the best indicator of risk followed by WC and WHR, and the authors advised against the use of BMI.[17] In a recent study of over 300,000 European subjects, both general adiposity, as represented by BMI, and abdominal adiposity, as represented by WC and WHR, were strong indicators of the risk of dying.[18] WC or WHR may still be more reflective of underlying pathophysiologic risk[19] in certain populations such as South Asians.[20] However, ethnic-specific ranges may not be deemed necessary if one accepts the evidence shown by one study, which indicated that the same low-risk BMI range applied to both European and Asian populations.[21] In addition, the value of using WHR in clinical practice is more difficult to assess because a clinically significant degree of loss of weight may not alter this measure significantly. Likewise, using a single measurement for WC without adjusting for height might underestimate the amount of fat in short subjects and overestimate it in tall subjects.[17] Despite its many caveats, BMI remains the most prevalent measurement of excess weight, among the other superior measures of obesity, because of its convenience (Table 8.1).

There is increasing recognition that a categoric or binary (obese, nonobese) variable with a definition based on a threshold does not reflect the biologic continuum.[22] That is, for many cardiovascular risk factors, there is a graded and continuous relation between risk and outcome. For not only this reason but also because cardiovascular disease is widely prevalent and available

resources to manage it are limited, there is a need to focus on the highest risk groups, for instance, when it comes to considering expensive treatment options, such as bariatric surgery. Therefore, three classes of obesity have been proposed by the American Heart Association: class I—BMI 30–35, class II—BMI > 35, and class III—BMI > 40; subjects with BMI between 30 and 35 are at moderate risk, those with BMI between 35 and 40 are at high risk, and those with BMI above 40 are at very high risk. In general, for each five-unit increase in BMI, there is a 29% increase in coronary heart disease (CHD) risk.[23]

Is Cardiovascular Risk Mediated by Obesity Itself or by Risk Factors?

The independence of obesity as a risk factor for cardiovascular disease has been examined in several studies. Framingham risk scoring in CHD originally excluded obesity because it was thought to be a mediator of risk rather than being independently related to it,[24] and one study from Germany indicated that the risk of death due to CHD associated with obesity could be accounted for by the presence of multiple cardiovascular risk factors, such as age, serum total and low-density lipoprotein (LDL) cholesterol, and systolic and diastolic blood pressure.[1] However, subsequent studies have indicated an independent effect: in the Nurses' Health Study of 115,195 subjects, rising BMI was continuously related to an increase in risk of death. For those with a BMI of >29 compared with that of <19, the relative risk was 2.2. Even for nurses who had never smoked and were deemed to be at low risk, the effect was more marked: for those with BMI above 32, the relative risk of cardiovascular death was 4.1.[3]

The Risk Continuum: Overweight, Obesity, Metabolic Syndrome, and *Diabesity*

Overweight and obesity have clear definitions based on body mass thresholds. The metabolic syndrome refers to the constellation of overweight (especially *abdominal* obesity), hypertension, insulin resistance, and raised serum insulin level and an atherogenic lipid profile (raised serum triglycerides and low high-density lipoprotein [HDL]). It is thought to confer a threefold increase in risk of developing stroke or CHD.[25]

Approximately half of those diagnosed with T2DM are obese,[26] and although not all obese subjects are diabetic (about 25% are deemed healthy by virtue of having normal insulin sensitivity[27]), the chance of developing diabetes increases with rising BMI. For those with a BMI greater than 35, the adjusted relative risk is 93 (95% confidence interval [CI]: 81–107) for

TABLE 8.1
Waist Circumference Measurements in Adult Asians and Caucasians and Associated Health Risk

	Men	Asian Men	Women	Asian Women
Waist circumference				
Increased risk	≥94 cm		≥80 cm	
Substantially increased risk	≥102 cm	90 cm	88 cm	80 cm
Waist/hip ratio	≥0.9		≥0.85	

From World Health Organisation. *Waist Circumference and Waist-Hip Ratio. Report of a WHO Expert Consultation.* www.who.int; 2008.

women[28] and 42 (95% CI: 22–81) for men.[29] The process begins early. Data from a large cohort of army personnel in Israel suggest that elevated BMI in early life predicts the development of not only T2DM in early adulthood but also atherosclerotic coronary artery disease (CAD) in later life.[30] These findings are consistent with preconceptions based on extrapolations from other data but nevertheless provide accurate numerical evidence of the long-term pernicious effects arising from obesity in early life. During follow-up over a mean of 17 years, for each one-unit increase in BMI, the multivariate adjusted risk of diabetes and CAD increased by 9.8% and 12%, respectively. This analysis of BMI as a continuous variable indicates that the increased risk of T2DM and CAD is evident from within a BMI range that is considered normal (at percentile 49.3 for CAD and 69.3 for diabetes on growth charts).[31]

Weight gain is associated with another cardiovascular morbidity apart from that mediated by diabetes. Data from the Framingham study indicate an increase of 5% in men and 7% in women in the risk of developing heart failure for each unit increase in BMI across all categories of BMI.[32] The particular tendency to develop a cardiomyopathy related to obesity seems to correlate with both the duration and degree of the excess weight: prevalence rates of 70% at 20 years and 90% at 30 years were noted by Alpert.[33]

The Obesity Paradox in Cardiovascular Disease

Despite the accepted view that obesity is related to *adverse* cardiovascular outcomes (Box 8.1), it is not universally demonstrated[34,35] and many studies have indicated a favorable effect among overweight and obese patients with heart failure,[36] CHD,[37] and hypertension.[38] In particular, overweight patients with diastolic dysfunction seem to enjoy a survival advantage.[39] In a metaanalysis of over 28,000 subjects followed for 2.7 years, when compared with heart failure subjects with a normal BMI, overweight or obese heart failure subjects had reduced rates of cardiovascular (19% and 40% lower, respectively) and all-cause (16% and 33% lower, respectively) mortality.[40] In a separate study of patients at the extreme end of the heart failure spectrum, i.e., hospitalized with decompensated heart failure, overweight and obesity also seemed to convey an advantage: for every five-unit increase in BMI, the risk of death was 10% lower.[41] For other heart-related disorders, although overweight and obesity are associated with a higher risk of first non-ST segment elevation myocardial infarction,[42] a paradoxical benefit is conferred on those overweight individuals who have

undergone revascularization.[37] The authors concluded that this apparent benefit was an aberration due to the poor predictive power of BMI, but others confirmed a similar finding by using percentage body fat rather than BMI in the analysis.[43] Furthermore, a recent metaanalysis of prospective data supports the existence of a paradoxical benefit among overweight patients with acute coronary events.[44] In over 22,000 treated hypertensive patients with established CAD, a 30% lower 2-year mortality rate among those who were obese or overweight was found.[38] Similarly, an apparent benefit was evident among overweight patients when compared with lean subjects in terms of stroke risk.[45]

In heart failure patients, the advantage conferred by the excess weight seems to exist irrespective of the degree of left ventricular dysfunction: in a multivariate analysis of a well-characterized group of patients in the CHARM trial, patients with ejection fractions above and below 40% had better outcomes if the BMI was between 30 and 34.9.[46] In addition, the advantage of being overweight conferred equal benefit on those with an ischemic or nonischemic cardiomyopathy.[47]

Although these large analyses may be prone to selection bias and the results appear counterintuitive, in terms of causation, there is a biologic plausibility to support this hypothesis of an obesity paradox. As advanced heart failure is considered to be a catabolic

---

BOX 8.1
Cardio Vascular and Metabolic Effects of Obesity

Increased insulin resistance ranging from glucose intolerance to type 2 diabetes mellitus

Structural heart disease: concentric remodeling and left ventricular hypertrophy

Hypertension

Atrial fibrillation

Coronary artery disease

Dyslipidemia:

  Raised serum total and LDL cholesterol and triglycerides, apolipoprotein B, small dense LDL particles

  Decreased apolipoprotein A1, decreased HDL

Heart failure with clinical and subclinical diastolic and systolic dysfunction

Endothelial dysfunction

Increased inflammatory activators

Prothrombosis

Obstructive sleep apnea

state, it is conceivable that overweight and obesity might confer a survival advantage through a variety of mechanisms. Heart failure is associated with activation of the neuroadrenergic and renin-angiotensin systems, but obese patients demonstrate reduced stimulation in these responses.[40] Obese patients also tend toward having higher systemic blood pressure and may be offered, and better tolerate, vasoactive medications that confer benefit in heart failure.[40] Obesity is associated with higher circulating levels of lipoproteins, which may bind and detoxify inflammatory cytokines,[48,49] and lower serum levels of atrial natriuretic peptides.[50] Equally, adipose cells may produce greater numbers of receptors for tumor necrosis factor-α, thus buffering the effect of this harmful cytokine.[51]

Genes, Gene-Lifestyle Interactions and Obesity

The contribution by inherited factors to the obesity epidemic is often cited as a reason for a "therapeutic nihilism" and for the long-term failure of dietary and lifestyle approaches in the effective management of obesity. Although there is strong evidence from twin[52] and family studies[53] of an inherited predisposition to develop cardiovascular disease and no doubt that monogenic factors increase the likelihood of developing coronary atherosclerosis, the phenotypic expression of genes is variable.[54] Furthermore, we inherit more than genes from our parents, and attitudes toward diet and food choices may become established in early life.[55] In one study of the effect of lifestyle changes on the cardiovascular risk conferred by genetic factors, a polygenic risk score was developed. More than 50 alleles, each associated with an increased risk of cardiovascular disease, were used to quantify the total genetic risk score, and although the risk of incident coronary events was 91% higher in the highest genetic risk stratum compared with that in the lowest genetic risk stratum, this effect was almost halved (46%) in subjects who had at least three of four favorable lifestyle factors, i.e., no current smoking, no BMI > 30, engagement in physical activity at least once a week, and a healthy diet. This observation of risk reduction by altering environmental factors fits with the fact that the global obesity epidemic is a relatively recent phenomenon. Although genetic influences are present, environmental aspects are worthy of our attention ranging from total caloric intake to complex qualitative aspects, such as the constitution of diet with potential effects mediated through inflammation,[56] the gut microbiome,[57] and gene-microbiome interactions.[58,59]

THERAPEUTIC STRATEGIES TO REDUCE CARDIOVASCULAR RISK IN OBESITY

Lifestyle Strategies to Reduce Weight and Cardiovascular Risk—Evidence

The most obvious manner by which obesity increases cardiovascular risk is by inducing diabetes. Combining diet and exercise therapies normalizes glucose metabolism and is effective in preventing diabetes.[60] However, it has been unclear to what extent diet, exercise, and weight loss each contributes toward prevention. Data gathered from a Caucasian population of overweight-obese and inactive postmenopausal women suggest that a significant reduction in insulin resistance is most noticeable in those adherent to dietary advice (24%) and to dietary and exercise advice (26%), whereas those who undertook exercise alone had a 9% reduction in insulin resistance; by comparison, controls had a 2% reduction.[61]

A common misconception is that substantial weight loss is required to achieve a reduction in cardiovascular risk. In a pioneering Finnish study of 523 men and women with impaired glucose tolerance randomized to either a combined dietary and exercise intervention (annual counseling on weight loss, reduction in total and saturated fat intake, increased intake of fiber and exercise) or usual care (verbal counseling and two pages of written information on diet and exercise at baseline and annually), the risk of developing diabetes was reduced by over half (11% vs. 23%) through achieving a net weight loss of 3.5 kg by the end of the second year.[62] Other effects observed included reductions in WC, fasting plasma glucose concentration, 2-h post–oral glucose tolerance test, and serum insulin concentration. The likelihood of averting diabetes was correlated with the degree of weight lost. Thus, it seems, a small weight reduction of the order of 5% body weight can lead to a significant reduction in the metabolic risk profile of a patient who is glucose intolerant (this 5% value is of interest as we will later see in relation to the effects of drug therapy). However, the size of this effect was considered likely to be an underestimate given that the analysis was by intention-to-treat and control subjects were also given advice on diet and lifestyle at baseline and at annual follow-up visits. More broadly, the results also suggest that the onset of an obesity epidemic need not be necessarily followed by an inevitable epidemic of T2DM.

Regarding other cardiovascular risk factors, no difference was evident between the two groups in serum total or HDL cholesterol, but serum triglyceride levels were significantly reduced by intensive lifestyle intervention. Similarly, systolic and, to a lesser extent, diastolic blood pressure was significantly reduced by the intervention in this trial.[62]

The proof of concept that weight loss can reduce insulin resistance seems clear from randomized controlled trials, such as the Diabetes Prevention Program[60] and Look AHEAD,[63] but could such an intervention with advice on diet, exercise, and lifestyle achieve this in the population at large and in routine medical practice? Implementing such a weight-loss program in primary care has indeed been found to achieve an approximate 2.5-kg weight loss over 6–18 months.[64–66] This result was considered modest by some and was attributed to the limited contact and interaction between the obese subject and primary care physicians.[67] Therefore, noting the methodology used in the Diabetes Prevention Program[60] and the potential expense of using primary care physicians, a trial was designed to test the effect of dietary and other counseling provided on a monthly basis by medical assistants rather than by doctors in a primary care setting over a 2-year period.[68] Three interventions were compared among 390 individuals: usual care, brief lifestyle counseling, and an "enhanced" lifestyle approach that used liquid meal replacements or weight-loss medication, i.e., orlistat or sibutramine. All participants were given the same goals in terms of diet and physical activity but received different levels of support to achieve these: if below a threshold weight of 113.4 kg, a balanced diet of 1200–1500 kcal/day was prescribed, and if above a threshold weight of 113.4 kg, a diet of 1500–1800 kcal/day was provided. All were instructed to gradually increase their physical activity to 180 min per week with provision of a pedometer, a calorie-counting book, and written information relating to diet. The three interventions differed in their intensity with a greater amount of time spent counseling those in the brief lifestyle counseling group (an extra 10–15 min *each month* provided by a lifestyle coach) than in the usual care cohort (5–7 min every 3 months for 2 years provided by the primary care physician).

The primary aim was to demonstrate that both brief and enhanced lifestyle counseling would achieve a weight loss greater than that achieved by "usual" care. Education attainment was high in this cohort, which constitutes 59% white and 39% black, and the mean BMI was 38.5. At 2 years, weight measurements were available for 86% of subjects and usual care achieved a weight loss of 1.7 kg compared with 2.9 and 4.6 kg for lifestyle and enhanced lifestyle approaches, respectively. In addition, improvements in serum HDL cholesterol and triglyceride values and WC were the greatest in the enhanced lifestyle group and the strength of the effect was not weakened when those taking sibutramine were excluded from analysis. However, smaller reductions were evident at 2 years in the enhanced lifestyle group and there was no difference in the blood pressure level between groups when compared with the baseline values. Importantly, no significant difference in adverse outcome was evident. Thus, the approach of providing an enhanced lifestyle program to the wider community seems feasible but with the caveat that lower educational attainment or application among ethnic groups not studied might have different effects. One might also conclude that even allowing for the difference in time allocated, physicians are not well suited to providing advice on lifestyle and diet, a deficiency that has often been attributed to inadequacies in medical school curricula.[69,70]

Recently, novel approaches to providing support to those in weight-management programs have been tested.[71] Sending text messages of semipersonalized advice four times each week proved highly acceptable (91%), easy to understand (97%), and effective at 6 months in altering the measured variables. The effect of such intervention was the strongest for blood pressure control (i.e., similar to standard blood pressure therapy vs. placebo), for smoking, and for BMI and exercise (equal to or greater than that achieved in cardiac rehabilitation) but also significantly effective in reducing serum LDL cholesterol levels.

The effect of lifestyle interventions among obese subjects are therefore measureable in terms of risk factor reduction, and although one might assume a benefit to arise therefrom in terms of reduction in adverse cardiovascular events, the demonstration of this has proved elusive. In the Look AHEAD trial,[63] initial and durable reductions in body weight (net difference between intervention and control: 7.9% at 1 year, 2.5% at 10 years) and WC, reductions in HBA1C, improvements in physical fitness, and reductions in all cardiovascular risk factors, except serum LDL cholesterol, were demonstrated (see Fig. 8.1). In addition, the use of insulin, blood pressure–lowering medication, and statins was also lower in the intervention group. However, no discernible benefit was evident in cardiovascular morbidity or mortality at 10 years.[63]

Lifestyle Strategies—Recommendations

Intensive and comprehensive lifestyle advice delivered by health personnel trained to do so should be offered to patients who are overweight or obese. Systematic and sufficiently frequent follow-up is essential to reinforce the initial message, provide encouragement, and support as well as measuring and documenting changes in risk factors. In the United Kingdom, NICE

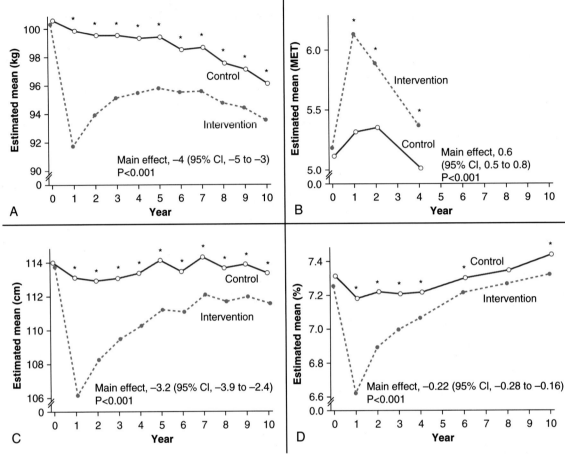

FIG. 8.1 Short- and long-term effects of intensive lifestyle intervention versus diabetes counseling (control) in obese and overweight patients with type 2 diabetes on body weight (panel A), physical fitness (panel B), waist circumference (panel C), and glycated hemoglobin (panel D). *CI,* confidence interval; *MET,* metabolic equivalent (one metabolic equivalent = the amount of oxygen consumed while sitting at rest and equals 3.5 mL oxygen per kg body weight per minute). (From The Look AHEAD Research Group. Cardiovascular effects of intensive lifestyle intervention in type 2 diabetes. *N Engl J Med.* 2013;369:145–154, with permission.)

has recommended the use of primary care and community-based multicomponent interventions to facilitate weight loss based on evidence from lifestyle data.[72]

Diet Alone—Evidence

Finding evidence in the literature of substantial benefit from dietary intervention is made especially difficult by the short-term nature of the studies and incomplete follow-up of subjects. A recent metaanalysis of the effect of dietary intervention among obese and overweight subjects[73] drew attention to a median follow-up of just 12–36 months and loss-to-follow-up rates of between 4% and 39% were cited. In 10 out of the 14 studies reviewed, loss-to-follow-up rates of 10% were evident.

In addition, no adjustment for this was made in the original analyses, but on the basis of a previous suggestion (Ware), the reviewers did correct for this by assuming these subjects had regained their original weight[73] as otherwise failure to adjust for those lost to follow up would have falsely inflated the reported weight loss. The metaanalysis therefore concluded that, after 3 years, a mean weight loss of 3.5% was evident and, after 4 years, it was 4.5%.

Dietary Strategies—Recommendations

As a guiding principle, dietary advice should be balanced, not disapproving or moralistic in tone and should avoid the hazard of inflicting nutritional deficiencies. Advance notice to the patient that weight regain is likely unless permanent changes in both lifestyle and caloric intake are made is warranted and, even if implemented, weight regain is still possible because, based on present evidence, it is difficult to predict in advance who will succeed. Weight stabilization may become an ultimate target rather than definitive weight loss.

Pharmacotherapy—Evidence

A variety of agents has been tested in obese subjects, yet only a few are currently available for use. While drug therapy can lower the risk of developing diabetes and reduce cardiovascular risk factor burden, only semaglutide has recently been found to reduce morbidity and mortality in a noninferiority trial of diabetes medication rather than one testing weight loss.[74] One aspect that undermines confidence in using any of these is the lack of long-term data on effectiveness. A recent meta-analysis found it difficult to establish the effectiveness of therapies beyond 1 year largely because four out of five of the agents included had been approved by the FDA only since 2012.[75] Among earlier agents to demonstrate promise, sibutramine was withdrawn from the market in 2010 because of reports of an increase in cardiovascular events in patients with established cardiovascular disease and the initially promising cannabinoid receptor blocker rimonabant,[76] which acts to suppress appetite centrally, was withdrawn within 2 years of approval after increased rates of suicide and depression were noted.[77] Reluctance on the part of physicians to prescribe such agents likely stems not only from the fear of inducing such harm but also from an awareness of ineffective outcomes in a significant proportion of those chosen for initial therapy.[78] A reluctance to pay for therapy at least in certain jurisdictions may also influence patients in their willingness to accept medication and the fact that weight regain is frequent after cessation of therapy also acts against uptake of agents.[78]

Pharmacotherapy—Recommendations

Pharmacotherapy is recommended for use in obesity management as an adjunct to other therapies. Together with multicomponent lifestyle modification as recommended by the U.S. Preventive Service Task Force and other bodies, significant weight loss can be achieved. Because of the potential for adverse effects from medication, it is recommended practice to overcome a threshold of achieving a weight loss of 5% at 12 weeks before suggesting suitability for long-term therapy. Drug therapy is not regarded as suitable for those who have failed to achieve this degree of initial weight loss

and merely results in exposure of an increased number of patients to potential harm without likely benefit. If weight loss at 12 weeks is not apparent, consideration should be given to drug cessation and referral for bariatric surgery.

Subjects with uncomplicated obesity

The details of the pharmacological treatment of obesity in this group of patients are discussed in Chapters 25 and 26.

Patients with comorbid conditions

Hypertension with or without LVH: Preference should be given toward using angiotensin converting enzyme (ACE) inhibitor therapy in patients who are hypertensive, especially given the favorable effect on regression of LVH.[79] Avoidance of agents that increase pulse and blood pressure is recommended.

Heart failure: In patients who have HFrEF, guidelines have traditionally suggested the use of ACE inhibitor therapy (ESC/ACC/AHA heart failure guidelines), whereas there is no evidence base for using these agents in patients with HFpEF unless hypertension coexists.

Type 2 diabetes: Metformin is used in clinical practice on the basis of its appetite-suppressing effect in overweight type 2 diabetic patients and in those who are at risk of developing diabetes.

Surgical Approaches to Obesity Management—Evidence

In general, surgical approaches to weight management are adopted when lifestyle modification and pharmacotherapy have failed. The threshold for considering surgery traditionally has not depended on BMI alone: patients with a BMI in excess of 40, or over 35, if there are coexisting obesity-related medical conditions, such as T2DM, or between 30 and 34.9 and recent-onset T2DM can be considered. National bodies have set guidelines on the selection of patients in whom bariatric surgery might be considered (BOMSS). Although long-term effects from nonrandomized studies suggest a sustainable effect from surgical intervention,[80] the evidence from randomized controlled trials of bariatric surgery points to improvements in insulin resistance, glucose control, ventricular function, blood pressure control, decreased leptin, and peroxisome proliferation-activated receptor-α–regulated genes. Two types of intervention have been studied in randomized trials: laparoscopic bypass and gastric banding. In the study by Dixon et al.,[81] 60 obese subjects (BMI 30–40) recently diagnosed (<2 years) with T2DM were randomized to either conventional lifestyle weight loss therapy alone or laparoscopic adjustable gastric banding and conventional diabetes care. 52 subjects completed the 2-year follow-up, and remission of T2DM was achieved by 22 subjects in the surgical group and 4 in the conventional therapy group. Thus, the chance of achieving remission was over five times greater for those treated by laparoscopic banding, and remission was directly related to weight loss and lower baseline HbA1c levels. There were no serious adverse outcomes in either group, but the study was not powered to examine mortality or other major cardiovascular outcomes. In addition, the significant benefit observed may not extend to all patients with T2DM. The fact that diabetes was *recently* diagnosed suggests a likely high residual pancreatic β cell function in these subjects.

In the recent STAMPEDE trial of 150 obese subjects with uncontrolled T2DM, the effects of medical therapy alone were compared against medical therapy with each of two surgical procedures at 12 months.[82] The primary end point of reaching a glycated hemoglobin of 6% or less 12 months after treatment was attained in 12% of subjects receiving medical therapy alone, 42% of those who underwent medical therapy/gastric bypass, and 37% of those receiving medical therapy/sleeve gastrectomy. Weight loss rates achieved for each group were 5.4 ± 8, 29.4 ± 9, and 25.1 ± 8.5 kg, respectively. A zero mortality rate was noted. In addition, the need to use drugs to control glucose, lipid, and blood pressure levels was reduced in patients undergoing surgery, whereas in those treated by medical therapy, the use of such medication increased. Compared with those patients in the trial by Dixon et al., patients in the STAMPEDE trial had well-established diabetes and a substantial prevalence of complications, e.g., retinopathy in 14%–22% and nephropathy with microalbuminuria in 29%. More than 60% of the surgical patients had biopsy-proven moderate to severe fatty liver.

Are the Effects Durable?

Although the evidence from the nonrandomized comparison of bariatric surgery with intensive medical therapy suggests an attenuation in the effect over time with no difference in the incidence of hypertension or hypercholesterolemia at 2- and 10-year follow-up,[80] the benefits/changes observed in randomized trials seem to be durable, at least to 5 years (Box 8.2).[83] Reduction in inflammatory markers, Apo-A, myeloperoxidase, leptin, and PAI-1 levels were noted, but there was no significant change in albuminuria, retinopathy, macular edema, or visual acuity. However, the intensity of the medical intervention has been criticized and it was noted that, by comparison, the frequency of visits in

---

BOX 8.2
Metabolic Effects of Weight Loss and Bariatric Surgery

Each 1 kg reduction in weight is associated with a reduction of:
1% in serum total cholesterol
0.7% in serum LDL cholesterol
1.9% triglycerides
1 mmHg systolic blood pressure
1 mmHg diastolic blood pressure
0.2 mmol/L serum glucose

---

the ACCORD trial was every 2 weeks for 4 months and monthly thereafter.[84] Other recent "real-world" registry data support that from randomized controlled trials; the effect is durable, at least until 4 years postsurgery. Primary care data from the United Kingdom on 3882 patients who underwent bariatric surgery were matched to obese patients who did not undergo surgery.[85] Rapid weight loss was evident in those who underwent surgery for the initial 4 months (4.98 kg per month) and at a slower rate by the end of year 4. Surgical patients were significantly less likely to develop T2DM, hypertension, angina, myocardial infarction, and obstructive sleep apnea. Resolution of T2DM and hypertension was also more likely. In addition, there was no association between bariatric surgery and risk of fractures, cancer, or stroke, and no effect on mortality was found. The likelihood of a favorable outcome was the strongest for those who had gastric bypass and sleeve gastrectomy with the weakest effect seen in gastric banding. The authors indicate that if the relationship between bariatric surgery, weight loss, and prevention of morbidity is causal, then with surgical therapy applied to the 1.4 million morbidly obese patients in England, T2DM could be averted in over 41,000 patients and resolved in 107,000 patients.

Surgical Approaches to Obesity Management—Recommendations

Although it is the most effective means by which weight loss in obese subjects can be achieved, careful selection of patients for a surgical approach to weight management is mandatory not least because of the need for long-term adherence to clinical guidance. A careful consideration of the psychological state of the patient is therefore required.

Advice to patients selected for bariatric surgery should include an awareness of potential complications and discussion regarding complication rates at the specific center in question:

- Average in-hospital mortality—0.07%
- Average postoperative length of stay—2.7 days
- Surgical complication rate—2.9% (anastomotic leakage, incisional herniation, stricture, obstruction, regurgitation)
- Revision surgery needed—1.4%; higher rates in banding
- Postoperative micronutrient deficiency (thiamine, vitamin A, iron)
- Potential for reduced bone mineral density and increased risk of fractures[86]
- Cardiovascular complications—0.3%

Support from an experienced nutritionist is essential in managing these problems, assessing levels of deficiency and prescribing appropriate replacement therapies. Multivitamin supplements may be required, and food intolerances develop including that to meat. Long-term behavioral change and adherence to a balanced diet will be essential in avoiding weight regain. More specifically and by way of illustrating the complexity of certain cases, for women of child-bearing age, avoiding pregnancy in the first 12–18 months after bariatric surgery is advised. If pregnancy is planned, it is essential to avoid vitamin A supplementation because of its adverse effects on the developing fetus.

CONCLUSION

The obesity epidemic constitutes an enormous challenge to the global health community. Much is already known about how this might be tackled, and numerous effective therapies have been proposed. Existing medical therapies for cardiovascular prevention in obesity can be effective in selected patients but are limited in their scope, and approaches to prevention, while essential and fundamental, are equally so. The scale of the problem means that bariatric surgery, the most effective therapy, cannot be regarded as the sole solution to the problem. Other research is needed to explore potential therapies in the arenas of nutrition, genetics, and their relationship with the gut microbiome.

USEFUL SOURCES OF INFORMATION

British Obesity and Metabolic Surgery Society (BOMSS) www.bomss.org.uk
British Obesity Surgery Patient Association (BOSPA) www.bospa.org
Dieticians in Obesity Management UK (DOMUK) www.domuk.org

ESC/AHA/ACC Guidelines on obesity
National Institute for Clinical Excellence www.org.uk/guidance

REFERENCES

1. Schulte H, Cullen P, Assmann G. Obesity, mortality and cardiovascular disease in the Munster heart study (PROCAM). *Atherosclerosis*. 1999;144:199–209.
2. Calle EE, Thun MJ, Petrelli JM, et al. Body mass index and mortality in a prospective cohort of US adults. *N Engl J Med*. 1999;341:1097–1105.
3. Manson JE, Willett WC, Stampfer MJ, et al. Body weight and mortality among women. *N Engl J Med*. 1995;333:677–685.
4. Garrison RJ, Castelli WP. Weight and thirty year mortality of men in the Framingham study. *Ann Intern Med*. 1985;103:1006–1009.
5. Empana JP, Ducimetiere P, Charles MA, Jouven X. Sagittal abdominal diameter and risk of sudden death in asymptomatic middle-aged men: the Paris prospective study I. *Circulation*. 2004;110:2781–2785.
6. DeMarco VG, Aroor AR, Sowers JR. The pathophysiology of hypertension in patients with obesity. *Nat Rev Endocrinol*. 2014;10(6):364–376.
7. Kannel WB, Brand N, Skinner Jr JJ, et al. The relation of adiposity to blood pressure and development of hypertension the Framingham study. *Ann Intern Med*. 1967;67:48–59.
8. Vangoitsenhoven R, Corbeels K, Mathieu C, et al. The inseverable link between obesity and glucose intolerance and how to break it? *Diabetes Res Metab*. 2016;2. OPEN ACCESS. (DRMOA-2-005).
9. Finucane MM, Stevens GA, Cowan MJ, et al. National, regional and global trends in body mass index since 1980. Systematic analysis of health examination surveys and epidemiological studies with 960 country-years and 9.1 million participants. *Lancet*. 2011;337(9765):557–567.
10. Ezatti M, Lopez AD, Rodgers A, et al. Selected major risk factors and global and regional burden of disease. *Lancet*. 2002;360:1347–1360.
11. Ogden CL, Flegal KM, Carroll MD, Johnson CL. Prevalence and trends in overweight among US children and adolescents, 1999-2000. *JAMA*. 2002;288(14):1728–1732. http://dx.doi.org/10.1001/jama.288.14.1728.
12. Flegal KM, Carroll MD, Ogden CL, Curtin LR. Prevalance and trends in obesity among US adults, 1999-2008. *JAMA*. 2010;303:235–241.
13. Ludwig DS, Ebbeling CB. Type 2 diabetes mellitus in children: primary care and public health considerations. *JAMA*. 2003;136:1427–1430.
14. Olshanksy SJ, Passaro DJ, Hershow RC, et al. A potential decline in life expectancy in the United States in the 21st Century. *N Engl J Med*. 2005;352:1138–1145.
15. *World Health Organisation Technical Report 894. Obesity: Preventing and Managing the Global Epidemic*. Geneva: WHO; 2000.

16. Futter JE, Cleland JGE, Clark AL. Body mass indices and outcome in patients with chronic heart failure. *Eur J Heart Fail.* 2011;(13):207–213.

17. Schneider HJ, Friedrich N, Klotsche J, et al. The predictive value of different measures of obesity for incident cardiovascular events and mortality. *J Clin Endocrinol Metab.* 2010;(95):1777–1785.

18. Pischon T, Boeing H, Hoffmann K, et al. General and abdominal adiposity and risk of death in Europe. *N Engl J Med.* 2008;359:2105–2120.

19. Lean MEJ, Han TS, Morrison CE. Waist circumference indicates the need for weight management. *BMJ.* 1995;311:158–161.

20. World Health Organisation 2004. Appropriate body mass index for Asian populations and its implications for policy and intervention strategies. *Lancet.* 2004;363:157–163.

21. Zheng W, Mc Lerran DF, Rolland B, et al. Association between body-mass index and risk of death in more than 1 million Asians. *N Engl J Med.* 2011;364:719–729.

22. Kelly AS, Barlow SE, Rao G, et al. Severe obesity in children and adolescents: identification, associated health risks, and treatment approaches: a scientific statement from the American Heart Association. *Circulation.* 2013;128:1689–1712.

23. Bogers RP, Bemelmans WJ, Hoogenveen RT, et al. Association of overweight with increased risk of coronary heart disease partly independent of blood pressure and cholesterol levels: a meta-analysis of 21 cohort studies including more than 300,000 persons. *Arch Intern Med.* 2007;167:1720–1728.

24. Wilson PWF, D'Agostino RB, Levy D, et al. Prediction of coronary heart disease using risk factor categories. *Circulation.* 1998;97:1837–1847.

25. Isomaa B, Almgren P, Tuomi T, et al. Cardiovascular morbidity and mortality associated with the metabolic syndrome. *Diabetes Care.* 2001;24:683–689.

26. Leibson CL, Williamson DF, Melton 3rd LJ, et al. Temporal trends in BMI among adults with diabetes. *Diabetes Care.* 2001;249:1584–1589.

27. Alam I, Ng TP, Larbi A. Does inflammation determine whether obesity is metabolically healthy or unhealthy? The aging perspective. *Mediat Inflamm.* 2012:456456. http://dx.doi.org/10.1155/2012/456456.

28. Colditz GA, Willett WC, Rotnitsky A, Manson JE. Weight gain a risk factor for clinical diabetes mellitus in women. *Ann Intern Med.* 1995;122(7):481–486.

29. Chan JM, Rimm EB, Colditz GA, Stampfer MJ, Willett WC. Obesity, fat distribution, and weight gain as risk factors for clinical diabetes in men. *Diabetes Care.* 1994;17(9):961–969.

30. Tirosh A, Shai I, Afek A, et al. Adolescent BMI trajectory and risk of diabetes versus coronary disease. *N Engl J Med.* 2011;364:1315–1325.

31. Twig G, Yaniv G, Levine H, et al. Body-mass index in 2.3 million adolescents and cardiovascular death in adulthood. *N Engl J Med.* 2016;374:2430–2440.

32. Kenchaiah S, Evans JC, Levy D, et al. Obesity and the risk of heart failure. *N Engl J Med.* 2002;347:305–313.

33. Alpert MA, Terry BE, Mulekar M, et al. Cardiac morphology and left ventricular function in morbidly obese patients with and without congestive heart failure and effect of weight loss. *Am J Cardiol.* 1997;80:736–740.

34. Pozzo J, Fournier P, Lairez O, et al. Obesity paradox: origin and best way to assess severity in patients with systolic HF. *Obesity (Silver Spring).* 2015;23:2002–2008.

35. Adamopoulos C, Meyer P, Desai RV, et al. Absence of obesity paradox in patients with chronic heart failure and diabetes mellitus: a propensity-matched study. *Eur J Heart Fail.* 2011;13:200–206.

36. Horwich TB, Fonarow GC, Hamilton MA, et al. The relationship between obesity and mortality in patients with heart failure. *J Am Coll Cardiol.* 2001;38:789–795.

37. Romero-Corral A, Montori VM, Somers VK, et al. Association of body weight with total mortality and with cardiovascular events in coronary artery disease: a systematic review of cohort studies. *Lancet.* 2006;368:666–678.

38. Uretsky S, Messerli FH, Bangalore S, et al. Obesity paradox in patients with hypertension and coronary artery disease. *Am J Med.* 2007;120:863–870.

39. Lam CS, Donal E, Kraigher-Krainer E, Vasan RS. Epidemiology and clinical course of heart failure with preserved ejection fraction. *Eur J Heart Fail.* 2011;13:18–28.

40. Oreopoulos A, Padwal R, Kalanatar-Zadeh K, et al. Body mass index and mortality in heart failure: a meta-analysis. *Am Heart J.* 2008;156:13–22.

41. Fonarow GC, Srikhanthan P, Costanzo MR, et al. An obesity paradox in acute heart failure: analysis of body mass index and in-hospital mortality for 108,927 patients in the acute decompensated heart failure national registry. *Am Heart J.* 2007;153:74–81.

42. Madala MC, Franklin BA, Chen AY, et al. Obesity and age of first non–ST-segment elevation myocardial infarction. *JACC.* 2008;52:979–985.

43. Lavie CJ, Milani RV, Artham SM, et al. The obesity paradox, weight loss and coronary disease. *Am J Med.* 2009;122(12):1106–1114.

44. Wang L, Liu W, He L, et al. Association of overweight and obesity with patient mortality after acute myocardial infarction. *Int J Obes.* 2015. http://dx.doi.org/10.138/ijo.2015.176.

45. Wassertheil-Smoller S, Fann C, Allman RM, et al. Relation of low body mass to death and stroke in the systolic hypertension in the elderly program. *Arch Intern Med.* 2000;160:494–500.

46. Kenchaiah S, Pocock SJ, Wang D, et al. Body mass index and prognosis in patients with chronic heart failure: insights from the Candesartan in Heart Failure Assessment of Reduction in Mortality and Morbidity (CHARM) program. *Circulation.* 2007;116:627–636.

47. Arena R, Myers J, Abella J, et al. Influence of etiology of heart failure on the obesity paradox. *Am J Cardiol.* 2009;104:1116–1121.

48. Lavie CJ, Mehra MR, Milani RV. Obesity and heart failure prognosis: paradox or reverse epidemiology. *Eur Heart J.* 2005;26:5–7.

49. Rauchhaus M, Coats AJC, Anker SD. The endotoxin-lipoprotein hypothesis. *Lancet.* 2000;356:930–933.

50. Mehra MR, Uber PA, Parh MH, et al. Obesity and suppressed B-type natriuretic levels in heart failure. *J Am Coll Cardiol.* 2004;43:1590–1595.

51. Mohamed-Ali V, Goodrick AS, Bulmer AK, et al. Production of soluble necrosis factor receptors by human subcutaneous adipose tissue in vivo. *Am J Physiol.* 1999;227:E971–E975.

52. Marenberg ME, Risch N, Berkman LF, Floderus B, de Faire U. Genetic susceptibility to death from coronary heart disease in a study of twins. *N Engl J Med.* 1994;330:1041–1046.

53. Lloyd-Jones DM, Nam B-H, D'Agostino RB, et al. Parental cardiovascular disease as a risk factor for cardiovascular disease in middle-aged adults a prospective study of parents and offspring. *JAMA.* 2004;291:2204–2211.

54. Sharifi M, Rakhit RD, Humphries SE, Nair D. Cardiovascular risk stratification in familial hypercholesterolaemia. *Heart.* 2016;0:1–6. http://dx.doi.org/10.1136/heartjnl-2015-308845. Also Heart Online First 2016.

55. Menella JA, Jagnow CP, Beauchamp GK. Prenatal and postnatal flavor learning by human infants. *Pediatrics.* 2001;107:E88.

56. Georgousopoulou EN, Kouli GM, Panagiotakos DB, et al. Anti-inflammatory diet and 10-year (2002-2012) cardiovascular disease incidence: the ATTICA study. *Int J Cardiol.* 2016;222:473–478.

57. Parekh PJ, Blart LA, Johnson DA. The influence of the gut microbiome on obesity, metabolic syndrome, and gastrointestinal disease. *Clin Transl Gastroenterol.* 2015;6:e91. http://dx.doi.org/10.1038/ctg.2015.16.

58. Karpe F, Lindgren CM. Obesity – on or off. *N Engl J Med.* 2016;374:1486–1488.

59. Hartstra AV, Bouter KEC, Bäckhed F, Nieuwdorp M. Insights into the role of the microbiome in obesity and type 2 diabetes. *Diabetes Care.* 2015;38:159–165.

60. Knowler WC, Barrett-Connor E, Fowler SF, et al. Reduction in the incidence of type 2 diabetes with lifestyle intervention or metformin. *N Engl J Med.* 2002;346:393–403.

61. Mason C, Foster-Schubert KE, Imayama I, et al. Dietary weight loss and exercise effects on insulin resistance in postmenopausal women. *Am J Prev Med.* 2011;41(4):366–375.

62. Tuomilehto J, Lindstrom J, Eriksson JG, et al. Prevention of type 2 diabetes by changes in lifestyle among subjects with impaired glucose tolerance. *N Engl J Med.* 2001;344(18):1343–1350.

63. The Look AHEAD Research Group. Cardiovascular effects of intensive lifestyle intervention in type 2 diabetes. *N Engl J Med.* 2013;369:145–154.

64. Martin PD, Dutton GR, Rhode PC, et al. Weight loss maintenance following a primary care intervention for low-income minority women. *Obesity (Silver Spring).* 2008;16:2462–2467.

65. Christian JG, Bessesen DH, Byers TE, et al. Clinic-based support to help overweight patients with type 2 diabetes increase physical activity and lose weight. *Arch Intern Med.* 2008;168:141–146.

66. Ockene IS, Hebert JR, Ockene JK, et al. Effect of physician-delivered nutrition counselling training and an office-support program on saturated fat intake, weight and serum lipid measurements in a hyperlipidemic population: Worcester Area Trial for Counselling in Hyperlipidemia (WATCH). *Arch Intern Med.* 1999;159:725–731.

67. Prevention Services Task Force. Screening for obesity in adults: recommendations and rationale. *Ann Intern Med.* 2003;139:930–932.

68. Wadden TA, Volger S, Sarwer DB, et al. A two-year randomised trial of obesity treatment in primary care practice. *N Engl J Med.* 2011;365:1969–1979.

69. Devries S, Dalen J, Eisenberg DM, et al. A deficiency of nutrition education in medical training. *Am J Med.* 2014. http://dx.doi.org/10.1016/j.amjmed.2014.04.003.

70. Kushner RF, Van Horn L, Rock CL, et al. Nutrition education in medical school: a time of opportunity. *Am J Clin Nutr.* 2014;99(suppl):1167S–1173S.

71. Chow CK, Redfern J, Hillis GS, et al. Effect of lifestyle-focused text messaging on risk factor modification in patients with coronary heart disease: a randomised clinical trial. *JAMA.* 2015;314:1255–1263.

72. Kirk SFL, Penney TL, McHugh TL, Sharma AM. Effective weight management practice: a review of the lifestyle intervention evidence. *Int J Obes.* 2012;36:178–185.

73. Langeveld M, DeVries JH. The long term effect of energy restricted diets for treating obesity. *Obesity.* 2015;23:1529–1538. http://dx.doi.org/10.1002/oby.21146.

74. Marso SP, Bain SC, Consoli A, et al. Semaglutide and cardiovascular outcomes in patients with type 2 diabetes. *N Engl J Med.* 2016;375:1834–1844.

75. Khera R, Murad MH, Chandar AK, et al. Association of pharmacological treatments for obesity with weight loss and adverse effects: a systematic review and meta-analysis. *JAMA.* 2016;315:2424–2434.

76. Pi-Sunyer FX, Aronne LJ, Heshmati HM, Devin J, Rosenstock J. Effect of rimonabant, a cannabinoid-1 receptor blocker, on weight and cardiometabolic risk factors in overweight or obese patients: RIO-North America: a randomized controlled trial. *JAMA.* 2006;295(7):761–775.

77. European Medicines Agency. *The European Medicines Agency Recommends Suspension of the Marketing Authorisation of Acomplia*; October 23, 2008.

78. Yanovski SZ, Yanovski JA. Long-term drug treatment for obesity: a systematic and clinical review. *JAMA.* 2014;311:74–86.

79. Dahlof B, Devereux RB, Kjeldsen SE, et al. Cardiovascular morbidity and mortality in the Losartan intervention for endpoint reduction in hypertension study (LIFE): a randomised trial against atenolol. *Lancet.* 2002;359:995–1003.

80. Sjostrum L, Lindroos A-K, Peltonen M, et al. Lifestyle, diabetes, and cardiovascular risk factors 10 years after bariatric surgery. *N Engl J Med.* 2004;351:2683–2693.

81. Dixon JB, O'Brien PE, Playfair J, et al. Adjustable gastric banding and conventional therapy for Type 2 diabetes. A randomised controlled trial. *JAMA.* 2008;299(3):316–323.

82. Schauer PR, Kashyap SR, Wolski K, et al. Bariatric surgery versus intensive medical therapy in obese patients with diabetes. *N Engl J Med*. 2012;366:1567–1576.

83. Schauer PR, Bhatt DL, Kirwan JP, et al. Bariatric surgery versus intensive medical therapy for diabetes—5-year outcomes. *N Engl J Med*. 2017;376:641–651.

84. The Action to Control Cardiovascular Risk in Diabetes Study Group. Effects of intensive glucose lowering in type 2 diabetes. *N Engl J Med*. 2008;358:2545–2559.

85. Douglas IJ, Bhaskaran K, Batterham RL, Smeeth L. Bariatric surgery in the United Kingdom: a cohort study of weight loss and clinical outcomes in routine clinical care. *PLOS Med*. 2015. http://dx.doi.org/10.1371/journal.pmed.1001925.

86. Rousseau C, Jean S, Gamache P, et al. Change in fracture risk and fracture pattern after bariatric surgery: nested case-control study. *BMJ*. 2016;354:i3794. http://dx.doi.org/10.1136/bmj.i3794.

FURTHER READING

1. Pi-Sunyer X, Astrup A, Fujioka K, et al. A randomised, controlled trial of 3.0 mg of liraglutide in weight management. *N Engl J Med*. 2015;373:11–22.

CHAPTER 9

Obesity and Nonalcoholic Fatty Liver Disease

NIMANTHA M.W. De ALWIS, MBBS, MD, FRCP, PHD

INTRODUCTION

The liver plays an important role in the metabolism and storage of lipids. In certain individuals, fat can be deposited in hepatocytes resulting in a "fatty liver," which can be associated with adverse cardiometabolic and liver-related disease. Obesity is a major risk factor for fatty liver. Nonalcoholic fatty liver disease (NAFLD) a spectrum of liver disease usually reserved for describing a chronic liver disease in the absence of significant alcohol consumption. Its close association with obesity and other cardiometabolic parameters has been confirmed and is now recognized as the commonest chronic liver disease worldwide. The healthcare burden of this disease has increased with the epidemics of obesity and diabetes.

THE HISTORICAL PERSPECTIVE OF FATTY LIVER DISEASE

In 1836 Thomas Addison from Newcastle first used the term "fatty liver" and was possibly describing an alcohol-related pathology.[1] Fatty liver associated with diabetes was described in 1884 by Pepper and its link to obesity and starvation was described in 1885 by Bartolow.[2] Since then, several authors described fatty liver similar to alcohol-related disease in those with diabetes and obesity who did not consume excess alcohol. However, the recent interest in NAFLD was not until 1980 when Ludwig et al. used the term nonalcoholic steatohepatitis (NASH) and described it as "a poorly understood and hitherto unnamed liver disease that histologically mimics alcoholic hepatitis and that may also progress to cirrhosis…." This was a cohort of 20 patients who were not alcohol misusers and had histologic evidence of steatohepatitis comprising of steatosis, hepatocyte ballooning, and fibrosis.[3]

THE SPECTRUM OF NONALCOHOLIC FATTY LIVER DISEASE

NAFLD is a spectrum of liver disease. Simple fatty deposition within hepatocytes (fatty liver) may be a benign, reversible condition. However, in some, this can lead to hepatic inflammation (NASH) and varying degrees of fibrosis and permanent liver damage. The latter can lead to cirrhosis and hepatocellular carcinoma (HCC).[4]

NAFLD is largely asymptomatic and most often diagnosed incidentally by the finding of unexpected abnormalities in liver blood tests or imaging, most often a bright liver on ultrasonography (US).[5,6] Case finding in high-risk groups has been suggested by some but not all guidelines published to date. Unfortunately, there are currently no simple, reliable, noninvasive tests in routine use for case finding, diagnosing, staging, and monitoring, although several biomarkers and imaging modalities have shown promise.[7] Despite being first described over 35 years ago, the lack of effective therapy continues to contribute to the current lack of enthusiasm among both primary and secondary care providers for case finding and diagnosing NAFLD.

EPIDEMIOLOGY

NAFLD is considered the liver component of the metabolic syndrome (MS) and is associated with several other cardiometabolic parameters including hyperlipidemia, insulin resistance, and coronary vascular disease.[8,9] NAFLD is now the commonest chronic liver disease in Western adults and is the second commonest cause of liver transplantation in the United States.

A recent large metaanalysis of over 300,000 patients reported that the prevalence of NAFLD in an obese population was 3.5 times that of nonobese. This also showed an incremental risk (per 1-unit increment in BMI: RR = 1.20) with a rising body mass index (BMI).[10] The current global prevalence of NAFLD is reported to be 25% with the highest prevalence in the Middle East and South America, although this figure can change depending on the screening method and population.[11] With the growing pandemic of obesity, the net population with NAFLD is likely to grow accordingly. NAFLD is an increasing indication for liver transplantation[5,11] and has been associated with increases in both liver- and cardiovascular-related mortality. The burden of NAFLD in an obese population is currently not recognized or addressed. Additionally, the worldwide prevalence of type 2 diabetes mellitus (T2DM) is increasing and is currently at 6%. These risk factors are contributing to a global rise in the risk of cardiovascular morbidity and mortality.[11] Strategies are required to prevent, diagnose, and manage NAFLD to reduce the disease burden.[12]

THE IMPORTANCE OF DIAGNOSING NONALCOHOLIC FATTY LIVER DISEASE

In the United States, NAFLD is now the second most common chronic liver disease among those awaiting a liver transplantation.[13] NAFLD is also the commonest cause of HCC in several countries.[4,14] Furthermore, in those who have T2DM, NAFLD increases the risk of atrial fibrillation, ischemic stroke, need for coronary revascularization, myocardial infarction, and cardiovascular death. The latter is the most common cause of mortality in NAFLD and is probably underestimated.[5,14] Given its contribution to liver and cardiovascular morbidity and mortality, it is clearly important to diagnose NAFLD at a stage where it may be reversible with lifestyle and/or pharmacologic management.

THE CLINICAL EVALUATION OF NONALCOHOLIC FATTY LIVER DISEASE

The diagnosis of NAFLD is usually following the incidental detection of a fatty liver on ultrasonography (US) or the exclusion of other causes of liver disease in an individual who does not consume excess alcohol and has abnormal liver blood tests.[6,15] This may lead to a review of clinical symptoms and signs.

Up to 80% of those with a fatty liver may have completely normal liver biochemistry. A raised alanine transaminase (ALT), aspartate transaminase (AST), alkaline phosphatase (ALP), and gamma-glutamyl transferase (GGT) are nonspecific. Ultrasound is possibly the commonest diagnostic tool used. Because of the lack of robust diagnostic markers, several collections of combined biophysical and biochemical parameters have been used. The fatty liver index (FLI) is one such. The FLI includes four variables: BMI, waist circumference, triglycerides, and GGT.[16] A score of 30 or less has a sensitivity of 87% and a score of 60 or more a specificity of 86% for steatosis. Other reports have shown a lower specificity in obese individuals of around 49%.[17]

DIAGNOSIS OF NONALCOHOLIC FATTY LIVER DISEASE
History and Examination

In an individual with suspected NAFLD due to biochemical or US abnormality (or a positive FLI test), a full clinical history is important to exclude other potential causes of steatosis and to look for conditions associated with this condition.[16] Most patients with NAFLD are asymptomatic—if symptoms are present, they tend to be nonspecific including fatigue, sleep disturbance, and/or right hypochondrial discomfort. Alternative causes of steatosis include excessive alcohol consumption (excluded by a consumption of <30 g alcohol per day for men and <20 g per day for women),[18] chronic hepatitis C infection (genotype 3), autoimmune liver disease, hemochromatosis, and Wilson's disease.[19] A careful drug history must also be taken, because a number of drugs have been associated with hepatic steatosis, including amiodarone, glucocorticoids, and methotrexate. In addition to features of the MS, other conditions associated with NAFLD include endocrine disorders, such as hypothyroidism, hypogonadism, hypopituitarism, and polycystic ovary syndrome. Examination is likely to be unremarkable apart from an enlarged liver and signs of portal hypertension in advanced fibrotic disease or cirrhosis. Clinical assessment should include a biophysical assessment for features of the MS including BMI, waist circumference, and blood pressure.

Biochemical Analysis

Although mildly deranged liver enzymes on routine testing often raise the first suspicion, clinicians must not overly rely on abnormal liver biochemistry to detect NAFLD because in over 80% of the patients the biochemistry remains normal, leading to patients remaining undiagnosed and untreated.[7,20,21] Important biochemical tests would include ALT, AST, prothrombin time, albumin and platelet count to assess liver activity, synthetic function, and the possibility of hypersplenism related to portal hypertension, respectively. The ALT is usually two to five times elevated in NAFLD. The ALT/AST ratio is greater than 1 unless there is advanced fibrosis or alcoholic liver disease. ALP is usually elevated but is not specific to NAFLD, and GGT can be raised in any metabolic disease.[22] Although there is some evidence that a raised ferritin (present in about 60% of NAFLD patients) is a marker of advanced fibrosis, it does not usually indicate a diagnosis of hemochromatosis, which relies on a raised transferrin saturation.[23] Anti–smooth muscle and α–smooth muscle actin-specific antibody levels can be positive at low titer in NAFLD and do not indicate a diagnosis of autoimmune hepatitis. HbA1C, urea and electrolytes, lipid profile, and thyroid-stimulating hormone should be measured to assess for related metabolic diseases. Cytokeratin 18 fragments are a marker of hepatocyte apoptosis and are used in some centers to diagnose NASH; however, this test has not come into widespread use because of uncertainties over its accuracy.[24]

BIOMARKERS AND IMAGING IN NONALCOHOLIC FATTY LIVER DISEASE

Liver Steatosis

Individual clinical features and biochemical tests have limited use in the diagnosis of steatosis, NASH, or liver fibrosis. Therefore several panels or "scores" consisting of combinations of parameters have been developed for the diagnosis and quantification of steatosis. The most studied panels thus far are the FLI (described above), the SteatoTest, and the NAFLD liver fat (NLF) score. SteatoTest is an algorithm based on α-2-macroglobulin, haptoglobin, apolipoprotein A1, GGT, total bilirubin, ALT, BMI, cholesterol, triglyceride, and glucose, adjusted for age and gender. A cutoff of 0.3 has a sensitivity of 85% to diagnose steatosis and a cutoff of 0.7 has a specificity of 80%.[25] The SteatoTest has an area under the receiver operating characteristic curve (AUROC) of 0.8 for diagnosing more than 30% steatosis in the liver.[26] The NLF score is based on the presence of MS; T2DM, fasting insulin, fasting AST, and AST/ALT ratio. A cutoff of −0.640 predicted increased liver fat with a sensitivity of 86% and a specificity of 71%.[16,27] Other indices include the liver accumulation product, which includes waist circumference, triglycerides, and gender, and the hepatic steatosis index, which includes AST/ALT ratio, BMI, and diabetes.[12] This has an AUROC of 0.812. A cutoff point less than 30 had sensitivity for a diagnosis of steatosis of 93%, and a cutoff of greater than 36 ruled out steatosis with a specificity of 92%. Unfortunately, none of these indices has gained much popularity or is used in routine clinical practice. The FLI may be the simplest and cheapest test showing the most promise for use in primary care or in case finding of liver steatosis. Combined biomarkers of steatosis are summarized in Table 9.1.

TABLE 9.1
Steatosis Indices and Parameters

Steatosis Index	Measured Parameters
Fatty liver index	Weight, height, waist, GGT, triglycerides
SteatoTest	α-2-Macroglobulin, haptoglobin, apolipoprotein A1, GGT, total bilirubin, ALT, BMI, cholesterol, triglyceride, and glucose
NAFLD liver fat (NFL) Score	Metabolic syndrome, T2DM, fasting insulin, AST, AST/ALT ratio
Liver accumulation product (LAP)	Waist circumference, triglycerides, gender
Hepatic steatosis index (HIS)	AST/ALT ratio, BMI, T2DM

ALT, alanine transaminase; *AST*, aspartate transaminase; *BMI*, body mass index; *GGT*, gamma-glutamyl transferase; *T2DM*, type 2 diabetes mellitus.

Imaging techniques for steatosis

Ultrasound is noninvasive, widely available, and the cheapest, most commonly used imaging modality for the diagnosis of NAFLD. US can detect increased fat in the liver (when >33% hepatocytes are affected) with a sensitivity of 64% and a specificity of 87%. Routine US does not enable the quantification of steatosis or fibrosis and cannot identify the presence of NASH.[28] US-based continued attenuation parameter may be used to quantify steatosis[29]; however, the reliability and reproducibility of this technique remains to be confirmed[30] and the clinical utility of accurately quantifying liver fat is unclear. Several magnetic resonance–based imaging modalities have been assessed for their ability to diagnose and quantify steatosis, but none is in routine use in clinical practice.[31] Magnetic resonance–determined proton density fat fraction seems to be the most accurate methodology developed thus far for diagnosing, grading, and monitoring steatosis.[32,33] It has the advantage over magnetic resonance spectroscopy of being able to assess the entire liver in a single measurement rather than a sample of it. At present, however, its expense and availability have restricted its use to research settings.

Liver Fibrosis

Advanced liver fibrosis (stage 3 or 4) is the strongest predictor of liver-related mortality in NAFLD,[34] and accordingly, considerable efforts have been made to identify noninvasive markers capable of accurately identifying its presence.[35] The presence of NASH seems to be less significant as a predictor of outcome and, as a result, noninvasive methods for its diagnosis have received less attention. Liver blood tests such as AST/ALT ratio (alone or including the AST to platelet ratio index), ferritin,[36] and procollagen-3-peptide[37] have all shown to identify the presence of advanced fibrosis with reasonable accuracy, although their negative predictive values are considerably better than their positive predictive values (PPVs). Several expanded laboratory tests have also shown utility in identifying stage 3 or 4 fibrosis with the NAFLD fibrosis score (NFS), Fibrosis-4 (FIB-4), BARD, and the enhanced liver fibrosis (ELF) score the best validated to date. Some of these have also been shown to predict cardiovascular- and liver-related mortality.[38]

The NFS uses six variables including age, BMI, T2DM, AST/ALT ratio, platelet count, and serum albumin. This has been validated in an international multicenter study with liver biopsy–confirmed NAFLD.[39] It carries a high accuracy for excluding advanced fibrosis with a negative predictive value (NPV) of 93 and 88% (score less than −1.455) in training and validation groups, respectively, and a PPV of 90 and 92% (score greater than 0.676). It was estimated to avoid liver biopsy in 75% of patients. Several subsequent studies have confirmed the high accuracy of the NFS in distinguishing patients with and without advanced fibrosis. The FIB-4 index has been suggested to be useful in excluding patients without advanced fibrosis with an NPP of 90% (cutoff less than 1.3) but a much lower PPV.[40] These two scores have been externally validated in different NAFLD populations using liver biopsy with consistent results. The European Liver Fibrosis group assessed the combination of age and serum markers, namely, hyaluronic acid, aminoterminal propeptide of type III collagen, and tissue inhibitor of matrix metalloproteinase 1 in predicting advanced fibrosis in a range of liver diseases.[41] The Enhanced Liver Fibrosis (ELF) score of 0.3576 had an AUROC of 0.93 with a sensitivity of 80% for detecting advanced fibrosis and a specificity of 90% in ruling out advanced fibrosis. However, the biochemical parameters in the ELF test are not in routine use in hospital biochemical panels, and adopting this would require the demonstration of significant cost-benefit. Combined biomarkers of liver fibrosis are summarized in Table 9.2.

Imaging techniques for fibrosis

Of the imaging techniques evaluated for their ability to detect advanced fibrosis, transient elastography (TE) has received the most attention and is being used in routine clinical practice.[42] This measures the elasticity of the liver in 1 × 4 cm cylinders and is measured in kilopascals. The advantages include being a relatively

TABLE 9.2
Hepatic Fibrosis Indices and Parameters

Fibrosis Index	Measured Parameters
NAFLD fibrosis score	Age, T2DM, BMI, platelet count, albumin, AST/ALT ratio
FIB-4 score	Age, AST, ALT
BARD score	BMI, AST/ALT ratio, T2DM
Enhanced liver fibrosis (ELF) score	Age, hyaluronic acid, aminoterminal propeptide of type III collagen, tissue inhibitor of metalloproteinase 1

ALT, alanine transaminase; *AST*, aspartate transaminase; *BMI*, body mass index; *T2DM*, type 2 diabetes mellitus.

quick (<5 min) procedure with immediate results that can be done at the bedside in a routine outpatient clinic. Although initially used in hepatitis C, its use in NAFLD is increasing. A recent large pool of 1047 patients from various ethnic backgrounds suggested a sensitivity of 79% and a specificity of 75% for detecting significant fibrosis in NAFLD. Obtaining accurate readings in the presence of obesity is a problem with using TE in NAFLD, although the introduction of the extra large probe for those with a higher BMI may circumvent this. Several other imaging modalities for liver elasticity are in development, including acoustic radiation force impulse Imaging (ARFI) and MR-based elastography. ARFI is likely to be better in obese subjects and further evaluation is awaited.[42–44] Currently, combinations of TE and serum biomarkers (NFS, FIB-4, and ELF) are widely used to stage NAFLD.

LIVER BIOPSY IN NONALCOHOLIC FATTY LIVER DISEASE

Because of the high prevalence of NAFLD, liver biopsy is clearly impractical for routine diagnosis and staging. However, a place for liver biopsy may still remain in certain settings: individuals may feel the need to know the accurate stage of their disease; noninvasive tests may produce an "indeterminate" result or there may be issue with differential diagnosis. Liver biopsy also remains important in the clinical trial setting and for research purposes. Brunt et al. suggested the initial grading for NAFLD[45,46] (Table 9.1). The NAFLD activity score developed by the NASH Clinical Research Network is based on this and is currently the most widely used measure of grading.[46] This score includes a numerical score for steatosis (0–3), hepatocyte ballooning (1–2), and lobular inflammation (0–3). The score thresholds of <3 and >5 correlate with the diagnosis of "not-NASH" and NASH, respectively. The NAS is mainly used in clinical trials to differentiate changes in individual key features of NASH and is not designed to differentiate between the various stages of the NAFLD spectrum. Recently, European Fatty Liver Inhibition of Progression Consortium developed an algorithm to aid in the histologic diagnosis of NASH.[47] This is another semiquantitative scoring of key features of NASH, including steatosis (S) (0–3), activity (A) (0–4), and fibrosis (F) (0–4). This score can differentiate between steatosis and NASH and the latter is only applied if all three features of steatosis, hepatocellular ballooning, and acinar inflammation are present. The SAF score also defines two categories of NAFLD severity: mild disease (A < 2 and/or F < 2) and significant disease (A > 2 and/or F > 2) depending on hepatocellular ballooning, acinar inflammation, and fibrosis. The impact of this score on NAFLD pathophysiology is yet to be defined in further studies.

SCREENING FOR HEPATOCELLULAR CARCINOMA

Because of the high risk of progression to HCC, those with NAFLD may warrant screening. HCC in NAFLD can occur without the presence of cirrhosis in nearly 50% of those with NAFLD progressing more aggressively compared with those with hepatitis C–related HCC.[48,49] Although it is a routine practice to screen those with cirrhosis for HCC in most etiologies, earlier screening in those with NASH may be warranted although the cost-effectiveness of this must be further analyzed.

THE DIAGNOSIS AND STAGING OF NONALCOHOLIC FATTY LIVER DISEASE IN THE FUTURE

Currently, routine case finding of NAFLD in those with metabolic risk factors is not universal and further guidance to physicians in primary and secondary care is required. Calculating the FLI is probably cost-effective and is relatively simple. The staging of NAFLD is recommended using NAFLD or FIB-4 to identify those with low or high risk combined with ELF or ARFI for those in the indeterminate category. Liver biopsy would only be recommended in a minority with a diagnostic dilemma. Recently identified genetic risk factors (PNPLA3, TM6SF2, GCKR, IGNL4) may be incorporated into clinical practice as these tests become more readily used. Oral glucose insulin sensitivity index has been shown to be associated with peripheral insulin

sensitivity in NAFLD and inversely associated with an increased risk of significant liver damage in nondiabetic subjects with NAFLD. It was shown to be better than the NFS in a recent study.[50] Some have also studied the usefulness of combining biochemical tests proven to be indicative of fatty liver with genetic variants such as PNPLA3 but have shown little contribution from the genetic analysis.[27] None has managed to show any correlation between genetic factors and risk of progression of NAFLD either. However, carrying the PNPLA3 rs738409C>G mutation may be indicative of a higher risk of HCC.[51] The role of epigenetics in transmission of risk of fibrosis has been studied in mice and may be a feature to look forward to in the future.[52] Recent studies and the future direction and utility of the use of the gut microbiota and relationship with the severity and NAFLD are also awaited with interest.[53]

PATHOPHYSIOLOGY OF NONALCOHOLIC FATTY LIVER DISEASE

The "two-hit" theory of NAFLD was a recognized one but is now largely superseded. While the pathophysiology continues to be debated, a few facts come about consistently. The association with insulin resistance is one of the key factors and thus up to 80% of those with T2DM seem to be effected by this condition. Nutritional, lifestyle, immunologic, genetic, and ethnic factors have been reported historically. Epigenetics and gut microbiota also seem to have been associated lately.

NAFLD correlates with hepatic and peripheral insulin resistance. In the liver, insulin resistance is associated with increased hepatic gluconeogenesis and reduced glycogen production. This results in increased hepatic fat deposition.[54-56] Peripheral insulin resistance results in less fat deposition in peripheral adipose tissue and forces liver fat accumulation. The liver gets fat from various sources including diet (15%), circulation (59%), and de novo lipogenesis (26%).[57] The latter can increase threefold in NAFLD and is related to stimulation by high levels of insulin, via the sterol regulatory element binding protein 1 c pathway, and by glucose, via the carbohydrate regulatory element binding protein. Therefore, insulin resistance and increased dietary fats can worsen hepatic fat deposition, i.e., fatty liver. Additionally, the hepatic free fatty acid pool is increased by reduced very low density lipoprotein–based lipid export from the liver.[54] Patients with NASH have also been shown to have various hepatic mitochondrial alterations, including depletion of mitochondrial DNA, abnormal redox homeostasis, and increased reactive oxygen species.[58,59] Mitochondria adapt to liver fat and inflammation, and when this capacity is exceeded, this results in lipid deposition and insulin resistance. Several hepatic proinflammatory cytokines, including interleukin 6 and tumor necrosis factor α, transcription factors (NF-KB), and extra hepatic cytokines, are activated in insulin resistance and play a significant role in the pathophysiology of NAFLD.[60]

FATTY LIVER AND TYPE 2 DIABETES MELLITUS

NAFLD is universally associated with insulin resistance. Therefore, it is no surprise that the risk of T2DM is extremely high in this population. Several large epidemiologic studies have demonstrated that a rise in ALT or GGT may predict the onset of diabetes.[61] This can be compounded by the fact that up to 80% of those with NAFLD may have normal liver enzyme levels.[21] In ultrasound-detected fatty liver, the risk of subsequent diabetes is increased by up to fivefold even after correction for other metabolic and lifestyle factors.[62] While the clearance of liver fat improves T2DM, increasing levels of liver fat seem to increase the incidence of T2DM. Initially, simple steatosis was thought to be a benign condition. However, it has been shown that in the case of those with insulin resistance and T2DM, there was progression to fibrosis even in patients with simple steatosis.[63] Therefore, it seems mandatory that screening for T2DM is undertaken periodically in those with NAFLD and not known to have T2DM, particularly if metabolic risk factors were to worsen.

NONALCOHOLIC FATTY LIVER DISEASE AND THE METABOLIC SYNDROME

Because NAFLD is considered to be the hepatic component of the MS, all components including increased waist circumference, low HDL, high triglycerides, elevated blood pressure, and T2DM are associated.[64] Therefore, it is logical that any person with positive parameters of the MS should be actively screened for NAFLD as well. The importance of the MS is that it is associated with increased cardiovascular morbidity and mortality. NAFLD itself has been shown to be an independent risk factor for cardiovascular disease.

NONALCOHOLIC STEATOHEPATITIS AND FIBROSIS WITH TYPE 2 DIABETES MELLITUS

Previously described cryptogenic cirrhosis is now thought to be due to NAFLD fibrosis. Several studies using different modalities have shown a high prevalence of fibrosis in patients with NAFLD and T2DM.[65]

Patients with T2DM have more severe forms of the NAFLD spectrum than those without T2DM with rates of up to 80% with NASH and 30%–40% with fibrosis.[66]

NONALCOHOLIC FATTY LIVER DISEASE AND HEPATOCELLULAR CARCINOMA

Although the commonest cause of death in those with NAFLD, obesity, and T2DM is cardiovascular disease, the burden of cirrhosis and HCC cannot be ignored. The prevalence of HCC is increasing in many Western countries. A report from Newcastle showed a 10-fold increase in 10 years between 2000 and 2010 in Newcastle. Additionally HCC has also been demonstrated in those with NASH without cirrhosis.[67] Many patients with NAFLD and HCC show a high incidence of obesity and hypertension. Smoking and alcohol may also have a synergistic effect on HCC.

MANAGEMENT OF NONALCOHOLIC FATTY LIVER DISEASE

Patient Education and Lifestyle Modification Including Diet and Exercise

One of the key elements in the management of NAFLD is patient education. Healthcare professionals are only just beginning to realize the presence of NAFLD as a common liver disease. The task of patient education seems daunting given how common this condition is. Those with risk factors are simply not aware of the potential development of liver cirrhosis or HCC and are often surprised and alarmed at being told they have a diagnosis with no contribution from alcohol. While we await the advent of a noninvasive, robust technique to diagnose NASH and those at risk of significant liver fibrosis, other risk assessment tools must be used to describe, at best, the risk of significant liver fibrosis. The NAFLD liver fibrosis score could be used. Some may take up the offer of a liver biopsy to be more informed of their condition, given there are no robust noninvasive markers.

Because there are no definitive treatment options on offer, it has been difficult to convince some patients and most healthcare professionals on the importance of patient education, investigation, and management. Because of the paucity of a pharmacologic treatment for NAFLD and, in particular NASH, lifestyle modifications are an important step in management.

The initial management of related T2DM and obesity is lifestyle modification through change in diet and exercise regimes. Reducing calorie intake, converting to a Mediterranean-type diet high in polyunsaturated fatty acids, increasing exercise, and modifying risk factors, such as smoking and excessive alcohol intake, are important. Weight reduction may be one of the most cost-effective modalities to reduce cardiovascular burden, given its beneficial effects on multiple risk factors. Studies in NAFLD have shown that up to 7% weight reduction may be required to show any histologic benefit, but any degree of weight loss and an active lifestyle must be encouraged.[68] A recent metaanalysis of studies investigating the effect of exercise with or without dietary modification on intrahepatic fat mobilization showed a 30.2% effect in the exercise-only group and 49.8% in the diet and exercise group. There was no difference between aerobic and resistance exercise. Most studies used hydrogen-magnetic spectroscopy.[69]

The management of hypertension, lipids, and diabetes using pharmacologic methods is also important.

Pharmacologic Treatment of Nonalcoholic Fatty Liver Disease

Currently, no medication has been proven to be effective independently in the treatment of liver inflammation and fibrosis. Given the pathophysiologic similarities between diabetes and NAFLD, several antidiabetic medications have been evaluated in the treatment of NAFLD.

Metformin is the first-line medical treatment in T2DM and is known to reduce insulin resistance, which is a key factor in NAFLD. However, no effect on fatty liver, inflammation or fibrosis has thus far been demonstrated.[70]

Thiazolidinediones, such as pioglitazone, also have an insulin-sensitizing effect via its action on adiponectin. In the PIVENS trial (pioglitazone, vitamin E, or placebo in the treatment of nonalcoholic steatohepatitis), pioglitazone showed a reduction in fatty liver and inflammation compared with vitamin E and placebo but did not show any improvement in liver fibrosis.[71] Several other studies have since been published using pioglitazone, but body weight gain, fluid retention with heart failure, and the risk of bladder cancer have dampened the widespread use of this drug in NAFLD.

Incretin-based therapy, primarily GLP-1 inhibitors such as liraglutide, has also shown some benefit over placebo in reducing histologic changes of NAFLD. But DPP4 inhibitors, which are also incretin based, have not shown any benefit. Weight loss is an additional advantage in the use of GLP-1 agonists and these remain an important treatment in diabetes and obesity.[72]

Several other agents, including elafibranor a PPAR-δ agonist, obeticholic acid, and pentoxyfyllin, have shown some promise and trials are ongoing.

CONCLUSION

The close association between obesity, insulin resistance, and NAFLD, with the latter presumed the liver component of the MS, is established. The contribution of NAFLD toward increasing the risk of cardiovascular disease risk and its impact on liver-related mortality is also recognized. However, a robust noninvasive diagnostic tool to identify those with significant risk of progression to NASH and related cardiovascular and hepatic mortality is not available. Furthermore, several genetic, epigenetic, and gut microbial contributors to NAFLD have been described, and new developments in the field of pathophysiology and treatment are promising.[73] However, currently our focus in clinical management of this high-risk cohort must include early suspicion and detection using available means in order that patients may be educated on this condition. Initial management of lifestyle, which would be beneficial in T2DM and obesity, must be encouraged. Pharmacologic treatments are hopefully imminent.

REFERENCES

1. Addison T. Observations on fatty degeneration of the liver. *Guys Hosp Rep.* 1836;1:476.
2. Bartolow P. Diseases of the liver. In: Pepper W, Starr L, eds. *System of Practical Medicine.* vol. II. Philedelphia, PA: Lea Brothers & Co; 1885:1050.
3. Ludwig J, Viggiano TR, McGill DB, Oh BJ. Nonalcoholic Steatohepatitis: mayo clinical experiences with a hitherto unnamed disease. *Mayo Clin Proc.* 1980;55(7):434–438.
4. Younossi ZM, Otgonsuren M, Henry L, et al. Association of nonalcoholic fatty liver disease (NAFLD) with hepatocellular carcinoma (HCC) in the United States from 2004 to 2009. *Hepatology.* 2015;62:1723–1730.
5. Adams LA, Lymp JF, St Sauver J, et al. The natural history of nonalcoholic fatty liver disease: a population-based cohort study. *Gastroenterology.* 2005;129:113–121.
6. Armstrong MJ, Houlihan DD, Bentham L, et al. Presence and severity of non-alcoholic fatty liver disease in a large prospective primary care cohort. *J Hepatol.* 2012;56(1):234–240.
7. Poynard T, Lassailly G, Diaz E, et al. Performance of biomarkers FibroTest, ActiTest, SteatoTest, and NashTest in patients with severe obesity: meta-analysis of individual patient data. *PLoS One.* 2012;7:e30325.
8. Alberti KG, Zimmet P, Shaw J, IDF Epidemiology Task Force Consensus Group. The metabolic syndrome — a new worldwide definition. *Lancet.* 2005;366:1059–1062.
9. Kotronen A, Yki-Järvinen H. Fatty liver: a novel component of the metabolic syndrome. *Arterioscler Thromb Vasc Biol.* 2008;28:27–38.
10. Li L, Liu DW, Yan HY, Wang ZY, Zhao SH, Wang B. Obesity is an independent risk factor for non-alcoholic fatty liver disease: evidence from a meta-analysis of 21 cohort studies. *Obes Rev.* June 2016;17(6):510–519.

11. Younossi ZM, Koenig AB, Abdelatif D, Fazel Y, Henry L, Wymer M. Global epidemiology of non-alcoholic fatty liver disease-meta-analytic assessment of prevalence, incidence and outcomes. *Hepatology*. 2016;64(1):73–84.

12. Corey KE, Klebanoff MJ, Tramontano AC, Chung RT, Hur C. Screening for nonalcoholic steatohepatitis in individuals with type 2 diabetes: a cost-effectiveness analysis. *Dig Dis Sci*. 2016;61(7):2108–2117.

13. Dyson J, Jaques B, Chattopadyhay D, et al. Hepatocellular cancer: the impact of obesity, type 2 diabetes and a multidisciplinary team. *J Hepatol*. 2014;60(1):110–117.

14. Torres DM, Harrison SA. Nonalcoholic fatty liver disease: fibrosis portends a worse prognosis. *Hepatology*. 2015;61:1462–1464.

15. Pendino GM, Mariano A, Surace P, et al. Prevalence and aetiology of altered liver tests: a population-based survey in a Mediterranean town. *Hepatology*. 2005;41:1151–1159.

16. Bedogni G, Bellentani S, Miglioli L, et al. The fatty liver index: a simple and accurate predictor of hepatic steatosis in the general population. *BMC Gastroenterol*. 2006;6:33.

17. Fedchuk L, Nascimbeni F, Pais R, et al. Performance and limitations of steatosis biomarkers in patients with nonalcoholic fatty liver disease. *Aliment Pharmacol Ther*. 2014;40:1209–1222.

18. Ratziu V, Bellentani S, Cortez-Pinto H, Day C, Marchesini G. A position statement on NAFLD/NASH based on the EASL 2009 special conference. *J Hepatol*. 2010;53:372–384.

19. Chalasani N, Younossi Z, Lavine JE, et al. The diagnosis and management of non-alcoholic fatty liver disease: practice guideline by the American Gastroenterological Association, American Association for the Study of Liver Diseases, and American College of Gastroenterology. *Gastroenterology*. 2012;142:1592–1609.

20. Wong RJ, Aguilar M, Cheung R, et al. Nonalcoholic steatohepatitis is the second leading aetiology of liver disease among adults awaiting liver transplantation in the United States. *Gastroenterology*. 2015;148(3):547–555.

21. Browning JD. Statins and hepatic steatosis: perspectives from the Dallas Heart study. *Hepatology*. 2006;44:466–471.

22. Fraser A, Harris R, Sattar N, Ebrahim S, Smith GD, Lawlor DA. Gamma-glutamyltransferase is associated with incident vascular events independently of alcohol intake: analysis of the British Women's Heart and Health study and meta-analysis. *Arterioscler Thromb Vasc Biol*. 2007;27:2729–2735.

23. Bugianesi E, Manzini P, D'Antico S, et al. Relative contribution of iron burden, HFE mutations, and insulin resistance to fibrosis in nonalcoholic fatty liver. *Hepatology*. 2004;39:179–187.

24. Bantel H, Ruck P, Gregor M, Schulze-Osthoff K. Detection of elevated caspase activation and early apoptosis in liver diseases. *Eur J Cell Biol*. 2001;80:230–239.

25. Poynard T, Ratziu V, Naveau S, et al. The diagnostic value of biomarkers (SteatoTest) for the prediction of liver steatosis. *Comp Hepatol*. December 23, 2005;4:10.

26. Lasailly G, Caiazzo R, Hollebecque A, et al. Validation of noninvasive biomarkers (FibroTest, SteatoTest, and NashTest) for prediction of liver injury in patients with morbid obesity. *J Gastroenterol Hepatol*. June 2011;23(6):499–506.

27. Kotronen A, Peltonen M, Hakkarainen A, et al. Prediction of non-alcoholic fatty liver disease and liver fat using metabolic and genetic factors. *Gastroenterology*. 2009;37:865–872.

28. Saadeh S, Younossi ZM, Remer EM, et al. The utility of radiological imaging in nonalcoholic fatty liver disease. *Gastroenterology*. 2002;123:745–750.

29. Shen F, Zheng RD, Mi YQ, et al. Controlled attenuation parameter for non-invasive assessment of hepatic steatosis in Chinese patients. *World J Gastroenterol*. 2015;20(16):4702–4711.

30. Sasso M, Beaugrand M, de Ledinghen V, et al. Controlled attenuation parameter (CAP): a novel VCTETM guided ultrasonic attenuation measurement for the evaluation of hepatic steatosis: preliminary study and validation in a cohort of patients with chronic liver disease from various causes. *Ultrasound Med Biol*. 2010;36:1825–1835.

31. Wu CH, Ho MC, Jeng YM, et al. Quantification of hepatic steatosis: a comparison of the accuracy among multiple magnetic resonance techniques. *J Gastroenterol Hepatol*. April 2014;29(4):807–813.

32. Tang A, Desai A, Hamilton G, et al. Accuracy of MR imaging-estimated proton density fat fraction for classification of dichotomized histologic steatosis grades in nonalcoholic fatty liver disease. *Radiology*. 2015;274:416–425.

33. Kühn J-P, Hernando D, Muñoz del Rio A, et al. Effect of multipeak spectral modeling of fat for liver iron and fat quantification: correlation of biopsy with MR imaging results. *Radiology*. 2012;265(1):133–142.

34. Ekstedt M, Hagstrom H, Nasr P, et al. Fibrosis stage is the strongest predictor for disease-specific mortality in NAFLD after up to 33 years of follow-up. *Hepatology*. 2015;61:1547–1554.

35. McPherson S, Stewart SF, Henderson E, Burt AD, Day CP. Simple non-invasive fibrosis scoring systems can reliably exclude advanced fibrosis in patients with non-alcoholic fatty liver disease. *Gut*. September 2010;59(9):1265–1269.

36. Kowdley KV, Belt P, Wilson LA, et al. Serum ferritin is an independent predictor of histologic severity and advanced fibrosis in patients with nonalcoholic fatty liver disease. *Hepatology*. 2012;55:77–85.

37. Tanwar S, Trembling PM, Guha IN, et al. Validation of terminal peptide of procollagen III for the detection and assessment of nonalcoholic steatohepatitis in patients with nonalcoholic fatty liver disease. *Hepatology*. 2013;57:103–111.

38. Castera L, Vilgrain V, Angulo P. Noninvasive evaluation of NAFLD. *Nat Rev Gastroenterol Hepatol*. 2013;10:666–675.

39. Angulo P, Hui J, Marchesini G, et al. The NAFLD fibrosis score: a noninvasive system that identifies liver fibrosis in patients with NAFLD. *Hepatology*. 2007;45:847–854.

40. Sterling RK, Lissen E, Clumeck N, et al. Development of a simple noninvasive index to predict significant fibrosis in patients with HIV/HCV coinfection. *Hepatology*. 2006;43:1317–1325.

41. Rosenberg WM, Voelker M, Thiel R, et al. Serum markers detect the presence of liver fibrosis: a cohort study. *Gastroenterology*. 2004;127:1704–1713.

42. Wong VW, Chu WC, Wong GL, et al. Prevalence of non-alcoholic fatty liver disease and advanced fibrosis in Hong

Kong Chinese: a population study using proton-magnetic resonance spectroscopy and transient elastography. *Gut.* 2012;61:409–415.

43. Palmeri ML, Wang MH, Nightingale KR, et al. Noninvasive evaluation of hepatic fibrosis using acoustic radiation force-based shear stiffness in patients with nonalcoholic fatty liver disease. *J Hepatol.* September 2011;55(3):666–672.

44. Dahl JJ, Pinton GF, Palmeri ML, et al. A parallel tracking method for acoustic radiation force impulse imaging. *IEEE Trans Ultrason Ferroelectr Freq Control.* 2007;54:301–312.

45. Brunt EM, Janney CG, Di Bisceglie AM, Neuschwander-Tetri BA, Bacon BR. Nonalcoholic steatohepatitis: a proposal for grading and staging histological the histological lesions. *Am J Gastroenterol.* 1999;94(9):2467–2474.

46. Kleiner DE, Brunt EM, Van Natta M, et al. Design and validation of a histological scoring system for nonalcoholic fatty liver disease. *Hepatology.* 2005;41:1313–1321.

47. Bedosa P, FLIP Pathology Consortium. Utility and appropriateness of the fatty liver inhibition of progression (FLIP) algorithm and steatosis, activity and fibrosis (SAF) score in evaluation of biopsies of non-alcoholic fatty liver disease. *Hepatology.* 2014;60(2):565–575.

48. Yasui K, Hashimoto E, Komorizono Y, et al. Characteristics of patients with nonalcoholic steatohepatitis who develop hepatocellular carcinoma. *Clin Gastroenterol Hepatol.* 2011;9(5):428–433.

49. Piscaglia F, Svegliati-Baroni G, Barchetti A, et al. Clinical patterns of hepatocellular carcinoma in nonalcoholic fatty liver disease: a multicenter prospective study. *Hepatology.* 2016;63:827–838.

50. Rosso C, Mezzabotta L, Gaggini M, et al. Peripheral insulin resistance predicts liver damage in nondiabetic subjects with nonalcoholic fatty liver disease. *Hepatology.* 2016;63:107–116.

51. Liu YL, Patman GL, Leathart JL, et al. Carriage of the *PNPLA3* rs738409 C >G polymorphism confers an increased risk of non-alcoholic fatty liver disease associated hepatocellular carcinoma. *J Hepatol.* 2014;61(1):75–81.

52. Zeybel M, Hardy T, Wong YK, et al. Multigenerational epigenetic adaptation of the hepatic wound-healing response. *Nat Med.* September 2012;18(9):1369–1377.

53. Boursier J, Mueller O, Barret M, et al. The severity of nonalcoholic fatty liver disease is associated with gut dysbiosis and shift in the metabolic function of the gut microbiota. *Hepatology.* 2016;63:764–775.

54. Roden M. Mechanisms of disease: hepatic steatosis in type 2 diabetes—pathogenesis and clinical relevance. *Nat Clin Pract Endocrinol Metab.* 2006;2:335–348.

55. Kotronen A, Westerbacka A, Bergholm R, Pietillainen KH, Yki-Jarvinen H. Liver fat in the metabolic syndrome. *J Clin Endocrinol Metab.* 2007;92:3490–3497.

56. Gaggini M, Morelli M, Buzzigoli E, DeFronzo RA, Bugianesi E, Gastadelli A. Non-alcoholic fatty liver disease (NAFLD) and its connection with insulin resistance, dyslipidemia, atherosclerosis and coronary heart disease. *Nutrients.* 2013;5:1544–1560.

57. Donnelly KL, Smith CI, Schwarzenberg SJ, Jessurun J, Boldt MD, Parks EJ. Sources of fatty acids stored in liver and secreted via lipoproteins in patients with nonalcoholic fatty liver disease. *J Clin Invest.* 2005;115:1343–1351.

58. Morris EM, Rector RS, Thyfault JP, Ibdah JA. Mitochondria and redox signaling in steatohepatitis. *Antioxid Redox Signal.* 2011;15:485–504.

59. Romestaing C, Piquet AM, Letexier D, et al. Mitochondrial adaptations to steatohepatitis induced by a methionine- and choline- deficient diet. *Am J Physiol Endocrinol Metab.* 2008;294:E110–E119.

60. Tilg H, Diehl AM. Cytokines in alcoholic and nonalcoholic steatohepatitis. *N Engl J Med.* 2000;343:1467–1476.

61. Lee DH, Ha MH, Kim JH, et al. Gamma-glutamyltransferase and diabetes—a 4 year follow-up study. *Diabetologia.* 2003;46:359–364.

62. Armstrong MJ, Adams LA, Canbay A, Syn WK. Extrahepatic complications of nonalcoholic fatty liver disease. *Hepatology.* 2014;59:1174–1197.

63. Pais R, Charlotte F, Fedchuck L, et al. A systematic review of follow-up biopsies reveals disease progression in patients with non- alcoholic fatty liver. *J Hepatol.* 2013;59:550–556.

64. Yki-Jarvinen H. Non-alcoholic fatty liver disease as a cause and a consequence of metabolic syndrome. *Lancet Diabetes Endocrinol.* 2014;2:901–910.

65. Poonawala A, Nair SP, Thuluvath PJ. Prevalence of obesity and diabetes in patients with cryptogenic cirrhosis: a case-control study. *Hepatology.* 2000;32:689–692.

66. Goh GB, Pagadala MR, Dasarathy J, et al. Clinical spectrum of non-alcoholic fatty liver disease in diabetic and non-diabetic patients. *BBA Clin.* 2015;3:141–145.

67. Zheng Z, Zhang A, Yan J, et al. Diabetes mellitus is associated with hepatocellular carcinoma: a retrospective case-control study in hepatitis endemic area. *PLoS One.* 2013;8:e84776.

68. Musso G, Cassader M, Rosina F, Gambino R. Impact of current treatments on liver disease, glucose metabolism and cardiovascular risk in non-alcoholic fatty liver disease (NAFLD): a systematic review and meta-analysis of randomised trials. *Diabetologia.* 2012;55:885–904.

69. Golabi P, Locklear CT, Austin P, et al. Effectiveness of exercise in hepatic fat mobilization in non-alcoholic fatty liver disease: systematic review. *World J Gastroenterol.* 2016;22(27):6318–6327.

70. Bugianesi E, Gentilcore E, Manini R, et al. A randomized controlled trial of metformin versus vitamin E or prescriptive diet in nonalcoholic fatty liver disease. *Am J Gastroenterol.* 2005;100:1082–1090.

71. Sanyal AJ, Chalasani N, Kowdley KV, et al. Pioglitazone, vitamin E, or placebo for nonalcoholic steatohepatitis. *N Engl J Med.* 2010;362:1675–1685.

72. Armstrong MJ, Gaunt P, Aithal GP, et al. Liraglutide safety and efficacy in patients with non-alcoholic steatohepatitis (LEAN): a multicentre, double-blind, randomised, placebo- controlled phase 2 study. *Lancet.* 2016;387:679–690.

73. Anstee QM, Day CP. The genetics of nonalcoholic fatty liver disease: spotlight on PNPLA3 and TM6SF2. *Semin Liver Dis.* August 2015;35(3):270–290.

CHAPTER 10

Lipid Disorders in Obesity

MANOJ WICKRAMASINGHE, MBBS •
JOLANTA U. WEAVER, MRCS, FRCP, PHD, CTLHE

INTRODUCTION

Obesity has numerous comorbidities with the increased cardiovascular risk being arguably the most significant. Fundamental to this increased risk is dyslipidemia, which is associated with adiposity.[1] Historically, adipose tissue was only known as an energy storage system in the form of lipids; however, advances in the last couple of decades have identified it as an endocrine organ with numerous different actions: one of these actions being the physiologic maintenance of triglycerides (TAGs) and free fatty acids (FFAs).[2]

Obesity, specifically increased visceral adiposity, has shown to increase FFAs in the circulation, thus creating lipotoxicity to other organs, such as the liver and muscle.[3] Furthermore, the link between dyslipidemia, specifically raised low-density lipoprotein (LDL), TAGs, and reduced high-density lipoprotein (HDL), and the development of atherosclerosis and subsequent cardiovascular disease (CVD) has been well known.[4]

Given the known adverse outcomes of dyslipidemia, it is critical that we can measure lipid levels, more specifically atherogenic fractions, accurately. This chapter will focus on measuring lipids in obesity and the optimal lipid biomarkers to monitor. Weight loss has been long proposed as a treatment for dyslipidemia—in this chapter we will discuss the different effects of weight on lipid profiles.

NORMAL LIPID METABOLISM

Lipid metabolism involves a number of key enzymes and subtypes of lipid fractions and lipoproteins. These include lipoprotein lipase (LPL), TAGs, cholesterol (CH), HDL, LDL, very-low-density lipoprotein (VLDL), and chylomicrons. TAGs are the main constituent of dietary lipids and their principal function is to act as energy reservoir stored in adipocytes. Lipids are insoluble in blood and are packaged in lipoproteins, which act to transport lipids in the blood. Lipoproteins are classified by their density and size.

To understand the pathogenesis of adiposity and lipid metabolism, it is critical to understand normal lipid metabolism. To do this it is helpful to look at three of the key pathways: the dietary component, endogenous component, and finally the reverse cholesterol transport pathway.

Exogenous Pathway

Following digestion and absorption of dietary fat, TAG and CH combine with protein and phospholipids to form chylomicrons in the epithelial layer of the small intestine.[5] These chylomicrons are then absorbed into the lymphatic system where they enter the circulation via the thoracic duct. Here they are transported to the rest of the body to be stored in adipose tissue. Endothelial LPL cleaves TAGs from chlylomicrons to form FFAs and glycerol, which can enter skeletal muscle and adipose tissue, leaving behind chylomicron remnants that are recycled by the liver (see Fig. 10.1).

Endogenous Pathway

VLDL is synthesized by the liver and released into the systemic circulation. In the tissues LPL cleaves TAGs from the VLDL to release fatty acids, which are taken up by myocytes for energy or by adipose tissue for storage. As LPL cleaves TAGs, the cholesterol concentration within the lipoprotein increases and becomes a smaller, denser lipoprotein named "intermediate density lipoproteins" (IDL)—the action of LPL may continue to form LDL, a smaller denser particle than IDL.

Reverse Cholesterol Transport

It involves the movement of cholesterol from nonhepatic peripheral tissues back to the liver. This is mainly regulated by the ATP-binding cassette transporter on HDL, which allows the transfer of cholesterol onto the HDL.

THE ROLE OF FREE FATTY ACIDS

The term FFA does not refer to its state in the blood, as most FFAs are albumin bound, but instead refers to the fact that they are nonesterified. Hence, the term nonesterified fatty acids (NEFA) has been preferred. There is a continual flux of NEFA entering and leaving adipose tissues.

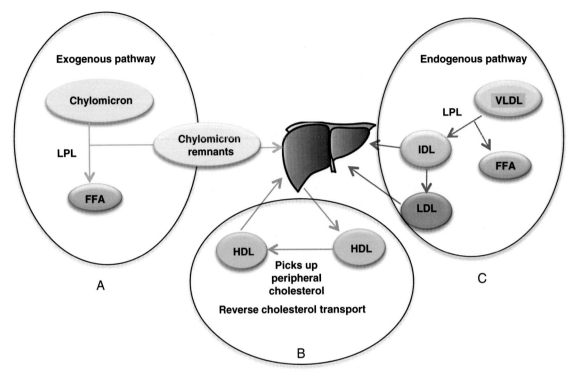

FIG. 10.1 Lipid Metabolism. Summary of the three key pathways of lipid metabolism: exogenous pathway, endogenous pathway, and reverse cholesterol transport. **(A)** The exogenous pathway: action of lipoprotein lipase (LPL) on chylomicrons to form free fatty acids (FFAs). **(B)** The reverse cholesterol transport pathway: action of high-density lipoprotein (HDL) in collecting peripheral cholesterol. **(C)** The endogenous pathway: role of LPL in cleaving very-low-density lipoproteins (VLDL) to form intermediate density lipoproteins (IDLs), taken up by the liver or low-density lipoproteins (LDLs) and FFAs.

In obesity the level of NEFA in the circulation is elevated because of the increased release from adipose tissue and associated insulin resistance. This elevation of NEFA is critical in the development of atherogenic dyslipidemia.

Increased NEFA in the circulation can cause increase in uptake in nonadipose tissues such as the liver (causing hepatosteatosis—a common finding in obesity). In addition to effects on nonadipose tissues, increased NEFA in the circulation has a direct effect on lipid profile by increasing hepatic secretion of VLDLs.[6]

THE ROLE OF INSULIN RESISTANCE
Dyslipidemia has an effect on insulin resistance and equally an insulin resistant state has an effect on lipids. Lipid-induced insulin resistance in skeletal muscle has been well documented in the past.[7] Insulin would normally upregulate LPL and inhibit adipocyte hormone–sensitive lipase; this has the combined effect of

trapping fatty acids within adipocytes. In the resistant state both of these actions are dampened, resulting in an increased postprandial lipid level as well as increased FFA levels.[3] This increases FFA levels thus promotes the liver to produce VLDL and TAGs (see Fig. 10.2).

THE ROLE OF FAT DISTRIBUTION
Over the years several studies have focused on the link between body fat distribution and its relation to comorbidities. An indisputable body of research exists, showing that there is a significant correlation between visceral adiposity and dyslipidemia.[8] There have been several different ways proposed to measure visceral adiposity. One way has been using waist-to-hip circumferences or waist-to-hip ratio (WHR), which is supposed to give a better indicator of abdominal and visceral adiposity. In fact, studies have shown that WHR is more correlated with the metabolic complications of obesity

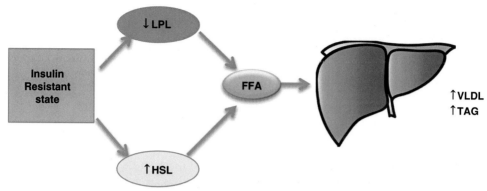

FIG. 10.2 **The Effect of Insulin Resistance on Lipid Metabolism.** The interrelationships between reduction of lipoprotein lipase (LPL) and increase in hormone-sensitive lipase (HSL) in the insulin resistant state. Insulin resistance subsequently increases the release of free fatty acids (FFAs), which promotes the liver to produce triglycerides (TAGs) and very-low-density lipoproteins (VLDLs).

than BMI.[9] However, several limitations of WHR have been identified such as its inability to distinguish between subcutaneous abdominal fat and visceral fat.[10] Therefore it has been suggested that WHR should be used alongside BMI to better determine a patient's atherogenic adiposity.

In recent years dual-energy X-ray absorptiometry (DEXA) measurement has become the gold standard method of evaluating body fat distribution.[11] However, currently not many centers across the world offer DEXA measurement routinely. In the future DEXA measurement and WHR together can give much better risk stratification for individuals compared with BMI alone.[3]

THE ROLE OF BROWN FAT

Brown adipose tissue (BAT) is ubiquitous in newborns and plays an important role in thermogenesis. Previously, it was thought that brown fat disappears in humans after infancy. The first suggestion that BAT was present in adults was in 2003 when clinical studies using flourodeoxyglucose-positron emission tomography (PET) detected uptake, which, with examinations with PET and CT, was identified to be BAT.[12] Its effects on lipids have since been of interest. Previous studies have highlighted the prevalence of BAT to be low (5%–10%); however, a recent critical appraisal looked the sensitivity, reproducibility, and accuracy of PET-CT scans to estimate the true prevalence of BAT to be of 64%.[13]

A recent study concluded that active BAT is an independent protective factor for CVD.[14] Studies have proven that increased activity of BAT causes an increased clearance of

TAGs. Residual hypertriglyceridemia has been proposed to be one of the reasons that cardiovascular events still occur with patients on statin treatment.[15] Increasing the activity of BAT hence can be seen as a therapeutic target for atherogenic dyslipidemia. Studies have shown increased activity of brown fat in adults by exposure to cold temperatures.[16]

Since the discovery of BAT in adults, there has been a wealth of research going into understanding BAT regulation and precursor cells. Studies have already identified potential pharmaceutic targets for activating BAT as well as suggest the potential of isolating progenitor cells in patients and treating them ex vivo with factors that stimulate BAT and then transplanting them back.[17]

Given the very recent discovery of BAT in adults and its potential as a therapeutic target for obesity, little is known about the efficacy, safety, and practicality of such pharmaceutic and ex vivo treatments. However, BAT remains an exciting prospect for tackling obesity and its correlated comorbidities.

MONITORING LIPID LEVELS IN OBESITY

There is an ongoing debate regarding the monitoring of lipids in obesity to provide prognostic information. Traditionally, calculation of fasting LDL levels has been the main lipid marker used in cardiovascular risk prediction. There is a wealth of research supporting the link with LDL cholesterol levels and CVD. Other parameters used have been HDL cholesterol, which is associated with beneficial cardiovascular effects, total cholesterol, non-HDL, and TAG levels.

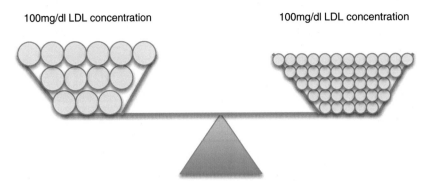

100mg/dl LDL concentration   100mg/dl LDL concentration

FIG. 10.3 Low-Density Lipoprotein (LDL) Particle Size and Concentration. The same concentration of LDL cholesterol can have different compositions of LDL particle size and number. The larger particles are known as pattern A, and the smaller denser particles are known as pattern B as described by others. (Data from Austin M, King M, Vranizan K, Krauss R. Atherogenic lipoprotein phenotype. A proposed genetic marker for coronary heart disease risk. *Circulation*. 1990;82(2):495–506. http://dx.doi.org/10.1161/01.cir.82.2.495.)

Low-Density Lipoprotein Particle Number and Apolipoprotein B (Apo-B) Versus Low-Density Lipoprotein Cholesterol

As discussed earlier the overall effect of obesity on lipids is to increase small, dense LDL, VLDL, and IDL concentrations and to reduce HDL concentrations. These changes, specifically, the increase in small, dense LDL particles, mean that an LDL cholesterol test may be incapable of fully capturing an increase in atherogenic particle numbers.[18] Thus, for many years, it has been hypothesized that apolipoproteins, which give a better picture of total lipoproteins, have a greater utility as a proatherogenic index in obese patients. Although LDL cholesterol has been proven to be a major predictor of CVD, it does not directly measure the cholesterol content within the LDL, nor take into account other TAG-rich lipoproteins. Hence, LDL cholesterol alone may not reflect the true atherogenic burden. Furthermore, at any given LDL concentration, there can be a different number of LDL particles (see Fig. 10.3). The Quebec Cardiovascular Study confirmed that CVD could be present when LDL levels themselves are low, but LDL particle number is high.[19]

One molecule of apolipoprotein B (Apo-B) is present in each atherogenic particle and hence represents the atherogenic potential of circulating particles. The majority of Apo-B is within LDL particles and thus Apo-B concentrations have been used to approximate the LDL particle number. LDL particle concentration has been a biomarker that has been proposed as a predictor of CVD. There has been mixed results from studies with some finding superiority of LDL particle number over other biomarkers and some finding no

differences.[21-23] However, where LDL particle number can be particularly useful is when metabolic syndrome is present and there is discordance between LDL cholesterol and Apo-B.

In terms of body weight the American Association of Clinical Endocrinologists use a BMI over 25 for diagnosis of metabolic syndrome. Metabolic syndrome, however, has several components and there are several different diagnostic criteria from different guidelines. Where metabolic syndrome is present, LDL cholesterol alone has been shown to underestimate CVD risk.[24,25] This suggests that in metabolic syndrome where LDL cholesterol alone may underestimate risk, clinicians may find it more beneficial to measure LDL particle number and measure Apo-B levels.

LDL particle number can be measured, directly in venous blood sample (LDL can be calculated in fasting stage or directly with nuclear magnetic resonance [NMR]), which has been shown to be the most accurate measure, or indirectly using Apo-B measurements as mentioned previously.[26] NMR is not widely available across centers and remains to be a relatively expensive test. Although Apo-B is less accurate than NMR at quantifying LDL particle number, it is a far more accessible test that can be done in a nonfasted state.

Non–High-Density Lipoprotein Cholesterol

Non-HDL comprises LDL, IDL, VLDL, VLDL remnants, chylomicron remnants, and lipoprotein(a). It is calculated by taking away HDL from total cholesterol. It has been proposed that non-HDL measurements are superior to LDL.[27]

Data from the Lipid Research Clinic program cohort study showed that non-HDL and HDL measurements were better predictors of CVD mortality than LDL.[28] Given that non-HDL has been proven to be a better tool at predicting CVD, it has been proposed that instead of LDL calculation, total cholesterol and HDL measurements are taken—thereby allowing the calculation of non-HDL.[29]

Non-HDL cholesterol has a stronger correlation with apolipoprotein B than LDL cholesterol, especially when TAGs are high, and hence represents a truer picture of total atherogenic burden.[30] This suggests that when TAGs are high, non-HDL levels can be particularly useful. Furthermore, a practical advantage of non-HDL over LDL is that non-HDL can be calculated using nonfasting samples, whereas LDL requires a fasting sample.

Non-HDL measurements are readily available tests that have CVD predictive benefits over standard LDL measurements while still having a good correlation with Apo-B and LDL particle number. These advantages have meant that in the newest annual summary of Clinical Lipidology, non-HDL remains to be the preferred treatment target for modification.[31]

High-Density Lipoprotein Cholesterol

Many decades of research have highlighted an inverse relationship with HDL and CVD risk. Low HDL levels are particularly apparent in obesity and metabolic syndrome. HDL cholesterol, especially large particles, acts to remove cholesterol from atherosclerotic plaques via reverse cholesterol transport. Therefore HDL is a useful measure alongside other lipid biomarkers.

Since the finding of HDL and its proposed atheroprotective functions, it has been postulated the HDL can be artificially raised for therapeutic benefits.[32] However, this has been fraught with many issues. Firstly, raising HDL cholesterol pharmacologically has proven to be very difficult, with only niacin increasing it substantially.[33] Furthermore, it has been suggested that instead of HDL particle number it is the quality of the HDL particles that is important.[34] A recent metaanalysis looking at all studies on increasing HDL pharmacologically found no reduction in mortality or CVD.[35] Therefore at the moment, there is no sufficient evidence to support targeted treatment to increase HDL levels with pharmacologic therapy.

Triglycerides

TAGs are elevated in obesity and are a key feature in metabolic syndrome. There is a strong correlation between increased abdominal circumference and hypertriglyceridemia. However, they become a primary target for therapy only when they are very high; at very high levels there is immediate risk of pancreatitis. In these cases, where TAGs are over 500 mg/dL (5.65 mmol/L) or even over 1000 mgd/L (11.3 mmol/L), treatment can be initiated with a very-low-fat diet, fibrates, niacin, statins, and fish oil supplements. Of these, niacin seems to be the most effective at lowering TAGs,[36] although it is no longer licensed for use in the United Kingdom. These drugs can be used in combination for severe hypertriglyceridemia.

There has been much debate regarding the measurement of TAGs and whether it is necessary to measure them fasted. TAGs remain high after meals with a peak at around 4–5 h. Historically, the variability with nonfasted samples has prompted the encouragement of fasted TAG measurements. However, fasting samples are harder to collect, and the need of a fasting sample can reduce the amount of people whoactually get tested because of practical reasons. Recent studies have also highlighted that nonfasting samples are adequate at predictive CVD.[37] This has prompted the use of nonfasted TAG samples in most cases, which is also where any abnormality will be most pronounced and hence detected. When TAG levels are particularly higher (over 4.5 mmol/L), clinicians may find it beneficial to monitor fasting samples because this can allow closer monitoring of treatment effects as well as more accurate assessment of LDL using the Friedewald equation.[38]

EFFECT OF WEIGHT LOSS ON LIPID PROFILE

There have been several studies looking at the effect of weight loss on different population groups.[39] These studies have found variable changes in lipid levels, which is expected as they have been on different population groups with different amounts of weight loss over different periods of time. The results of metaanalysis of 70 studies examining the effect of weight loss on lipid profiles are provided in Table 10.1.

TAGs seem to be the most sensitive and responsive lipid biomarker to weight loss.[3]

It has been proven that the people benefiting the most from weight loss are ones who have a high baseline lipid level—and therefore have the greatest improvement in lipid profile with dietary and/or exercise interventions. On the other hand, people with normal lipid levels at baseline seem to not have any significant improvement on their lipid profile with weight loss. Clinically, a weight loss of 5%–10% in obese patients with dyslipidemia shows an improvement in lipid profile.[29]

TABLE 10.1
Weight Loss Metaanalysis Findings

	Total Cholesterol	Low-Density Lipoprotein	High-Density Lipoprotein (Active)	High-Density Lipoprotein (Stable)	Triglycerides
Average change per kilogram of weight loss	−1.93 mg/dL (0.05 mmol/L)	−0.77 mg/dL (0.02 mmol/L)	−0.27 mg/dL (0.01 mmol/L)	+0.35 mg/dL (0.01 mmol/L)	−1.33 mg/dL (0.03 mmol/L)

Summary findings from a metaanalysis looking at data from 70 different studies on weight loss and effects on lipid profile.
Data from Dattilo AM, Kris-Etherton PM. Effects of weight reduction on blood lipids and lipoproteins: a meta-analysis. *Am J Clin Nutr.* 56:320–328.

Some studies in the past have suggested that improving lipid profile with weight loss is not a sustainable option because they have found that the benefits last only during the hypocaloric weight loss period and return near to baseline during the weight maintenance phase.[41] However, many studies have disputed this theory, showing data highlighting sustained improvement in lipid profile following weight loss.[42]

When discussing the effect of weight loss on lipid profile, it is important to recognize that there are different strategies of weight loss; it can be achieved through diet, exercise, medication, or surgery.

DIETARY INTERVENTIONS

Within the dietary side, there are different proportions of the three macronutrients (carbohydrate, protein, and fat) that one can consume. Over the years there have been several studies looking into the most effective diets in loosing weight and modifying cardiovascular risk factors. A recent metaanalysis found that a high-protein diet, compared with a low-protein diet, provided greater reductions in TAGs.[43] Lower-carbohydrate diet compared with a higher-carbohydrate diet also induces greater reductions in TAGs with weight loss.[44] Another metaanalysis in 2012 looked at 23 trials with 2788 participants comparing low-carbohydrate versus low-fat diets.[45] This study found that low-carbohydrate and low-fat diets induced a similar amount of weight loss but found that the low-carbohydrate group had a slight, but statistically significant, reduction in total cholesterol and LDL and an increase in HDL compared with low-fat diets. Therefore it was concluded that low-carbohydrate diets were at least as good as low-fat diets at reducing metabolic risk and weight loss. There seems to be some conflicting evidence; however, the majority of evidence and randomized controlled trials seem to

be in favor of low-carbohydrate diets for atherogenic dyslipidemia in obesity.

Despite all of these findings from various pieces of research, it is widely accepted that weight loss on most forms of conventional diets produces favorable changes to lipid profile. In fact, it has been proposed that diet adherence is far more important than specific type of diet to achieve weight loss and subsequent favorable metabolic changes.[46]

ROLE OF EXERCISE IN LIPID PROFILE

As with other weight loss interventions, exercise has created varied responses in lipid levels. Some studies show favorable increases in HDL and decreases in LDL as well as decreasing fasting TAGs.[47,48] Interestingly, studies have highlighted that exercise can positively modify lipids independent of weight loss; substantial reduction in LDL particle numbers has been seen while the total LDL cholesterol remains largely similar.[49] A normal lipid measurement in this scenario would show no improvement in lipid levels while in reality the reduction in LDL particle number might signify a step toward reducing cardiovascular risk. This begs the question whether the standard lipid markers tested give enough information on overall dyslipidemia. Exercise has been shown to reduce adiposity even without weight loss, which has a positive effect on lipid profile.[50] This shows that although the weight loss seen with exercise is not as substantial as with diet restriction there are added benefits of exercising for lipid profiles independent of actual weight loss.

As to the type of exercise training, the salient factor seems to be the volume of exercise as opposed to the intensity.[51] Studies also suggest that there is a preferential loss of visceral adipose tissue with exercise-induced weight loss compared with caloric restriction.[52]

TABLE 10.2 Effectiveness of Orlistat			
	Low-Risk Cardiovascular Disease Patients	**High-Risk Cardiovascular Disease Patients**	**Type 2 Diabetes Mellitus Patients**
Total cholesterol reduction with orlistat after 1 year	12 mg/dL (0.31 mmol/L)	9.3 mg/dL (0.24 mmol/L)	9.7 mg/dL (0.25 mmol/L)

Summary of data from a metaanalysis in 2004 examining the effectiveness of orlistat in reducing total cholesterol.
Data from Hutton B, Fergusson D. Changes in body weight and serum lipid profile in obese patients treated with orlistat in addition to a hypocaloric diet: a systematic review of randomized clinical trials. *Am J Clin Nutr.* 2004;80:1461–1468.

TABLE 10.3 1-Year Follow-Up After Bariatric Surgery				
	Total Cholesterol	**Low-Density Lipoprotein**	**Triglycerides**	**High-Density Lipoprotein**
Changes at 1 year follow-up after bariatric surgery	−28.5 mg/dL (0.74 mmol/L)	−22.0 mg/dL (0.57 mmol/L)	−61.6 mg/dL (1.60 mmol/L)	+6.9 md/dL (0.18 mmol/L)

Summary from a recent metaanalysis looking at changes in lipid profile at 1-year follow-up after bariatric surgery.
Data from Heffron S, Parikh A, Volodarskiy A, et al. Changes in lipid profile of obese patients following contemporary bariatric surgery: a metaanalysis. *Am J Med.* 2016;129(9):952–959.

PHARMACEUTIC INTERVENTIONS

A metaanalysis in 2012 looked into the effectiveness of antiobesity medications in changing cardiovascular risk factors.[53] Orlistat, phentermine, lorcaserin, phentermine/topiramate controlled release, and naltrexone sustained release (SR)/bupropion SR have all been shown to improve lipid biomarkers as well as reduce weight.[3] The effectiveness of orlistat treatment on lipid profile has been studied in metaanalysis of several trials (Table 10.2).

Thus there is a place for antiobesity medication for weight loss and improving dyslipidemia while balancing it with the safety of these medications.

SURGICAL INTERVENTIONS

The weight loss benefits of bariatric surgery have been well proven and will be discussed in this book. The SOS (Swedish Obese Subjects Study) found beneficial effects on TAG and HDL levels 10 years postsurgery.[55] In addition to the obvious benefit of weight loss on lipid profile, there seems to be hormonal changes that have favorable effects—specifically changes to GLP-1, PYY, leptin, and ghrelin were found postoperatively.[56] Roux-en-Y gastric bypass seems to have the best effect on weight loss and lipid changes compared with other forms of bariatric surgery.[57,58]

The effectiveness of bariatric surgery has been studied in the recent metaanalysis (Table 10.3).

Overall, the effect of weight loss on lipid profile is substantial and should be actively encouraged. The method of weight loss is of significance. Low-carbohydrate diets seem to be the most beneficial type of diet for altering lipid profiles. The evidence seems to point toward low-carbohydrate diets and shows that Atkins-type diets are more beneficial for atherogenic dyslipidemia compared with low-fat diets.[60] Exercise and surgery have important effects on lipid profile independent of weight loss. Despite safety concerns, pharmaceutic therapies for weight loss have also got proven benefits for lipid profile. Therefore all these strategies should be considered and catered for the individual patient, while keeping in mind that the most benefits are seen in patients with higher baseline lipid levels.

CONCLUSION

Dyslipidemia is arguably the biggest contributing factor to the development of atherosclerosis and subsequent CVD in obesity. The link between obesity and dyslipidemia is one that is complex in nature and is directly affected by body fat distribution, insulin resistance, and brown fat.

The increasing prevalence of obesity in the world makes the ideal monitoring of lipids even more important. Recent advances in research suggest moving away from looking at LDL and looking more into apolipoprotein B and non-HDL, which give a better picture of the true atherogenic burden.

Given the ubiquitous nature of dyslipidemia and obesity and the magnitude of its importance for healthcare, there will be an abundance of research in the future—specifically looking into new therapeutic targets for dyslipidemia.

REFERENCES

1. Yu Y. Adipocyte signaling and lipid homeostasis: sequelae of insulin-resistant adipose tissue. *Circ Res.* 2005;96(10):1042–1052. http://dx.doi.org/10.1161/01.res.0000165803.47776.38.
2. Kershaw EE, Flier JS. Adipose tissue as an endocrine organ. *J Clin Endocrinol Metab.* 2004;89(6):2548–2556. http://dx.doi.org/10.1210/jc.2004-0395.
3. Bays H, Toth P, Kris-Etherton P, et al. Obesity, adiposity, and dyslipidemia: a consensus statement from the National Lipid Association. *J Clin Lipidol.* 2013;7(4):304–383. http://dx.doi.org/10.1016/j.jacl.2013.04.001.
4. Yusuf S, Hawken S, Ounpuu S. Effect of potentially modifiable risk factors associated with myocardial infarction in 52 countries (The Interheart Study). *J Cardiopulm Rehabil.* 2005;25(1):56–57. http://dx.doi.org/10.1097/00008483-200501000-00013.
5. Kingsbury KJ, Bondy G. Understanding the essentials of blood lipid metabolism. *Prog Cardiovasc Nurs.* 2003;18(1):13–18. http://dx.doi.org/10.1111/j.0889-7204.2003.01176.x.
6. Ebbert JO, Jensen MD. Fat depots, free fatty acids, and dyslipidemia. *Nutrients.* 2013;5(2):498–508. http://dx.doi.org/10.3390/nu5020498.
7. Schmitz-Peiffer C. Protein kinase C and lipid-induced insulin resistance in skeletal muscle. *Ann N Y Acad Sci.* 2006;967(1):146–157. http://dx.doi.org/10.1111/j.1749-6632.2002.tb04272.x.
8. Sam S, Haffner S, Davidson M, et al. Relationship of abdominal visceral and subcutaneous adipose tissue with lipoprotein particle number and size in type 2 diabetes. *Diabetes.* 2008;57(8):2022–2027. http://dx.doi.org/10.2337/db08-0157.
9. Noble R. Waist-to-hip ratio versus BMI as predictors of cardiac risk in obese adult women. *West J Med.* 2001;174(4):240–241. http://dx.doi.org/10.1136/ewjm.174.4.240-a.
10. Despres J. Body fat distribution and risk of cardiovascular disease: an update. *Circulation.* 2012;126(10):1301–1313. http://dx.doi.org/10.1161/circulationaha.111.067264.
11. Shepherd J, Fan B, Lu Y, et al. A multinational study to develop universal standardization of whole-body bone density and composition using GE Healthcare Lunar and Hologic DXA systems. *J Bone Miner Res.* 2012;27(10):2208–2216. http://dx.doi.org/10.1002/jbmr.1654.
12. Cohade C, Osman M, Pannu HK, Wahl RL. Uptake in supraclavicular area fat ("USA-Fat"): description on 18F-FDG PET/CT. *J Nucl Med.* 2003;44(2):170–176.
13. Lee P, Greenfield J, Ho K, Fulham M. A critical appraisal of the prevalence and metabolic significance of brown adipose tissue in adult humans. *Am J Physiol Endocrinol Metab.* 2010;299(4):E601–E606. http://dx.doi.org/10.1152/ajpendo.00298.2010.
14. Shao X, Yang W, Shao X, Qiu C, Wang X, Wang Y. The role of active brown adipose tissue (aBAT) in lipid metabolism in healthy Chinese adults. *Lipids Health Dis.* 2016;15(1). http://dx.doi.org/10.1186/s12944-016-0310-8.
15. Efficacy and safety of cholesterol-lowering treatment: prospective meta-analysis of data from 90 056 participants in 14 randomised trials of statins. *Lancet.* 2005;366(9493):1267–1278. http://dx.doi.org/10.1016/s0140-6736(05)67394-1.
16. van der Lans A, Hoeks J, Brans B, et al. Cold acclimation recruits human brown fat and increases nonshivering thermogenesis. *J Clin Invest.* 2013;123(8):3395–3403. http://dx.doi.org/10.1172/jci68993.
17. Cypess AM, Kahn CR. Brown fat as a therapy for obesity and diabetes. *Curr Opin Endocrinol Diabetes Obes.* 2010;17(2):143–149. http://dx.doi.org/10.1097/med.0b013e328337a81f.
18. Sniderman A, St-Pierre A, Cantin B, Dagenais G, Després J, Lamarche B. Concordance/discordance between plasma apolipoprotein B levels and the cholesterol indexes of atherosclerotic risk. *Am J Cardiol.* 2003;91(10):1173–1177. http://dx.doi.org/10.1016/s0002-9149(03)00262-5.
19. Lamarche B, Despres J, Moorjani S, Cantin B, Dagenais G, Lupien P. Prevalence of dyslipidemic phenotypes in ischemic heart disease (prospective results from the Quebec cardiovascular study). *Am J Cardiol.* 1995;75(17):1189–1195. http://dx.doi.org/10.1016/s0002-9149(99)80760-7.
20. Austin M, King M, Vranizan K, Krauss R. Atherogenic lipoprotein phenotype. A proposed genetic marker for coronary heart disease risk. *Circulation.* 1990;82(2):495–506. http://dx.doi.org/10.1161/01.cir.82.2.495.
21. Blake G. Low-density lipoprotein particle concentration and size as determined by nuclear magnetic resonance spectroscopy as predictors of cardiovascular disease in women. *Circulation.* 2002;106(15):1930–1937. http://dx.doi.org/10.1161/01.cir.0000033222.75187.b9.
22. Mora S, Buring J, Ridker P. Discordance of low-density lipoprotein (LDL) cholesterol with alternative LDL-related measures and future coronary events. *Circulation.* 2013;129(5):553–561. http://dx.doi.org/10.1161/circulationaha.113.005873.
23. Mora S, Otvos J, Rifai N, Rosenson R, Buring J, Ridker P. Lipoprotein particle profiles by nuclear magnetic resonance compared with standard lipids and apolipoproteins in predicting incident cardiovascular disease in women. *Circulation.* 2009;119(7):931–939. http://dx.doi.org/10.1161/circulationaha.108.816181.

24. Sniderman A. Differential response of cholesterol and particle measures of atherogenic lipoproteins to LDL-lowering therapy: implications for clinical practice. *J Clin Lipidol*. 2008;2(1):36–42. http://dx.doi.org/10.1016/j.jacl.2007.12.006.

25. Sniderman A. Targets for LDL-lowering therapy. *Curr Opin Lipidol*. 2009;20(4):282–287. http://dx.doi.org/10.1097/mol.0b013e32832ca1d6.

26. Cromwell WC, Otvos JD. Low-density lipoprotein particle number and risk for cardiovascular disease. *Curr Atheroscler Rep*. 2004;6(5):381–387. http://dx.doi.org/10.1007/s11883-004-0050-5.

27. Frost P, Havel R. Rationale for use of non–high-density lipoprotein cholesterol rather than low-density lipoprotein cholesterol as a tool for lipoprotein cholesterol screening and assessment of risk and therapy. *Am J Cardiol*. 1998;81(4):26B–31B. http://dx.doi.org/10.1016/s0002-9149(98)00034-4.

28. Grover S. Serum lipid screening to identify high-risk individuals for coronary death. The results of the Lipid Research Clinics prevalence cohort. *Arch Intern Med*. 1994;154(6):679–684. http://dx.doi.org/10.1001/archinte.154.6.679.

29. Cui Y, Blumenthal R, Flaws J, et al. Non–high-density lipoprotein cholesterol level as a predictor of cardiovascular disease mortality. *Arch Intern Med*. 2001;161(11):1413. http://dx.doi.org/10.1001/archinte.161.11.1413.

30. Ballantyne C, Andrews T, Hsia J, Kramer J, Shear C. Correlation of non-high-density lipoprotein cholesterol with apolipoprotein B: effect of 5 hydroxymethylglutaryl coenzyme A reductase inhibitors on non-high-density lipoprotein cholesterol levels. *Am J Cardiol*. 2001;88(3):265–269. http://dx.doi.org/10.1016/s0002-9149(01)01638-1.

31. Bays H, Jones P, Orringer C, Brown W, Jacobson T. National lipid association annual summary of clinical lipidology 2016. *J Clin Lipidol*. 2016;10(1):S1–S43. http://dx.doi.org/10.1016/j.jacl.2015.08.002.

32. High density lipoprotein as a protective factor against coronary heart disease. The Framingham study. *Am J Med*. 1977;62(5):A77. http://dx.doi.org/10.1016/0002-9343(77)90899-3.

33. Carlson L. Nicotinic acid: the broad-spectrum lipid drug. A 50th anniversary review. *J Intern Med*. 2005;258(2):94–114. http://dx.doi.org/10.1111/j.1365-2796.2005.01528.x.

34. Tall A. Cholesterol efflux pathways and other potential mechanisms involved in the athero-protective effect of high density lipoproteins. *J Intern Med*. 2008;263(3):256–273. http://dx.doi.org/10.1111/j.1365-2796.2007.01898.x.

35. Keene D, Price C, Shun-Shin M, Francis D. Effect on cardiovascular risk of high density lipoprotein targeted drug treatments niacin, fibrates, and CETP inhibitors: meta-analysis of randomised controlled trials including 117 411 patients. *BMJ*. July 18, 2014;349:g4379. http://dx.doi.org/10.1136/bmj.g4379.

36. McKenney J. New perspectives on the use of niacin in the treatment of lipid disorders. *Arch Intern Med*. 2004;164(7):697. http://dx.doi.org/10.1001/archinte.164.7.697.

37. Bansal S, Buring J, Rifai N, Mora S, Sacks F, Ridker P. Fasting compared with nonfasting triglycerides and risk of cardiovascular events in women. *JAMA*. 2007;298(3):309. http://dx.doi.org/10.1001/jama.298.3.309.

38. Nordestgaard B, Langsted A, Mora S, et al. Fasting is not routinely required for determination of a lipid profile: clinical and laboratory implications including flagging at desirable concentration cut-points—a joint consensus statement from the European Atherosclerosis Society and European Federation of Clinical Chemistry and Laboratory Medicine. *Eur Heart J*. 2016;37(25):1944–1958. http://dx.doi.org/10.1093/eurheartj/ehw152.

39. Franz M, VanWormer J, Crain A, et al. Weight-loss outcomes: a systematic review and meta-analysis of weight-loss clinical trials with a minimum 1-year follow-up. *J Am Diet Assoc*. 2007;107(10):1755–1767. http://dx.doi.org/10.1016/j.jada.2007.07.017.

40. Dattilo AM, Kris-Etherton PM. Effects of weight reduction on blood lipids and lipoproteins: a meta-analysis. *Am J Clin Nutr*. 1992;56:320–328.

41. Wadden T, Anderson D, Foster G. Two-year changes in lipids and lipoproteins associated with the maintenance of a 5% to 10% reduction in initial weight: some findings and some questions. *Obes Res*. 1999;7(2):170–178. http://dx.doi.org/10.1002/j.1550-8528.1999.tb00699.x.

42. Marckmann P, Toubro S, Astrup A. Sustained improvement in blood lipids, coagulation, and fibrinolysis after major weight loss in obese subjects. *Eur J Clin Nutr*. 1998;52(5):329–333. http://dx.doi.org/10.1038/sj.ejcn.1600558.

43. Wycherley T, Moran L, Clifton P, Noakes M, Brinkworth G. *Am J Clin Nutr*. 2012;96(6):1281–1298. http://dx.doi.org/10.3945/ajcn.112.044321.

44. Vernon M, Kueser B, Transue M, Yates H, Yancy W, Westman E. Clinical experience of a carbohydrate-restricted diet for the metabolic syndrome. *Metab Syndr Relat Disord*. 2004;2(3):180–186. http://dx.doi.org/10.1089/met.2004.2.180.

45. Hu T, Mills K, Yao L, et al. Effects of low-carbohydrate diets versus low-fat diets on metabolic risk factors: a meta-analysis of randomized controlled clinical trials. *Am J Epidemiol*. 2012;176(suppl 7):S44–S54. http://dx.doi.org/10.1093/aje/kws264.

46. Dansinger M, Gleason J, Griffith J, Selker H, Schaefer E. Comparison of the Atkins, Ornish, Weight Watchers, and Zone diets for weight loss and heart disease risk reduction. *JAMA*. 2005;293(1):43. http://dx.doi.org/10.1001/jama.293.1.43.

47. Mestek ML. Physical activity, blood lipids, and lipoproteins. *Am J Lifestyle Med*. 2009;3(4):279–283.

48. Durstine J, Grandjean P, Davis P, Ferguson M, Alderson N, DuBose K. Blood lipid and lipoprotein adaptations to exercise. *Sports Med*. 2001;31(15):1033–1062. http://dx.doi.org/10.2165/00007256-200131150-00002.

49. Kraus WE, Houmard JA, Duscha BD, et al. Effects of the amount and intensity of exercise on plasma lipoproteins. *N Engl J Med*. 2002;347(19):1483–1492.

50. Kelley G. Walking, lipids, and lipoproteins: a meta-analysis of randomized controlled trials. *Prev Med*. 2004;38(5):651–661. http://dx.doi.org/10.1016/j.ypmed.2003.12.012.

51. Donnelly J, Blair S, Jakicic J, Manore M, Rankin J, Smith B. Appropriate physical activity intervention strategies for weight loss and prevention of weight regain for adults. *Med Sci Sports Exerc*. 2009;41(2):459–471. http://dx.doi.org/10.1249/mss.0b013e3181949333.

52. Murphy J, McDaniel J, Mora K, Villareal D, Fontana L, Weiss E. Preferential reductions in intermuscular and visceral adipose tissue with exercise-induced weight loss compared with calorie restriction. *J Appl Physiol*. 2011;112(1):79–85. http://dx.doi.org/10.1152/japplphysiol.00355.2011.

53. Zhou Y, Ma X, Wu C, et al. Effect of anti-obesity drug on cardiovascular risk factors: a systematic review and meta-analysis of randomized controlled trials. *PLoS One*. 2012;7(6):e39062. http://dx.doi.org/10.1371/journal.pone.0039062.

54. Hutton B, Fergusson D. Changes in body weight and serum lipid profile in obese patients treated with orlistat in addition to a hypocaloric diet: a systematic review of randomized clinical trials. *Am J Clin Nutr*. 2004;80:1461–1468.

55. Kennedy L. Effects of bariatric surgery on mortality in Swedish obese subjects. *Yearb Endocrinol*. 2008;2008:20–21. http://dx.doi.org/10.1016/s0084-3741(08)79142-x.

56. Beckman L, Beckman T, Sibley S, et al. Changes in gastrointestinal hormones and leptin after Roux-en-Y gastric bypass surgery. *J Parenter Enteral Nutr*. 2011;35(2):169–180. http://dx.doi.org/10.1177/0148607110381403.

57. Waitman J, Aronne L. Obesity surgery: pros and cons. *J Endocrinol Invest*. 2002;25(10):925–928. http://dx.doi.org/10.1007/bf03344059.

58. Iannelli A, Anty R, Schneck A, Tran A, Gugenheim J. Inflammation, insulin resistance, lipid disturbances, anthropometrics, and metabolic syndrome in morbidly obese patients: a case control study comparing laparoscopic Roux-en-Y gastric bypass and laparoscopic sleeve gastrectomy. *Surgery*. 2011;149(3):364–370. http://dx.doi.org/10.1016/j.surg.2010.08.013.

59. Heffron S, Parikh A, Volodarskiy A, et al. Changes in lipid profile of obese patients following contemporary bariatric surgery: a meta-analysis. *Am J Med*. 2016;129(9):952–959. http://dx.doi.org/10.1016/j.amjmed.2016.02.004.

60. Foster G, Wyatt H, Hill J. A randomized trial of a low-carbohydrate diet for obesity. *ACC Curr J Rev*. 2003;12(4):29. http://dx.doi.org/10.1016/s1062-1458(03)00265-4.

CHAPTER 11

Obesity and the Effects on the Respiratory System

DR. ANINDO BANERJEE, PHD, FRCP • DR. EMILY HEIDEN, BM, MRCP

The effects of obesity on the respiratory system are far-reaching and the consequences directly lead to increased morbidity and mortality. The link between increased body mass index (BMI) and systemic conditions, such as diabetes and cardiovascular disease are well documented. While there is a clear link between obesity and certain respiratory diseases, for example, obesity hypoventilation syndrome (OHS) and obstructive sleep apnea (OSA), there is an increasing understanding of its association with airway diseases and pulmonary vascular disorders.

Documented observations of the link between obesity and respiratory disease can be found as early as the ancient Greeks; Dionysius, an oppressor of Heraclea, was described as being very obese, and "through daily gluttony and intemperance, increased to an extraordinary degree of Corpulency and Fatness, by reason whereof he had much adoe to take breath."[1] In more recent history, Charles Darwin's description of an obese character who suffered with daytime somnolence in the Pickwick papers led to the description of Pickwickian syndrome, later named OHS.

This chapter will review the effects of obesity on respiratory physiology and explore the relationship between high BMI and common respiratory disorders, in particular those with sleep-related conditions.

RESPIRATORY PHYSIOLOGY
Normal Quiet Breathing
In a non-obese individual, for inspiration to occur the diaphragm contracts inferiorly and external intercostal muscles pull the chest wall outward, increasing the volume of the thoracic cavity.[2] This change in thoracic volume reduces intrapleural pressure to approximately 8 cmH_2O below atmospheric pressure and also reduces alveolar pressure to a subatmospheric level. This negative pressure draws air into the lungs, increasing their volume until alveolar pressure returns to atmospheric level, when the inspiratory pressure gradient ceases. For expiration, the muscles of inspiration relax and the elastic recoil of the respiratory system results in lung deflation.

Inspiration requires the inspiratory muscles to overcome airway resistance and compliance. Lung compliance is the lung's ability to stretch and expand as a result of a change in intrapleural pressure and comprises the distensibility of the lungs, chest wall, and abdominal viscera.[3] With increased compliance, the lungs are able to inflate more easily, whereas a decrease in compliance means the lungs are stiffer and require increased energy to move a given volume of air.

Airway resistance is the impedance to the flow of air during inspiration and expiration, caused by forces of friction. The main influences for resistance are the properties of airflow (laminar or turbulent) and the size of the airway. Turbulent airflow can be caused by bronchospasm, excessive secretions, or any other insult that increases the peak pressure of flow.

Effects of Obesity on Respiratory Physiology
Total lung capacity, the total effective size of the lungs, tends to be preserved, or only slightly reduced in morbidly obese individuals. In obese individuals, the increased volume of adipose tissue around the rib cage and abdomen loads the chest wall, restricting diaphragm mobility and rib movement and results in a reduction in chest wall compliance. Chest wall compliance has been shown to reduce by up to two-thirds in obese individuals[4] and the reduction in compliance is exponentially related to BMI.[5,6] Chest wall compliance varies between individuals depending on fat distribution. Mass loading of the upper abdomen and thorax leads to larger changes in chest wall compliance than mass loading of the upper thorax alone.[7,8] The pressures causing deflation of the lung (i.e., breathing out) rise because obesity increases intraabdominal pressure, which in turn impacts on the diaphragm. This change in the relationship between chest wall stiffness (inflationary pressure) and intra-abdominal pressure (deflationary pressure) results in a reduction in the total amount of air in the lungs at the end of normal expiration; in other words,

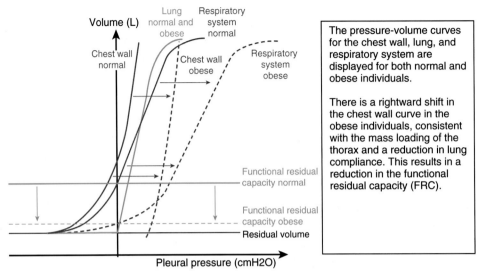

FIG. 11.1 Pressure-volume curves for normal and obese individuals.

Text within the figure:

Volume (L)

Lung normal and obese

Respiratory system normal

Chest wall normal

Chest wall obese

Respiratory system obese

Functional residual capacity normal

Functional residual capacity obese

Residual volume

Pleural pressure (cmH2O)

The pressure-volume curves for the chest wall, lung, and respiratory system are displayed for both normal and obese individuals.

There is a rightward shift in the chest wall curve in the obese individuals, consistent with the mass loading of the thorax and a reduction in lung compliance. This results in a reduction in the functional residual capacity (FRC).

the functional residual capacity (FRC) and expiratory reserve volume (ERV) occur at a lower lung volume than in the non-obese individual. The stiffened chest wall changes the slope of the respiratory pressure-volume curve (Fig. 11.1); individuals tend to breathe on the flatter and less efficient part of the curve, which increases the work of breathing. As a result of the increased work of breathing, obese individuals tend to develop a rapid and shallow pattern of tidal breathing, which is more pronounced during exercise when individuals tend to further increase their respiratory rate rather than their tidal volume (volume of each individual breath).

Reductions in FRC and ERV are detectable even at a modest increase in weight.[9] The reduction in FRC and ERV means that obese individuals breathe at lower lung volumes, which increases the likelihood of expiratory flow limitation and airway closure during quiet breathing. This can lead to the development of intrinsic positive end-expiratory pressure (PEEP), especially in the supine position. The work of breathing rises because of the intrinsic PEEP and the airway closure causing a threshold load on the respiratory muscles, which results in dyspnea,[10] and is particularly prominent when supine.[11] The reduction in FRC and ERV can lead to ventilation distribution abnormalities, with closure of airways in the dependent zones of the lungs and subsequent ventilation-perfusion mismatch and gas exchange abnormalities.[10] The lung bases tend to be particularly susceptible to ventilation-perfusion mismatch; they tend to be poorly ventilated because of early airway closure while receiving normal perfusion. The resultant

hypoxemia is further exacerbated by hypoventilation (low tidal volume), which lowers the partial pressure of oxygen in the alveoli. In obese subjects the partial pressure of oxygen in the blood (pO_2) is relatively well maintained, but the alveolar-arterial oxygen gradient ($AaDO_2$) increases.[12-14] The carbon monoxide transfer factor is relatively normal, resulting in a high carbon monoxide transfer coefficient when the transfer factor is corrected for alveolar volume ($TLco/VA$, the K_{CO}).

The largest study to demonstrate the effect of obesity on spirometry involved nearly 20,000 patients and revealed an inverse linear correlation between waist-to-hip ratio and forced expiratory volume in 1 s (FEV1) and forced vital capacity (FVC).[8] Fat distribution is thought to influence spirometric values, with a better correlation between waist circumference and waist-hip ratio than the BMI alone.[15,16] However, other studies have shown only a minimal effect on the FEV1 and FVC except in morbidly obese individuals.[17,18] When affected, the FEV1 and FVC fall proportionately, and therefore the FEV1/FVC ratio is unaffected (Table 11.1).[15,17,19]

The fall in FRC in obesity results in a reduction in airway caliber.[4] Airway resistance has been shown to rise significantly with obesity and seems to be inversely related to changes in FRC, but airway resistance is normal when corrected for the reduction in FRC. This increase in airway resistance is due to a reduction in lung volumes rather than airway obstruction. Upper airway resistance also increases in obesity; increased adiposity increases the load on the pharynx with consequent

TABLE 11.1
Interpretation of Lung Function Tests

Test	Result Expected in Obese Patients	What the Result Suggests
FEV1	Normal	Airflow obstruction, e.g., asthma or chronic obstructive pulmonary disease
FVC	Normal	Causes of restrictive ventilatory defect
FEV1/FVC ratio	Normal	Airflow obstruction, e.g., asthma or chronic obstructive pulmonary disease
Carbon monoxide gas transfer	Normal	Parenchymal lung disease
Carbon monoxide gas transfer coefficient	Normal or raised	Parenchymal lung disease
Fraction of exhaled nitric oxide (FeNO)	Normal	Asthma or eosinophilic lung disease
Total lung capacity	Normal	Chest wall, pleural, or parenchymal lung disease
Residual volume	Normal	Gas trapping, e.g., asthma or chronic obstructive pulmonary disease
Forced oscillation/tests of airway resistance	Raised	Expected in obesity
Reversibility tests/challenge tests	Normal	Asthma
Partial pressure of oxygen (PaO$_2$)	Normal/slightly reduced	Other causes of hypoxemia
Partial pressure of carbon dioxide (PaCO$_2$)	Normal	Obesity hypoventilation, obstructive sleep apnoa, chest wall or neuromuscular disease

FEV1, forced expiratory volume in 1 s; *FVC*, forced vital capacity.

pharyngeal collapse. The heightened demand for ventilation, elevated work of breathing, respiratory muscle inefficiency, and diminished respiratory compliance all contribute to the respiratory morbidity associated with obesity.

Recently, questions have been raised about a potential correlation between length of sleep and obesity; although the precise physiologic functions of sleep are still unknown, the contribution of sleep to physical and psychologic health and its social and economic significance is being increasingly recognized. There is increasing evidence that short sleep duration results in metabolic changes that may contribute to the development of obesity, insulin resistance, diabetes, and cardiovascular disease.[20,21]

> **Practice point**: Lung function can be used to assess and diagnose respiratory disease in obese individuals and can differentiate pathologic from obesity effects on the respiratory system.

CARDIOPULMONARY EXERCISE TESTING

The use of cardiopulmonary exercise testing (CPET) in the evaluation of the causes of breathlessness and exercise limitation is increasing. The test involves pedaling on a static exercise bicycle at a fixed rate (usually 60 rpm). The bicycle is programmed to increase the resistance to pedaling to increase the workload of cycling progressively through the test. The "ramp," or increase in resistance to pedaling, is chosen so that the patient reaches maximum symptoms and stops the test between 8 and 12 minutes of exercise. This ensures the optimum rate of exercise and produces the most reliable and reproducible results.

In obese patients, the oxygen cost of unloaded cycling is higher than normal, causing a greater rise in the oxygen uptake curve than expected during the warm-up phase of the test.[22] The VO$_2$-work rate curve is displaced upward by ~5.8 mL/min/kg of body weight and so varies with the degree of obesity. The slope of the VO$_2$-work rate curve is not altered and remains ~10.3 mL/min/W. The maximum oxygen uptake and anaerobic threshold are low when adjusted for body weight (VO$_{2max}$ in mL/min/kg) but are normal when the predicted value is derived from height or lean body mass equations. Typically, the corrected VO$_{2max}$ and anaerobic threshold are normal, but with low peak work capacity. As seen in Fig. 11.2, ventilation-perfusion relationships normalize in exercise in obese patients,

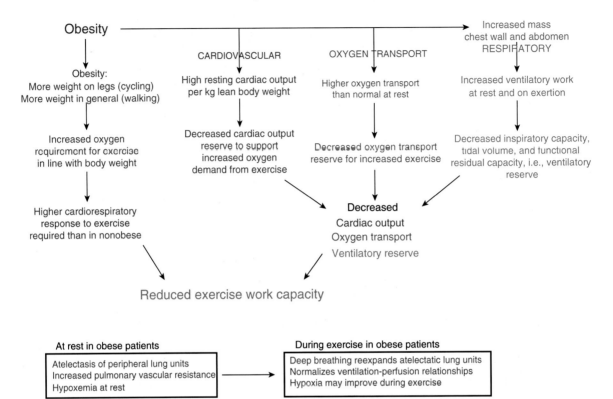

FIG. 11.2 Flow chart showing the physiologic changes in obese patients that impact on exercise function.

and therefore the ventilatory dead space-tidal volume relationship, alveolar-arterial oxygen pressure gradient, and arterial-end tidal oxygen relationship are usually normal. The arterial partial pressure of oxygen is low at rest and normalizes during exercise. The oxygen pulse is normal when the predicted normal weight is used to calculate the predicted oxygen pulse. The minute ventilation increases linearly with exercise, but there is a failure of the normal ventilatory compensation for metabolic acidosis, which may result in a degree of metabolic acidosis at peak exercise. This means that the CPET can be used to differentiate pathologic limitation of function from the effects of obesity in individuals with exercise limitation.

> **Practice point:** CPET can be used to determine the causes of breathlessness in obese individuals and can differentiate pathologic causes from fitness and obesity effects.

SLEEP-DISORDERED BREATHING
Obesity is an important risk factor for the development of sleep-related breathing disorders, of which obstructive sleep apnea syndrome (OSAS), obstructive sleep apnea/hypopnea (OSAH), and obesity hypoventilation (OHS) contribute significantly to morbidity and mortality in affected individuals. There is accumulating evidence that sleep-related breathing disorders have an adverse effect on a variety of cardiovascular and metabolic disorders. Although there have been major advances in the investigation and management of this diverse group of conditions, weight gain remains one of the most important modifiable risk factors for the occurrence of OSAS and OHS, and obese individuals are strongly encouraged to lose weight as part of their treatment. The financial burden of OSAS on society is significant; individuals with OSA have been shown to have had increased healthcare use up to 10 years before diagnosis and reduced productivity; evidence suggests that treating OSAS improves patients' productivity at work and could reduce the cost of work-related injuries to the United Kingdom by £491 million.[23]

OBSTRUCTIVE SLEEP APNEA SYNDROME
OSAS is characterized by dynamic upper airway obstruction during sleep, due to a reduction in airway

muscle tone. This results in episodes of significant decrease (hypopnea) or complete cessation (apnea) of airflow through the upper airway, leading to hypoxemia and transient arousals, in which the individual moves from deep sleep to a lighter sleep phase, or full wakefulness. On moving to a lighter sleep phase, airway tone is restored, the obstruction resolves, and the individual returns to a deeper sleep state. The effect is a cycle of sleep and arousal that occurs throughout the night. When this occurs without daytime sleepiness, it is termed OSAH. When the episodes are of sufficient frequency to fragment sleep and cause daytime sleepiness, the disorder is termed "obstructive sleep apnea syndrome". OSAS is less common than OSAH and typically occurs between the ages of 30 and 60.[24]

Obesity predisposes to and often potentiates OSAS. Patients typically present on the account of excessive tiredness and loud snoring, usually reported by partners or relatives. Information regarding weight gain, which is usually rapid over a period of time, should be obtained. Often, an increase in collar size or clothing size will be reported. The diagnosis should be suspected in obese patients exhibiting further uncontrollable weight gain. There will be signs of reduced concentration, including failure to complete tasks, such as the crossword or puzzles, or the inability to watch whole television programs. There may be reports of excessive daytime sleepiness and falling asleep in unusual circumstances, such as in the cinema or theatre, or in public places such as shopping centers or restaurants. In extreme circumstances, there may be reports of individuals falling asleep during conversations or in the car while driving. Morning headaches may occur in those developing respiratory failure at night, due to a rise in nocturnal blood carbon dioxide levels. In all patients suspected of OSAS, the Epworth Sleepiness Score Questionnaire should be administered; those with a score of 10 or more should be referred for further evaluation (Box 11.1).[24]

The definition of an apnea is of breath cessation for longer than 10 s, while a 50% reduction in airflow for longer than 10 s, with a subsequent drop in oxygen saturations by 4%, is termed a hypopnea.[25] The apnea-hypopnea index (AHI) is the average number of disordered breathing events per hour. OSAS is defined as an AHI of at least five events per hour, with associated daytime symptoms of excessive sleepiness, impaired cognition, and fatigue. It can be further stratified according to the degree of AHI: mild being between 5 and 15 events per hour, moderate 15 to 30, and severe greater than 30 events per hour.

BOX 11.1
Epworth Sleepiness Score Questionnaire

The Epworth Sleepiness Score is calculated using eight questions, which assess the likelihood of a person falling asleep in different conditions. The patient can score a total of 24 points.

The person is asked "How likely are you to doze or fall asleep in the following situations, in contrast to just feeling tired?"
- Sitting and reading
- Watching television
- Sitting, inactive in a public place (for example, at the theater or in a meeting)
- As a passenger in a car for an hour without a break
- Lying down to rest in the afternoon when circumstances permit
- Sitting and talking to someone
- Sitting quietly after lunch without alcohol
- In a car, while stopped for a few minutes in traffic

Each question is answered using one of the following options:
Would never doze (0 points)
Slight chance of dozing (1 point)
Moderate chance of dozing (2 points)
High chance of dozing (3 points)

Diagnosis requires overnight polysomnography; a detailed analysis of oximetry (looking for desaturation of 4%), chest wall, and abdominal movement; and electroencephalogram (EEG) (to show sleep stage and wakefulness). Limited sleep studies have become the usual first-line investigation in most centres because of cost and availability of equipment. In these studies, oximetry is performed with some analysis of hypopnea and apnea (either by video or chest wall and abdominal movement analysis). EEG and sleep stage analysis is not performed in these studies. The tests are interpreted in conjunction with evidence of daytime symptoms, using a validated and objective assessment tool such as the Epworth Sleepiness Scale, which assesses the individual's tendency to fall asleep during various activities.

Epidemiology and Risk Factors

It is estimated that OSAS has a prevalence of 4% in men and 2% in women in the Western world[26]; these figures are expected to rise as the obesity pandemic worsens. In the United Kingdom, it is estimated that OSAS affects 1.5 million people, although a considerable further number remain undiagnosed.[27]

Central obesity is the strongest risk factor for the development and progression of OSAS.[26] In the United Kingdom, approximately 40% people who are obese have OSAS, while 77% of people who are morbidly obese have OSAS.[27] Other risk factors include increasing age, heritable factors such as abnormal craniofacial structures, and male sex; men are two to three times more affected than premenopausal women, likely because of hormonal influences on breathing during sleep.[28]

Anatomic causes include pharyngeal encroachment due to tonsillar and adenoid hypertrophy, chronic nasal obstruction, and retrognathia, all of which can cause upper airway obstruction. Individuals with OSA have been found to have anatomically smaller upper airways, due to the deposition of fat and lateral wall folding, making them more susceptible to airway obstruction.[29] Furthermore, during sleep, the effect of gravitational force and supine positioning causes retroposition of the tongue and soft palate, resulting in a reduction in the cross-sectional area of the upper airway. Functional abnormalities of muscle tone in the upper airways may be caused by neurodegenerative disorders, bulbar palsies, and the use of sedative drugs or alcohol.

Associated Comorbidities

OSAS is associated with hypertension due to neural, humoral, and cellular factors, although the exact mechanisms are not fully known. Intermittent activation of the sympathetic nervous system in response to hypoxia plays an important role in the development of high blood pressure, both in the systemic and pulmonary circulations. The increase in sympathetic drive tends to persist during the day; theories for this include the development of baroreflex dysfunction, chemoreflex dysfunction, and endothelin dysfunction.[1] Large cross-sectional studies have confirmed the link between OSAS and hypertension, and OSAS remains a key element in the treatment of hypertension in the context of OSAS. OSAS and hypertension are associated with cardiovascular morbidity and the incidence of ischemic heart disease is raised in this population.[30]

OSAS is associated with a reduction in quality of life as well as a range of neurocognitive function defects. Individuals often struggle to maintain concentration, have impairments in their memory, and can have significant reductions in their executive function.[31] Individuals with OSA often report difficulties maintaining relationships, poor work performance, and fatigue; the use of continuous positive airway pressure (CPAP) has been shown to increase quality of life in these patients.[32]

Treatment

Treatment approaches for the long-term management of OSAS focus on mechanical tools to splint open the airway during sleep, particularly mandibular advancement devices and CPAP therapy. These therapeutic approaches are used in conjunction with interventions to target the behavioral and lifestyle factors, which contribute to the development of OSAS.

Advice regarding weight loss is of utmost importance and remains a highly effective treatment for OSAS. All overweight patients should be advised to lose weight; in a longitudinal study, there was a 26% reduction in AHI associated with a 10% loss in weight,[33] while for some individuals with milder OSA, there may be complete resolution of symptoms. Attempts to reduce weight are best achieved through dietary modification and exercise, although for individuals with morbid obesity for whom physical activity is more difficult, bariatric surgery has been used to improve their sleep-disordered breathing, as well as having many other far-reaching consequences. Although the number of studies is limited, all those evaluating the effect of substantial weight loss on polysomnography have revealed significant improvements in AHI. Alongside weight loss, general measures to improve upper airway tone include the avoidance of alcohol and the positional therapy, to avoid sleep positions that precipitate symptoms, such as sleeping on one's back.

CPAP is the mainstay of treatment to support the upper airway during sleep; the continuous pressure delivered through either a nasal or full face mask increases lateral airway dimensions, thereby preventing intermittent airway obstruction. There is good evidence for its efficacy; it reduces the number of apneic and hypopneic episodes and subsequently reduces daytime symptoms of somnolence. It is indicated for all patients with an AHI greater than 15 events per hour and for those patients with a lower AHI but associated daytime symptoms. The CPAP device typically delivers between 5 and 20 cm H_2O to abolish apneas, snoring, and oxygen desaturation during rapid eye movement (REM) sleep. There are a number of different CPAP systems on the market. Some require titration and setting to the correct pressure with regular checks to ensure the appropriate pressure is delivered; this requires a number of visits to hospital. Other systems titrate the pressures automatically during sleep and can be monitored from the treating center remotely. Current NICE guidelines state that decisions on the make and type of CPAP device to be used should be made on the basis of the requirements of the individual.[34]

The CPAP mask can be difficult to wear, and issues can arise regarding the selection of the interface between the machine and the patient. It is important to ensure adequate mask fit and comfort; the noise of a leaking mask may itself impair sleep, although modern machines are considerably quieter than their older contemporaries. The machines are also more portable than previously, allowing them to be taken on holiday and therefore avoiding breaks in treatment. Nevertheless, there is accumulating evidence that, on average, CPAP machines are only used for 4–5 h per night, despite a quoted sleep time of 6–8 h, although there is no clear evidence of impact on daytime functioning or Epworth Sleepiness Score.[35]

Over the last two decades, there has been an expansion in the number of devices that increase upper airway caliber, particularly in response to the often poor tolerance of CPAP. Mandibular advancement devices and dental splints augment the position of the upper airway, thereby enlarging airway caliber and reducing the risk of airway obstruction.

Surgical options are also available, in particular, when enlarged tonsils or adenoids are encroaching into the upper airway and contributing to the obstruction. Less often, individuals may undergo more invasive procedures, including genioglossus advancement and uvulopalatopharyngoplasty,[36] although the role of upper airway surgery remains largely unknown, because of small sample sizes in trials and a lack of consensus on a clear definition of surgical success.[37]

> **Practice point:** Practitioners should be alert to the possibility of OSAS in the context of obesity. At each review, there should be inquiry regarding the symptoms of OSAS and a low threshold for referral for investigation. A multidisciplinary approach to the management of OSA in the context of obesity is important in the management of this complex condition.

OBESITY HYPOVENTILATION SYNDROME

OHS is defined as daytime hypercapnia ($PaCO_2 >$ 45 mmHg or 6 kPa) in an obese individual where no other cause can be implicated (such as neuromuscular disease or underlying lung disease), with associated sleep-related breathing disorder.[38] Hypoventilation (i.e., insufficient ventilation of alveoli to clear carbon dioxide) in patients with obesity occurs when the normal compensatory ventilatory mechanisms that maintain adequate ventilation fail.[39] Complex interactions between obesity, altered respiratory drive, and sleep-disordered breathing combine to cause OHS, a condition with significant medical and societal repercussions.

Pathophysiology

Excess body mass causes an increase in oxygen consumption and carbon dioxide production, compared with individuals with normal body weight, due to increased body surface area. As a consequence, metabolism can be significantly increased in morbidly obese individuals.[40] Chest wall compliance is reduced in obese individuals, meaning the stiffness of the chest wall is increased and therefore the work of breathing is increased, even at rest. The increased stiffness of the chest wall results in breathing at a flatter and less efficient part of the respiratory pressure-volume curve (as seen in the physiology section above), which further increases the work of breathing. The decreased chest wall compliance means that the individual breathes at a low FRC and ERV, causing the smaller airways to close, particularly in the lung bases. The consequence is an even further increased work of breathing. The standard compensatory mechanism is to increase minute ventilation (the total amount of air inspired in 1 min) to maintain a normal blood carbon dioxide level. The narrowed airways also induce a degree of ventilation-perfusion mismatch, which reduces blood and tissue oxygenation and thereby the functional capacity of the ventilatory system.

There is blunting of the central respiratory drive in the context of the altered respiratory mechanics described in the preceding paragraph. Individuals with OHS do not hyperventilate in response to a hypercapnic challenge in the same way as obese individuals without the condition. Obese individuals have higher levels of circulating leptin, a satiety hormone produced by adipocytes, which has a stimulatory effect on ventilatory drive. Several studies have implicated leptin resistance in the pathophysiology of OHS; genetically obese leptin-deficient mice demonstrate many of the characteristics of human OHS including reduced ventilatory response to hypercapnia and impaired respiratory muscle mechanics.[41] The increased levels of leptin in obese individuals may be a direct result of the increased CO_2 burden or may be a compensatory response to underlying leptin resistance. The blunting of the central respiratory drive further reduces the capacity of the ventilatory system, in the context of an increased work of breathing.

This imbalance between a significantly increased work of breathing, a need to increase minute ventilation further, and reduction in the functional capacity of the ventilatory system results in ventilatory failure and therefore failure of alveolar ventilation and carbon dioxide clearance. Obese individuals can experience an increase in their work of breathing of up to 30%, which considerably contributes to their feeling of dyspnea.[1] Despite this increase in work of breathing, a proportion of these individuals will develop daytime hypercapnia. For those with a BMI > 35 kg/m^2, there is a 30% risk of developing daytime hypercapnia; this risk increases to 50% for those with a BMI > 50 kg/m^2. Many individuals will display features of both OHS and OSAS; approximately 90% of individuals with OHS will have concurrent OSAS.[42]

Diagnosis

A proportion of patients with OHS will present acutely to hospital with acute respiratory failure. In this circumstance, the patient will be acutely ill with dyspnea, hypoventilation, a flapping tremor, confusion, and a history of weight gain and/or daytime somnolence. Often the history will be of deteriorating functioning and exercise limitation due to breathlessness with or without long-term weight gain. There may a precipitant such as an infection (acute bronchitis or pneumonia, viral or bacterial) or pulmonary embolism that induces a change from chronic to acute ventilatory failure.

In an outpatient setting, OHS is characterized by progressive ventilatory failure with carbon dioxide retention, leading to deterioration in functioning and increasing breathlessness. The presenting features are of breathlessness, decreased exercise tolerance, daytime sleepiness and poor concentration, and further weight gain. Because 90% of patients with OHS have concomitant OSAS, OHS may present with clinical features of OSAS.

In obese patients, OHS is a diagnosis of awareness and recognition. All patients should be questioned regarding limitation of functioning and symptoms of breathlessness. The clinical signs of flapping tremor, bounding pulse, and warm peripheries should be sought. The Epworth Sleepiness Score is a useful tool to determine daytime sleepiness. If the diagnosis is suspected, an arterial blood gas will show a high plasma partial pressure of carbon dioxide (PaCO$_2$) with renal compensation leading to high plasma bicarbonate. In the early stages, there may be increased ventilatory drive and function through the day with normalization of the PaCO$_2$, but the plasma bicarbonate will typically be raised. The diagnosis may further be confirmed by overnight oximetry (or polysomnography). This will show either OSAS or persistent overnight hypoxia, and an early morning arterial blood gas analysis will confirm a rise in PaCO$_2$ overnight, with a high morning PaCO$_2$. The plasma bicarbonate will be raised.

OHS is associated with chronic hypoxia, particularly overnight and chronic hypercapnia, which worsens with sleep overnight. This is associated with the development of pulmonary hypertension (PH). PH is associated with an adverse prognosis and a deterioration in breathlessness and functioning.

Management and Prognosis

In the acute setting, the underlying cause of the deterioration should be sought and treated. In the case of infection, this should be treated with appropriate antibiotics, or antivirals in the case of influenza. Bronchospasm, if present, may be treated with nebulized bronchodilators and oral corticosteroids if there are signs of chronic obstructive pulmonary disease (COPD).

Ventilation may be supported with non-invasive ventilation. Non-invasive ventilation involves the use of a bilevel ventilator connected to a face mask or nasal pillows, although a variety of different interfaces are available. The ventilator is synchronized to deliver support to inspiration and expiration to reduce the load on the ventilatory system and relieve some of the work of breathing. This allows treatment of the underlying cause of the deterioration and recovery to the preacute ventilatory failure state. On inspiration, the ventilator senses the change in airflow and delivers a mixture of air and entrained oxygen to a set inspiratory oxygen concentration at a pressure set to generate an adequate tidal volume (normal depth of inspiration). On expiration, the ventilator generates a PEEP to keep the airways open and allow full expiration. The PEEP opens the partially narrowed and collapsed airways and alveoli, facilitating oxygenation. Thus the ventilator compensates for the increased work of breathing and improves the functional capacity of the ventilatory system.

In the outpatient setting, weight reduction is the first-line intervention for individuals with OHS. For those with chronic ventilatory failure, with or without PH, nocturnal domiciliary non-invasive ventilation may be used to treat ventilatory failure. At night during REM sleep, there is loss of tone of the ventilatory muscles, resulting in worsening of ventilatory failure. Support for ventilation overnight can reduce the symptoms of loss of daytime functioning, daytime sleepiness, and breathlessness. A bilevel ventilator similar to that used in the acute setting is used, with regular monitoring to ensure the efficacy of the ventilatory support. Considerable support for the individual patient at home is required to deliver this treatment. The face mask pressures generated by the ventilator may be uncomfortable and the treatment is not tolerated by all patients.

The average hours of daily use of the non-invasive ventilator over a period of 1 month directly correlates with improved arterial blood gas results. Non-adherence to treatment is the main reason for a lack of improvement in symptoms and blood gas results. Different ventilatory settings can be tried to improve compliance to treatment; effective treatment can reduce healthcare costs, hospital admissions, and the associated morbidity and mortality. The prognosis for individuals with OHS is considerably worse than for that for obese individuals with OSA alone, and mortality is usually due to cardiovascular disease, particularly PH.

> **Practice point**: Patients with obesity should be observed and questioned for signs of sleep-disordered breathing and chronic ventilatory failure. Patients suspected of OHS require arterial blood gas analysis and overnight oximetry or polysomnography. On diagnosis, the patient may be offered long-term non-invasive ventilation.

THE EFFECT OF OBESITY ON RESPIRATORY DISEASE

Asthma

Obesity is the most common asthma comorbidity, and obese patients with asthma often pose a therapeutic challenge.[43] Multiple studies and metaanalyses suggest a correlation between increased body weight and the development of asthma, and obesity is associated with a unique asthma phenotype. This is characterized typically by adult-onset disease, altered pulmonary function, and noneosinophilic airway inflammation with a poor response to treatment (in particular biologic therapies) and more severe disease. In the Severe Asthma Research Program (SARP) cluster study, clinical characteristics associated with the highest BMI cluster, which were consistently described, included having late onset asthma, lower fractional exhaled nitric oxide (FeNO) levels, less airway eosinophils, and reduced atopy.[44]

The correlation between the two conditions is likely multifactorial and includes immunologic pathways, chemical responses, and hormonal influences. The incidence of asthma is 1.47 times higher in obese individuals than in non-obese individuals, and a three-unit increase in BMI is associated with a 35% increase in the risk of asthma.[45] The change in airway diameter as a result of a reduction in FRC can result in the development of bronchial hyperresponsiveness even in nonasthmatic individuals. There is also growing understanding of the link between prenatal nutrition and diet in early childhood with the development of both asthma and obesity, through influences of the central endocrine regulatory systems and programming the development of adipose tissue. A recent prospective study of the effects of bariatric surgery on airway hyperresponsiveness, asthma control, and inflammation revealed a reduction in airway hyperresponsiveness in obese asthmatic patients with normal serum IgE levels.[46]

Pathophysiology

Metabolically active adipose tissue is a key source of cytokine production, and obese individuals sustain a chronic, low-grade proinflammatory state. In particular, significantly elevated levels of proinflammatory cytokines, namely IL-1, IL-6, TNF-α, and plasminogen-activator inhibitor 1 (PAI-1) may affect the airways directly or through other cell-mediated pathways.[47] These cytokines promote the generation of reactive oxygen and nitrogen species by macrophages and monocytes, making obese individuals more susceptible to oxidative damage. However, the relationship between systemic and airway inflammation in asthma remains incompletely understood; obese asthmatic individuals do not exhibit increased eosinophilic or neutrophilic inflammation in their airways, and weight loss in obese asthmatics does not alter airway cellular inflammation.

Adipocytes also have a major endocrine function, by producing a variety of hormones. In particular, adiponectin and leptin have an effect on asthma, because of their immunomodulatory functions. Raised leptin levels result in an increase in T-helper cells, which subsequently increase circulating levels of TNF-α and IL-6. In animal models, leptin infusions increase allergen-induced airway hyperreactivity in normal-weight mice, whereas adiponectin infusions decrease allergen-induced airway hyperreactivity.[47] Most human studies have shown a positive relationship between serum leptin and a negative association between serum adiponectin and the risk of asthma. While the obesity-asthma association does not appear to be explained completely by these hormones, more studies are required to investigate this link further, to help direct future therapies.

Treatment

The mainstay of treatment for patients with asthma as a consequence of obesity is weight loss; because of the reduction in FRC in obese individuals, there is effective permanent airflow limitation as a result of breathing at lower lung volumes. Studies have shown how a reduction in weight improves asthma control and reduces bronchial hyperreactivity (Table 11.2).[46]

For patients with asthma secondary to obesity, it is prudent to consider small-particle inhaled therapies,

---

TABLE 11.2
A Comparison of Approaches to the Investigation and Management of Asthma Depending on Etiology

Diagnosis	Asthma With Concurrent Obesity	Asthma Secondary to Obesity
Airway features	Airway eosinophilia	No demonstrable airway eosinophilia or neutrophilia
Atopy features	Often a predominant feature	Less of a predominant feature
FeNO	Tends to be raised in uncontrolled disease	Less likely to be raised in uncontrolled disease
Treatment	Responds well to inhaled corticosteroids	Responds less well to inhaled corticosteroids. Weight loss mainstay of treatment

FeNO, fraction of exhaled nitric oxide.

---

and avoidance of high-dose inhaled corticosteroid is also important. Although there are no pharmacologic strategies designed to specifically treat obese asthmatics, weight loss interventions, both surgical and nutritional, have been tested and shown to have varying degrees of effectiveness in improving the respiratory health of these patients.[48] However, the effectiveness of this intervention may depend on other phenotypical factors and the degree of weight loss.

> **Practice point**: Obese asthmatic patients may not respond to conventional therapies as expected. In those patients with late-onset asthma, with low FeNO levels, who are poor responders to inhaled and oral corticosteroids, consider weight loss early in the treatment strategy. Avoid high-dose inhaled corticosteroids in this group of patients because of lack of efficacy and likely resultant weight gain.

CHRONIC OBSTRUCTIVE PULMONARY DISEASE

COPD is increasingly being recognized as a heterogenous condition with many systemic features. The relationship between obesity and COPD has become increasingly identified, although the exact connection remains unclear. The risk of developing obesity is increased in patients with COPD as a result of a reduced level of physical activities in daily life when compared with healthy age-matched controls.[49] Additionally, individuals with COPD who require repeated courses of oral corticosteroids are at increased risk of developing truncal obesity. An epidemiologic study of 650,000 patients revealed that the prevalence of obesity was significantly higher in patients with COPD than in those without COPD over a 13-year observation period, and the presence of obesity in COPD was associated with significantly higher risk of severe activity limitation and increased healthcare utilization.[50] A

recent multicenter prospective cohort study of COPD identified a prevalence of obesity of approximately one-third in those patients with GOLD stage 2–4 and revealed an increased risk of severe acute exacerbations of COPD, theorized to be due to the increased prevalence of comorbidities in obese individuals compared with their normal-weight counterparts.[51]

The role of adipose tissue in the pathogenesis of systemic inflammation in COPD has not yet been studied, although the same potential deleterious effects of increased levels of proinflammatory cytokines from adipose tissue on systemic and airway inflammation may occur in COPD as they do in asthma. Interestingly however, the relative risk for mortality seems to be decreased in overweight and obese patients with COPD in GOLD stage 3–4, compared with underweight individuals with the same degree of airway disease.[52] A possible protective role for obesity in COPD may arise; low BMI is associated with increased all-cause and COPD-related mortality. This phenomenon, referred to as the "obesity paradox," has been identified in several other chronic disease states such as chronic heart failure, end-stage chronic kidney disease, and rheumatoid arthritis. The pathophysiologic mechanisms of the "obesity paradox" are yet to be determined; in obese men with COPD the annual decline in FEV_1 is significantly lower than in men of normal BMI range; however, this effect is not seen in women.[53] A BMI greater than 30 has been shown to be protective in COPD while extremes of BMI are related to an increased risk of death, despite the individual's smoking history.[54] The BODE registry (an ongoing prospective multicenter cohort study of COPD patients attending outpatient pulmonary clinics at one of the five BODE study centers) has recently concluded that different BMI categories are associated with distinct clinical expressions of COPD and comorbidity patterns and that the relationship between mortality and BMI remains unclear.[54]

Pulmonary rehabilitation (PR) is an evidence-based intervention shown to improve outcomes in COPD.[55]

The role of PR for obese patients with COPD is of particular importance. Vagaggini et al. showed it to be an independent predictor of efficacy,[56] while a retrospective analysis revealed a similarity in health outcomes between obese and nonobese individuals following completion of a PR program.[57] Questions remain unanswered as to the potential role of PR to improve morbidity and mortality through a reduction in systemic inflammation.

> **Practice point:** Obesity increases the risk for patients with COPD developing ventilatory failure. This should be considered early in the presence of hypercapnic symptoms.

PULMONARY VASCULAR DISEASE

PH is a potentially life-threatening condition arising from a wide variety of pathophysiologic mechanisms. Although risk factors for pulmonary arterial hypertension are poorly defined, recent studies indicate that obesity may be an important risk factor for the condition. The mechanisms leading to this association are largely unknown, but proinflammatory mediators secreted from adipose tissue have been implicated in this process.

Obesity and PH frequently coexist in clinical practice and the symptoms of both conditions often overlap. Multiple mechanisms link obesity to PH and more than one may simultaneously operate in an individual patient. Sleep-disordered breathing is found in Group 3 of the WHO Classification of PH.[58]

> **Practice point:** In obese breathless patients with otherwise normal chest radiology and normal lung function tests, investigations to exclude PH should always be performed.

CONCLUSION

The direct consequences of obesity on the respiratory system are wide-ranging and often associated with considerable morbidity and mortality; however, they remain underrecognized and undertreated. Recognition is of utmost importance, particularly as the prevalence of obesity continues to increase at such a concerning rate. Identifying the potential impact of obesity on respiratory conditions is vital; although standard treatments are often less successful, effective therapies targeting role of obesity on the condition can significantly improve the success of treatment and the health of the patient.

REFERENCES

1. Dixon AE, Clerisme-Beaty EM. Obesity and lung disease: a guide to management. *Respir Med.* 2013. 72–110, 248.
2. Koo P, Gartman EJ, Sethi JM, McCool FD. Physiology in medicine: physiological basis of diaphragmatic dysfunction with abdominal hernias-implications for therapy. *J Appl Physiol.* 2015;118(2):142. Available from: http://go.libproxy.wakehealth.edu/login?url=http://search.proquest.com/docview/1647734957?accountid=14868%5Cnhttp://uv7gq6an4y.search.serialssolutions.com/?ctx_ver=Z39.88-2004&ctx_enc=info:ofi/enc:UTF-8&rfr_id=info:sid/ProQ:pqrl&rft_val_fmt=info:ofi/fmt:k.
3. Nikischin W, Gerhardt T, Everett R, Bancalari E. A new method to analyze lung compliance when pressure-volume relationship is nonlinear. *Am J Respir Crit Care Med.* 1998;158(4):1052–1060.
4. Parameswaran K, Todd DC, Soth M. Altered respiratory physiology in obesity. *Can Respir J.* 2006;13:203–210.
5. Jones RL, Nzekwu MM. The effects of body mass index on lung volumes. *Chest.* 2006;130(3):827–833. Available from: http://www.ncbi.nlm.nih.gov/pubmed/16963682.
6. Pelosi P, Croci M, Ravagnan I, et al. The effects of body mass on lung volumes, respiratory mechanics, and gas exchange during general anesthesia. *Anesth Analg.* 1998;87(3):654.
7. Sharp JT, Henry JP, Sweany SK, Meadows WR, Pietras RJ. Effects of mass loading the respiratory system in man. *J Appl Physiol.* 1964;19:959–966 (Bethesda, Md. : 1985).
8. Lazarus R, Sparrow D, Weiss ST. Effects of obesity and fat distribution on ventilatory function: the normative aging study. *Chest.* 1997;111(4):891–898.
9. Mafort TT, Rufino R, Costa CH, Lopes AJ. Obesity: systemic and pulmonary complications, biochemical abnormalities, and impairment of lung function. *Multidiscip Respir Med.* 2016;11(1):28. Available from: http://mrmjournal.biomedcentral.com/articles/10.1186/s40248-016-0066-z.
10. Lin CK, Lin CC. Work of breathing and respiratory drive in obesity. *Respirology.* 2012;17(3):402–411.
11. Zerah F, Harf A, Perlemuter L, Lorino H, Lorino AM, Atlan G. Effects of obesity on respiratory resistance. *Chest.* 1993;103(5):1470–1476.
12. Vaughan RW, Cork RC, Hollander D. The effect of massive weight loss on arterial oxygenation and pulmonary function tests. *Anesthesiology.* 1981;54(4):325–328. Available from: http://www.ncbi.nlm.nih.gov/pubmed/7212333.
13. Holley HS, Milic-Emili J, Becklake MR, Bates DV. Regional distribution of pulmonary ventilation and perfusion in obesity. *J Clin Invest.* 1967;46(4):475–481. Available from: http://www.pubmedcentral.nih.gov/articlerender.fcgi?artid=442031&tool=pmcentrez&rendertype=abstract.
14. Douglas F, Chong PY. Influence of obesity on peripheral airways patency. *J Appl Physiol.* November 1972;33:559–563.
15. Canoy D, Luben R, Welch A, et al. Abdominal obesity and respiratory function in men and women in the EPIC-Norfolk Study, United Kingdom. *Am J Epidemiol.* 2004;159(12):1140–1149.

16. Chen Y, Rennie D, Cormier YF, Dosman J. Waist circumference is associated with pulmonary function in normal-weight, overweight, and obese subjects. *Am J Clin Nutr.* 2007;85(1):35–39.

17. Biring MS, Lewis MI, Liu JT, Mohsenifar Z. Pulmonary physiologic changes of morbid obesity. *Am J Med Sci.* 1999;318(5):293–297. Available from: http://journals.lww.com/amjmedsci/Abstract/1999/11000/Pulmonary_Physiologic_Changes_of_Morbid_Obesity.2.aspx%5Cnhttp://www.ncbi.nlm.nih.gov/pubmed/10555090.

18. Watson RA, Pride NB. Postural changes in lung volumes and respiratory resistance in subjects with obesity. *J Appl Physiol.* 2005;98(2):512–517.

19. Collins LC, Hoberty PD, Walker JF, Fletcher EC, Peiris AN. The effect of body fat distribution on pulmonary function tests. *Chest.* 1995;107(5):1298–1302.

20. Agras WS, Hammer LD, McNicholas F, Kraemer HC. Risk factors for childhood overweight: a prospective study from birth to 9.5 years. *J Pediatr.* 2004;145(1):20–25. Available from: http://www.ncbi.nlm.nih.gov/pubmed/15238901.

21. Gangwisch JE, Malaspina D, Boden-Albala B, Heymsfield SB. Inadequate sleep as a risk factor for obesity: analyses of the NHANES I. *Sleep.* 2005;28(10):1289–1296. Available from: https://www.researchgate.net/profile/Dolores_Malaspina/publication/7473864_Inadequate_sleep_as_a_risk_factor_for_obesity_analyses_of_the_NHANES_I/links/53f4d99f0cf2888a74912841.pdf.

22. Ofir D, Laveneziana P, Webb KA, O'Donnell DE. Ventilatory and perceptual responses to cycle exercise in obese women. *J Appl Physiol.* 2007;102(6):2217–2226.

23. Hillman DR, Murphy AS, Pezzullo L. The economic cost of sleep disorders. *Sleep.* 2006;29(3):299–305.

24. NICE. *NICE Clinical Knowledge Summaries Obstructive Sleep Apnoea Syndrome*; April 2015. https://cks.nice.org.uk/obstructive-sleep-apnoea-s.

25. Dauglas N. Sleep apnoea. In: *Harrisons Principles of Internal Medicine.* ; 2008:1665–1667.

26. Young T, Palta M, Dempsey J, Skatrud J, Weber S, Badr S. The occurrence of sleep-disordered breathing among middle-aged adults. *N Engl J Med.* 1993;328(17):1230–1235. Available from: http://www.nejm.org/doi/abs/10.1056/NEJM199304293281704.

27. Moore A. The big sleep problem. *Health Sci J.* 2013 Nov 22; 123(6376):Suppl 2–3.

28. Marks S. *Oxford Desk Reference: Respiratory.* Oxford Med Publ; 2009. xxii, 754. Available from: http://discovery.ucl.ac.uk/89826/.

29. Kuna ST, Bedi DG, Ryckman C. Effect of nasal airway positive pressure on upper airway size and configuration. *Am Rev Respir Dis.* 1988;138(4):969–975. Available from: http://www.atsjournals.org/doi/abs/10.1164/ajrccm/138.4.969.

30. Punjabi NM, Caffo BS, Goodwin JL, et al. Sleep-disordered breathing and mortality: a prospective cohort study. *PLoS Med.* 2009;6(8).

31. Quan SF, Wright R, Baldwin CM, et al. Obstructive sleep apnea-hypopnea and neurocognitive functioning in the sleep heart health study. *Sleep Med.* 2006;7(6):498–507.

32. Engleman H, Martin S, Douglas N, Deary I. Effect of continuous positive airway pressure treatment on daytime function in sleep apnoea/hypopnoea syndrome. *Lancet.* 1994;343(8897):572–575. Available from: http://www.sciencedirect.com/science/article/pii/S0140673694915229.

33. Peppard PE, Young T, Palta M, Dempsey J, Skatrud J. Longitudinal study of moderate weight change and sleep-disordered breathing. *JAMA.* 2000;284(23):3015–3021.

34. NICE. *Continuous Positive Airway Pressure for the Treatment of Obstructive Sleep Apnoea/Hypopnoea Syndrome*; 2008. https://www.nice.org.uk/guidance/TA139/chapter/4-E.

35. Weaver TE, Maislin G, Dinges DF, et al. Relationship between hours of CPAP use and achieving normal levels of sleepiness and daily functioning. *Sleep.* June 2007;30:711–719.

36. Mehra P, Wolford LM. Surgical management of obstructive sleep apnea. *Proc (Bayl Univ Med Cent).* 2000;13(4):338–342. Available from: http://www.pubmedcentral.nih.gov/articlerender.fcgi?artid=1312227&tool=pmcentrez&rendertype=abstract.

37. Khan A, Ramar K, Maddirala S, Friedman O, Pallanch JF, Olson EJ. Uvulopalatopharyngoplasty in the management of obstructive sleep apnea: the mayo clinic experience. *Mayo Clin Proc.* 2009;84(9):795–800. Available from: http://www.pubmedcentral.nih.gov/articlerender.fcgi?artid=2735429&tool=pmcentrez&rendertype=abstract.

38. Mokhlesi B, Kryger MH, Grunstein RR. Assessment and management of patients with obesity hypoventilation syndrome. *Proc Am Thorac Soc.* 2008;5(2):218–225. Available from: http://www.pubmedcentral.nih.gov/articlerender.fcgi?artid=2645254&tool=pmcentrez&rendertype=abstract.

39. Piper A. Obesity hypoventilation syndrome – the big and the breathless. *Am J Sleep Med Rev.* 2011;15(2):79–89.

40. Gilbert R. Respiratory control and work of breathing in obese subjects. *J Appl Physiol.* January 1961;16:21–26.

41. O'Donnell CP, Schaub CD, Haines AS, et al. Leptin prevents respiratory depression in obesity. *Am J Respir Crit Care Med.* 1999;159(5 I):1477–1484.

42. Mokhlesi B. Obesity hypoventilation syndrome: a state-of-the-art review. *Respir Care.* 2010;55(10):1347–1362.

43. Baffi CW, Winnica DE, Holguin F. Asthma and obesity: mechanisms and clinical implications. *Asthma Res Pract.* 2015;1(1):1. Available from: Missingcontent/1/1/1.

44. Moore WC, Meyers DA, Wenzel SE, et al. Identification of asthma phenotypes using cluster analysis in the severe asthma research program. *Am J Respir Crit Care Med.* 2010;181(4):315–323.

45. Brumpton BM, Leivseth L, Romundstad PR, et al. The joint association of anxiety, depression and obesity with incident asthma in adults: the HUNT study. *Int J Epidemiol.* 2013;42(5):1455–1463.

46. Dixon AE, Pratley RE, Forgione PM, et al. Effects of obesity and bariatric surgery on airway hyperresponsiveness, asthma control, and inflammation. *J Allergy Clin Immunol.* 2011;128(3).

47. Dixon AE, Holguin F, Sood A, et al. An official American Thoracic Society Workshop report: obesity and asthma.

Proc Am Thorac Soc. 2010;7(5):325–335. Available from: http://pats.atsjournals.org/content/7/5/325.full.pdf%5Cnhttp://pats.atsjournals.org/content/7/5/325.long.

48. Maniscalco M, Zedda A, Faraone S, et al. Weight loss and asthma control in severely obese asthmatic females. *Respir Med.* 2008;102(1):102–108.

49. Pitta F, Troosters T, Spruit MA, Probst VS, Decramer M, Gosselink R. Characteristics of physical activities in daily life in chronic obstructive pulmonary disease. *Am J Respir Crit Care Med.* 2005;171(9):972–977.

50. Vozoris NT, O'Donnell DE. Prevalence, risk factors, activity limitation and health care utilization of an obese, population-based sample with chronic obstructive pulmonary disease. *Can Respir J.* 2012;19(3):e18–24. Available from: http://eutils.ncbi.nlm.nih.gov/entrez/eutils/elink.fcgi?dbfrom=pubmed&id=22679617&retmode=ref&cmd=prlinks%5Cnhttp://www.ncbi.nlm.nih.gov/pubmed/22679617%5Cnhttp://www.pubmedcentral.nih.gov/articlerender.fcgi?artid=PMC3418099.

51. Allison A. Obesity is associated with increased morbidity in moderate to severe COPD. *Chest.* 2017;151(1):68–77.

52. Landbo C, Prescott E, Lange P, Vestbo J, Almdal TP. Prognostic value of nutritional status in chronic obstructive pulmonary disease. *Am J Respir Crit Care Med.* 1999;160(6):1856–1861.

53. Watson L, Vonk JM, Löfdahl CG, et al. Predictors of lung function and its decline in mild to moderate COPD in association with gender: results from the Euroscop study. *Respir Med.* 2006;100(4):746–753.

54. Divo MJ, Cabrera C, Ciro C, et al. Comorbidity distribution, clinical expression and survival in COPD patients with different body mass index. *J COPD Found.* 2014;1(2):229–238.

55. Spruit MA, Singh SJ, Garvey C, et al. An official American Thoracic Society/European Respiratory Society Statement: key concepts and advances in pulmonary rehabilitation. *Am J Respir Crit Care Med.* 2013;188:13–64.

56. Vagaggini B, Costa F, Antonelli S, et al. Clinical predictors of the efficacy of a pulmonary rehabilitation programme in patients with COPD. *Respir Med.* 2009;103(8):1224–1230.

57. Ramachandran K, McCusker C, Connors M, Zuwallack R, Lahiri B. The influence of obesity on pulmonary rehabilitation outcomes in patients with COPD. *Chron Respir Dis.* 2008;5(4):205–209. Available from: http://www.ncbi.nlm.nih.gov/entrez/query.fcgi?cmd=Retrieve&db=PubMed&dopt=Citation&list_uids=19029231.

58. Simonneau G, Galie N, Rubin LJ, et al. Clinical classification of pulmonary hypertension. *J Am Coll Cardiol.* 2004;43(12 suppl S):S5–S12. Available from: http://www.ncbi.nlm.nih.gov/pubmed/15194173.

CHAPTER 12

The Effect of Obesity on Reproductive Health

IAN A. AIRD, MBCHB, DA, FRCOG • YITKA GRAHAM, PhD, BSc

INTRODUCTION

Obesity was once considered to be a problem of more affluent developed nations, but there is increasing evidence of a rise in the level of obesity in low- and middle-income countries.[1]

Obesity adversely affects reproductive health; although many women with obesity do not have problems with conceiving, the time taken to conception is increased if either the female or male partner in a relationship is obese.[2,3] In the female, obesity is also associated with oligomenorrhea and amenorrhea due to disturbance in the hypothalamic-pituitary-ovarian (HPO) axis, leading to irregular or absent ovulation. However, fecundity has also been found to be reduced in obese women with regular menses,[2] suggesting that obesity in the female affects more than just ovulation.[4]

Obesity in the male has also been associated with reduced fertility. There are less research data available concerning how obesity affects male fertility although abnormalities in semen parameters and sperm function have been reported.[5]

The adverse effect of obesity on fecundity has led to an increase in the number of couples where one or both partners are obese and seeking help with their fertility treatment. Unfortunately, there is increasing evidence that the outcome of assisted reproductive treatments (ARTs) is also negatively impacted on where obesity is present.[6,7]

Not only will obesity increase the time to conception, but once pregnant there is an also an association with early pregnancy failure and miscarriage for both spontaneous and assisted conceptions.[6,8,9]

Obesity is also associated with increased obstetric and fetal complications such as gestational diabetes, preeclampsia. Preterm birth, operative delivery, shoulder dystocia postpartum hemorrhage, infection, congenital abnormality, fetal macrosomia, and intrauterine fetal death.[10]

Weight loss through lifestyle modification, medical or surgical treatment can improve the chances of both spontaneous and assisted conception.[11–13]

EFFECT OF OBESITY ON MALE REPRODUCTIVE FUNCTION

There is evidence that the rise in the levels of adult obesity has been mirrored by a reported decline in the quality of semen over a similar period. This decline in semen quality was not evident in countries with lower levels of adult obesity,[14] suggesting a possible causal relationship between obesity and impaired male fertility.[15]

The adverse effect that obesity exerts on male fertility has been assessed in epidemiologic studies. Two studies carried out in 2007 revealed a significant increase in the number of couples who had not conceived within 2 years of trying where the male partner was obese.[3,16] These two studies were combined in a recent meta-analysis that revealed such couples were significantly more likely to experience infertility than couples with a normal-weight male partner (odds ratio = 1.66, 95% CI 1.53–1.79).[7]

Although there is increasing and consistent evidence of the adverse effect of male obesity on reproductive function, the underlying cause of the impaired fertility is less clear. Possible areas where obesity can cause adverse effects include disruption in the hormonal control of spermatogenesis, production of adipocytokines by adipose tissue, and also impaired spermatogenesis leading to abnormalities in semen quality and sperm function.[17]

Male Obesity and the Hypothalamic-Pituitary-Gonadal Axis

Spermatogenesis is a highly complex process in which healthy fertile sperms are produced from testicular germ cells. This process is controlled via a strict regulatory mechanism in which the hypothalamic-pituitary-gonadal (HPG) axis plays a central role.

Male obesity has been shown to produce a hypogonadotropic state with reduced levels of testosterone and elevated levels of estrogen. This can, in turn, lead to dysregulation of the HPG axis with adverse effects on testicular function, spermatogenesis, and male libido.[17]

Elevated levels of estrogen can arise from increased peripheral aromatase activity in which the cytochrome P450 enzyme plays an important role. White adipose tissue expresses high levels of cytochrome P450 enzyme. In obese individuals, this increase in aromatase activity leads to increased conversion of androgens to estrogens.[15]

The elevated levels of estrogen can exert negative feedback on the HPG axis via kisspeptin neurons,[18] resulting in reduced gonadotropin-releasing hormone (GnRH) and consequently luteinizing hormone (LH) secretion and testosterone production from the testicles. Evidence from animal studies has shown that estrogens may also exert a direct effect on the testicle, resulting in reduced gonad size and decreased sperm count and quality.[19]

The lower levels of testosterone found in obese men may also have a direct effect on Sertoli cell function, leading to retention and phagocytosis of mature spermatids.[20]

Male obesity is also associated with insulin resistance, which can lead to other endocrine effects with adverse consequences for spermatogenesis. The increased insulin levels can have a direct inhibitory effect on spermatogenesis.[17] Hyperinsulinemia may also lead to a suppression of hepatic sex hormone–binding globulin (SHBG) production. SHBG binds sex hormones including testosterone and estrogen; reduced levels can thus lead to an increase in unbound and therefore biologically active estrogen with further suppression of the HPG axis. Hyperinsulinemia in obese males has also been associated with higher levels of nuclear and mitochondrial DNA damage in the sperm.[21]

Production of Adipokines

In addition to producing increased levels of estrogen via aromatase activity, adipose tissue may also exert endocrine effects through the production of other hormones—the adipokines.

Leptin is an adipokine secreted during the fed state and has several functions including stimulation of the satiety center, regulation of the neuroendocrine system, energy expenditure, puberty, and reproduction.

Although low levels of leptin due to a mutation in the gene controlling leptin production can cause obesity, paradoxically an elevated level of leptin is a common finding in obese infertile men.[15] The effect of leptin on the hypothalamus in normal-weight individuals would be to stimulate GnRH levels; however, the excess leptin seen in obese individuals causes the HPG axis to become resistant to leptin.[18]

Elevated levels of leptin in obesity have been associated with reduced testosterone levels via an inhibition of gonadotropic stimulation of Leydig cells. Leptin receptors have also been found to be present on the plasma membrane of the sperm, indicating a possible effect of leptin on spermatogenesis independent of the HPG axis.[22]

Obesity is also associated with increased production of proinflammatory cytokines, which may also exert an inhibitory effect on the hypothalamus, leading to further dysregulation of the HPG axis.[17]

Inhibin B production by Sertoli cells is an effective marker for spermatogenesis. It acts within the testis to inhibit follicle-stimulating hormone (FSH) production and stimulate testosterone production by Leydig cells. Reduced levels of Inhibin B have been reported in obese males and are indicative of seminiferous tubule dysfunction and may be related to a reduced number of Sertoli cells in the testis of obese males.[23]

Impairment of Spermatogenesis

Studies investigating the effect of male obesity on conventional parameters of semen quality have produced conflicting results. A review article by Davidson et al. in 2015 referenced 13 studies in which there was no relationship between increased BMI and one or more of the following semen parameters: sperm concentration, count, morphology, motility, and ejaculate volume. However, the paper also referenced nine studies showing that raised BMI was associated with abnormalities in one of more of the following: sperm concentration, count, motility, or ejaculate volume.[17]

A systematic review and metaanalysis of available studies investigating the effect of paternal obesity on reproductive potential in 2015[7] found a significant increase in percentage of sperm with abnormal morphology in samples from obese men but no other clinically significant differences for other conventional semen parameters.

Suggested reasons for this conflicting evidence include the possibility that BMI may be a poor measure of body fatness. The study populations also varied between obese men within the general population and those attending fertility clinics, which may have introduced bias toward a population of subfertile men. Confounding variables that could affect semen quality, including smoking, alcohol consumption, recreational drug use, or the presence of medical comorbidities, may not have been controlled for in all studies.[17]

Spermatogenesis and Oxidative Stress

Increased production of proinflammatory cytokines can lead to a chronic low-grade inflammation, which in turn can lead to insulin resistance, the metabolic syndrome, and type 2 diabetes mellitus.[24]

Alongside this, obesity can lead to higher metabolic rates, which are required to maintain normal biologic processes. The net effect of these changes is to produce an increase in the formation of reactive oxygen species (ROS). ROS are thought be responsible for damaging DNA in the nucleus of the sperm and also the sperm plasma membrane.[17]

There is evidence for altered DNA integrity within the sperm of obese males from a number of studies. The systematic review by Campbell et al.[7] reported a significant increase in the percentage of sperm with DNA fragmentation in obese men compared with normal-weight men. Reduced DNA integrity has been negatively correlated with successful pregnancies after both spontaneous and assisted conception.[25,26]

Alterations in DNA methylation and histone acetylation and changes in the sperm content and function of RNA and small noncoding RNA between the sperm from obese men and lean individuals have all been suggested as potential consequences of increased oxidative stress caused by male obesity. It is beyond the scope of this chapter to discuss in more detail the potential differences in the molecular aspects of spermatogenesis between obese and lean males; for a more detailed account, the reader is directed to Palmer et al.[5]

Obesity-induced reduction in sperm DNA integrity could lead to an adverse effect on childhood and adult health in the offspring of obese fathers, a phenomenon termed "transgenerational epigenetic inheritance."

There is evidence that obese fathers are more likely to have an obese child,[27,28] although it is not possible to separate out the individual contributions of environmental, genetic, and epigenetic factors from epidemiologic studies. Animal models of paternal obesity have been created to address this issue and have found evidence of altered metabolic and reproductive health in the first and second generation offspring where there was paternal obesity. Alterations in the sperm caused by obesity-induced molecular changes have been implicated as the likely mediator for this effect.[5]

Physical Factors

In addition to the hormonal and genetic factors discussed above, there are potential physical factors that have been implicated in reduced fertility potential in the obese male.

Increased scrotal adiposity may raise the testicular temperature. Spermatogenesis is acutely sensitive to heat, and increased scrotal temperature has been associated with reduced sperm motility, increased sperm

DNA damage, and increased sperm oxidative stress.[5] Surgical removal of scrotal fat has also been reported to lead to an improvement in sperm parameters.[29]

Erectile dysfunction is also more prevalent in obese males. The dysfunction has been linked to hormonal dysfunction and cardiovascular disease—both conditions being more common in the obese.

Sleep apnea, in which there is intermittent nocturnal upper airway obstruction, is frequently linked to obesity. The disrupted sleep pattern can adversely affect the nighttime rise in testosterone, and the reduced levels of testosterone and LH subsequent to this have been associated with decreased pituitary-gonadal function with consequent abnormal spermatogenesis and reduced male reproductive potential.[15]

Obesity can therefore be seen to exert an adverse effect on male reproductive potential in a number of different areas including hormonal, genetic, and physical (see Fig. 12.1). Treatment of the obesity can lead to significant improvement in all of these areas with consequent improvement in reproductive potential.

EFFECT OF OBESITY ON FEMALE REPRODUCTIVE FUNCTION

Female obesity is thought to impair reproductive function by exerting an adverse effect on the regulation of ovulation, oocyte development, embryo development, endometrial development, implantation, and pregnancy loss.[4]

Obesity has been reported to more than double the risk of anovulatory infertility,[30] but reduced fecundity has also been reported in obese women with normal menstrual cycles,[2] highlighting the adverse effect of obesity on fertility other than ovulatory disorders.

Central distribution of body fat has also been linked to impairment of fertility. Raised waist circumference and waist-to-hip ratios have been associated with delayed conception and reduced fecundability, even after controlling for BMI.[31,32]

Obesity is frequently associated with menstrual cycle disturbance and irregular or absent ovulation largely through a disruptive effect on the HPO axis. Indeed the rate menstrual cycle disturbance has been found to be 3.1 times higher in grossly obese women than normal-weight women.[33] Weight loss has also been shown to restore regular menstrual cycles and improve spontaneous conception rates and response to ovulation induction.[11]

Obesity is associated with significant imbalance in the hormones important for normal reproductive function, including sex steroid hormones, gonadotropins, and insulin.

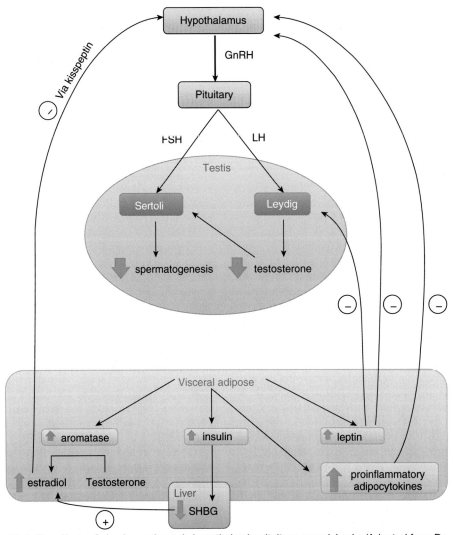

FIG. 12.1 The effects of obesity on the male hypothalamic-pituitary-gonadal axis. (Adapted from Davidson LM, Millar K, Jones C, Fatum M, Coward K. Deleterious effects of obesity upon the hormonal and molecular mechanisms controlling spermatogenesis and male fertility. *Hum Fertil*. 2015;18(3):184–193, with permission.)

Far from being an inert tissue, white adipose tissue is an active endocrine organ secreting a large number of hormones—the adipokines that can have both direct and indirect effects on female fertility. White adipose tissue is also a metabolically active organ.

The net result of this hormonal imbalance, adipokine production, and metabolic activity is an adverse effect on female fecundity not just at the HPO axis level but also on ovarian follicles, oocytes, endometrial, and early embryo development.

Obesity and Sex Steroid Metabolism

Obesity, especially central obesity, is associated with a relative excess of bioavailable sex steroid hormones. This includes both estrogens and androgens. This excess arises as a result of increased production and reduced protein binding. Adipose tissue can also affect the balance of sex hormone availability by acting as a reservoir of lipid-soluble steroid hormones.[34]

Increased estrogen production arises as a result of aromatase activity in adipose tissue responsible for the conversion of androgens to estrogen. Increased androgen production arises through the activity of 17β-hydroxydehydrogenase and 3β-dehydrogenase enzymes.

Obesity also has an effect on the bioavailability of sex steroids through its effect on SHBG. Obesity, particularly central obesity, can lead to a decrease in SHBG production largely through reduced hepatic synthesis as a result of hyperinsulinemia.[35]

Changes in SHBG concentration lead to an alteration of androgen and estrogen delivery to target tissues.

The overall effect of increased production and bioavailability of sex steroids leads to an inflated steroid pool in obese women compared with normal-weight controls,[36] with the overall effect on androgen metabolism leading to a relative functional hyperandrogenism.[34]

Alterations in sex steroid metabolism may produce adverse effects on the regulation of the HPO axis, affecting the control of ovulation and folliculogenesis. The altered availability of estrogen at target organ level may also affect endometrial development with consequent effects on implantation.[37]

Gonadotropins

The level of LH and the ratio of LH to FSH (LH:FSH ratio) have been reported to be increased in obese women. This finding is also common in both obese and nonobese women with polycystic ovarian syndrome (PCOS). The hypersecretion of LH has been linked to disturbance of the HPO axis, resulting in exaggerated GnRH pulsatility[38] and enhanced pituitary sensitivity of LH secretion to GnRH.[39]

The relative excess of LH to FSH represents an unfavorable environment for normal follicular development. Weight loss had been shown to normalize the LH to FSH ratio, allowing FSH predominance favoring folliculogenesis.[40]

Insulin

Obesity is linked to insulin resistance and consequent hyperinsulinemia. Deposition of adipose tissue centrally is associated with production of nonesterified fatty acids (NEFA) by adipocytes. This in turn induces local macrophages to produce high levels of tumor necrosis factor alpha (TNF-α). The TNF-α induces the adipocytes to produce proinflammatory cytokines and chemokines, resulting in inflammation of visceral adipose tissue as well as systematic low-grade inflammation affecting multiple tissues.[24]

This chronic low-grade metabolic inflammation leads to the development of insulin resistance, diabetes mellitus, and metabolic syndrome.

As a response to the insulin resistance, there is increased production of insulin from the pancreas.

Insulin has a direct effect on the ovary where it acts on insulin receptors, which are widely distributed through all ovarian compartments. Stimulation of the insulin receptors leads to increased ovarian steroidogenesis. Insulin excess may adversely affect ovulation via enhanced ovarian androgen production or via a leptin-mediated effect on the HPO axis.[41]

Insulin has also an effect on the pituitary by upregulation of gonadotropin receptors and increasing the sensitivity to GnRH, leading to further stimulation of ovarian steroidogenesis.

Insulin also has an amplifying effect on insulin-like growth factor (IGF-1) via upregulation of IGF-1 receptors as well as inhibiting hepatic insulin-like growth factor binding protein type 1.[42]

Hyperinsulinism also leads to suppression of SHBG production by the liver, with consequent increased bioavailability of sex steroids.[34]

The combined effect of insulin resistance and hyperinsulinism on increased ovarian steroidogenesis, increased sex steroid bioavailability, hyperandrogenism, and the effect on the HPO axis and IGF system is to increase the likelihood of ovulatory and menstrual disturbance in obese women.

Adipokines

Far from being an inert organ, adipose tissue is now well recognized to have a crucial endocrine function involving the secretion of many hormones—the adipokines[43] and also several immune effectors including cytokines and chemokines.[24] Some of the adipokines are secreted uniquely by adipose tissue, whereas others are produced more widely with adipose tissue contributing to the circulating pool.[41]

Adipose tissue is an important homeostatic organ. It is involved in the regulation of several vital physiologic processes including food intake and energy balance via its effects on hunger and satiety centers. It has been more recently discovered that adipose tissue plays an important role in the regulation of the HPG axis with an essential role in the onset of puberty and fertility and their adaptation to the availability of energy and the size of fat deposits. Adipokines, cytokines, and chemokines mediate the effect of adipose tissue on the HPG axis.[24]

The exact role of the adipokines, chemokines, and cytokines on fertility and reproductive function remains to be fully elucidated as does any perturbation in the roles produced by excess adiposity. Much of the research into their effects has been carried out in animal models, the result of which may not be directly transferrable to the human model.[4]

Leptin

Leptin was identified as a product of adipose tissue in 1994.[44] It is expressed solely by adipose tissue where it is coded by the *ob* gene. Leptin is a potent appetite suppressant, its secretion increases with food intake, and it is a key signaling protein relaying the magnitude of peripheral energy stores through its effects at the hypothalamic level. Paradoxically, levels of leptin are high in obesity because of the development of leptin resistance, which in turn is mediated by the chronic low-grade inflammation associated with obesity.

Low leptin levels are associated with sexual immaturity. Females who are leptin deficient are known to have delayed puberty.[45] Low leptin levels may also be associated with exercise-induced and weight-related amenorrhea, where leptin levels are reduced as a result of low adipose store and body mass.[46]

Leptin levels fluctuate throughout the menstrual cycle with the lowest levels during the early follicular phase and the highest levels occurring during the luteal phase.

At normal serum concentrations of leptin, the effect at the hypothalamic level is to stimulate expression of GnRH.[47] This is thought to be mediated via the kisspeptin neurons. Conversely, the increased leptin levels seen in obesity can exert an inhibitory effect on the control of folliculogenesis.

At an ovarian level, leptin receptors and leptin receptor mRNA expression have been identified in theca and granulosa cells. In vitro studies have found a dose-dependent antagonistic effect of leptin on ovarian growth factors and gonadotropins with high leptin levels, leading to suppressed estradiol synthesis and possible interference with follicular development and oocyte maturation.[48] Results from animal studies have also shown that high levels of leptin can impair ovulation via a direct effect on the ovary.[49] Leptin, through its effect on growth factors including vascular endothelial growth factor, may also have an effect on endothelial cell proliferation and angiogenesis. Elevated levels of leptin, such as those seen in obesity, may induce oxidative damage in endothelial cells via ROS.[50] Elevated follicular levels of leptin have been associated with reduced intrafollicular oxygen levels in patients undergoing in vitro fertilization (IVF).[51] The elevated intrafollicular leptin levels could exert a local effect on perifollicular angiogenesis, leading to impaired delivery of nutrients and oxygen with consequent adverse effects on oocyte maturation.[52]

Leptin and its receptors have also been detected in preimplantation embryos and the endometrium in a mouse model, the level of leptin in the uterus being higher in pregnant rather than in nonpregnant mice.[53] Abnormally high levels of leptin as seen in obese women could impair embryo development and endometrial receptivity.

Adiponectin

Adiponectin is the most abundantly secreted protein from white adipose tissue, and in contrast to leptin, its levels are reduced in obesity.[54] Circulating levels of adiponectin are two- to threefold higher in females than in males[55] and are inversely correlated with hyperinsulinemia and insulin resistance.[56] Adiponectin improves insulin sensitivity, inhibits hepatic gluconeogenesis, and inhibits vascular inflammation.[54] Weight loss leads to an increase in adiponectin levels.[57]

The effects of adiponectin are exerted through two receptors, AdipoR1 and AdipoR2, and one or both of these receptors are present in all peripheral reproductive tissues. The role of adiponectin in peripheral reproductive tissues remains unclear. Studies using the mouse model have shown that mice that are deficient in either adiponectin or one or both of the receptors do not seem to be infertile.[58] The role of adiponectin in ovarian function has not been fully elucidated. Expression of the hormone or its receptors in ovarian and granulosa cells has been linked to steroidogenesis within these cells although findings are inconsistent.[54] Any effect of obesity on changes in adiponectin levels and ovarian function remains controversial. Deficient adiponectin levels have been implicated in the pathogenesis of PCOS, with affected patients showing a disordered response to adiponectin.[59]

Other adipokines, including resistin, visfatin, and chemerin, have been found in animal studies to affect ovarian steroidogenesis and follicular development. Any direct role of these hormones in the human and any adverse effect in obese individuals remain unclear.[59]

Cytokines and Chemokines

Adipose tissue also produces a number of proinflammatory substances implicated in the systemic chronic low-grade inflammatory state that leads to insulin resistance and hyperinsulinism.

Interleukin 6 (IL-6) is a key mediator of inflammation and levels are increased in obesity and weight loss through diet and exercise,[60] or bariatric surgery[61] has been shown to reduce levels. Elevated IL-6 levels are associated with increased insulin resistance. Animal studies have also revealed possible adverse effects on LH secretion, LH-induced ovulation, and reduced estrogen production in granulosa cells.[62]

Plasminogen activator inhibitor type 1 (PAI-1) regulates blood fibrinolytic activity and is primarily produced by white adipose tissue, especially visceral fat.[41] Plasma concentrations correlate strongly with metabolic syndrome. Excess levels of PAI-1 may impair implantation and have been implicated as a potential contributor to miscarriage in women with PCOS.[63] Again weight loss has been shown to lower levels of PAI-1.[61]

TNF-α is also produced by adipose tissue with plasma concentrations correlating with BMI and hyperinsulinemia. Women with PCOS have higher circulating levels of TNF-α. TNF-α has been shown to inhibit insulin signaling and also stimulate increased secretion of leptin and PAI-1 while decreasing adiponectin secretion.[41] Putative reproductive roles of TNF-α include regulation of progesterone production by the corpus luteum, LH secretion, ovarian steroidogenesis, ovulation, and corpus luteum regression.[41] TNF-α has also been implicated as a potential factor in miscarriage.[64]

Unlike the other cytokines, studies investigating the effect of weight loss on TNF-α concentrations have found inconsistent findings.[41]

Effect of Obesity on Expression of Polycystic Ovarian Syndrome

PCOS affects approximately 5%–10% of women of reproductive age. Approximately 80% of women with anovulatory infertility have PCOS. About 50% of PCOS patients are obese and, although not required as part of the diagnostic criteria for PCOS, obesity can exert a profound effect on how the syndrome is expressed.[59]

Obese women with PCOS are more likely to suffer menstrual disturbance than nonobese women with PCOS.[65]

Obesity further exaggerates the insulin resistance and hyperinsulinism associated with PCOS with consequent worsening of the hormonal disturbance and subsequent dysregulation of the HPO axis leading to more severe impairment of ovulation.[4]

As evidence for these, obese women with PCOS are more likely to exhibit the clinical manifestations of hyperinsulinism such as acanthosis nigricans.[34]

The elevated insulin levels stimulate ovarian androgen production by theca cells, which in turn can exert a local effect, resulting in follicular atresia with increased likelihood of impaired ovulation.[34,66] Obese women with PCOS are less likely to conceive naturally[33] or following fertility treatment[67] and have a higher risk of miscarriage.[68]

In summary, obesity can be seen to have a significant adverse impact on female fertility. The most significant effect is on the hormonal control of ovulation and the menstrual cycle brought about by the hormonal disturbance, leading to increased production and bioavailability of sex steroids, insulin resistance, and hyperinsulinism. Obesity also exacerbates the adverse effects of PCOS on female fertility.

Adipose tissue is also an important source of adipokines, chemokines, and cytokines, which can also exert an effect on fertility through alterations in insulin sensitivity, and dysregulation of the HPO axis. The effects of adipokines and chemokines on peripheral reproductive tissues are less clear. Animal studies have shown effect at ovarian, follicular, and endometrial levels although such effects in humans are more controversial.

Even modest weight loss, by whatever means, has been shown to improve the hormonal disturbance caused by obesity allowing resumption of regular menstruation and improvement in fertility.[69]

Assisted conception treatments such as IVF have allowed assessment of the effects of obesity in terms of oocyte quality and embryo development. Implantation rates following assisted conception also allows some degree of assessment of the effect of obesity on functional capacity on the endometrium. This will be discussed more fully in the next section.

OBESITY AND ASSISTED REPRODUCTIVE TREATMENTS

The rising levels of obesity and the adverse effects it has on both male and female fertility mean that an increasing number of couples where one or both of the partners may be obese will approach fertility clinics requesting assistance to help them conceive. A recent survey of UK fertility clinics revealed in nearly half of the responding clinics more than 20% of women referred for fertility treatment had a body mass index (BMI) above 30 kg/m^2.[70]

In general, there are a number of reasons how obesity may affect fertility treatment. Obesity can affect drug pharmacodynamics involving distribution and clearance of fertility drugs. Physiologic changes associated with obesity could also alter how the drug is delivered to the target organ.[71]

Many fertility treatments involve ovarian stimulation, which may require ultrasound monitoring of follicular development. Obesity can make ultrasound monitoring more challenging and less precise. Obesity may also increase the difficulty and risks of procedures requiring ultrasound guidance.[72]

General anesthesia or conscious sedation may be required for procedures such as egg collection; obesity can create problems with airway management increasing the risks of such procedures.[73]

Ovulation Induction

Studies investigating the effect of raised BMI in women undergoing ovulation induction have produced conflicting results. Clomifene, which is commonly used as the first-line drug in anovulatory infertility, has been associated with lower rates of ovulation[74] and lower pregnancy rates in obese women.[75]

Ovulation induction using aromatase inhibitors (AIs) has shown to be effective in women with elevated BMI, it may also have the advantage of causing fewer antiestrogenic side effects and lower rates of multiple pregnancy than clomifene.[76]

For women who fail to ovulate with oral therapy, ovarian stimulation with gonadotropins is frequently used as a second-line therapy. Obesity and insulin resistance have been shown to be predictors of suboptimal outcomes for such treatment. Women with higher BMI have been reported to require higher dosage of FSH to achieve ovulation and have a higher risk of cycle cancellation and lower rates of ovulation.[77] Other studies, however, have shown that, although it may require higher dosages of FSH, rates of ovulation and clinical pregnancy rates (CPRs) were not significantly different from women with a normal BMI.[78]

It may be that it is the altered pharmacodynamics seen in obese women that causes the threshold for serum FSH concentration required for follicular recruitment to be higher in women with elevated BMI. Other possibilities to explain the relative resistance to gonadotropins include an association with insulin resistance or higher follicular leptin concentrations.[4]

Whatever the cause of the relative gonadotropin resistance, using higher doses of gonadotropins may have other adverse effects including impairment of embryonic development potential and implantation.[79]

Intrauterine Insemination

The strong association between obesity and anovulation means that the majority of women undergoing intrauterine insemination treatment also need to undergo ovarian stimulation with either oral or injectable ovarian stimulants. Studies into the effect of increasing BMI on the outcome of superovulated intrauterine insemination (IUI) have revealed that women with a higher BMI require larger dosages of medication, have reduced peak estradiol levels, but have similar conception and miscarriage rates to women with normal BMI.[80,81]

Interestingly, studies have reported a negative correlation between increasing BMI and pregnancy rates where insemination with donor sperm was carried out.[82] Waist-to-hip ratio (WHR) has also been shown to be more sensitive than BMI in predicting the outcome of donor insemination cycles with a 0.1 increase in WHR, resulting in a 30% reduction in the probability of conception per cycle.[83]

In Vitro Fertilization and Intracytoplasmic Sperm Injection

IVF involves a coordinated sequence of processes, all of which have the potential to be affected by obesity. The procedures involved include ovarian stimulation, oocyte collection, fertilization—with or without intracytoplasmic sperm injection (ICSI), embryo culture, and transfer.

Obesity may also have an effect on the miscarriage rate. Any adverse effects of obesity on the above processes could have a detrimental effect on the outcome of ART as measured in terms of CPR and live birth rate (LBR).

1. Ovarian stimulation: The majority of studies show increasing requirement for gonadotropin for ovarian stimulation during IVF. Systematic reviews on the effect of obesity on the outcome of ART have found higher doses of gonadotropin stimulation were required in overweight and obese women compared with women with a normal BMI, and also gonadotropin requirement was higher for women with a BMI over 30 compared with those with a BMI < 30.[6,84]

2. Oocyte collection: The surgical procedure to remove eggs can be more challenging in obese women because of difficult ovarian access. There is conflicting evidence as to whether obesity adversely affects the number of eggs collected. Some studies have shown that overweight women undergoing ovarian stimulation for IVF produce fewer oocytes compared with women with normal BMI.[44] This finding was supported in a systematic review.[84] However, a later systematic review failed to find any significant differences in the number of oocytes retrieved in the different study groups.[6]

3. Oocyte quality: The number of mature metaphase II oocytes collected has been used to assess differences in oocyte quality between women with normal and raised BMI. A number of studies have shown significant reductions in metaphase II oocytes in women with BMI > 25.[85–87] A nonsignificant reduction in metaphase II oocytes was found in obese women in a prospective analysis of IVF outcome. This study also found a significantly reduced concentration of intrafollicular of human chorionic gonadotropin (hCG) in obese women, suggesting a possible mechanism of reduced maturity being reduced hCG delivery to the follicle.[88] In contrast to this no weight-related

reduction in the number and maturity of oocytes was noted in a large retrospective analysis of 6500 IVF cycles. Interestingly in this study a larger number of women followed a GnRH antagonist protocol as opposed to the more commonly used GnRH agonist cycle followed by patients in the other studies, which may have accounted for the difference in findings.[89] Similarly, using the number of oocytes inseminated and fertilization rate as a marker of oocyte quality, Metwally et al. found no difference comparing obese with nonobese patients.[90]

Although the evidence for an effect of raised BMI on oocyte maturity is conflicting, there are other mechanisms via which obesity may affect oocyte quality. Obesity can lead to lipotoxicity in other tissues, leading to endoplasmic reticulum stress, mitochondrial dysfunction, and apoptosis. It has been suggested that lipotoxicity may impact on oocyte quality in obese women and this may contribute to the detrimental effects on pregnancy rates following spontaneous and assisted conception in obese women.[91]

4. Oocyte fertilization: The fertilization rate has also been used as a surrogate marker of oocyte quality. Evidence from published studies also does not provide a clear indication as to whether the fertilization rate during IVF/ICSI treatment is affected in obese women. A number of studies have shown a reduction in the fertilization rate during IVF/ICSI cycles in overweight or obese women,[92–94] whereas others have noticed no difference in women with raised or normal BMI.[79,85–87,89,95] A large degree of heterogeneity in these studies suggests significant differences in design and study populations, which may account for the lack of consensus, highlighting the need for properly designed prospective trials to clarify the picture. Because of the association between obesity and PCOS, a significant number of women with obesity included in studies will also be suffering from PCOS and indeed some studies have found different IVF outcomes when the obese women have been subdivided into those with and without PCOS.[96]

A prospective study looking at any alterations in the cytoskeletal and chromosomal organization of oocytes that failed to fertilize after IVF in women with severe obesity and normal BMI found a greater prevalence of spindle anomalies and nonaligned chromosomes in failed fertilized oocytes from severely obese women compared with normal BMI patients, suggesting a possible mechanism for altered reproductive outcome in obese women.[97]

5. Embryo quality: Adverse effects of obesity on embryo quality may contribute to an increase in miscarriage. Parameters of embryo quality that have been used in studies include functional, such as cleavage rate, progression to blastocyst stage, number of embryos suitable for cryopreservation, and embryo utilization or morphologic-involving grading according to microscopic physical appearance or genetic using embryo biopsy followed by chromosomal analysis.

The available evidence for obesity producing an adverse effect on embryo quality is conflicting. Some studies have reported reduced cleavage rates, reduced numbers of high-grade embryos, and reduced numbers of embryos for cryopreservation in obese patients compared with those of normal weight.[44,90] Others have found poorer quality embryos in women with a BMI > 30 compared with those with a BMI between 20 and 30.[88] Interestingly, Metwally in 2007 found the mean embryo quality, number of embryos suitable for cryopreservation and embryo utilization was significantly reduced in obese women compared with nonobese women but only in women aged less than 35 years. In contrast to this, other studies have shown no differences in embryo quality or numbers of embryos suitable for cryopreservation in women who are overweight or obese compared with women of normal weight.[89] Similarly, other studies found no difference in the quality of embryos used for embryo transfer according to BMI.[98–100]

In many of the quoted studies, embryo assessment has been carried out on cleavage stage embryos 2 or 3 days postfertilization. With the development of prolonged embryo culture technique to the day 5 or blastocyst stage, more information is becoming available. A recent study has reported a significant reduction in the number of embryos reaching the blastocyst stage in obese and overweight women with metabolic dysfunction compared with women of normal weight.[101] The authors suggest that it is the metabolic environment caused by the increased body weight that has a significant effect on blastocyst formation and that this contributes to the poorer reproductive outcome in women with raised BMI.

Embryonic aneuploidy is probably the commonest cause of early pregnancy failure and miscarriage. A recent study involving trophectoderm biopsy followed by 24 chromosome preimplantation genetic screening found no statistically significant relationship between BMI and embryonic euploidy in a cohort of patients undergoing IVF, suggesting that the negative impact of overweight and obesity on IVF and reproductive outcomes may not be related to aneuploidy.[102]

6. Treatment outcome: Early studies into the effect of obesity on the outcome of assisted conception treatments came largely from smaller observational studies. Results from these studies were conflicting with some showing lower rates of embryo transfer, pregnancy, and higher rates of miscarriage.[98,103] Other studies were unable to find any negative impact of obesity on the outcome of assisted conception.[87,94,100,104]

A systematic review performed in 2007 found that women with a BMI > 25 kg/m² had a lower chance of pregnancy compared with women with a normal BMI; however, there was insufficient evidence on the effect of BMI on LBR.[84]

Similar findings were reported from a further systematic review in 2008, which also found insufficient evidence to describe the effect of obesity on miscarriage in specific groups such as those conceiving after assisted conception.[9]

A larger review of 33 studies involving 47,967 treatment cycles in 2011 found that women with a BMI > 25 kg/m² had a significantly lower clinical pregnancy and LBR but a significantly higher miscarriage rate compared with women with a normal BMI. Subgroup analysis also showed that women who were overweight also had significantly lower clinical pregnancy and LBRs and higher miscarriage rates.[6]

The results of a very large retrospective cohort study involving the outcome of 239,127 fresh IVF cycles from the 2008–10 Society for Assisted Reproductive Technology registry in the United States has recently been published.[105] In this study the cycles were stratified into cohorts according to the WHO BMI guidelines. Cycles in women with a normal BMI were used as the reference group. The main outcome measures were implantation rate, CPR, pregnancy loss rate, and LBR. The findings revealed that success rates were higher in women with low or normal BMI (see Table 12.1). There was a progressive and statistically significant worsening of outcomes in groups with higher BMIs. Interestingly, in this study, subgroup analysis on cycles reporting purely PCOS-related infertility and pure male factor infertility also found a significantly increased pregnancy loss rate and a trend toward worsening pregnancy rates that was not at a significant level. The obvious strengths of this study are its size and that by isolating subgroups with PCOS and male factor–related infertility it was possible to isolate female obesity

from other underlying pathologies. The authors concluded that the results suggest that it is obesity rather than underlying pathologies that contribute to worsening outcomes with increasing BMI.

Successful implantation requires a genetically competent embryo embedding within a receptive endometrium. In an attempt to isolate the possible effects of obesity on the endometrium in IVF cycles, it has been proposed that the oocyte donation model, although not perfect, provides the best human model. Studies using this model have produced conflicting results; some studies have shown no difference in success rates with increasing BMI when donor oocytes were used.[106] Similarly, results of a systematic review including 4758 women published in 2013 reported no difference in the chance of pregnancy after IVF in obese donor oocyte recipients compared with those with a normal BMI.[107] In contrast to this a retrospective cohort analysis of the outcome of ovum donation cycles using normal-weight donors over 12 years involving 9857 first cycles of treatment reported that obesity was associated with a significant reduction in implantation, pregnancy, clinical pregnancy, twin pregnancy, and LBRs as BMI increased. The authors concluded that the impaired reproductive outcome was probably due to reduced uterine receptivity.[108] Similarly, a further recent retrospective cohort study involving 22,317 donor oocyte cycles from the 2008–10 Society for Assisted Reproductive Technology Clinic Outcome Reporting System (SARTCORS) in which the cycles were stratified into groups based on WHO BMI guidelines found that implantation rates, CPRs, pregnancy loss rates, and LBRs were all most favorable in cohorts of recipients with low and normal BMIs, but progressively worsened as BMI increased.[109] (see Table 12.2)

Considering the interest shown in the effect of female obesity on the outcome of assisted conception, any adverse effect caused by obesity in the male partner has received relatively little attention. Available studies have produced conflicting results. A retrospective study involving 290 cycles of IVF in 2010 found significantly reduced CPR after cycles involving IVF but not ICSI when the male partner's BMI was >25 kg/m². The authors suggest that ICSI may overcome some obesity-related impairment of sperm-egg interaction.[110]

In contrast to this a prospective study by Colaci et al. in 2012 found higher fertilization rates in obese men compared with normal-weight men in conventional IVF cycles. There was also no association found between male BMI and embryo quality, pregnancy rate, or LBR

TABLE 12.1

Outcome of Fresh Autologous In Vitro Fertilization Cycles by Body Mass Index (BMI) Category From 2008–10 Society for Assisted Reproductive Technology Registry

Parameter		BMI (KG/M²)						
	<18.5	18.5-24.9	25-25.9	30-34.9	35-35.9	40-44.9	45-49.9	>50
Parameter n	7,149	134,588	54,822	24,922	11,747	4,084	1,292	463
Implantation rate %	30.4	29.5	28.3	26.9	25.8	23.6	22.9	20.3
aOR (95% CI)	0.99 (0.98-1.00)	REF	0.99 (0.99-0.996)	0.98 (0.97-0.99)	0.96 (0.95-0.97)	0.95 (0.93-0.07)	0.91(0.88-0.95)	0.91 (0.88-0.95)
P value	.26		<.001	<.001	<.001	<.001	<.001	<.001
Clinical pregnancy rate %	37.7	37.9	36.8	35.7	33.7	32.0	30.6	30.0
aOR(95% CI)	0.93 (0.88-0.99)	REF	0.97 (0.95-0.99)	0.90 (0.87-0.93)	0.81 (0.76-0.85)	0.80 (0.74-0.87)	0.75 (0.65-0.85)	0.66 (0.53-0.82)
P value	.06		.013	<.001	<.001	<.001	<.001	.002
Pregnancy loss rate	11.4	11.3	12.7	14.6	15.3	14.8	17.6	20.3
aOR (95% CI)	1.11 (0.97-1.28)	REF	1.14 (1.08-1.21)	1.33 (1.23-1.43)	1.40 (1.26-1.56)	1.26 (1.06-1.51)	1.59 (1.19-2.14)	1.87 (1.18-2.95)
P value	.21		<.001	<.001	<.001	.009	.002	.007
Live birth rate %	31.2	31.4	29.8	28.0	26.3	24.3	22.8	21.2
aOR (95% CI)	0.92 (0.86-0.97)	REF	0.94 (0.91-0.96)	0.84(0.81-0.87)	0.76 (0.72-0.79)	0.73 (0.67-0.77)	0.67 (0.58-0.77)	0.52 (0.41-0.66)
P value	.022		<.001	<.001	<.001	<.001	<.001	<.001

aOR, adjusted odds ratio; *CI*, confidence intervals.

All outcomes are quoted as percentages of cycles started except for pregnancy loss (percentage of clinical pregnancies).

Data from Luke B, Brown M.B, Stern J.E., et al. Female obesity adversely affects assisted reproductive technology (ART) pregnancy and live birth rates. *Hum Reprod.* 2011;26(1): 245–252.

TABLE 12.2
In Vitro Fertilization Outcome of Fresh Donor/Egg Recipient Cycles by Recipient Body Mass Index (BMI) Category From 2008–10 Society for Assisted Reproductive Technology Registry

Characteristic	BMI (KG/M²)								
	<18.5	18.5–24.9	25–25.9	30–34.9	35–35.9	40–44.9	45–49.9	>50	Combined >40
No. of patients	637	13,058	5,394	2,016	823	280	77	32	389
Implantation rate %	49.3	49.3	47.9	42.6	45.6	40.9	39.3	39.7	40.7
Embryos transferred	1.9	2.0	2.0	2.1	2.0	2.1	2.2	2.0	2.1
Mean fetal heartbeats	0.92	0.93	0.92	0.84	0.89	0.80	0.84	0.79	0.81
aOR (95% CI)	0.99 (0.96–1.03)	REF	0.99 (0.98–1.01)	0.95 (0.92–0.97)	0.98 (0.95–1.02)	0.94 (0.89–1.00)	0.95 (0.86–1.05)	0.86 (0.74–1.02)	0.94 (0.89–0.99)
P value	.71		.33	<.001	.28	.06	.30	.08	.010
Clinical pregnancy rate %	59.7	59.6	57.7	53.6	56.9	52.9	48.0	53.1	52.1
aOR (95% CI)	1.00 (0.82–1.22)	REF	0.93 (0.86–1.01)	0.78 (0.69–0.87)	0.88 (0.74–1.04)	0.83 (0.63–1.09)	0.65 (0.40–1.06)	0.46 (0.21–0.99)	0.74 (0.59–0.94)
P value	.99		.08	<.001	.14	.19	.08	.047	.013
Pregnancy loss rate	8.5	8.6	10.2	11.2	12.3	15.9	8.3	7.1	13.5
aOR (95% CI)	0.92 (0.59–1.40)	REF	1.18 (1.00–1.39)	1.25 (0.99–1.58)	1.30 (0.92–1.83)	1.95 (1.17–3.25)	0.95 (0.29–0.311)	1.19 (0.15–9.50)	1.67 (1.05–2.63)
P value	.68		.04	.06	.14	.01	.93	.87	.03
Live birth rate %	51.2	51.4	48.6	43.9	46.7	40.0	42.9	40.6	40.7
aOR (95% CI)	1.03 (0.86–1.24)	REF	0.90 (0.83–0.97)	0.75 (0.67–0.84)	0.87 (0.73–1.03)	0.65 (0.49–0.85)	0.74 (0.46–1.21)	0.41 (0.18–0.93)	0.64 (0.51–0.81)
P value	.75		.005	<.001	.1	.002	.23	.03	<.001

aOR, adjusted odds ratio with 95% confidence intervals (CI).

All outcomes are per transfer except for pregnancy loss (per clinical pregnancy).

Data from Keltz J, Zapantis A, Jindal S.K, Lieman H.J, Santoro N, Polotsky A.J. Overweight men: clinical pregnancy after ART is decreased in IVF but not in ICSI cycles. *J Assist Reprod Genet.* 2010;27(9–10);539–544. 2016;105(2):364–368.

per embryo transfer. However, among couples undergoing ICSI, the odds of a live birth in couples with obese male partners was 84% lower than the odds in couples with normal BMI.[111]

A recent systematic review involving five studies found a nonsignificant decrease in CPR but statistically significant decrease in LBR for obese men compared with normal-weight men. Additionally, further analysis revealed a significant increase in the odds of having a nonviable pregnancy in couples with an obese male partner.[7]

It is clear from the available evidence that further properly designed trials are required to elucidate the extent and causes of any adverse effects of obesity in either the male or female partner on the chances of a spontaneous conception or the success of assisted conception. Currently available evidence suggests that obesity in either partner increases the time taken to achieve a spontaneous pregnancy or an assisted conception and that it has the potential to exert its effect on conception and implantation through a cumulative impairment of several processes.[4]

TREATMENT OPTIONS AND EFFECT ON REPRODUCTIVE FUNCTION

The first line in the management of obese patients with reduced fertility should be to lose weight because this has been shown to reverse the effects of obesity on reproductive function. The British Fertility Society recommends deferring fertility treatment until the BMI is less than $35 \, kg/m^2$ and ideally for younger women (<37 years) less than $30 \, kg/m^2$.[112]

Weight loss is associated with improvements in the hormonal disturbance associated with reduced fertility and also improved outcome following assisted conception. Weight loss of 5%–10%, particularly a reduction in central obesity, has been shown to improve insulin sensitivity, improve SHBG concentrations, reduce androgenicity, and reduce leptin levels.[40,113–116] As a consequence of this, weight loss also leads to restoration of menstrual cyclicity and an improvement in spontaneous conception rates.[11]

Although there is less research into the effect of weight loss on male fertility, some studies have shown that weight loss induced by lifestyle modification in men has led to improvement in androgen levels, inhibin B, and semen parameters.[15,29]

Lifestyle Modification

In obese females, lifestyle modifications can produce impressive improvements in both spontaneous conception rates and response to fertility treatment. A prospective study by Clark et al. found that in 67 women who completed a 6-month program of lifestyle changes involving diet and exercise, average weight loss was 10.2 kg with 60 women resuming spontaneous ovulation and 52 achieving a pregnancy (18 spontaneously) with 45 live births. Miscarriage rates were also lower following the intervention.[12] Further studies have confirmed the beneficial effects of weight loss on fertility through lifestyle modification.[69,117]

In light of the improved fertility produced by weight loss and exercise, this is now recognized as the first-line management option for obese women with reproductive issues.[112,118,119]

The optimum diet to adopt for improved fertility remains unclear. The most important factor is to reduce energy input by adopting a reduced caloric intake. Various claims have been made for different types of diet including low-carbohydrate, high-protein diets, which have been claimed to produce better therapeutic outcomes or low-fat, high-carbohydrate diets, which may be more effective in producing longer-term weight loss. The evidence to support these claims is inconsistent and lacking.[120]

Increasing energy expenditure through increased aerobic capacity has been found to be effective in improving reproductive function either alone or in combination with dietary modification. The combination of both diet and exercise as part of improved lifestyle changes may be better in terms of producing longer-term weight maintenance.[121] Both aerobic and resistance exercise have been found to be beneficial in terms of improved body composition and insulin sensitivity. The combination of aerobic and resistance exercise has been reported to be more effective in improving insulin sensitivity and glycemic control and reducing abdominal fat compared with either form of exercise alone.[122,123]

Maintenance of weight loss is an important issue in the longer-term management of obesity. By combining dietary modification with an exercise program, the achieved weight loss is more likely to be maintained.[124] The support provided for participants on lifestyle modification programs by a group environment may also improve achieving and maintaining weight loss.[11,120]

Pharmacologic Intervention

For subjects who struggle to achieve or maintain satisfactory levels of weight loss, pharmacologic therapy may be considered as an option. Dietary agents that have been studied in the past include orlistat, sibutramine, and rimonabant; all three have been shown to be effective in assisting weight loss,[125] but because of side effects the latter two have been withdrawn from the market.[126] In obese females with PCOS, orlistat in combination with lifestyle changes induced substantial weight loss and improvements in insulin resistance, hyperandrogenemia, and cardiovascular risk factors.[126]

Fertility issues in obese males with increased estrogen levels and reduced testosterone levels have been treated with AIs.[127] There have been case reports where this type of therapy has been used to improve semen quality with subsequent improved fertility.[128] Further research is required to investigate this promising pharmacologic intervention in the management of obesity-induced male infertility with increased estradiol to testosterone ratio.[129]

Bariatric Surgery and Management of Infertility

Because of the effectiveness of bariatric surgery in providing sustained weight loss, it is becoming an increasing option for an increasing number of women with more severe levels of obesity or those who have struggled to achieve or maintain sufficient weight loss through lifestyle modification, in addition to improving the metabolic conditions associated with an obese state, such as PCOS and type 2 diabetes.[130,131]

In the United Kingdom and generally in the rest of the world, bariatric surgery is offered provided the following criteria are met:

BMI ≥ 40 kg/m²

BMI ≥ 35–40 kg/m² with the presence of disease such as type 2 diabetes, which could be improved through weight loss

Consideration of access for patients with a BMI ≥ 30–34.9 kg/m² with recent onset of type 2 diabetes

Patients with a BMI 50 kg/m², bariatric surgery should be considered first

Other methods of weight loss have been attempted, but weight loss has not been maintained[132]

Globally, more females than males undergo bariatric surgery, with an estimated ratio of 3:1.[133] In the United Kingdom, over 70% of females presenting for bariatric surgery are in their prime reproductive years.[131] Compared with other weight loss methods such as diet and exercise, bariatric surgery offers rapid and sustained weight loss.[134] Bariatric surgery requires lifelong commitment to lifestyle modification such as different eating patterns, vitamin and mineral supplementation, and physical activity to supplement and maintain the effects of bariatric surgery.[132] Given the demographics of the bariatric surgical–seeking population, and the negative impact of obesity on fecundity, many women are likely to view bariatric surgery as a means of improving fertility. The link between bariatric surgery and fertility is an emergent area of research, but the role of bariatric surgery within infertility management has not been clearly elucidated.[135] Studies have shown that bariatric surgery may improve menstrual patterns[136] and symptoms of metabolic diseases such PCOS,[137] which may lead to improved rates of pregnancy in this cohort. A consensus on the optimum time to conceive following bariatric surgery has not been agreed to date.[138] The British Obesity and Metabolic Surgery Society recommends waiting for 12–18 months after surgery[139]; however, the American College of Obstetricians and Gynaecologists recommends waiting for 12–24 months.[140] The first 2 years following bariatric surgery are the time of the most weight loss,[133] and there is potential for nutrient deficiencies to occur, particularly after gastric bypass, owing to its malabsorptive effects.[141] The theoretical risks of these factors to a woman and the developing fetus have not been accurately determined[142]; this is an emerging area of research, but the problems in early pregnancy, such as miscarriage, in women with obesity[143,144] are well evidenced.

This waiting time may be a source of anxiety to women experiencing infertility, because current UK guidelines for fertility treatment are determined by both age and weight status. If the latter is improved through bariatric surgery, the waiting time for assisted reproduction may cause further delay and, for older women, may render them ineligible for treatment. Therefore, it is recommended that women with obesity over the age of 30 meeting the eligibility criteria for bariatric surgery are considered for referral early on to increase the efficacy of future assisted reproduction treatments.[145] Clearly, there is a need for communication between assisted conception and bariatric surgical teams to support and manage women with obesity who may be experiencing infertility.

There is an emerging body of research on bariatric surgery and pregnancy. A systematic review found that compared with pregnant women with obesity, women who become pregnant after bariatric surgery tend to have fewer maternal complications in three matched cohort studies.[146] A further review found a small number of case-control or cohort studies comparing the same populations with lower rates of gestational diabetes, macrosomia, and hypertension.[147] The authors suggest that the increased risk of fetal growth restriction and the risks of preterm labor or miscarriage compared with women with comparable BMI who had not undergone bariatric surgery needed further investigation.

The AURORA study is an ongoing multicenter prospective cohort study, which will examine reproductive outcomes before and after bariatric surgery,[148] which should provide information on this cohort of women.

Bariatric Surgery and Assisted Reproduction Treatment

The effect of bariatric surgery on assisted reproduction outcomes is an ongoing area of research. Currently, there is only a small body of research about bariatric surgery and assisted reproduction outcomes.

Excess abdominal skin as a result of weight loss following bariatric surgery may affect the absorption of drugs by subcutaneous injection resulting in poor ovarian response.[149] A retrospective study of seven women before and after bariatric surgery (five sleeve gastrectomy, two gastric banding) found a decrease in the amount of gonadotropins required during stimulation.[150] By comparing women with obesity (n = 57) and patients undergoing assisted reproduction because of male factor infertility (n = 94), statistically significant differences were found in follicles observed by ultrasound, retrieved, and matured in women who had undergone bariatric surgical procedures (n = 29), suggesting that bariatric surgery may have an impact on the formation of follicles and ooctyes.[151]

The role of bariatric surgery in infertility in males with obesity has not been determined.[152] Three case studies found worsening of semen parameters after bariatric surgery, with one showing reversal after 2 years[153] but no azoospermia. Two of the three cases were treated with ICSI, with resulting successful clinical pregnancies.

SUMMARY

Levels of obesity among males and females of reproductive age are increasing. Obesity has a significant adverse effect on both spontaneous and assisted conception. Obesity in males leads to a state of hypogonadotropic hyperestrogenic hypoandrogenemia with adverse effects on spermatogenesis and testicular function. Obesity in the female leads to hyperinsulinemia and hyperandrogenemia with reduced frequency of ovulation and anovulatory infertility. Adipokines, chemokines, and cytokines may also adversely affect fertility, but the exact role in humans needs to be fully elucidated. Obesity may exert a transgenerational effect affecting the metabolic and reproductive health of offspring. Obesity adversely affects the outcome of assisted conception treatment, and BMI has been used as a means to restrict access to funding for fertility treatment. Weight loss through lifestyle modification is the first-line management of obesity-induced reproductive morbidity. The role of bariatric surgery in the management of obesity affecting male and female fertility requires further research. Effective management of the adverse effects of obesity on reproductive health requires a multidisciplinary approach.

REFERENCES

1. World Health Organisation. *Obesity and Overweight. Fact Sheet*; 2016. Available at: http://www.who.int/mediacentre/factsheets/fs311/en/.
2. Gesink Law DC, Maclehose RF, Longnecker MP. Obesity and time to pregnancy. *Hum Reprod.* 2007;22(2):414–420.
3. Ramlau-Hansen CH, Thulstrup AM, Nohr EA, Bonde JP, Sørensen TI, Olsen J. Subfecundity in overweight and obese couples. *Hum Reprod.* 2007;22(6):1634–1637.
4. Brewer CJ, Balen AH. The adverse effects of obesity on conception and implantation. *Reproduction.* 2010;140(3):347–364.
5. Palmer NO, Bakos HW, Fullston T, Lane M. Impact of obesity on male fertility, sperm function and molecular composition. *Spermatogenesis.* 2012;2(4):253–263.
6. Rittenberg V, Seshadri S, Sunkara SK, Sobaleva S, Oteng-Ntim E, El-Toukhy T. Effect of body mass index on IVF treatment outcome: an updated systematic review and meta-analysis. *Reprod Biomed Online.* 2011;23(4):421–439.
7. Campbell JM, Lane M, Owens JA, Bakos HW. Paternal obesity negatively affects male fertility and assisted reproduction outcomes: a systematic review and meta-analysis. *Reprod Biomed Online.* 2015;31(5):593–604.
8. Boots C, Stephenson MD. Does obesity increase the risk of miscarriage in spontaneous conception: a systematic review. *Semin Reprod Med.* 2011;29(6):507–513.
9. Metwally M, Ong KJ, Ledger WL, Li TC. Does high body mass index increase the risk of miscarriage after spontaneous and assisted conception? A meta-analysis of the evidence. *Fertil Steril.* 2008;90(3):714–726.
10. Leddy MA, Power ML, Schulkin J. The impact of maternal obesity on maternal and fetal health. *Rev Obstet Gynecol.* 2008;1(4):170–178.
11. Clark AM, Ledger W, Galletly C, et al. Weight loss results in significant improvement in pregnancy and ovulation rates in anovulatory obese women. *Hum Reprod.* 1995;10(10):2705–2712.
12. Clark AM, Thornley B, Tomlinson L, et al. Weight loss in obese infertile women results in improvement in reproductive outcome for all forms of fertility treatment. *Hum Reprod.* 1998;13(6):1502–1505.
13. Norman RJ, Chura LR, Robker RL. Effects of obesity on assisted reproductive technology outcomes. *Fertil Steril.* 2008;89(6):1611–1612.
14. Swan SH, Elkin EP, Fenster L. The question of declining sperm density revisited: an analysis of 101 studies published 1934-1996. *Environ Health Perspect.* 2000;108(10):961–966.

15. Du Plessis SS, Cabler S, McAlister DA, Sabanegh E, Agarwal A. The effect of obesity on sperm disorders and male infertility. *Nat Rev Urol.* 2010;7(3):153–161.

16. Nguyen RH, Wilcox AJ, Skjaerven R, Baird DD. Men's body mass index and infertility. *Hum Reprod.* 2007;22(9):2488–2493.

17. Davidson LM, Millar K, Jones C, Fatum M, Coward K. Deleterious effects of obesity upon the hormonal and molecular mechanisms controlling spermatogenesis and male fertility. *Hum Fertil.* 2015;18(3):184–193.

18. Rao PM, Kelly DM, Jones TH. Testosterone and insulin resistance in the metabolic syndrome and T2DM in men. *Nat Rev Endocrinol.* 2013;9(8):479–493.

19. Akingbemi BT. Estrogen regulation of testicular function. *Reprod Biol Endocrinol.* 2005;3:51.

20. Kerr JB, Millar M, Maddocks S, Sharpe RM. Stage-dependent changes in spermatogenesis and Sertoli cells in relation to the onset of spermatogenic failure following withdrawal of testosterone. *Anat Rec.* 1993;235(4):547–559.

21. Agbaje IM, Rogers DA, McVicar CM, et al. Insulin dependant diabetes mellitus: implications for male reproductive function. *Hum Reprod.* 2007;22(7):1871–1877.

22. Jope T, Lammert A, Kratzsch J, Paasch U, Glander HJ. Leptin and leptin receptor in human seminal plasma and in human spermatozoa. *Int J Androl.* 2003;26(6):335–341.

23. Winters SJ, Wang C, Abdelrahaman E, Hadeed V, Dyky MA, Brufsky A. Inhibin-B levels in healthy young adult men and prepubertal boys: is obesity the cause for the contemporary decline in sperm count because of fewer Sertoli cells? *J Androl.* 2006;27(4):560–564.

24. Tsatsanis C, Dermitzaki E, Avgoustinaki P, Malliaraki N, Mytaras V, Margioris AN. The impact of adipose tissue-derived factors on the hypothalamic-pituitary-gonadal (HPG) axis. *Hormones.* 2015;14(4):549–562.

25. Kumar K, Deka D, Singh A, Mitra DK, Vanitha BR, Dada R. Predictive value of DNA integrity analysis in idiopathic recurrent pregnancy loss following spontaneous conception. *J Assist Reprod Genet.* 2012;29(9):861–867.

26. Bakos HW, Thompson JG, Feil D, Lane M. Sperm DNA damage is associated with assisted reproductive technology pregnancy. *Int J Androl.* 2008;31(5):518–526.

27. Li L, Law C, Lo Conte R, Power C. Intergenerational influences on childhood body mass index: the effect of parental body mass index trajectories. *Am J Clin Nutr.* 2009;89(2):551–557.

28. Lane M, Zander-Fox DL, Robker RL, McPherson NO. Peri-conception parental obesity, reproductive health, and transgenerational impacts. *Trends Endocrinol Metab.* 2015;26(2):84–90.

29. Kasturi SS, Tannir J, Brannigan RE. The metabolic syndrome and male infertility. *J Androl.* 2008;29(3):251–259.

30. Rich-Edwards JW, Goldman MB, Willett WC, et al. Adolescent body mass index and infertility caused by ovulatory disorder. *Am J Obstet Gynecol.* 1994;171(1):171–177.

31. Wise LA, Palmer JR, Rosenberg L. Body size and time to pregnancy in black women. *Hum Reprod.* 2013;28(10):2856–2864.

32. McKinnon CJ, Hatch EE, Rotman KJ, et al. Body mass index, physical activity and fecundability in a North American preconception cohort study. *Fertil Steril.* 2016;106(2):451–459.

33. Hartz AJ, Barboriak PN, Wong A, Katayama KP, Rimm AA. The association of obesity with infertility and related menstural abnormalities in women. *Int J Obes.* 1979;3(1):57–73.

34. Pasquali R, Gambineri A. Metabolic effects of obesity on reproduction. *Reprod Biomed Online.* 2006;12(5):542–551.

35. von Schoultz B, Carlström K. On the regulation of sex-hormone-binding globulin–a challenge of an old dogma and outlines of an alternative mechanism. *J Steroid Biochem.* 1989;32(2):327–334.

36. Gambineri A, Pelusi C, Vicennati V, Pagotto U, Pasquali R. Obesity and the polycystic ovary syndrome. *Int J Obes Relat Metab Disord.* 2002;26(7):883–896.

37. Tamer Erel C, Senturk LM. The impact of body mass index on assisted reproduction. *Curr Opin Obstet Gynecol.* 2009;21(3):228–235.

38. Balen A. The pathophysiology of polycystic ovary syndrome: trying to understand PCOS and its endocrinology. *Best Pract Res Clin Obstet Gynaecol.* 2004;18(5):685–706.

39. Dafopoulos K, Venetis C, Pournaras S, Kallitsaris A, Messinis IE. Ovarian control of pituitary sensitivity of luteinizing hormone secretion to gonadotropin-releasing hormone in women with the polycystic ovary syndrome. *Fertil Steril.* 2009;92(4):1378–1380.

40. Bützow TL, Lehtovirta M, Siegberg R, et al. The decrease in luteinizing hormone secretion in response to weight reduction is inversely related to the severity of insulin resistance in overweight women. *J Clin Endocrinol Metab.* 2000;85(9):3271–3275.

41. Gosman GG, Katcher HI, Legro RS. Obesity and the role of gut and adipose hormones in female reproduction. *Hum Reprod Update.* 2006;12(5):585–601.

42. Poretsky L, Cataldo NA, Rosenwaks Z, Giudice LC. The insulin-related ovarian regulatory system in health and disease. *Endocr Rev.* 1999;20(4):535–582.

43. Kershaw EE, Flier JS. Adipose tissue as an endocrine organ. *J Clin Endocrinol Metab.* 2004;89(6):2548–2556.

44. Zhang D, Zhu Y, Gao H, et al. Overweight and obesity negatively affect the outcomes of ovarian stimulation and in vitro fertilisation: a cohort study of 2628 Chinese women. *Gynecol Endocrinol.* 2010;26(5):325–332.

45. von Schnurbein J, Moss A, Nagel SA, et al. Leptin substitution in the induction of menstrual cycles in an adolescent with leptin deficiency and hypogonadotrophic hypogonadism. *Horm Res Paediatr.* 2012;77(2):127–133.

46. Mallinson RJ, Williams NI, Olmstead MP, Scheid JL, Riddle ES, De Souza MJ. A case report of recovery of menstrual function following a nutritional intervention in two exercising women with amenorrhoea of varying duration. *J Int Soc Sports Nutr.* 2013;10:34.

47. Burcelin R, Thorens B, Glauser M, Gaillard RC, Pralong FP. Gonadotrophin-releasing hormone secretion from hypothalamic neurons: stimulation by insulin and potentiation by leptin. *Endocrinology.* 2003;144(10):4484–4491.

48. Moschos S, Chan JL, Mantzoros CS. Leptin and reproduction: a review. *Fertil Steril.* 2002;77(3):433–444.

49. Duggal PS, Van Der Hoek KH, Milner CR, et al. The in vivo and in vitro effects of exogenous leptin on ovulation in the rat. *Endocrinology.* 2000;141(6):1971–1976.

50. Cao R, Brakenhielm E, Wahlestedt C, Thyberg J, Cao Y. Leptin induces vascular permeability and synergistically stimulates angiogenesis with FGF-2 and VEGF. *Proc Natl Acad Sci USA.* 2001;98(11):6390–6395.

51. Bouloumie A, Marumo T, Lafontan M, Busse R. Leptin induces oxidative stress in human endothelial cells. *FASEB J.* 1999;13(10):1231–1238.

52. Brannian JD, Hansen KA. Leptin and ovarian folliculo-genesis: implications for ovulation induction and ART outcomes. *Semin Reprod Med.* 2002;20(2):103–112.

53. Kawamura K, Sato N, Fukuda J, et al. The role of leptin during the development of mouse preimplantation embryos. *Mol Cell Endocrinol.* 2003;202(1–2):185–189.

54. Kawwass JF, Summer R, Kallen CB. Direct effects of leptin and adiponectin on peripheral reproductive tissues: a critical review. *Mol Hum Reprod.* 2015;21(8):617–632.

55. Pajvani UB, Du X, Combs TP, et al. Structure-function studies of the adipocyte-secreted hormone Acrp30/adiponectin. Implications fpr metabolic regulation and bioactivity. *J Biol Chem.* 2003;278(11):9073–9085.

56. Stefan N, Stumvoll M. Adiponectin–its role in metabolism and beyond. *Horm Metab Res.* 2002;34(9):469–474.

57. Yang WS, Lee WJ, Funahashi T, et al. Weight reduction increases plasma levels of an adipose-derived anti-inflammatory protein, adiponectin. *J Clin Endocrinol Metab.* 2001;86(8):3815–3819.

58. Qiao L, Yoo HS, Madon A, Kinney B, Hay WW, Shao J. Adiponectin enhances mouse fetal fat deposition. *Diabetes.* 2012;61(12):3199–3207.

59. Chen X, Jia X, Qiao J, Guan Y, Kang J. Adipokines in reproductive function: a link between obesity and polycystic ovary syndrome. *J Mol Endocrinol.* 2013;50(2):R21–R37.

60. Ryan AS, Nicklas BJ. Reductions in plasma cytokine levels with weight loss improve insulin sensitivity in overweight and obese postmenopausal women. *Diabetes Care.* 2004;27(7):1699–1705.

61. Vázquez LA, Pazos F, Berrazueta JR, et al. Effects of changes in body weight and insulin resistance on inflammation and endothelial function in morbid obesity after bariatric surgery. *J Clin Endocrinol Metab.* 2005;90(1):316–322.

62. Deura I, Harada T, Taniguchi F, Iwabe T, Izawa M, Terakawa N. Reduction of estrogen production by interleukin-6 in a human granulosa tumor cell line may have implications for endometriosis-associated infertility. *Fertil Steril.* 2005;83(suppl 1):1086–1092.

63. Glueck CJ, Wang P, Bornovali S, Goldenberg N, Sieve L. Polycystic ovary syndrome, the G1691A factor V Leiden mutation, and plasminogen activator inhibitor activity: associations with recurrent pregnancy loss. *Metabolism.* 2003;52(12):1627–1632.

64. Berman J, Girardi G, Salmon JE. TNF-alpha is a critical effector and a target for therapy in antiphospholipid antibody-induced pregnancy loss. *J Immunol.* 2005;174(1):485–490.

65. Balen AH, Conway GS, Kaltsas G, et al. Polycystic ovary syndrome: the spectrum of the disorder in 1741 patients. *Hum Reprod.* 1995;10(8):2107–2111.

66. Dunaif A. Insulin resistance and the polycystic ovary syndrome: mechanism and implications for pathogenesis. *Endocr Rev.* 1997;18(6):774–800.

67. Jungheim ES, Lanzendorf SE, Odem RR, Moley KH, Chang AS, Ratts VS. Morbid obesity is associated with lower clinical pregnancy rates after in vitro fertilization in women with polycystic ovary syndrome. *Fertil Steril.* 2009;92(1):256–261.

68. Hamilton-Fairley D, Kiddy D, Watson H, Paterson C, Franks S. Association of moderate obesity with a poor pregnancy outcome in women with polycystic ovary syndrome treated with low dose gonadotrophin. *Br J Obstet Gynaecol.* 1992;99(2):128–131.

69. Crosignani PG, Colombo M, Vegetti W, Somigliana E, Gessati A, Ragni G. Overweight and obese anovulatory patients with polycystic ovaries: parallel improvements in anthropometric indices, ovarian physiology and fertility rate induced by diet. *Hum Reprod.* 2003;18(9):1928–1932.

70. Aird I, Evbuomwan I, Green A, et al. Management of obese women in UK assisted conception units; a survey of current practice. In: *British Fertility Society Annual Meeting.* ; 2016. Gateshead, UK.

71. Hanley MJ, Abernethy DR, Greenblatt DJ. Effect of obesity on the pharmacokinetics of drugs in humans. *Clin Pharmacokinet.* 2010;49(2):71–87.

72. Martinuzzi K, Ryan S, Luna M, Copperman AB. Elevated body mass index (BMI) does not adversely affect in vitro fertilization outcome in young women. *J Assist Reprod Genet.* 2008;25(5):169–175.

73. Jirapinyo P, Thompson CC. Sedation challenges: obesity and sleep apnea. *Gastrointest Endosc Clin N Am.* 2016;26(3):527–537.

74. Al-Azemi M, Omu FE, Omu AE. The effect of obesity on the outcome of infertility management in women with polycystic ovary syndrome. *Arch Gynecol Obstet.* 2004;270(4):205–210.

75. Imani B, Eijkemans MJ, te Velde ER, Habbema JD, Fauser BC. Predictors of patients remaining anovulatory during clomiphene citrate induction of ovulation in normogonadotropic oligoamenorrheic infertility. *J Clin Endocrinol Metab.* 1998;83(7):2361–2365.

76. McKnight KK, Nodler JL, Cooper Jr JJ, Chapman VR, Cliver SP, Bates Jr GW. Body mass index-associated differences in response to ovulation induction with letrozole. *Fertil Steril.* 2011;96(5):1206–1208.

77. Mulders AG, Laven JS, Eijkemans MJ, Hughes EG, Fauser BC. Patient predictors for outcome of gonadotrophin ovulation induction in women with normogonadotrophic anovulatory infertility: a meta-analysis. *Hum Reprod Update.* 2003;9(5):429–449.

78. Balen AH, Platteau P, Andersen AN, et al. The influence of body weight on response to ovulation induction with gonadotrophins in 335 women with World Health Organization group II anovulatory infertility. *BJOG.* 2006;113(10):1195–1202.

79. Fedorcsák P, Dale PO, Storeng R, Tanbo T, Abyholm T. The impact of obesity and insulin resistance on the outcome of IVF or ICSI in women with polycystic ovarian syndrome. *Hum Reprod.* 2001;16(6):1086–1091.

80. Dodson WC, Kunselman AR, Legro RS. Association of obesity with treatment outcomes in ovulatory infertile women undergoing superovulation and intrauterine insemination. *Fertil Steril.* 2006;86(3):642–646.

81. Souter I, Baltagi LM, Kuleta D, Meeker JD, Petrozza JC. Women, weight, and fertility: the effect of body mass index on the outcome of superovulation/intrauterine insemination cycles. *Fertil Steril.* 2011;95(3):1042–1047.

82. Koloszár S, Daru J, Kereszturi A, Závaczki Z, Szöllosi J, Pál A. Effect of female body weight on efficiency of donor AI. *Arch Androl.* 2002;48(5):323–327.

83. Zaadstra BM, Seidell JC, Van Noord PA, et al. Fat and female fecundity: prospective study of effect of body fat distribution on conception rates. *BMJ.* 1993;306(6876):484–487.

84. Maheshwari A, Stofberg L, Bhattacharya S. Effect of overweight an obesity on assisted reproductive technology – a systematic review. *Hum Reprod Update.* 2007;13(5):433–444.

85. Esinler I, Bozdag G, Yarali H. Impact of isolated obesity on ICSI outcome. *Reprod Biomed Online.* 2008;17(4):583–587.

86. Dokras A, Baredziak L, Blaine J, Syrop C, VanVoorhis BJ, Sparks A. Obstetric outcomes after in vitro fertilization in obese and morbidly obese women. *Obstet Gynecol.* 2006;108(1):61–69.

87. Wittemer C, Ohl J, Bailly M, Bettahar-Lebugle K, Nisand I. Does body mass index of infertile women have an impact on IVF procedure and outcome? *J Assist Reprod Genet.* 2000;17(10):547–552.

88. Carrell DT, Jones KP, Peterson CM, Aoki V, Emery BR, Campbell BR. Body mass index is inversely related to intrafollicular HCG concentrations, embryo quality and IVF outcome. *Reprod Biomed Online.* 2001;3(2):109–111.

89. Bellver J, Ayllon Y, Ferrando M, et al. Female obesity impairs invitro fertilization outcome without affecting embryo quality. *Fertil Steril.* 2010;93(2):447–454.

90. Metwally M, Cutting R, Tipton A, Skull J, Ledger WL, Li TC. Effect of increased body mass index on oocyte and embryo quality in IVF patients. *Reprod Biomed Online.* 2007;15(5):532–538.

91. Wu LL, Norman RJ, Robker RL. The impact of obesity on oocytes: evidence for lipotoxicity mechanisms. *Reprod Fertil Dev.* 2011;24(1):29–34.

92. van Swieten EC, van der Leeuw-Harmsen L, Badings EA, van der Linden PJ. Obesity and clomiphene challenge test as predictors of outcome of in vitro fertilisation and itracytoplasmic sperm injection. *Gynecol Obstet Invest.* 2005;59(4):220–224.

93. Salha O, Dada T, Sharma V. Influence of body mass index and self administration of hCG on the outcome of IVF cycles: a prospective cohort study. *Hum Fertil.* 2001;4(1):37–42.

94. Matalliotakis I, Cakmak H, Sakkas D, Mahutte N, Koumantakis G, Arici A. Impact of body mass index on IVF and ICSI outcome: a retrospective study. *Reprod Biomed Online.* 2008;16(6):778–783.

95. Schliep KC, Mumford SL, Ahrens KA, et al. Effect of male and female body mass index on pregnancy and live birth rate success after in vitro fertilisation. *Fertil Steril.* 2015;103(2):388–395.

96. Bailey AP, Hawkins LK, Missmer SA, Correia KF, Yanushpolsky EH. Effect of body mass index on in vitro fertilisation outcomes in women with poly cystic ovary syndrome. *Am J Obstet Gynecol.* 2014;211(2):163.

97. Machtinger R, Combelles CM, Missmer SA, Correia KF, Fox JH, Racowsky C. The association between severe obesity and characterisitics of failed fertilized oocytes. *Hum Reprod.* 2012;27(11):3198–3207.

98. Fedorcsak P, Dale PO, Storeng R, et al. Impact of overweight and underweight on assisted reproduction treatment. *Hum Reprod.* 2004;19(11):2523–2528.

99. Spandorfer SD, Kump L, Goldschlag D, Brodkin T, Davis OK, Rozenwaks Z. Obesity and in vitro fertilisation: negative influences on outcome. *J Reprod Med.* 2004;49(12):973–977.

100. Dechaud H, Anahory T, Reyftmann L, Loup V, Hamamah S, Hedon B. Obesity does not adversely affect results in patients who are undergoing in vitro fertilisation and embryo transfer. *Eur J Obstet Gynecol Reprod Biol.* 2006;127(1):88–93.

101. Comstock IA, Kim S, Behr B, Lathi RB. Increased body mass index negatively impacts blastocyst formation rate in normal responders undergoing in vitro fertilisation. *J Assist Reprod Genet.* 2015;32(9):1299–1304.

102. Goldman KN, Hodes-Werz B, McCulloch DH, Flom JD, Grifo JA. Association of body mass index with embryonic aneuploidy. *Fertil Steril.* 2015;103(3):744–748.

103. Wang JX, Davies M, Norman RJ. Body mass index and probability of pregnancy during assisted reproduction treatment; retrospective study. *BMJ.* 2000;321(7272):1320–1321.

104. Lashen H, Ledger W, Bernal AL, Barlow D. Extremes of body mass do not adversely affect the outcome of superovulation and in-vitro fertilisation. *Hum Reprod.* 1999;14(3):712–715.

105. Provost MP, Acharya KS, Acharya CR, et al. Pregnancy outcomes decline with increasing body mass index: analysis of 239,127 fresh autologous in vitro fertilization cycles from the 2008-2010 Society for Assisted Reproductive Technology registry. *Fertil Steril.* 2016;105(3):663–669.

106. Luke B, Brown MB, Stern JE, et al. Female obesity adversely affects assisted reproductive technology (ART) pregnancy and live birth rates. *Hum Reprod.* 2011;26(1):245–252.

107. Jungheim ES, Schon SB, Schulte MB, DeUgarte DA, Fowler SA, Tuuli MG. IVF outcomes in obese donor oocyte recipients: a systematic review and meta-analysis. *Hum Reprod.* 2013;28(10):2720–2727.

108. Bellver J, Pellicer A, Garcia-Velasco JA, Ballesteros A, Remohi J, Mesequer M. Obesity reduces uterine receptivity: clinical experience from 9587 first cycles of ovum donation with normal weight donors. *Fertil Steril.* 2013;100(4):1050–1058.

109. Provost MP, Acharya KS, Acharya KS, et al. Pregnancy outcomes decline with increasing body mass index: an analysis of 22,317 fresh donor/recipient cycles from the 2008-2010 Society for Assisted Reproductive Technology Clinic Outcome Reporting System registry. *Fertil Steril.* 2016;105(2):364–368.

110. Keltz J, Zapantis A, Jindal SK, Lieman HJ, Santoro N, Polotsky AJ. Overweight men: clinical pregnancy after ART is decreased in IVF but not in ICSI cycles. *J Assist Reprod Genet.* 2010;27(9–10):539–544.

111. Colaci DS, Afeiche M, Gaskins AJ, et al. Mens body mass index in relation to embryo quality and clinical outcomes in couples undergoing in vitro fertilization. *Fertil Steril.* 2012;98(5):1193–1199.

112. Balen AH, Anderson RA, Policy and Practice Committee of the BFS. Impact of obesity on female reproductive health: British Fertility Society, Policy and Pracice Guidelines. *Hum Fertil.* 2007;10(4):195–206.

113. Leenen R, vander Kooy K, Seidell JC, Deurenberg P, Koppeschaar HP. Visceral fat accumulation in relation to sex hormones in obese men and women undergoing weight loss therapy. *J Clin Endocrinol Metab.* 1994;78(6):1515–1520.

114. Moran LJ, Hutchison SK, Norman RJ, Teede HJ. Lifestyle changes in women with polycystic ovary syndrome. *Cochrane Database Syst Rev.* 2011;6(7):CD007506.

115. Considine RV, Sinha MK, Helman ML, et al. Serum immunoreactive-leptin concentrations in normal-weight and obese humans. *N Engl J Med.* 1996;334(5):292–295.

116. Rubino F, Gagner M, Gentileschi P, et al. The early effect of the Roux-en-Y gastric bypass on hormones involved in body weight regulation and glucose metabolism. *Ann Surg.* 2004;240(2):236–242.

117. Palomba S, Falbo A, Valli B, et al. Physical activity before IVF and ICSI cycles in infertile obese women: an observational cohort study. *Reprod Biomed Online.* 2014;29(1):72–79.

118. Norman RJ, Davies MJ, Lord J, Moran LJ. The role of lifestyle modification in polycystic ovary syndrome. *Trends Endocrinol Metab.* 2002;13(6):251–257.

119. National Institute for Health and Clinical Excellence. *Fertility Problems: Assessment and Treatment Clinical Guideline No 156;* 2013. Available at: https://www.nice.org.uk/guidance/cg156/resources/fertility-problems-assessment-and-treatment-35109634660549/.

120. Norman RJ, Noakes M, Wu R, Davies MJ, Moran L, Wang JX. Improving reproductive performance in overweight/obese women with effective weight management. *Hum Reprod Update.* 2004;10(3):267–280.

121. Thomson RL, Buckley JD, Brinkworth GD. Exercise for the treatment and management of overweight women with polycystic ovary syndrome: a review of the literature. *Obes Rev.* 2011;12:e202–e210.

122. Park SK, Park JH, Kwon YC, Kim HS, Yoon MS, Park HT. The effect of combined aerobic and resistance exercise training on abdominal fat in obese middle-aged women. *J Physiol Anthropol Appl Hum Sci.* 2003;22(3):129–135.

123. Schwingshackl L, Dias S, Strasser B, Hoffmann G. Impact of different training modalities on anthropometric and metabolic characteristics in overweight/obese subjects: a systematic review and network meta-analysis. *PLoS One.* 2013;8(12):e82853.

124. Frost G, Lyons F, Bovill-Taylor C, Carter L, Stuttard J, Dornhorst A. Intensive lifestyle intervention combined with the choice of pharmacotherapy improves weight loss and cardiac risk factors in the obese. *J Hum Nutr Diet.* 2002;15(4):287–295. Quiz 297–289.

125. Rubio MA, Gargallo M, Isabel Millan A, Moreno B. Drugs in the treatment of obesity: sibutramine, orlistat and rimonabant. *Public Health Nutr.* 2007;10(10A):1200–1205.

126. Panidis D, Tziomalos K, Papadakis E, et al. The role of orlistat combined with lifestyle changes in the management of overweight and obese patients with polycystic ovary syndrome. *Clin Endocrinol.* 2014;80(3):432–438.

127. Raman JD, Schlegel PN. Aromatase inhibitors for male infertility. *J Urol.* 2002;167(2 Pt 1):624–629.

128. Roth MY, Amory JK, Page ST. Treatment of male infertility secondary to morbid obesity. *Nat Clin Pract Endocrinol Metab.* 2008;4(7):415–419.

129. Schlegel PN. Aromatase inhibitors for male infertility. *Fertil Steril.* 2012;98(6):1359–1362.

130. Spritzer PM, Motta AB, Sir-Petermann T, Diamanti-Kandarakis E. Novel strategies in the management of polycystic ovary syndrome. *Minerva Endocrinol.* 2015;40(3):195–212.

131. Welbourn R, Small PK, Finlay I, Sareela A, Somers S, Mahawar K. *The UK National Bariatric Surgery Registry: Second Registry Report.* Henley-on-Thames: Dendrite Clinical Systems Limited; 2014.

132. National Institute for Health and Care Excellence. *Obesity: Identification, Assessment and Management. Clinical Guideline No. 189*; 2014. Available at: https://www.nice.org.uk/guidance/cg189/chapter/1-recommendations/.

133. Sjöström L, Narbro K, Sjöström CD, et al. Effects of bariatric surgery on mortality in Swedish obese subjects. *N Engl J Med.* 2007;357(8):741–752.

134. Sjöström L. Review of the key results from the Swedish Obese Subjects (SOS) trial – a prospective controlled intervention study of bariatric surgery. *J Intern Med.* 2013;273(3):219–234.

135. Royal College of Obstetricians and Gynaecologists. *The Role of Bariatric Surgery in the Management of Female Infertility.* London: RCOG; 2010.

136. Teitelman M, Grotegut CA, Williams NN, Lewis JD. The impact of bariatric surgery on menstrual patterns. *Obes Surg.* 2006;16(11):1457–1463.

137. Eid GM, Cottam DR, Velcu LM, et al. Effective treatment of polycystic ovarian syndrome with Roux-en-Y gastric bypass. *Surg Obes Relat Dis.* 2005;1(2):77–80.

138. Mahawar KK, Graham Y, Small PK. Optimum time for pregnancy after bariatric surgery. *Surg Obes Relat Dis.* 2016;12(5):1126–1128.

139. O'Kane M, Pinkney J, Aashiem K, Barth J, Batterham R, Welbourn R. *BOMSS Guidelines on the Perioperative and Postoperative Biochemical Monitoring and Micronutrient Replacement for Patients Undergoing Bariatric Surgery*; 2014. London.

140. American College of Obstetricians and Gynecologists. ACOG Practice bulletin; bariatric surgery and pregnancy 105. *Obstet Gynecol.* 2009;113:1405–1413.

141. Mechanick JI, Youdim A, Jones DB, et al. Clinical practice guidelines for the perioperative nutritional, metabolic, and nonsurgical support of the bariatric surgery patient–2013 update: cosponsored by American Association of Clinical Endocrinologists, the Obesity Society, and American Society for Metabolic & Bariatric Surgery. *Surg Obes Relat Dis.* 2013;9(2):159–191.

142. Graham Y, Wilkes S, Mansour D, Small PK. Contraceptive needs of women following bariatric surgery. *J Fam Plann Reprod Health Care.* 2014;40(4):241–244.

143. Raatikainen K, Heiskanen N, Heinonen S. Transition from overweight to obesity worsens pregnancy outcome in a BMI-dependent manner. *Obesity (Silver Spring).* 2006;14(1):165–171.

144. Lash MM, Armstrong A. Impact of obesity on women's health. *Fertil Steril.* 2009;91(5):1712–1716.

145. Royal College of Obstetricians and Gynaecologists. *The Role of Bariatric Surgery in Improving Reproductive Health.* London: RCOG; 2015.

146. Maggard MA, Yermilov I, Li Z, et al. Pregnancy and fertility following bariatric surgery: a systematic review. *JAMA.* 2008;300(19):2286–2296.

147. Guelinckx I, Devlieger R, Vansant G. Reproductive outcome after bariatric surgery: a critical review. *Hum Reprod Update.* 2009;15(2):189–201.

148. Jans G, Matthys C, Bel S, et al. AURORA: bariatric surgery registration in women of reproductive age – a multicenter prospective cohort study. *BMC Pregnancy Childbirth.* 2016;16(1):195.

149. Hirshfeld-Cytron J, Kim HH. Empty follicle syndrome in the setting of dramatic weight loss after bariatric surgery: case report and review of available literature. *Fertil Steril.* 2008;90(4). 1199.e1121-1193.

150. Tsur A, Orvieto R, Haas J, Kedem A, Machtinger R. Does bariatric surgery improve ovarian stimulation characteristics, oocyte yield, or embryo quality? *J Ovarian Res.* 2014;7:116.

151. Christofolini J, Bianco B, Santos G, Adami F, Christofolini D, Barbosa CP. Bariatric surgery influences the number and quality of oocytes in patients submitted to assisted reproduction techniques. *Obesity (Silver Spring).* 2014;22:939–942.

152. Reis LO, Dias FG. Male fertility, obesity and bariatric surgery. *Reprod Sci.* 2012;19(8):778–785.

153. Sermondade N, Massin N, Boitrelle F, et al. Sperm parameters and male fertility after bariatric surgery: three case series. *Reprod Biomed Online.* 2012;24(2):206–210.

CHAPTER 13

Obesity and Pregnancy

EMMA SLACK, BSC (HONS), MSC • HELENE BRANDON, MBCHB, FRCOG •
DR. NICOLA HESLEHURST, BSC (HONS), MSC, PHD

Obesity prevalence is increasing among women of childbearing age, which has an impact on pregnancy. Maternal obesity has been described as the biggest challenge maternity services face in contemporary society.[1] Delivery of health services to manage maternal obesity is challenging because of the high prevalence and impact on multiple adverse outcomes for both the mother and the developing fetus. Health professionals face clinical challenges of managing and preventing adverse pregnancy outcomes to ensure the safety of the mother and her baby, while simultaneously promoting public health recommendations for healthy diet and physical activity behaviors and managing gestational weight gain (GWG). This chapter will give an overview of the scientific evidence base relating to maternal obesity and GWG (Part 1) and a reflective account of the challenges health professionals face when providing care for women with obesity in routine practice (Part 2).

PART 1: THE EVIDENCE BASE

This section will discuss the current evidence base relating to maternal obesity and GWG, including definitions, population trends and inequalities, risks to mother and offspring, guidelines on GWG, excessive GWG, and the potential mechanisms linking maternal obesity and GWG with adverse outcomes of pregnancy.

Defining Maternal Obesity

There is an absence of pregnancy-specific body mass index (BMI) criteria to define maternal weight status during pregnancy. The World Health Organization (WHO) BMI categories for nonpregnant populations are usually applied to research, guidelines, and clinical practice[2]: underweight ($<18.5\,\mathrm{kg/m^2}$), recommended weight ($18.5-24.9\,\mathrm{kg/m^2}$), overweight ($25-29.9\,\mathrm{kg/m^2}$), and obese ($\geq30\,\mathrm{kg/m^2}$). The obesity category can also be further subdivided into class I ($30-34.9\,\mathrm{kg/m^2}$), class II ($35-39.9\,\mathrm{kg/m^2}$), and class III obesity ($\geq40\,\mathrm{kg/m^2}$). There is an additional obesity subgroup often used

in pregnancy research to define women with extreme obesity ($\mathrm{BMI}\geq50\,\mathrm{kg/m^2}$) and the highest degree of risk. As these criteria were developed based on risk information for nonpregnant populations, such as diabetes and cardiovascular disease, their use is limited to the early stages of pregnancy because the measures do not account for the naturally incurred weight gain in pregnancy including the fetus, placenta, fluid, and adipose tissue.[3] Guidelines recommend that weight and height are measured in early pregnancy, usually the first trimester, to calculate maternal BMI and plan maternity care.[4]

Population Trends in Maternal Obesity

Maternal obesity has been increasing over time internationally. Published incidence data from Europe, the United States, and Australia show that around 2%–8% of women had an obese BMI in pregnancy in the 1980s, with an increase in incidence observed in the 2000s of 10%–15% in Europe and Australia, and 20%–30% in the United States.[5-10] In the United Kingdom, overweight among women of childbearing age increased from 25% in 1993 to 29% in 2013, and obesity increased from 12% to 19%.[11,12] In pregnancy, first trimester obesity in England doubled from 7.6% in 1989 to 15.6% in 2007,[13] and more recent data estimate 21% of pregnancies in August 2016 were among obese women.[14] There is regional variation in maternal obesity in England, United Kingdom, with above average incidence in the West Midlands, Yorkshire and the Humber, and the North East regions.[13] Therefore, maternity services in certain regions will have disproportionate impact of the increasing incidence of maternal obesity over time.

Much of the regional differentiation in maternal obesity can be linked to sociodemographic and socioeconomic inequalities. A study of nationally representative pregnancies in England identified that maternal overweight or obesity was significantly associated with increasing maternal parity and age.[13] Women with class III obesity were also significantly more likely to be unemployed than women with a recommended BMI.[13]

The strongest association was observed with socioeconomic status, where women with obesity were more than twice as likely as women with a recommended BMI to be residing in areas of highest deprivation following adjustment for potential confounders (adjusted odds ratio [AOR] 2.20; 95% confidence interval [CI] 2.13–2.28). There was also a pattern of socioeconomic disadvantage with increasing obesity class, which remained after adjusting for confounding sociodemographic factors (such as maternal age and ethnicity). Women with class III obesity were significantly more likely to be residing in areas of highest deprivation (BMI 40.0–49.9 kg/m^2 AOR 2.97 [95% CI 2.69–3.29]; BMI ≥ 50 kg/m^2 AOR 4.69 [95% CI 3.20–6.87]), or to be unemployed (BMI ≥50 kg/m^2 AOR 1.50 [95% CI 1.12 2.02]), compared with women with a BMI in the recommended range.[13] There are also associations with maternal obesity and ethnic groups in the United Kingdom with a significantly increased adjusted odds of obesity among black women (AOR 1.70 95% CI 1.62–1.78) or South Asian women (AOR 1.72 95% CI 1.66–1.79) compared with white women.[15] For South Asian women, the associations were most pronounced for Pakistani women (AOR 2.08 95% CI 2.08–2.31) compared with Indian (AOR 1.49 95% CI 1.39–1.60), or Bangladeshi women (AOR 1.15 95% CI 1.15 95% CI 1.06–1.24).[15]

Maternal Obesity Risks to Mother and Child

International research has highlighted that maternal obesity has implications for both mother and child.[16,17] Of all maternal deaths in the United Kingdom between 2006 and 2008, 49% occurred in overweight or obese women, and 27% in obese women.[18] Additional maternal risks include preeclampsia, thromboembolic complications, cesarean section, and gestational diabetes, which have been linked to an increased risk of the future development of type 2 diabetes.[1,19–22] Increased risks to the infant include macrosomia, shoulder dystocia, late fetal death (after 28 weeks gestation), preterm (<37 weeks) and postterm birth (>42 weeks gestation), and congenital anomalies.[16,23–26] There is evidence that maternal obesity contributes to subsequent obesity development and the associated life course morbidities in offspring.[27]

There is an increased risk of complications during labor and the need for more induced and operative deliveries when mothers have an obese BMI.[16] As a result, women may experience limited choices relating to where and how they can give birth, and an increased need for pain relief and general anesthesia, which also contributes to risk.[4] There are also complications associated with maternal obesity after birth such as difficulties establishing breastfeeding, slower wound healing, and risk of infection.[17,28] Because of the increased morbidity during pregnancy and labor, women with obesity are also more likely to be hospitalized and to spend longer time in hospital following pregnancy,[28] and there is an increased risk of mental health disorders including antenatal and postnatal depression.[29] Prevention and management of the increased health risks for both mother and infant requires additional care and resources from healthservice providers.[28] In the United Kingdom there are national guidelines for the management of obesity in pregnancy published by the Royal College of Obstetricians and Gynaecologists (RCOG) and the Centre for Maternal and Child Enquiries (CMACE).[30] These guidelines include recommendations for both risk prevention and risk management, such as the need for consultant-led care, anesthetic reviews, screening for gestational diabetes and venous thromboembolism (VTE), thromboprophylaxis treatment, and equipment requirements.[30]

Gestational Weight Gain

In addition to the impact of prepregnancy obesity on pregnancy outcomes, pregnancy itself is a significant life course time in the development of obesity among women. The weight a woman gains between the time of conception and the onset of labor is known as GWG.[31] Excessive GWG and postnatal weight retention are significant predictors of long-term obesity development in women. Excessive GWG can also incur additional risks to the mother and child. This section will give an overview of the existing evidence base on GWG including definitions, the associated risks, and current guidelines.

Defining gestational weight gain

GWG is a complex and unique biologic phenomenon, which supports the growth and development of the fetus.[32] GWG is made up of maternal components (including fat mass, fat-free mass, and total body water), placenta components (including placental weight, placental growth, placental development, and placental composition), and fetal components (amniotic fluid and fetal growth; both fat mass and fat-free mass).[32] The total amount of weight gained in normal-term pregnancies differs from woman to woman.[32] However, some generalizations can be made about the patterns of GWG and the impact on pregnancy outcome. Data from singleton pregnancies in the United States suggested that adult women with a recommended BMI who delivered at full term had a GWG ranging from 10.0 to 16.7 kg, whereas adolescents had a higher GWG

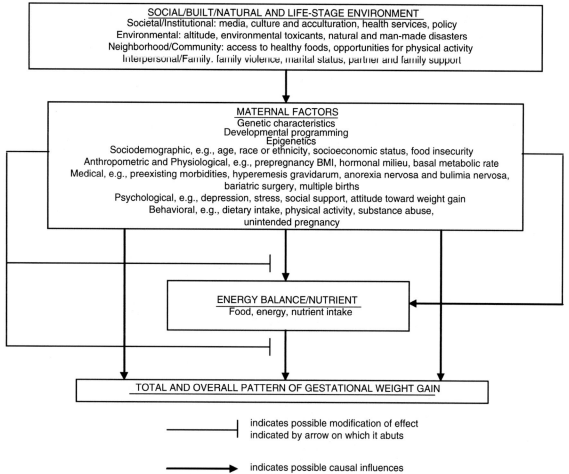

FIG. 13.1 Schematic summary of factors influencing gestational weight gain. (From Institute of Medicine. *Weight Gain During Pregnancy: Reexamining the Guidelines*. Washington DC: National Academic Press; 2009, with permission.)

(14.6–18.0 kg).[32] There was also an inverse association between maternal prepregnancy BMI and GWG; the higher the BMI, the lower the total GWG.[32] The pattern of GWG also differs by trimester of pregnancy and is generally higher in the second trimester.[32]

There are multiple factors that contribute to the amount of weight gained during pregnancy, which may explain some of the differences observed in the patterns of weight gain between subgroups of the population. Potential determinants of gestational weight gain include social and environmental factors (e.g., culture, family, and living environments), maternal factors (e.g., genetics, ethnicity, and comorbidities), and energy balance.[32] A summary of the determinants, and interactions between determinants, is shown in Fig. 13.1.

Excessive gestational weight gain

In Europe and the United States, 20%–40% of women gain more than the recommended weight during pregnancy.[33] Excessive GWG increases the risk of adverse outcomes of pregnancy for the mother, including abnormal or impaired glucose tolerance, pregnancy-induced hypertension, cesarean delivery, unsuccessful breastfeeding, and longer hospital stay; and for the offspring, including high birth weight (large for gestational age and macrosomia), very preterm birth, low Apgar score, seizure, hypoglycemia, meconium aspiration syndrome, and polycythemia.[32,34–36] Excessive GWG has also been associated with longer-term risks, including postnatal weight retention and long-term development of overweight and obesity in women and

TABLE 13.1
2009 Institute of Medicine Gestational Weight Gain Recommendations

Prepregnancy Weight Category	BMI (kg/m²)	Recommended GWG Range, kg	Recommended Rate of Weight Gain in Second and Third Trimesters Mean (Range) kg/week
Underweight	<18.5	12.5–18	0.51 (0.44–0.58)
Recommended weight	18.5–24.9	11.5–16	0.42 (0.35–0.50)
Overweight	25.0–29.9	7.5–11.5	0.28 (0.23–0.33)
Obese	≥30.0	5–9	0.22 (0.17–0.27)

BMI, body mass index; *GWG*, gestational weight gain.
Data from Institute of Medicine. *Weight Gain During Pregnancy: Reexamining the Guidelines.* Yaktine A, Rasmussen K, eds. Washington DC: National Academic Press; 2009.

offspring.[37,38] There are challenges to interpreting the evidence base on GWG and adverse pregnancy outcomes, such as inconsistent methods and timing of measurements, and definitions of appropriate GWG[39–42] making it difficult to compare results across studies. However, there seems to be a consensus that GWG is a modifiable risk factor that may influence both long- and short-term pregnancy outcomes for both mother and infant.

Gestational weight gain guidelines

There is a lack of international agreement on appropriate GWG for optimal pregnancy outcomes for the mother and offspring. However, many countries have developed national GWG guidelines,[43] which are predominantly based on the recommendations made by the Institute of Medicine (IoM) in the United States for GWG stratified by prepregnancy BMI category (Table 13.1).[32] The recommendations aim to improve maternal outcomes while minimizing harm to the infant, and vice versa. Low GWG can benefit the mother but increase risks to the infant, whereas a high GWG improved outcomes for the infant but increased risks for the mother.[32] The pregnancy outcomes considered in the development of the IoM weight gain recommendations were postnatal weight retention, cesarean delivery, small or large for gestational age, and childhood obesity. Despite rigorous systematic review methods to inform the development of recommendations, the evidence base was limited by inconsistent use of GWG categories, and a lack of data on GWG and childhood obesity among offspring, or the influence of population subgroups, such as ethnicity.[32]

There has been criticism of the IoM recommendations from physicians who believe that the GWG ranges are very high for women with a BMI ≥ 25 kg/m² and the lack of recommendations for obesity classes.[44] As the risks of adverse pregnancy outcomes differ across obesity classes, a single GWG recommendation for all obesity classes may be inappropriate to minimize risk, especially among the higher obesity classes with the highest degree of risk. However, there are also concerns about increasing the risk to the infant if the GWG is too low. A recent systematic review and meta-analysis explored the safety of recommending GWG below the IoM guidelines for women with obesity.[45] Following adjustment for confounding factors, the analyses identified that a reduced GWG was associated with significantly increased odds of preterm birth and small for gestational age. However, there were significantly decreased odds of large for gestational age, macrosomia, gestational hypertension, preeclampsia, and cesarean delivery.[45] The review concluded that GWG below the IoM guidelines may be beneficial for some women if advice was individualized, taking into account their excising comorbidities. However, this could not be a routine recommendation for all women without better risk prediction models.[45] The United Kingdom does not currently have evidence-based recommendations for GWG. National guidelines for weight management before, during, and after pregnancy instead focus on supporting women to lose weight in the preconception and postnatal periods and on healthy dietary and physical activity behaviors during pregnancy.[4]

Potential Mechanisms Linking Maternal Obesity and Gestational Weight Gain to Adverse Pregnancy Outcomes

Currently, the mechanisms by which maternal obesity and excess GWG cause adverse pregnancy outcomes are unclear and are likely to be different for different pregnancy outcomes. For example, mechanisms linking obesity and post-term birth could include mechanical and hormonal interactions between the mother, fetus, and placenta. Hormones (such as corticotrophin-releasing hormone and oxytocin),[46] plus obesity-associated insulin resistance, inflammation, circulating leptin concentrations, lipolysis, and dyslipidemia, may impact on the onset of labor and uterine contractility.[46] Insulin resistance is thought to be caused by excess adipose tissue and to play a vital role in the development of adverse maternal and fetal outcomes, including gestational diabetes, and the subsequent development of type 2 diabetes.[32] During pregnancy, insulin resistance develops in the mother to provide the growing fetus with vital nutrients.[47] It has been suggested that in mothers with greater amounts of adipose tissue during pregnancy, either as a result of being overweight at the start of pregnancy or through excessive GWG (or both), delivery of nutrients to the fetus is exaggerated through further increased insulin resistance and possible interference with maternal hormones that regulate placental nutrient transporters.[47] Greater concentrations of glucose and fatty acids cross the placenta to the fetus, leading to increased fetal production of insulin and fetal growth: the "fetal overnutrition hypothesis."[48] The increased fetal insulin in utero may also influence longer-term outcomes for the infant, such as adiposity in adult life, through permanent changes to pancreatic islet cells, hypothalamus, and adipose tissue.[49] However, the association between maternal and offspring obesity may also be explained by shared genetic and environmental exposures of the mother and her offspring.[50] Lawlor et al. found that most of the association between maternal BMI, gestational weight gain, and offspring obesity could be explained by shared familial characteristics, such as lifestyle and environment, when maternal BMI was in the recommended range.[50] However, when mothers were overweight or obese, there was a contribution to offspring obesity development through mechanisms in utero.[50]

PART 2: A CLINICIAN'S PERSPECTIVE

This reflection is based on my experience of working in the United Kingdom, in the specialty of obstetrics, particularly maternal medicine, since 2003. I describe my experience of the challenges posed when caring for overweight and obese pregnant women antenatally, peripartum, and postnatally. My experience is in the context of a small district general hospital in Gateshead with 2000 deliveries a year. The population accessing antenatal care at this NHS Trust live in a deprived area of the North East of England and are mainly white ethnic group, with low income and a high prevalence of adult obesity.

At Gateshead, a local clinical pathway was developed, drawing on evidence-based national guidance, to aid decision-making and management of clinical risk (Table 13.2). The pathways include care required for different stages of pregnancy, and the level of intervention required increases with increasing obesity class. In addition to the pregnancy requirements, the pathways also include preconception and postnatal care. Preconception, women with a BMI greater than 30 kg/m² should be advised of the increased risks associated with pregnancy, prescribed an increased dose (5 mg) of folic acid daily for at least 1 month, and supported to lose weight. Postnatally, there are several interventions to alleviate risks including early mobilization plus thromboprophylaxis and screening for type 2 diabetes for women who developed gestational diabetes during pregnancy. Breastfeeding should be encouraged and supported, and the lifestyle advice and ongoing weight management support should be provided.

The pathway characterizes the risks, as well as the challenges that are faced in the clinical care of obese women and their babies, and the decisions to be made along the way to alleviate these (in obstetrics not all risks can be eliminated entirely). The challenges of maternal obesity care arise preconceptually, antenatally, intrapartum, and postnatally. Ideally, women with obesity would have a planned pregnancy, access preconception advice about preparing for pregnancy, and embark on weight loss to minimize the impact of obesity in pregnancy. But in my experience this rarely happens, and the low engagement with preconception care among this population reflects the challenge we face engaging the wider population with preconception care, which is important for all women but especially those with preexisting comorbidities such as diabetes, or behavioral/social challenges such as smoking, alcohol, or domestic violence.

Throughout the pregnancy there are equipment issues, which need to be addressed in anticipation of need to ensure that women's health and safety of the need are prioritized, as well as the health and safety of health professionals (e.g., manual handling). Equipment requirements include larger armchairs and wheelchairs, suitably sized beds safe for women's weight, and larger blood pressure cuffs that more accurately measure blood pressure. This is particularly important in order not to miss preeclampsia, which is a known risk for women with obesity. The preferable mode of delivery is spontaneous labor and a vaginal birth to reduce surgical risk and achieve full mobility more quickly after delivery, thus reducing the risk of postnatal thromboembolic disease and potential pressure-associated skin damage.

TABLE 13.2
Summary of Gateshead Health NHS Foundation Trust Obesity Pathway of Care

BMI (kg/m^2)	Booking/First Trimester	Throughout Pregnancy	Third Trimester	Labor and Delivery
≥30	• Measure weight and height; calculate BMI • Use appropriate size BP cuff • 5 mg folic acid daily up to 12 weeks • 10 µg vitamin D daily throughout pregnancy • 75 mg aspirin daily if risk for preeclampsia • Assess VTE risk and treat if indicated • Provide obesity risk management; verbal information and leaflet	• Assess VTE risk and treat if indicated • Use appropriate size BP cuff • Encourage breast-feeding, discuss benefits, and provide information leaflet • Reweigh at 28 weeks • Refer to WHC for re-view of care pathway if required	• 75 g OGTT (24–28 weeks) • Offer antenatal infant feeding session • Give breastfeed-ing advice and support (benefits, initiation, and maintenance)	• Risk assessment for planned place of birth • Recommend active management of third stage of labor and document in notes Cesarean sections: • Single dose prophy-lactic antibiotics • Suture subcutane-ous tissue space if >2 cm subcutane-ous fat
≥35: as above plus	• Refer to specialist care if one or more ad-ditional risk factors for preeclampsia		• Fetal presentation and growth scan at 34 weeks	• Advise birth in con-sultant led unit • Alert theatre staff if weight >120 kg and needs operative intervention • Consider surgical adjuncts at caesar-ean section
≥40: as above plus	• Arrange antenatal anesthetic review and management plan for labor and delivery at 36 weeks	Monitor for preeclampsia • Every 3 weeks between 24 and 32 weeks • Every 2 weeks from 32 weeks to delivery	• Remeasure ma-ternal weight at 34 weeks • Assess risk for VTE • Anesthetic review; document labor and delivery plan • Risk assessment for manual han-dling	• Continuous 1:1 midwifery care • Inform duty anes-thetist if operative intervention antici-pated • Establish early venous access • Consider early epidural in labor • Senior obstetrician and anesthetist to review on ward round

BMI, body mass index; *BP*, blood pressure; *OGTT*, oral glucose tolerance test; *VTE*, venous thromboembolism; *WHC*, women's health clinic (consultant obstetrician led clinic).

There are also additional equipment requirements in labor such as extra-long elastic belts to accommodate fetal heartrate and Doppler transducers for fetal moni-toring. An obstetrician should always remain nearby in case of shoulder dystocia (when the head has been delivered, but the fetal shoulders do not follow). This is an obstetric emergency more common in obese women. When cesarean section cannot be avoided (either elective or emergency), then there are surgical challenges. Given the difficulty of an emergency cesarean, there is currently a debate, as yet unresolved, as to whether women with extreme obesity should have a surgical delivery planned electively, in daylight hours, with plenty of additional assistance, rather than risking an emergency section, potentially in the middle of the night, in a hurry. On delivery suite in our unit, the beds have a weight-bearing load of 227 kg. In the operating theater the table will bear up to 450 kg and additional equipment has been purchased to deal with surgical difficulties that may be encountered: a larger retractor to gain adequate surgical access to the abdomen, lateral extensions to the operating table to accommodate greater girth, and a state-of-the-art operating table with a weight limit we hope we will never need. Anesthetic issues include a difficult airway risk in addition to moving and handling risks, and for elective delivery all this can be planned for.

The increasing incidence of maternal obesity, and associated risks, makes it a challenging priority for clinical practice. Maternity services need to be prepared for further increases in maternal obesity over time, particularly ensuring that they are adequately equipped and staff are appropriately trained to provide safe and supportive care for women and their babies, as well as ensuring the health and safety of the health professionals caring for women with class III obesity. The highest BMI I have ever encountered in labor was 64 kg/m², and no doubt readers will soon encounter this or more.

SUMMARY

The evidence base shows that maternal obesity poses significant risks to women and their offspring, and the challenges to practice identified in the reflective account are not uncommon. Prepregnancy obesity is increasing over time, internationally, and is now part of routine daily practice for clinicians. Data suggest that incidence of class III obesity is increasing more rapidly than classes I and II.[13] Therefore, the clinician experience of managing the care of women with a BMI of 64 kg/m² is a regular occurrence, particularly among maternity services in regions of highest obesity prevalence, socioeconomic deprivation, and ethnic diversity. Given the health and social inequalities associated with maternal obesity, and the potential impact on women's and future generations' lifelong health, prevention and management is both a public health and clinical priority. There is a substantial evidence base reporting health professionals' experiences of managing maternal obesity or providing weight management support during pregnancy, including limitations with equipment, lack of weight management support service availability, health professional training needs, and barriers to engaging women with preconception care.[51,52] However, pregnancy is also a time of increased motivation for behavior change among pregnant women, and an opportunity to capitalize on routine antenatal contacts to support women weight management, their diet, and physical activity behaviors and to promote their own health and the health of their developing baby.

ACKNOWLEDGMENTS

The authors would like to acknowledge Andrea Barber, public health midwife at Gateshead Health NHS Foundation Trust, the lead author for Gateshead Obesity in Pregnancy Care Pathway, and other contributing authors. Emma Slack has PhD funding from the Medical Research Council, supervised by Dr. Nicola Heslehurst, Professor Judith Rankin, and Professor Steven Rushton from Newcastle University, United Kingdom.

REFERENCES

1. Centre for Maternal and Child Enquiries (CMACE). *Maternal Obesity in the UK: Findings from a National Project.* London: CMACE; 2010.
2. World Health Organisation. *Obesity: Preventing and Managing the Global Epidemic*; 2000. Geneva.
3. Heslehurst N. Symposium I: consequences of obesity and overweight during pregnancy identifying 'at risk' women and the impact of maternal obesity on National Health Service maternity services. *Proc Nutr Soc.* 2011;70(4): 439–449.
4. National Institute for Health and Clinical Excellence. *Weight Management before, during and after Pregnancy*; 2010. Department of Health.
5. Bhattacharya S, Campbell DM, Liston WA, Bhattacharya S. Effect of body mass index on pregnancy outcomes in nulliparous women delivering singleton babies. *BMC Public Health.* 2007;7(1):168.
6. Scholz R, Voigt M, Schneider KTM, et al. Analysis of the German perinatal survey of the years 2007–2011 and comparison with data from 1995–1997: maternal characteristics. *Geburtshilfe Frauenheilkd.* 2013;73(12):1247–1251.
7. Brynhildsen J, Sydsjö A, Ekholm-Selling K, Josefsson A. The importance of maternal BMI on infant's birth weight in four BMI groups for the period 1978–2001. *Acta Obstet Gynecol Scand.* 2009;88(4):391–396.
8. Kanagalingam MG, Forouhi NG, Greer IA, Sattar N. Changes in booking body mass index over a decade: retrospective analysis from a Glasgow Maternity Hospital. *BJOG.* 2005;112(10):1431–1433.
9. Fisher SC, Kim SY, Sharma AJ, Rochat R, Morrow B. Is obesity still increasing among pregnant women? Prepregnancy obesity trends in 20 states, 2003–2009. *Prev Med.* 2013;56(6):372–378.
10. Hinkle SN, Sharma AJ, Kim SY, et al. Prepregnancy obesity trends among low-income women, United States, 1999–2008. *Matern Child Health J.* 2012;16(7):1339–1348.
11. Health and Social Care Information Centre Lifestyle Statistics. *Statistics on Obesity, Physical Activity and Diet: England, 2013*; 2013. https://catalogue.ic.nhs.uk/publications/public-health/obesity/obes-phys-acti-diet-eng-2013/obes-phys-acti-diet-eng-2013-rep.pdf.
12. Moody A. *Adult Anthropometric Measures, Overweight and Obesity.* The Health and Social Care Information Centre; 2014.

13. Heslehurst N, Rankin J, Wilkinson JR, Summerbell CD. A nationally representative study of maternal obesity in England, UK: trends in incidence and demographic inequalities in 619 323 births, 1989–2007. *Int J Obes.* 2010;34(3):420–428.

14. NHS Digital. *Maternity Services Monthly Statistics, England – August 2016, Experimental Statistics*; 2017. http://www.content.digital.nhs.uk/catalogue/PUB23047.

15. Heslehurst N, Sattar N, Rajasingam D, Wilkinson J, Summerbell CD, Rankin J. Existing maternal obesity guidelines may increase inequalities between ethnic groups: a national epidemiological study of 502,474 births in England. *BMC Pregnancy Childbirth.* 2012;12(1):156.

16. Andreasen KR, Andersen ML, Schantz AL. Obesity and pregnancy. *Acta Obstet Gynecol Scand.* 2004;83(11):1022–1029.

17. Guelinckx I, Devlieger R, Beckers K, Vansant G. Maternal obesity: pregnancy complications, gestational weight gain and nutrition. *Obes Rev.* 2008;9(2):140–150.

18. Centre for Maternal and Child Enquiries (CMACE). Saving mothers' lives: reviewing maternal deaths to make motherhood safer: 2006–08. The eighth report on confidential enquiries into maternal deaths in the United Kingdom. *BJOG.* 2011;118(suppl 1):1–203.

19. CMACE. The confidential enquiry into maternal and child health (CEMACH) saving mothers' lives: reviewing maternal deaths to make motherhood safer-2003-2005. In: *CEMACH.* London: CEMACH; 2007.

20. Heslehurst N, Simpson H, Ells LJ, et al. The impact of maternal BMI status on pregnancy outcomes with immediate short-term obstetric resource implications: a meta-analysis. *Obes Rev.* November 2008;9(6):635–683.

21. Torloni MR, Betrán AP, Horta BL, et al. Prepregnancy BMI and the risk of gestational diabetes: a systematic review of the literature with meta-analysis. *Obes Rev.* 2009;10(2):194–203.

22. Bellamy L, Casas J-P, Hingorani AD, Williams D. Type 2 diabetes mellitus after gestational diabetes: a systematic review and meta-analysis. *Lancet.* 2009;373(9677):1773–1779.

23. Aune D, Saugstad OD, Henriksen T, Tonstad S. Maternal body mass index and the risk of fetal death, stillbirth, and infant death: a systematic review and meta-analysis. *JAMA.* 2014;311(15):1536–1546.

24. McDonald SD, Han Z, Mulla S, Beyene J, Knowledge Synthesis Group. Overweight and obesity in mothers and risk of preterm birth and low birth weight infants: systematic review and meta-analyses. *Br Med J.* July 20, 2010;341.

25. Heslehurst N, Vieira R, Hayes L, Crowe L, Jones D, Robalino S, Slack E, Rankin, J. Maternal body mass index and post-term birth: a systematic review and meta-analysis. *Obesity Reviews.* 2017;18:293–308.

26. Stothard KJ, Tennant PWG, Bell R, Rankin J. Maternal overweight and obesity and the risk of congenital anomalies: a systematic review and meta-analysis. *JAMA.* 2009;301(6):636–650.

27. Ramachenderan J, Bradford J, McLean M. Maternal obesity and pregnancy complications: a review. *Aust N Z J Obstet Gynaecol.* 2008;48(3):228–235.

28. Heslehurst N, Lang R, Rankin J, Wilkinson JR, Summerbell CD. Obesity in pregnancy: a study of the impact of maternal obesity on NHS maternity services. *BJOG.* 2007;114(3):334–342.

29. Molyneaux E, Poston L, Ashurst-Williams S, Howard LM. Obesity and mental disorders during pregnancy and postpartum: a systematic review and meta-analysis. *Obstet Gynecol.* 2014;123(4):857.

30. Centre for Maternal, Child Enquiries, Royal College of Obstetricians and Gynaecologists. *CMACE/RCOG Joint Guideline: Management of Women with Obesity in Pregnancy.* Centre for Maternal and Child Enquiries and the Royal College of Obstetricians and Gynaecologists; 2010.

31. Viswanathan M, Siega-Riz AM, Moos M-K, et al. *Outcomes of Maternal Weight Gain*; 2008.

32. Institute of Medicine. *Weight Gain during Pregnancy: Reexamining the Guidelines.* Washington DC: National Academic Press; 2009.

33. Thangaratinam S, Jolly K. Obesity in pregnancy: a review of reviews on the effectiveness of interventions. *BJOG.* 2010;117(11):1309–1312.

34. Diesel JC, Eckhardt CL, Day NL, Brooks MM, Arslanian SA, Bodnar LM. Is gestational weight gain associated with offspring obesity at 36 months? *Pediatr Obes.* 2015 Aug;10(4):305–310.

35. Mamun AA, Callaway LK, O'Callaghan MJ, et al. Associations of maternal pre-pregnancy obesity and excess pregnancy weight gains with adverse pregnancy outcomes and length of hospital stay. *BMC Pregnancy Childbirth.* 2011;11(1):62.

36. Stotland NE, Cheng YW, Hopkins LM, Caughey AB. Gestational weight gain and adverse neonatal outcome among term infants. *Obstet Gynecol.* 2006;108(3, Part 1):635–643.

37. Nehring I, Schmoll S, Beyerlein A, Hauner H, von Kries R. Gestational weight gain and long-term postpartum weight retention: a meta-analysis. *Am J Clin Nutr.* 2011;94(5):1225–1231.

38. Lau EY, Liu J, Archer E, McDonald SM, Liu J. Maternal weight gain in pregnancy and risk of obesity among offspring: a systematic review. *J Obes.* 2014;2014.

39. Dietz PM, Callaghan WM, Sharma AJ. High pregnancy weight gain and risk of excessive fetal growth. *Am J Obstet Gynecol.* 2009;201(1). 51. e51–51. e56.

40. Gunderson EP, Abrams B, Selvin S. The relative importance of gestational gain and maternal characteristics associated with the risk of becoming overweight after pregnancy. *Int J Obes Relat Metab Disord.* 2000;24(12):1660–1668.

41. Amorim AR, Rössner S, Neovius M, Lourenço PM, Linné Y. Does excess pregnancy weight gain constitute a major risk for increasing long-term BMI? *Obesity.* 2007;15(5):1278–1286.

42. Margerison Zilko CE, Rehkopf D, Abrams B. Association of maternal gestational weight gain with short-and long-term maternal and child health outcomes. *Am J Obstet Gynecol.* 2010;202(6). 574. e571–574. e578.

43. Alavi N, Haley S, Chow K, McDonald SD. Comparison of national gestational weight gain guidelines and energy intake recommendations. *Obes Rev.* 2013;14(1):68–85.

44. The American College of Obstetricians, Gynecologists. *Committee Opinion: Weight Gain during Pregnancy*; 2013. http://www.acog.org/Resources-And-Publications/Committee-Opinions/Committee-on-Obstetric-Practice/Weight-Gain-During-Pregnancy.

45. Kapadia MZ, Park CK, Beyene J, Giglia L, Maxwell C, McDonald SD. Can we safely recommend gestational weight gain below the 2009 guidelines in obese women? A systematic review and meta-analysis. *Obes Rev*. 2015;16(3).

46. Bogaerts A, Witters I, Van den Bergh BR, Jans G, Devlieger R. Obesity in pregnancy: altered onset and progression of labour. *Midwifery*. 2013;29(12):1303–1313.

47. Ryan EA. Hormones and insulin resistance during pregnancy. *Lancet*. 2003;362(9398):1777–1778.

48. Wu Q, Suzuki M. Parental obesity and overweight affect the body-fat accumulation in the offspring: the possible effect of a high-fat diet through epigenetic inheritance. *Obes Rev*. 2006;7(2):201–208.

49. Oken E, Gillman MW. Fetal origins of obesity. *Obes Res*. 2003;11(4):496–506.

50. Lawlor DA, Lichtenstein P, Fraser A, Långström N. Does maternal weight gain in pregnancy have long-term effects on offspring adiposity? A sibling study in a prospective cohort of 146,894 men from 136,050 families. *Am J Clin Nutr*. 2011;94(1):142–148.

51. Poels M, Koster MPH, Boeije HR, Franx A, van Stel HF. Why do women not use preconception care? A systematic review on barriers and facilitators. *Obstet Gynecol Surv*. 2016;71(10):603–612.

52. Heslehurst N, Newham J, Maniatopoulos G, Fleetwood C, Robalino S, Rankin J. Implementation of pregnancy weight management and obesity guidelines: a meta-synthesis of healthcare professionals' barriers and facilitators using the Theoretical Domains Framework. *Obes Rev*. 2014;15(6):462–486.

CHAPTER 14

Genetics of Obesity

BÉATRICE DUBERN, MD, PHD • KARINE CLÉMENT, MD, PHD • CHRISTINE POITOU, DM, PHD

Obesity, defined as an excess of fat mass having an impact on body's health, is a complex and multifactorial disease. The World Health Organization (http://www.who.int) has estimated that 1.5 billion adults are overweight (body mass index [BMI] > 25 kg/m^2), among which 500 million are obese (BMI > 30 kg/m^2). In children, the worldwide prevalence of overweight and obesity has increased from 4.2% in 1990 to 6.7% in 2010, but has stabilized in recent years.[1] Obesity results from the interaction of numerous environmental factors (such as overeating and/or reduction in physical activity) with genetic factors. The understanding of the molecular mechanisms contributing to obesity has quickly progressed in recent years focusing on the genetic study of obese individuals and their families. The development of new genetic screening tools applied to cohorts was also instrumental in this progress.

Several clinical presentations are described in obesity depending on the genes involved[2,3]:

- **Syndromic obesity** corresponds to severe obesity associated with additional phenotypes (endocrine disorders or mental retardation, dysmorphic features, and organ-specific developmental abnormalities). Prader-Willi (PWS) and Bardet-Biedl (BBS) syndromes are the two most frequently described syndromes, but more than 100 syndromes are now associated with obesity. Genetic mutations of the leptin/melanocortin axis involved in food intake regulation (genes of leptin [LEP], the leptin receptor [LEPR], proopiomelanocortin [POMC], proconvertase 1 [PCSK1]) or targeted genes involved in these pathways are also responsible for syndromic obesity. These severe diseases are characterized by rare and severe early-onset obesity associated with endocrine disorders.
- **Melanocortin 4 receptor (MC4R)-linked obesity** is characterized by the development of obesity, but the phenotypic expression varies partly because of dependence on environmental factors. Thus, there is no specific phenotype associated with MC4R-linked obesity, which is responsible for 2%–3% of obesity in adults and children.
- **These rare forms of monogenic obesity distinguish themselves from the polygenic obesity**, which is the most common clinical situation (>95% of cases). In polygenic obesity, each susceptibility gene, taken individually, would only have a slight effect on weight. Furthermore, the cumulative contribution of these genes would become significant only in an obesogenic environment (such as overfeeding, sedentary living, stress, etc.).

POLYGENIC OBESITY

Polygenic obesity is caused by multiple gene defects with modest effects that interact with the environment[3] Several approaches, such as linkage/positional cloning, candidate gene, and genomewide scan (GWAS), have been used to identify genes associated with polygenic obesity. For example, using linkage analysis, a three-SNP (single-nucleotide polymorphism) haplotype in ectonucleotide pyrophosphate/phosphodiesterase 1 (ENPP1) was found to contribute to childhood and adult obesity as well as several variants in PCSK1 (N221D, Q665E, and S690T).[4,5] These genetic variations all induce in vitro functional alterations, and one example of these effects is the impairment in the N221D-mutant PC1/3 protein's catalytic activity.

A candidate gene approach was also undertaken to examine the role of a putative candidate in the pathogenesis of obesity. Using this approach, the V66M polymorphism in BDNF was associated to BMI in adults.[6] Intriguingly, a −13910 C>T polymorphism, located upstream from the lactase (LCT) gene was associated with a higher BMI in several European populations as well.[7] This finding suggests a relationship between lactose digestion and BMI and could be in accordance with the high selection of this allele observed in areas with extensive dairy farming. Thus lactase persistence may confer an evolutionary advantage contributing to higher weight.

The rapid development of GWAS contributed to the identification of other important genetic variants. Identification of variants in fat mass and obesity (FTO) gene was the first example of discovery of a new gene associated with corpulence. In children, the most significant variant (rs9939609) was strongly associated with BMI. Children (and adults) carrying two copies (16% of the sample) of this variant allele had ~1.67 more risk to be obese than noncarriers. Metaanalyses of several large GWAS in European populations confirmed the strong association of this variant with BMI and identified 35 additional SNPs in 33 loci robustly associated with BMI.[8,9] However, altogether, the loci identified by GWAS explained only 1.45% of the variance in BMI, suggesting that many additional common genetic variants associated with BMI remain to be discovered.[10] To date, GWAS has identified 135 gene variants including 21 loci associated with only obesity. Interestingly, SNPs in several genes found implicated in syndromic/monogenic obesities (such as *BDNF, NTRK2, LEPR, MC4R, PCSK1, POMC, SH2B1, TUB*) also have been shown to contribute to corpulence in more common forms of obesity. Although some preliminary studies predicted that SNPs could explain around 30% of BMI variance, genetic screening in large populations in the world revealed that currently identified SNPs explain only 3% of BMI variance. More variants or other genetic changes still remain to be discovered in obesity diseases.[3]

As such, epigenetics or copy number variants (CNVs) likely contribute to the variability of obesity phenotype as well. Epigenetics is defined as changes in gene transcription and expression that occur without altering the DNA sequence (such as methylation). Recent studies described associations between different DNA methylation status and variable expression of genes involved in obesity such as POMC or FTO[11] For example, the obesity risk allele of FTO is associated with higher methylation sites within the FTO gene and methylation of other genes.[12] CNVs are chromosomal segments encompassing large replications or deletions in genes. Several CNVs have also been associated with obesity, but differential associations found within the same ethnicity of studied populations suggest epistasis (interaction between nonallelic genes in which one combination of such genes has a dominant effect over other combinations).

SYNDROMIC OBESITIES

Syndromic obesity is defined by severe obesity associated with additional clinical phenotypes (intellectual disability, endocrine and organ-specific developmental abnormalities, dysmorphic features). More than 50 syndromes are now associated with the development of obesity (Table 14.1).

The most frequent forms of syndromic obesity with intellectual disability are PWS and BBS. PWS (1 in 15,000 to 20,000 births and a population prevalence of 1/50,000 people) is characterized by severe neonatal hypotonia, eating disorders evolving in several phases. This consists of failure to thrive with suckling disorders in the first months of life and hyperphagia with major food impulsiveness beginning at 4–8 years of age.[13] Furthermore, PWS is characterized by body composition abnormalities with increased fat mass endocrine anomalies (such as growth hormone [GH] deficiency, hypogonadism), variable intellectual disability or behavioral difficulties, and dysmorphy.[14] The cause of PWS is physical or functional absence of the paternal chromosomal segment 15q11-q13. While the most frequent molecular abnormality is a paternal deletion (60%–65%), the remainder of cases are due to maternal uniparental disomy (33%–35%) and imprinting defects or translocation (<5%). At least five genes, located in the PWS chromosomal region and expressed in the hypothalamus, have been identified, but their functions are incompletely understood. These genes include *MRKN3* (makorin 3), *MAGEL2* (MAGE-like 2), *NDN* (necdin), *NPAP1* (nuclear pore associated protein 1), and the complex *SNURF-SNRPN* (SNRPN upstream reading frame—small nuclear ribonucleoprotein polypeptide N) and several clusters of small nucleolar RNAs that encompass the small nuclear RNA C/D box 116 cluster (SNORD 116).[15] The mechanisms involving these genes at the 15q11-q13 chromosomal segment, which underlie the development of early-onset and severe obesity, remain unresolved. Similarly, recent studies suggest that point mutations in the imprinted MAGEL2 and SNORD116 genes can also contribute to several aspects of the PWS neuroendocrine phenotypes[16–18] with mechanisms yet to be precisely defined.

BBS is a heterogeneous disease characterized by severe early-onset obesity, retinal dystrophy, malformed extremities (syndactyly, polydactyly), kidney diseases, hypogonadism, dysmorphy, and sometimes mental disabilities. At least 19 different genes are implicated in BBS and mapped on various chromosomes, but all are involved in primary cilium function.[19] Thus, BBS is now defined as a ciliopathy (primary cilium dysfunction)[20] as well as Alstrom syndrome characterized by blindness, truncal obesity, type 2 diabetes, cardiomyopathy, and other organ dysfunctions.[21] The precise mechanisms leading to

TABLE 14.1
Main Syndromic Forms of Obesity

Name of Syndrome/ Gene	Clinical Features in Addition to Obesity	Prevalence	Genetic
With Mental Disability			
Prader-Willi	Neonatal hypotonia, hyperphagia, facial dysmorphy, hypogonadism, short stature	1/20000 births	Lack of the paternal segment 15q11-q13 (microdeletion, maternal disomy, imprinting defect, or reciprocal translocation)
Bardet-Biedl	Retinal dystrophy or pigmentary retinopathy, dysmorphic extremities, hypogonadism, kidney dysfunction	1/125000 to 1/175000 births	BBS1 (11q13); BBS2 (16q12.2); BBS3 (*ARL6*, 3q11); BBS4 (15q24.1); BBS5 (2q31.1); BBS6 (*MKKS*, 20p12); BBS7 (4q27); BBS8 (*TTC8*, 14q31); BBS9 (*PTHB1*, 7p14); BBS10 (*C12ORF58*, 12q21.2); BBS 11 (*TRIM32*, 9q33.1); BBS12 (*FLJ35630*, 4q27); BBS13 (*MKS1*, 17q23); BBS14 (*CEP290*, 12q21.3); BBS15 (*WDPCP*, 2p15); BBS16 (*SDCCAG8*, 1q43); BBS17 (*LZTFL1*, 3p21); BBS18 (*BBIP1*, 10q25); BBS19 (*IFT27*, 22q12)
Alström	Retinal dystrophy, neurosensory deafness, type 2 diabetes, dilated cardiomyopathy	Diagnosed in about 950 patients worldwide	Autosomal recessive *ALMS1* gene (chr 2p13-p14)
Cohen	Retinal dystrophy, prominent central incisors, dysmorphic extremities, microcephaly, cyclic neutropenia, joint laxity	Diagnosed in fewer than 1000 patients worldwide	Autosomal recessive *COH1* gene (chr 8q22-q23)
X fragile	Hyperkinetic behavior, macroorchidism, large ears, prominent jaw	1/2500 births	X-linked *FMR1* gene (Xq27.3)
Smith-Magenis	Sleep disorders, craniofacial and skeletal anomalies, behavioral disorders, motor retardation, and language delay	1/15000–25000 births	De novo RAI1
Borjeson-Forssman-Lehmann	Hypotonia, hypogonadism, short stature facial dysmorphy with large ears, epilepsy	Approximately 50 reported patients	X-linked *PHF6* gene (Xq26-q27)
Albright hereditary osteodystrophy	Short stature, skeletal defects, facial dysmorphy, endocrine anomalies	1/1000000 births	*GNAS1* gene (20q13.2)
Carpenter/acrocephalopolysyndactyly type II	Craniofacial malformations, syndactyly, short stature, cardiopathy, hypogenitalism, umbilical hernia	1/1000000 births	Autosomal recessive RAB23
WAGRO	Wilms tumor, aniridia, genitourinary anomalies	1/100000 births	11p13 deletion including PAX6 Possible haploinsufficiency of BDNF (11p14.1)
Kinase suppressor of Ras2 (KSR) variants	Low heartrate, reduced basal metabolic rate, severe insulin resistance	Approximately 65 reported patients	Rare *KSR2* variants (12q24.22-q24.23)

Continued

TABLE 14.1
Main Syndromic Forms of Obesity—cont'd

Name of Syndrome/ Gene	Clinical Features in Addition to Obesity	Prevalence	Genetic
TUB mutation	Night blindness, decreased visual acuity and electrophysiological features of a rod-cone dystrophy	Identified in three affected sibs from a consanguineous Caucasian family	Homozygous *TUB* mutation (11p15.4)
ACP1, TMEM18, MYT1L deletion	Hyperphagia, intellectual deficiency, severe behavioral difficulties	Approximately 13 reported patients	Paternal deletion encompassing the *ACP1, TMEM18, MYT1L* genes (2p25)
Neurotrophic tyrosine kinase receptor type 2 (NTRK2 or TrkB)	Developmental delay, behavioral disturbance, blunted response to pain	Diagnosed in fewer than 10 patients worldwide	De novo heterozygous mutation
16p11.2 deletion syndrome	Developmental delay, autism spectrum disorders, impaired communication, socialization skills	Approximately 3/10000 births	Microdeletion of 16p11.2 encompassing SH2B adaptor protein 1
6q16.1 deletion syndrome			Encompassing *POU3F2*
Single-minded 1 (SIM1)	Inconstantly, neurobehavioral abnormalities (including emotional lability or autism-like behavior)	Diagnosed in fewer than 50 patients worldwide	Translocation between chr 1p22.1 and 6q16.2 in the *SIM1* gene
MAGEL 2	Hypotonia, autism spectrum disorder, poor suck, contracture, dysmorphic features	Diagnosed in fewer than 30 patients worldwide	De novo heterozygous mutation
Without Mental Disability			
Leptin (LEP)	Gonadotropic and thyrotropic insufficiency Alteration in immune function	Diagnosed in fewer than 100 patients worldwide	Homozygous mutation
Leptin receptor (LEPR)	Gonadotropic, thyrotropic and somatotropic insufficiency Alteration in immune function	2%–3% of patients with severe early-onset obesity	Homozygous mutation
Proopiomelanocortin (POMC)	ACTH insufficiency, mild hypothyroidism and ginger hair if the mutation leads to the absence of POMC production	Diagnosed in fewer than 10 patients worldwide	Homozygous or compound heterozygous
Proprotein convertase subtilisin/kexin type 1 (PCSK1)	Adrenal, gonadotropic, somatotropic and thyrotropic insufficiency, postprandial hypoglycemia severe malabsorptive neonatal diarrhea, central diabetes insipidus	Diagnosed in fewer than 20 patients worldwide	Homozygous or compound heterozygous
Melanocortin 4 receptor (MC4R)	Increased lean body mass and bone density, increased linear growth in infancy,	Diagnosed in fewer than 10 patients worldwide	Homozygous mutation

denoted a central origin relating to BBS obesity, which involved alterations in the hypothalamic regulation of food intake. In particular, BBS proteins are required for leptin receptor localization in the hypothalamus.[22] Other hypotheses suggest a peripheral origin involving

is also suggested as a factor involved in this complex disease (reviewed by Refs. 21,23).

Syndromic obesity with endocrine abnormalities without mental disability (<5% of obesities) is mainly due to mutations in human genes encoding LEP, LEPR,

POMC, and PC1[2] (Table 14.1). Patients carrying these mutations show a very quick, early, and severe increase in weight soon after birth, which is illustrated by the weight curve of LEPR-deficient subjects.[24] With a few exception, feeding behavior is typically characterized by severe hyperphagia and ravenous hunger.[25]

Associated with the severe early-onset obesity, hypogonadotropic hypogonadism completes the phenotype of patients carrying mutations in the *LEP* or *LEPR* gene. The absence of pubertal development was observed in some individuals with *LEP* or *LEPR* mutations, while in others there was evidence of spontaneous but delayed pubertal development suggesting a recovery of hormonal functions with time.[26] Insufficient somatotropic secretion and thyrotropic insufficiency are also described in some patients with a *LEPR* mutation.[24] *LEPR* mutations in severely obese subjects are not extremely rare with an estimated prevalence of 2%–3%, which denotes the need to search for these mutations in cases of extreme obesity associated with endocrine abnormalities. Recently, a congenital LEP deficiency with high circulating levels of biologically inactive leptin was described in a young boy presenting with typical clinical phenotype.[27] We recently reported obese patients carrying homozygous *LEPR* mutations display slightly increased circulating leptin.[24] Thus, circulating levels of leptin in accordance with BMI and fat mass do not rule out *LEP* or *LEPR* mutations if other clinical features are present.

Obese children with complete POMC deficiency have ACTH deficiency, mild central hypothyroidism,[2] and sometimes alterations in the somatotropic and gonadotropic axes as well as red hair. The modifications in hair color, adrenal function, and body weight are consistent with the lack of POMC-derived ligands for the melanocortin receptors MC1R, MC2R, and MC4R respectively. Patients carrying a rare mutation in the proprotein convertase subtilisin/kexin type 1 (*PCSK1*) gene leading to proconvertase 1 (PC1) deficiency, an enzyme also involved in the maturation of insulin, display postprandial hypoglycemic malaises, hypogonadotropic hypogonadism, central hypothyroidism, and adrenal insufficiency in addition to severe obesity. Importantly severe and unorthodox diarrhea, secondary to lack in mature GLP-1 (glucagon-like peptide-1), is also described in case of PC1 deficiency,[28,29] as well as persistent polydipsia and polyuria due to central diabetes insipidus.[30]

Other rare obesities, due to mutations in several genes involved in the development of hypothalamus and central nervous system, have also been described in humans, allowing the identification of new pathways underlying the obese phenotype. Deletions of the *SIM1*

(single-minded homolog 1) gene encoding a transcriptional factor involved in the development of the hypothalamic paraventricular nucleus have been identified in subjects with early-onset obesity associated with hyperphagia and food impulsivity and PWS-like features.[31,32] Likewise, mutations in the *NTRK2* (neurotrophic tyrosine kinase receptor type 2) gene were described in subjects with severe early-onset obesity and mental retardation.[2] This gene encodes for BDNF (brain-derived neurotropic factor) and its associated tyrosine kinase receptor (TRKB), which is involved in feeding regulation via a role downstream from MC4R signaling. Other mutations in *NTRK2* were found in patients with early-onset obesity and developmental delay, but their functional consequences and implication in obesity are yet to demonstrate.[2]

Obesity related to **MC4R mutations** are between the exceptional forms of monogenic obesity and common polygenic obesity and represent approximately 2%–3% of childhood and adult obesity.[33] To date, hundreds of mutations have been identified and are associated with many functional alterations. They are mainly characterized by an autosomal dominant transmission with incomplete penetrance and a lack of additional obvious phenotypes. The severity of the obese phenotype is variable (moderate to severe obesity), denoting the role of environment and other potential genetic factors. Subjects carrying *MC4R* mutations are usually heterozygous with homozygous or compound heterozygous carriers of *MC4R* mutations being very rare and their phenotype more severe.[2,34,35] In addition to obesity, children carrying *MC4R* mutations have a marked hyperphagia that decreases with age.

Genetic Diagnosis

If a rare genetic form of obesity is suspected, genetic diagnosis must be discussed and confided to specialists in the clinical reference centers. In cases of obesity associated with mental disability and/or behavioral difficulties, genetic tests should include at least high-resolution karyotype, investigation of DNA methylation on chromosome 15, fragile X search, and study by CGH (comparative genomic hybridization) array. The specific research for other monogenic anomalies (*SIM1*, *MAGEL2*, *NTRK2* etc.) must also be considered depending on the clinical phenotype. Furthermore, in patients with obesity and retinal dystrophy, ciliopathy should be searched, in particular BBS.

In cases of severe early-onset obesity associated with endocrine irregularities, suggesting a monogenic obesity, direct sequencing of the candidate gene (*LEP*, *LEPR*, *POMC*, *PCSK1*, *MC4R*) is necessary to confirm the diagnosis. This method detects homozygous or compound heterozygous mutations responsible for interruptions of the leptin-melanocortin axis. Family members also must be tested for segregation analysis and to evaluate the risk of recurrence.

Finally, with early-onset, severe, and isolated obesity, *MC4R* mutations can be detected by direct sequencing of the *MC4R* gene.

Treatment in Genetic Obesity

It is important to diagnose genetic forms of obesity because specific management, provided by specialized and multidisciplinary teams, is needed as soon as possible in early infancy. Indeed, early intervention and global and multidisciplinary management (diet and physical activity, psychomotricity, adapted physical activities, hormone substitution, etc.) have a pivotal role in the care and outcome of patients with genetic obesity. For example, in PWS, GH therapy with doses typically used for childhood growth, started before 1 year of age, can greatly improve growth, body composition, muscle thickness, physical strength and agility, motor performance, fat utilization, and lipid metabolism in children and in adults with PWS (reviewed by Ref. 36). GH treatment in childhood and adolescence also lead to better body composition and metabolic status during adulthood.[37]

The use of bariatric surgery and its potential efficacy may be viewed a viable treatment in patients with genetic obesity. Today, bariatric surgery, a comprehensive term comprising several operative methods (laparoscopic gastric bypass, gastric banding, or sleeve gastrectomy), is the only long-term efficient treatment for severe obesity (as reviewed in Ref. 38). However, bariatric surgery should be approached with caution for patients with genetic obesity because of data on this being limited and controversial. As the author of a recent review, we consider that bariatric surgery performed on individuals with mental disability should be imperatively accompanied with intensive multidisciplinary approaches and integrated social support system during pre- and postoperative periods.[39]

In PWS, the indication of bariatric surgery is highly discussed due to early-onset morbid obesity. A retrospective review examined 60 cases of PWS patients who underwent bariatric surgery (mean age at the time of bariatric procedure 19.7 ± 6.4 years). The findings of this review were that various bariatric procedures have been used with poor results in PWS patients compared with individuals with common obesity. In addition to poor results on weight outcomes, a variety of postoperative issues were reported in PWS patients, including death, pulmonary embolus, postoperative wound infection,

and gastric perforation.[40] In a recent publication examining 24 adolescents with PWS (mean age 10.7 years), bariatric surgery was reported to be beneficial. After laparoscopic sleeve gastrectomy, BMI loss was 14.7% (n = 22 patients) and 10.7% (n = 7 patients), at the first and fifth annual visits, respectively. 95% of comorbidities (obstructive sleep apnea, dyslipidemia, hypertension, type 2 diabetes) were in remission or improved as well, and no postoperative complications occurred.[41] One can ask whether these results can be extrapolated to an adult population. Finally, in a recent review, 48 surgical interventions in PWS patients were examined and the findings showed that the mean excess weight loss is highly inconsistent between individuals (from 12% to 86%).[39] Furthermore, only one study included a postoperative follow-up period longer than 3 years. In conclusion, indication of this therapeutic option in PWS needs to be discussed in depth in specialist centers for PWS and bariatric surgery. Surgery should not replace the multidisciplinary medical management (i.e., early diagnosis and multidisciplinary care with GH treatment, reduced-energy diets with restricted access to food, and regular physical activity) because this has proven effectiveness and safety in PWS patients. In BBS, the indication of bariatric surgery has also been discussed. In one case, a morbidly obese 16-year-old patient with BBS underwent a laparoscopic Roux-en-Y gastric bypass. The postoperative period was uneventful, and BMI decreased from 52.28 to 34.85 kg/m^2 42 months after surgery with significant improvements in his hypertension and mobility.[42] In another study, a 33-year-old morbidly obese BBS woman underwent a sleeve gastrectomy without significant postoperative complications. In this example, weight loss was 23.9% at 12 months.[43] In contrast, a gastric banding performed in a 35-year-old morbidly obese man with BBS resulted in little weight loss (9%) without an effect on type 2 diabetes.[43] Thus, increased and longer follow-up is required to evaluate long-term safety and efficacy of bariatric surgery in patients with BBS.

In the case of two LEPR-deficient patients, vertical gastroplasty seems to be beneficial, inducing a 40-kg weight loss (–20% of the initial weight) over 8 years of regular follow-up in the first 16-year-old patient to receive this treatment.[44] Additionally, in a second 18-year-old patient, significant initial weight loss (–44% of weight loss after 9 months) was observed.[24] However, it is important to mention that this second patient remained severely obese. In contrast to these two examples, relative failure of bariatric surgery efficacy was illustrated in a 26-year-old LEPR-deficient morbidly obese woman with rapid weight regain 1 year after bypass. However, this patient with low socioeconomic status was noncompliant to the recommendations provided in this type of surgery and had very irregular medical follow-up.[44] In another 36-year-old LEPR-deficient patient, gastric bypass did not induce significant weight loss long term (−7% at 5 years after surgery).[24] Laparoscopic adjustable gastric banding in one 17-year-old teenager with homozygous *MC4R* mutation resulted in the absence of long-term weight loss (12 months postoperatively).[45]

Overall, because of the limited number of cases, the long-term efficacy and safety of bariatric surgery in genetic forms of obesity need further evaluation. A multidisciplinary team approach should always be undertaken to discuss the opportunity of bariatric surgery in this context. Additionally, severe eating disorders are a common argument against performing bariatric surgery in obese patients. To this end, the position of the French Reference Center of Prader-Willi Syndrome is cautious and does not recommend the use of surgery in cases of syndromic obesity with major hyperphagia.

In addition to surgical and dietary intervention, current active research on several molecules (oxytocin, topiramate, desacylated ghrelin) is very promising for the future in PWS. Individuals with PWS have a significant reduction in the number of oxytocin-producing neurons in the hypothalamic paraventricular nucleus, and a number of the PWS features, such as hyperphagia, obesity, and behavioral anomalies, may be due to consequent hypothalamic hyposecretion of oxytocin. Preliminary studies in mice and humans have investigated the capacity of exogenous oxytocin to improve physical, behavioral, and cognitive aspects of PWS and food-related behavior, but future research is necessary to better understand the exact effects of oxytocin on syndrome-specific behaviors in patients with PWS.[46–48]

In monogenic obesity due to the leptin/melanocortin pathway alteration, therapeutic development now provides hope for the patients. Subcutaneous injection of leptin in children and adults with *LEP* mutations results in weight loss, mainly due to decreased fat mass, with a major effect on reducing food intake.[27,34] Leptin treatment also induces features of puberty, even in adults.[49] Novel pharmacologic MC4R agonists have been tested in vitro as well and can restore normal activity in mutated MC4R receptor.[50] In vivo, treatment with a highly selective novel MC4R agonist (RM-493) in an obese animal model resulted in decreased food intake, increased total energy expenditure, weight loss, and weight-independent improvement of insulin sensitivity after 8 weeks of treatment. Importantly, no side effect on blood pressure or heart rate, was observed

in these studies.[51,52] In humans, RM-493 was able to increase resting energy expenditure without cardiovascular side effects in obese subjects as well.[53] In a recent study, RM-493 treatment led to weight loss in two homozygous POMC deficiency obesity patients with early-onset extreme obesity.[54] RM-493 also demonstrated an impact on appetite and metabolism in Magel2-null mice.[55] Further studies are now needed to establish whether RM-493 could be efficacious in PWS and other rare monogenic forms of obesity exhibiting impaired function of POMC neurons. Finally, knowing that RM-493 stimulates the MC1R, the long-term side effects concerning chronic melanocyte stimulation should be closely monitored.

CONCLUSION AND PERSPECTIVES

Genetic forms of obesity are important to diagnose, because a specific management exists depending on multidisciplinary teams, to be set up as soon as possible. Innovative treatments have recently emerged, particularly for PWS and leptin/melanocortin pathway mutations, which could change the prognosis for these rare severe forms of obesity. Yet, to date, causal therapy is not available for most forms of obesity. Moreover, progress in understanding the underlying mechanisms of genetic obesity by using whole-exome sequencing, in particular, will likely help physicians to identify new molecular abnormalities in patients with severe early-onset obesity in the near future. As such, this will aid in better understanding the pathophysiology of the more common forms of obesity and ultimately improving patient care management.

REFERENCES

1. De Onis M, Blossner M, Borghi E. Global prevalence and trends of overweight and obesity among preschool children. *Am J Clin Nutr.* 2010;92(5):1257–1264. http://dx.doi.org/10.3945/ajcn.2010.29786.
2. Huvenne H, Dubern B, Clément K, Poitou C. Rare genetic forms of obesity: clinical approach and current treatments in 2016. *Obes Facts.* 2016;9(3). http://dx.doi.org/10.1159/000445061.
3. Pigeyre M, Yazdi FT, Kaur Y, Meyre D. Recent progress in genetics, epigenetics and metagenomics unveils the pathophysiology of human obesity. *Clin Sci.* 2016;130(12):943–986. http://dx.doi.org/10.1042/CS20160136.
4. Wang R, Zhou D, Xi B, et al. ENPP1/PC-1 gene K121Q polymorphism is associated with obesity in European adult populations: evidence from a meta-analysis involving 24,324 subjects. *Biomed Environ Sci.* 2011;24(2):200–206. http://dx.doi.org/10.3967/0895-3988.2011.02.015.

5. Benzinou M, Creemers JWM, Choquet H, et al. Common nonsynonymous variants in PCSK1 confer risk of obesity. *Nat Genet.* 2008;40(8):943–945. http://dx.doi.org/10.1038/ng.177.

6. Gunstad J, Schofield P, Paul RH, et al. BDNF Val66Met polymorphism is associated with body mass index in healthy adults. *Neuropsychobiology.* 2006;53(3):153–156. http://dx.doi.org/10.1159/000093341.

7. Corella D, Arregui M, Coltell O, et al. Association of the LCT-13910C>T polymorphism with obesity and its modulation by dairy products in a Mediterranean population. *Obesity (Silver Spring).* 2011;19(8):1707–1714. http://dx.doi.org/10.1038/oby.2010.320.

8. Frayling TM, Timpson NJ, Weedon MN, et al. A common variant in the FTO gene is associated with body mass index and predisposes to childhood and adult obesity. *Science.* 2007;316(5826):889–894. http://dx.doi.org/10.1126/science.1141634.

9. Hinney A, Nguyen TT, Scherag A, et al. Genome wide association (GWA) study for early onset extreme obesity supports the role of fat mass and obesity associated gene (FTO) variants. Kronenberg F, ed. *PLoS One.* 2007;2(12):e1361. http://dx.doi.org/10.1371/journal.pone.0001361.

10. Speliotes EK, Willer CJ, Berndt SI, et al. Association analyses of 249,796 individuals reveal 18 new loci associated with body mass index. *Nat Genet.* 2010;42(11):937–948. http://dx.doi.org/10.1038/ng.686.

11. Yeo GSH. Genetics of obesity: can an old dog teach us new tricks? *Diabetologia.* December 2016. http://dx.doi.org/10.1007/s00125-016-4187-x.

12. Bell CG, Finer S, Lindgren CM, et al. Integrated genetic and epigenetic analysis identifies haplotype-specific methylation in the FTO type 2 diabetes and obesity susceptibility locus. Sorensen TIA, ed. *PLoS One.* 2010;(11):e14040. http://dx.doi.org/10.1371/journal.pone.0014040.

13. Miller JL, Lynn CH, Driscoll DC, et al. Nutritional phases in Prader–Willi syndrome. *Am J Med Genet A.* 2011;155(5):1040–1049. http://dx.doi.org/10.1002/ajmg.a.33951.

14. Driscoll DJ, Miller JL, Schwartz S, Cassidy SB. Prader-Willi syndrome. In: Pagon RA, Adam MP, Ardinger HH, et al., eds. *GeneReviews(®).* Seattle, WA: University of Washington; 1993. http://www.ncbi.nlm.nih.gov/books/NBK1330/. Accessed March 9, 2017.

15. Cheon CK. Genetics of Prader-Willi syndrome and Prader-Willi-like syndrome. *Ann Pediatr Endocrinol Metab.* 2016;21(3):126–135. http://dx.doi.org/10.6065/apem.2016.21.3.126.

16. Schaaf CP, Gonzalez-Garay ML, Xia F, et al. Truncating mutations of MAGEL2 cause Prader-Willi phenotypes and autism. *Nat Genet.* 2013;45(11):1405–1408. http://dx.doi.org/10.1038/ng.2776.

17. Bieth E, Eddiry S, Gaston V, et al. Highly restricted deletion of the SNORD116 region is implicated in Prader–Willi syndrome. *Eur J Hum Genet.* 2015;23(2):252–255. http://dx.doi.org/10.1038/ejhg.2014.103.

18. Burnett LC, LeDuc CA, Sulsona CR, et al. Deficiency in prohormone convertase PC1 impairs prohormone processing in Prader-Willi syndrome. *J Clin Invest.* 2017;127(1):293–305. http://dx.doi.org/10.1172/JCI88648.

19. Khan SA, Muhammad N, Khan MA, Kamal A, Rehman ZU, Khan S. Genetics of human Bardet–Biedl syndrome, an updates. *Clin Genet.* 2016;90(1):3–15. http://dx.doi.org/10.1111/cge.12737.

20. Zaghloul NA, Katsanis N. Mechanistic insights into Bardet-Biedl syndrome, a model ciliopathy. *J Clin Invest.* 2009;119(3):428–437. http://dx.doi.org/10.1172/JCI37041.

21. Mariman ECM, Vink RG, Roumans NJT, et al. The cilium: a cellular antenna with an influence on obesity risk. *Br J Nutr.* 2016;116(4):576–592. http://dx.doi.org/10.1017/S0007114516002282.

22. M'hamdi O, Ouertani I, Chaabouni-Bouhamed H. Update on the genetics of Bardet-Biedl syndrome. *Mol Syndromol.* 2014;5(2):51–56. http://dx.doi.org/10.1159/000357054.

23. Chennen K, Scerbo MJ, Dollfus H, Poch O, Marion V. Syndrome de Bardet-Biedl : cils et obésité - De la génétique aux approches intégratives. *Médecine/Sciences.* 2014;30(11):1034–1039. http://dx.doi.org/10.1051/medsci/20143011018.

24. Huvenne H, Le Beyec J, Pépin D, et al. Seven novel deleterious LEPR mutations found in early-onset obesity: a Δexon6-8 shared by subjects from Reunion Island, France, suggests a founder effect. *J Clin Endocrinol Metab.* 2015;100(5). http://dx.doi.org/10.1210/jc.2015-1036.

25. Fischer-Posovszky P, von Schnurbein J, Moepps B, et al. A new missense mutation in the leptin gene causes mild obesity and hypogonadism without affecting T cell responsiveness. *J Clin Endocrinol Metab.* 2010;95(6):2836–2840. http://dx.doi.org/10.1210/jc.2009-2466.

26. Nizard J, Dommergues M, Dommergue M, Clément K. Pregnancy in a woman with a leptin-receptor mutation. *N Engl J Med.* 2012;366(11):1064–1065. http://dx.doi.org/10.1056/NEJMc1200116.

27. Wabitsch M, Funcke J-B, Lennerz B, et al. Biologically inactive leptin and early-onset extreme obesity. *N Engl J Med.* 2015;372(1):48–54. http://dx.doi.org/10.1056/NEJMoa1406653.

28. Jackson RS, Creemers JW, Ohagi S, et al. Obesity and impaired prohormone processing associated with mutations in the human prohormone convertase 1 gene. *Nat Genet.* 1997;16(3):303–306. http://dx.doi.org/10.1038/ng0797-303.

29. Martín MG, Lindberg I, Solorzano-Vargas RS, et al. Congenital proprotein convertase 1/3 deficiency causes malabsorptive diarrhea and other endocrinopathies in a pediatric cohort. *Gastroenterology.* 2013;145(1):138–148. http://dx.doi.org/10.1053/j.gastro.2013.03.048.

30. Frank GR, Fox J, Candela N, et al. Severe obesity and diabetes insipidus in a patient with PCSK1 deficiency. *Mol Genet Metab.* 2013;110(1–2):191–194. http://dx.doi.org/10.1016/j.ymgme.2013.04.005.

31. Michaud JL, Boucher F, Melnyk A, et al. Sim1 haploinsufficiency causes hyperphagia, obesity and reduction of the paraventricular nucleus of the hypothalamus. *Hum Mol Genet.* 2001;10(14):1465–1473.

32. Izumi K, Housam R, Kapadia C, et al. Endocrine phenotype of 6q16.1-q21 deletion involving SIM1 and Prader-Willi syndrome-like features. *Am J Med Genet A*. 2013;161A(12):3137–3143. http://dx.doi.org/10.1002/ajmg.a.36149.

33. Hinney A, Volckmar A-L, Knoll N. Melanocortin-4 receptor in energy homeostasis and obesity pathogenesis. In: *Progress in Molecular Biology and Translational Science*. Vol. 114. 2013:147–191. http://dx.doi.org/10.1016/B978-0-12-386933-3.00005-4.

34. Farooqi IS, Keogh JM, Yeo GSH, Lank EJ, Cheetham T, O'Rahilly S. Clinical spectrum of obesity and mutations in the melanocortin 4 receptor gene. *N Engl J Med*. 2003;348(12):1085–1095. http://dx.doi.org/10.1056/NEJMoa022050.

35. Dubern B, Bisbis S, Talbaoui H, et al. Homozygous null mutation of the melanocortin-4 receptor and severe early-onset obesity. *J Pediatr*. 2007;150(6). http://dx.doi.org/10.1016/j.jpeds.2007.01.041.

36. Grugni G, Marzullo P. Diagnosis and treatment of GH deficiency in Prader–Willi syndrome. *Best Pract Res Clin Endocrinol Metab*. 2016;30(6):785–794. http://dx.doi.org/10.1016/j.beem.2016.11.003.

37. Coupaye M, Lorenzini F, Lloret-Linares C, et al. Growth hormone therapy for children and adolescents with Prader-Willi syndrome is associated with improved body composition and metabolic status in adulthood. *J Clin Endocrinol Metab*. 2013;98(2):E328–E335. http://dx.doi.org/10.1210/jc.2012-2881.

38. Nguyen NT, Varela JE. Bariatric surgery for obesity and metabolic disorders: state of the art. *Nat Rev Gastroenterol Hepatol*. 2017;14(3):160–169. http://dx.doi.org/10.1038/nrgastro.2016.170.

39. Gibbons E, Casey AF, Brewster KZ. Bariatric surgery and intellectual disability: furthering evidence-based practice. *Disabil Health J*. 2017;10(1):3–10. http://dx.doi.org/10.1016/j.dhjo.2016.09.005.

40. Scheimann AO, Butler MG, Gourash L, Cuffari C, Klish W. Critical analysis of bariatric procedures in Prader-Willi syndrome. *J Pediatr Gastroenterol Nutr*. 2008;46(1):80–83. http://dx.doi.org/10.1097/01.mpg.0000304458.30294.31.

41. Alqahtani AR, Elahmedi MO, Qahtani ARA, Lee J, Butler MG. Laparoscopic sleeve gastrectomy in children and adolescents with Prader-Willi syndrome: a matched-control study. *Surg Obes Relat Dis*. 2016;12(1):100–110. http://dx.doi.org/10.1016/j.soard.2015.07.014.

42. Daskalakis M, Till H, Kiess W, Weiner RA. Roux-en-Y gastric bypass in an adolescent patient with Bardet–Biedl syndrome, a monogenic obesity disorder. *Obes Surg*. 2010;20(1):121–125. http://dx.doi.org/10.1007/s11695-009-9915-6.

43. Mujahid S, Huda MSB, Beales P, Carroll PV, McGowan BM. Adjustable gastric banding and sleeve gastrectomy in Bardet-Biedl syndrome. *Obes Surg*. 2014;24(10):1746–1748. http://dx.doi.org/10.1007/s11695-014-1379-7.

44. Le Beyec J, Cugnet-Anceau C, Pépin D, et al. Homozygous leptin receptor mutation due to uniparental disomy of chromosome 1: response to bariatric surgery. *J Clin Endocrinol Metab*. 2013;98(2):E397–E402. http://dx.doi.org/10.1210/jc.2012-2779.

45. Aslan IR, Ranadive SA, Ersoy BA, Rogers SJ, Lustig RH, Vaisse C. Bariatric surgery in a patient with complete MC4R deficiency. *Int J Obes*. 2011;35(3):457–461. http://dx.doi.org/10.1038/ijo.2010.168.

46. Einfeld SL, Smith E, McGregor IS, et al. A double-blind randomized controlled trial of oxytocin nasal spray in Prader Willi syndrome. *Am J Med Genet A*. 2014;164(9):2232–2239. http://dx.doi.org/10.1002/ajmg.a.36653.

47. Meziane H, Schaller F, Bauer S, et al. An early postnatal oxytocin treatment prevents social and learning deficits in adult mice deficient for Magel2, a gene involved in Prader-Willi syndrome and autism. *Biol Psychiatry*. 2015;78(2):85–94. http://dx.doi.org/10.1016/j.biopsych.2014.11.010.

48. Kuppens RJ, Bakker NE, Siemensma EPC, et al. Beneficial effects of GH in young adults with Prader-Willi syndrome: a 2-year crossover trial. *J Clin Endocrinol Metab*. 2016;101(11):4110–4116. http://dx.doi.org/10.1210/jc.2016-2594.

49. Licinio J, Caglayan S, Ozata M, et al. Phenotypic effects of leptin replacement on morbid obesity, diabetes mellitus, hypogonadism, and behavior in leptin-deficient adults. *Proc Natl Acad Sci USA*. 2004;101(13):4531–4536. http://dx.doi.org/10.1073/pnas.0308767101.

50. Fani L, Bak S, Delhanty P, van Rossum EFC, van den Akker ELT. The melanocortin-4 receptor as target for obesity treatment: a systematic review of emerging pharmacological therapeutic options. *Int J Obes*. 2014;38(2):163–169. http://dx.doi.org/10.1038/ijo.2013.80.

51. Kumar KG, Sutton GM, Dong JZ, et al. Analysis of the therapeutic functions of novel melanocortin receptor agonists in MC3R- and MC4R-deficient C57BL/6J mice. *Peptides*. 2009;30(10):1892–1900. http://dx.doi.org/10.1016/j.peptides.2009.07.012.

52. Kievit P, Halem H, Marks DL, et al. Chronic treatment with a melanocortin-4 receptor agonist causes weight loss, reduces insulin resistance, and improves cardiovascular function in diet-induced obese rhesus macaques. *Diabetes*. 2013;62(2):490–497. http://dx.doi.org/10.2337/db12-0598.

53. Chen KY, Muniyappa R, Abel BS, et al. RM-493, a melanocortin-4 receptor (MC4R) agonist, increases resting energy expenditure in obese individuals. *J Clin Endocrinol Metab*. 2015;100(4):1639–1645. http://dx.doi.org/10.1210/jc.2014-4024.

54. Kühnen P, Clément K, Wiegand S, et al. Proopiomelanocortin deficiency treated with a melanocortin-4 receptor agonist. *N Engl J Med*. 2016;375(3):240–246. http://dx.doi.org/10.1056/NEJMoa1512693.

55. Bischof JM, Van Der Ploeg LHT, Colmers WF, Wevrick R. Magel2-null mice are hyper-responsive to setmelanotide, a melanocortin 4 receptor agonist. *Br J Pharmacol*. 2016;173(17):2614–2621. http://dx.doi.org/10.1111/bph.13540.

CHAPTER 15

Childhood Obesity

CRISTINA G. MATEI, MD, MSc • PHILIPPE BAREILLE, MD

INTRODUCTION

In the last 40 years the prevalence of obesity in children and adolescents has increased worldwide in both developed and developing countries and has become a major global public health issue. The obesity epidemic is well established in many different epidemiologic studies irrespective of the definitions used to define obesity.[1] It is not unusual now to see adolescents with complications such as type 2 diabetes, which is a disease considered extremely rare in this age group in the past. Childhood obesity is not only associated with a higher risk of morbidity later in adulthood, but it also increases the risk of weight-related medical complications in childhood. Obesity poses perhaps a greater challenge in children than in adults for various reasons: it involves an additional layer of complexity, because often parents underestimate their child's body weight, children fall more easily victim to targeted marketing from the food industry, and the appropriate diet in a growing child is not always easy to define. Long-term consequences may be more serious given the young age of the subject, and pharmacologic treatments are usually not recommended in children. It is not easy to distinguish between those most likely to remain obese into adulthood and those unlikely to do so and less at risk of complications. Ideally, obesity should be prevented early because it is very difficult to treat once established. Tackling obesity effectively does not involve only the individual but also the family, school, society in general, and a multitude of other factors sometimes difficult to control or change, such as the environment.

DEFINING OVERWEIGHT AND OBESITY IN CHILDREN

Obesity can simply be defined as excess of body fat, often associated with health risks, the most serious being cardiovascular diseases and type 2 diabetes.[2] In practice, overweight and obesity in children are assessed by measuring the body mass index (BMI) and then plotting it on appropriate age- and sex-specific growth charts.[3] BMI is obtained by dividing weight (in kilograms) by height squared (square meters). There are a number of BMI reference charts in use. In the United Kingdom, in clinical settings, the National Institute for Health and Care Excellence (NICE) recommends the UK 1990 growth charts, whereby the cutoffs are 91st centile for overweight and 98th centile for obesity (Fig. 15.1A).

In the United States, the Centers for Disease Control (CDC) defines overweight as BMI 85th to 95th percentile and obesity as greater than 95th percentile (Fig. 15.1B), and the World Health Organization (WHO) defines overweight as 85th to 97th centile and obesity as greater or equal to 97th percentile. There is no agreed definition for severe and very severe obesity, but it is suggested that severe obesity is defined as BMI>99.6th centile (>2.5 standard deviation [SD] above the mean) and extreme obesity is defined as a BMI>3.5 SD.[4,5]

ETIOLOGY OF OBESITY

Childhood obesity is a complex condition that involves the interplay of genetics and the environment (diet, physical activity, socioeconomic factors). Less than 10% of cases have an identified cause, with a fraction of those having an effective cure (e.g., hypothyroidism).

Hypothalamus

The hypothalamus plays a central role for regulating energy expenditure and satiety (see Fig. 15.2).[6] Any insult to the hypothalamus results in disturbance of energy homeostasis and leads to being overweight and obesity. The hypothalamus can be affected by a physical injury (tumor, inflammation, radiotherapy, trauma, surgery) or by functional disruption. The latter includes genetic disorders, often monogenic or part of complex syndromes. Most of the identified monogenic or syndromic forms of obesity interfere with hypothalamic function. It can also be caused by a variety of drugs. Hypothalamic obesity should be suspected when (1) the weight gain is rapid and massive, (2) there is excessive hyperphagia, (3) it occurs in infants or very young children, (4) it is at odds with parent's weight, or (5) it is associated with other signs such as developmental delay, dysmorphic features, or hormonal disorders.

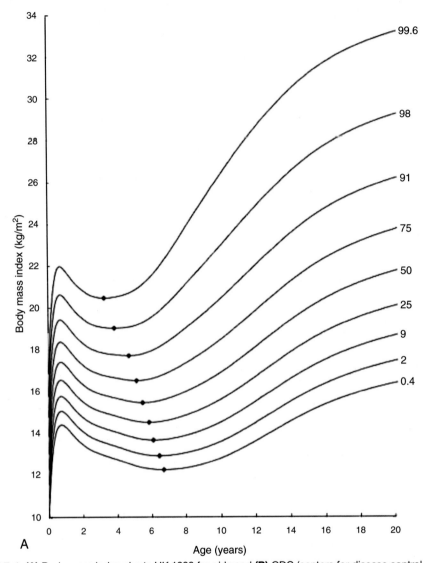

FIG. 15.1 **(A)** Body mass index charts UK 1990 for girls and **(B)** CDC (centers for disease control and prevention) girls. (From Royal College of Paediatrics and Child Health Copyright (c) 2009 and Kuczmarski RJ, Ogden CL, Guo SS, et al. 2000 CDC growth charts for the United States: Methods and development. National Center for Health Statistics. *Vital Health Stat 11.* 2002 (246).)

Intrauterine Environment

Fetal and postnatal environment can significantly influence the development of childhood obesity and its associated risks. During pregnancy, excessive weight gain and gestational diabetes can influence fetal growth and metabolism, leading to high adiposity in the offspring. Delivery by cesarean may also be associated with an increased risk of obesity. A prospective Dutch study in 2641 children among whom 236 were born

by cesarean delivery found a 1.52 times higher risk of being overweight throughout childhood [1.52 (95% [confidence interval] CI 1.18, 1.96)].[7] This study confirmed other published data,[8] although the magnitude of effect is variable and controversial.[9] Short sleep duration in infancy has also been suspected of being associated with increased risk of obesity later in life.[10]

In a pilot study, there was an attempt to prevent obesity by prolongation of sleep duration combined

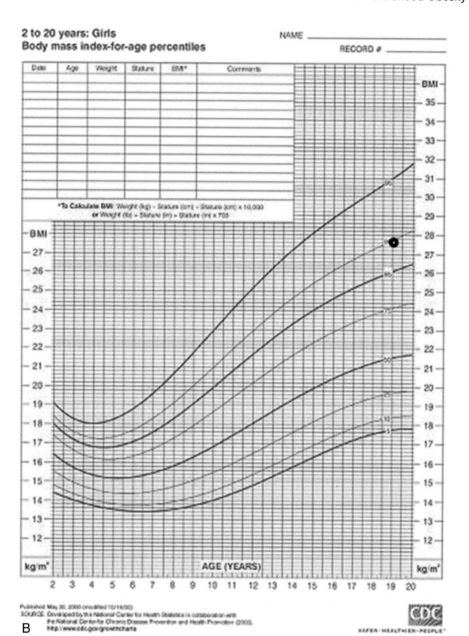

FIG. 15.1, cont'd

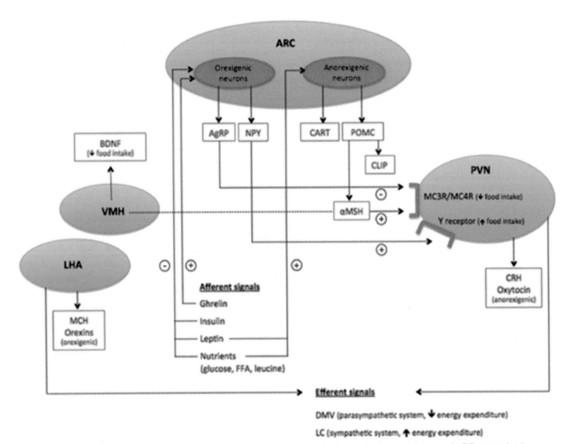

FIG. 15.2 Simplified scheme of regulation of energy homeostasis by the hypothalamus. *AgRP*, agouti-related peptide; *ARC*, arcuate nucleus; *BDNF*, brain-derived neurotrophic factor; *CART*, cocaine-amphetamine-related transcript; *CLIP*, corticotropin-like-intermediate lobe peptide; *CRH*, corticotropin releasing hormone; *DVM*, dorsal motor nucleus of the vagus; *FFA*, free fatty acid; *LC*, locus coeruleus; *LHA*, lateral hypothalamic area; *MCH*, melanin concentrating hormone; *NPY*, neuropeptide Y; *POMC*, proopiomelanocortin; *PVN*, paraventricular nucleus; *VMH*, ventromedial hypothalamus; *α-MSH*, alpha-melatonin stimulating hormone. (From Haliloglu B, Bereket A. Hypothalamic obesity in children: pathophysiology to clinical management. *J Pediatr Endocrinol Metab*. 2015;28(5–6):503–513. http://dx.doi.org/10.1515/jpem-2014-0512, with permission.)

with a change in feeding frequency in infancy. The results of this pilot study showed some evidence for effects of multiple behavioral intervention components (sleep, feeding frequency, and introduction of solids) delivered during the first year after birth on weight status at 1 year.[11] However, this pilot study was a short-term study in first-time mothers who intended to breastfeed. A longitudinal study over 13 years (895 children) did not confirm these findings and found that this association depends on the definition of sleep disturbance.[12] Maternal smoking has also been suspected as an independent risk factor affecting appetite regulation in the developing brain.[13] It has also been demonstrated that exclusive breastfeeding

for the first 4–6 months of life has a protective effect against childhood obesity.[14]

Endocrine Causes

A basic hormonal screening should exclude hypothyroidism, pseudohypoparathyroidism, Cushing's syndrome, and growth hormone (GH) deficiency because these endocrine disorders are commonly associated with being overweight/obese and slowed growth. However, one should be aware that a hormonal disorder such as GH deficiency or hypothyroidism when present may not be the only reason for the excessive weight gain and is often the consequence of a pituitary hypothalamic disorder. The hormone leptin produced at the

TABLE 15.1 Causes of Hypothalamic Obesity			
Physical Causes	**Genetic Causes (Monogenic)**	**Syndromes**	**Drug Induced**

Tumors: e.g., craniopharyngioma glioma/hamartoma/meningioma/histiocytosis Inflammatory: e.g., sarcoidosis, TB, encephalitis Trauma: e.g., radiotherapy, neurosurgery	e.g.,
	• Leptin promoter
	• Leptin receptor
	• Melanocortin 4 receptor(MC4R)
	  • SIM-1
	• Proopiomelanocortin (POMC)
	  • SH2B1
	• Brain-derived neurotrophic factor (BDNF)
		• *Prader-Willi syndrome* (loss of function of specific genes on chromosome 15)
		• ROHHAD (rapid-onset obesity with hypothalamic dysfunction, hypoventilation, and autonomic dysregulation)
		• Bardet-Biedl syndrome
			• Antipsychotics
			• Antidepressants

adipocyte level induces satiety at the hypothalamus level and is increased in obesity. As with the mechanism of insulin resistance (IR), leptin resistance occurs with increased adiposity, leading to reduced satiety and further weight gain (Table 15.1).[3]

Simple Exogenous Obesity

While genetic and in utero environment have an important role to play, for obesity to develop, there has to be an energy imbalance between energy intake and energy expenditure. This becomes more important as the child gets older.[2]

Risk factors for increased energy intake include high calorie–low nutrition processed foods, eating rapidly, eating alone (absence of family at meal times), sugar-sweetened drinks, reduced intake of fruit and vegetables, not eating breakfast, and large portion size.

Watching TV and playing video games are associated with sedentary behavior and obesity in childhood.

Family socioeconomic status, parental weight, education, nutritional knowledge, and modeling, as well as community factors such as school activity programs and recreational facilities, all contribute to forming personal behaviors and lifestyle that will reduce future risks of developing obesity.

Reduced sleep in older children (9–12 years)[15] and chronic stress, with adverse events described in childhood,[16] are also linked with a higher risk of developing obesity.

Key Messages

• The overwhelming majority of common obesity is primarily caused by excessive food intake and reduced physical activity as reflected in the increase in prevalence over the past decades. Some genetic predisposition (often multigenic) can make some individuals more prone to excessive weight gain than others.

• Associated hormonal disturbances, developmental delay, excessive satiety, massive obesity, or very rapid weight gain should point to the suspicion of a hypothalamic disorder and/or monogenic obesity.

HOW EARLY COULD OBESITY BE PREVENTED?

Obesity in childhood is a health hazard associated notably with increased cardiovascular risk (CR). Common obesity-related morbidities in Children are summarized in Table 15.2. Impaired glucose tolerance is highly prevalent in obese children and adolescents. In a US study conducted in 55 children (4–10 years) and 112 adolescents (11–18 years) impaired glucose tolerance after oral glucose tolerance test (OGTT) was detected in 25% of the obese children and 21% of obese adolescents. Type 2 diabetes was detected in 4% of the adolescents.[17] Other complications seen in adults are also common such as dyslipidemia, hypertension, fatty liver disease, obstructive sleep apnea, or orthopedic problems. Type 2 diabetes, which is called "adult-onset diabetes," has now become far more common in the pediatric population with a significant increase in referrals of newly diagnosed type 2 diabetes (e.g., from 2% to 33% in some areas).[18] Metabolic syndrome, associated with IR is also increasingly present in pediatric population.

Although there is a lot of evidence to suggest that childhood obesity will continue into adulthood, there is a proportion of obese children who will no longer be obese as adults; it seems that obese children who became nonobese as adults do not increase their risk of cardiovascular diseases in adulthood.[19]

A comprehensive review and metaanalysis was performed to investigate what was the proportion of obese children and adolescents who became obese adults.[20] The authors found that obese children and adolescents

TABLE 15.2
Common Obesity-Related Morbidities in Children

Cardiovascular	Endocrine	Pulmonary	Gastrointestinal	Orthopedic	Psychosocial
• Hypertension • Dyslipidemia • Atherosclerosis	• Insulin resistance • Early puberty • PCOS	Obstructive sleep apnea	• Fatty liver disease • GE reflux • Cholelithiasis • Vitamin D deficiency • Iron deficiency	• Slipped femoral epiphysis • Blount's disease	• Quality of life • Bullying • Anxiety • Eating disorders

PCOS, polycystic ovarian syndrome.

were five times more likely to become obese as adults than those who were not obese. A total of 65% of obese or overweight adolescents were obese or overweight at a younger age and 37% were already obese in earlier childhood. A majority (66%) of obese or overweight adolescents remain obese in early adulthood; however, childhood obesity does not appear to persist so strongly in adolescence as just over half (55%) of obese children are still obese in adolescence and only 32% of overweight children. Furthermore, in this review it was found that 70% of obese adults were not obese in childhood or adolescence. The authors concluded that reducing obesity in childhood is unlikely to have a major impact on adult obesity. Therefore the identification of the overweight and obese children who should be treated more aggressively is becoming more important.

Several studies tried to address the best predictors of adult obesity[21]: birth weight, adiposity rebound (AR), socioeconomic status, and genetic factors have all been considered. The exact role of these factors is difficult to define because they are often intertwined and confounded. The prenatal period is critical because the environment in utero influences the weight later on in life,[22,23] Both low birth weight and high birth weight are associated with a higher prevalence of obesity (U-shaped relationship).

What is the AR phenomenon? There is a rapid increase in BMI during the first year of life, followed by a drop to reach a minimum at approximately the age of 6 years and then a gradual increase (see Fig. 15.1). The point of minimal BMI is the start of the AR. Some authors have shown that the earlier the AR, the higher the BMI in early adulthood.[24,25] This association may be caused by an early increase in adipocyte numbers although this has not been consistently demonstrated across studies.[26] The BMI at the age of 6 or 7 is probably a more a reliable predictor of adult BMI[27] because the evidence regarding the AR is difficult to establish.[28]

Metabolic syndrome is a complex disorder defined by a constellation of CR factors, including high blood pressure, glucose intolerance, dyslipidemia, elevated waist circumference, and IR. The clinical utility of identifying the presence of metabolic syndrome before adulthood is the subject of intense debate, especially regarding to its predictive value in the development of adult metabolic syndrome. However, it is worth distinguishing between children who are at a higher risk of developing metabolic syndrome and those who are more likely to remain healthy. A cross-sectional study (prospective and retrospective collection data) was conducted to identify the demographic, adiposity, and lifestyle predictors of metabolically healthy obesity (MHO) in children.[29] A total of 181 children between 8 and 17 years were enrolled in this study. The author's classification rested on two independent systems based either on IR or on other CRs. IR was determined based on HOMA-IR—subjects with a HOMA-IR score <3.16 were considered MHO. The CR system was based on the presence or absence of common CR factors (blood pressure, triglycerides, high-density lipoprotein [HDL] cholesterol, and glucose)—MHO was defined as the absence of any risk factors. When using the IR system, 31.5% were metabolically healthy, and when using the CR system, 21.5% were metabolically healthy. Using the IR system, waist circumference was the strongest independent adiposity marker of MHO status. For every unit of SD score increase in waist circumference, there was a 67% reduction in the odds of being in the MHO group. Dietary fat intake was also a strong predictor of the MHO status. Using the CR system, moderate-to-vigorous exercise was the strongest independent predictor related to the metabolic status.

However, some authors believe that obese children who do not meet the criteria for metabolic syndrome may still show an independent effect on adult metabolic risk. All overweight and obese children should therefore be encouraged to have an appropriate BMI.[30]

Early identification of children at risk of becoming obese later in life has become of great importance to address the current obesity epidemics. Greece currently has the highest prevalence of childhood overweight and obesity in Europe (44.1% and 38.1% in school-aged boys and girls, respectively). Some Greek specialists have proposed a "Childhood Obesity Risk Evaluation (CORE)" index as a screening tool for the early prediction of obesity in childhood and adolescence.[31] The scoring system is based on pregnancy medical records, anthropometric and sociodemographic data: mother's prepregnancy weight, maternal smoking during pregnancy, maternal educational model, gender and infant weight gain in the first 6 months of life. The authors created the index after conducting a cross-sectional study, which retrospectively collected data from a representative sample of 5946 Greek children and adolescents. The scale of the CORE index ranged from 0 to 11 units. The authors found that the likelihood of children becoming obese between the ages of 6–15 years increased by 30% for each unit increase. Although the results are encouraging, the system needs to be validated prospectively and to include other populations.

Key Messages
- Approximately half of obese children become obese adolescents.
- Most obese adolescents continue to be obese as adults.
- Obesity can lead to complications early in life similar to those seen in adults.
- There are some adiposity and lifestyle risks factors that can predict if a child has a low risk of developing a cardiometabolic risk.
  - e.g., waist circumference and dietary fat intake are two important factors usually strongly associated with an increased risk of developing metabolic syndrome.
- Metabolically healthy obese children may not require the same aggressive approach as those with a high metabolic risk but should still be encouraged to lose weight.
- Adolescents no longer obese as adults will show a significant reduction of their CR in adulthood (similar to adults who were never obese).
- The relationship between obesity and metabolic risk from childhood to adulthood remains controversial.

We should not underestimate the psychosocial impact obesity can have. An inverse relationship between health-related quality of life and BMI has been reported.[4,32] Childhood obesity increases risks of bullying and teasing, social isolation, anxiety, depression, lower self-esteem, stigmatization, eating disorders (bulimia, binge eating), and poor academic performance. Obese boys have been shown to be more vulnerable to emotional and behavioral problems.[33]

FIRST CONSULTATION WITH AN OBESE CHILD

The initial consultation of an overweight or obese child should define the degree of obesity, identify possible causes for the obesity (secondary obesity), and exclude the presence of comorbidities. It should include at least the following:
- Comprehensive medical history and examination
- Social background.
- Child and family history including BMI of parents.
- Accurate calculation of BMI and plot height and weight since birth on appropriate charts (e.g., CDC charts for the United States).
- Pattern of obesity: generalized, central, or upper body.
- Pubertal assessment.
- Neurologic and psychomotor assessment.
- Dysmorphic features that could be suggestive of an obesity syndrome.
- Acanthosis nigricans indicative of IR.
- Signs of an endocrine disorder such as goiter, abnormal growth velocity, fatigue, hirsutism, sign of hypo/hyperthyroidism/hypoparathyroidism.
- Obstructive sleep apnea.
- Concomitant medication.
- Hypertension.
- Nutrition and physical activity.

The first line of investigations should include at least the following
- Thyroid function.
- Fasting glucose and insulin. Calculate HOMA as a measure of IR (HOMA = fasting insulin [mU/L] × fasting glucose [mmol/L]/22.5).
- Fasting HDL, low-density lipoprotein cholesterol, triglycerides, and liver function (ALT). The second line of investigations will be guided by the degree of obesity, the presence of comorbidities, the associated clinical signs, and generally the results of the first line of investigations. The additional tests are more likely to be requested by a specialist (i.e., obesity endocrinology service and/or geneticist). These investigations may include potential investigations for etiology purposes: genetic studies, GH stimulation tests, 3-day 24-h urine cortisol, and brain MRI.

- Further specialist investigations to identify other potential comorbidities: OGTT, sleep studies, pelvic ultrasound, androgens, follicle-stimulating hormone, luteinizing hormone (see Fig. 15.3).

TREATMENT
Lifestyle Modifications

Once established, childhood obesity is hard to treat. To have a significant BMI reduction, it should be at least −0.25 or −0.5 BMI z-score, as at this level a reduction in CR has been observed and IR is improved.[33]

Lifestyle modifications are the foundation of all obesity treatments. They are perhaps more fundamental in children because pharmacologic interventions should be limited to severe obesity (>99.6 centile or 2.5 SD). Because obesity occurs when energy intake is greater than energy expenditure, reducing calorie intake (diet) and increasing energy expenditure (physical activity) are essential to manage obesity irrespective of the level of obesity. This approach involves the child, parents, school, and the whole community to promote healthy eating and increase physical activity.

There has been a wealth of reviews assessing the impact of various interventions for preventing or treating obesity in children and adolescents.[34] However, there is a disappointing lack of good quality data.[34,35]

Some guidelines provide good guidance to prevent and/or treat obesity in children and adolescents. They include a stepwise approach with different levels of intervention, including a combination of diet, exercise, and behavioral changes (*Guidelines from the American Academy of Pediatrics, CDC guidelines, NICE guidelines [UK]*).

Even modest decreases in BMI z-score (0.5 or 0.25) are considered beneficial in terms of improvement in cardiometabolic risk factors in overweight and obese children and adolescents. A study is ongoing (2016) to establish what change in BMI is required to achieve clinically meaningful improvements in metabolic health status in obese children and adolescents attending lifestyle treatment interventions.[36]

Another important aspect is policy related to public health. In the United Kingdom the NICE guideline PH47 (2013) and NG7 (2015) refer to lifestyle management in children up to age 18 years.

Public Health England published the report "Sugar Reduction: The Evidence for Action" in October 2015, recommending sugar no more than 5% of total dietary intake. A tax was proposed on full sugar soft drinks to increase price by up to 20%.[33]

Pharmacologic Management of Obesity in Children and Adolescents

Medications are not recommended in children. Currently, only a lipase inhibitor "orlistat" has been approved for treating obesity in pediatric patients over the age of 12 years. Most treatments prescribed in adults have not been tested in children in randomized placebo-controlled trials. Only treatments that have demonstrated both an acceptable safety profile and efficacy over at least a year are worth considering. Some of the adult treatments have been given open-label or tested for periods of time too short to be validated and recommended.

So far obesity drugs have limited efficacy or have unacceptable adverse effects that preclude their use. The difficulty in conducting long-term clinical trials lies in the low rate of compliance and completion in this kind of study. Thus no long-term data are available.

Experts agree that medications should be restricted to extremely obese children (>3.5 SD) and exhibiting comorbidities such as fatty liver disease, hypertension, or glucose intolerance. No medications should be prescribed in isolation without concomitant lifestyle modifications. When, after initiating lifestyle modifications, should pharmacologic treatment be considered as additional therapy has not been clearly established. It is, however, reasonable to have at least 6 months of lifestyle management before considering additional pharmacologic treatment.[37]

Orlistat

Orlistat inhibits gastrointestinal lipases, hence reducing the absorption of 30% of ingested dietary fat. Because it acts locally with minimum absorption, systemic adverse effects are limited. It was approved by the FDA in 2003 for treating obesity in 12-year and above adolescents, at a dose of 120 mg three times daily. Several clinical trials have been conducted from 3-month to 1-year (54-week) duration.[38–42] Only two were placebo-controlled[41,42] and one was open-label but used placebo.[40] The Chanoine study[41] randomized 539 patients 12–16 years with a BMI ≥ 2 units above the 95th centile either to orlistat 120 mg three times daily or placebo coupled with lifestyle improvement. After 12 weeks, BMI decreased in both groups. After 54 weeks the orlistat group maintained an average of 0.55 kg/m² BMI reduction (95% CI not specified in the paper), whereas the placebo group showed a 0.310 kg/m² BMI increase (95% CI not specified) over baseline. The most common adverse events were oily stools (50%), oily spotting (29%), oily evacuation (23%), abdominal pain (22%), and fecal urgency (21%). This study showed a medium-term benefit, but

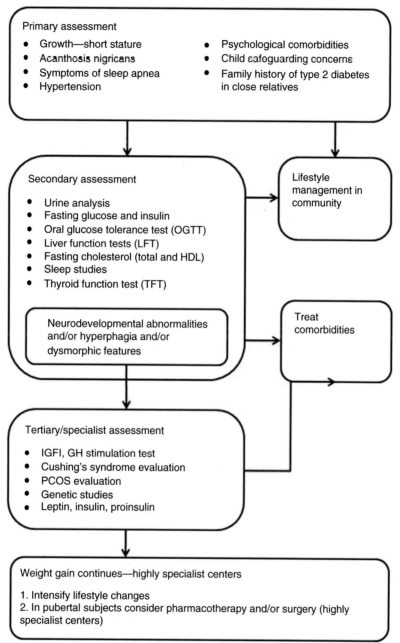

FIG. 15.3 Assessment of Children with Obesity (BMI > 98th centile)—adapted from OSCA (Obesity Services for Children and Adolescents). *GH*, growth hormone; *HDL*, high-density lipoprotein; *IGF1*, insulin growth factor 1; *PCOS*, polycystic ovarian syndrome.

the degree of improvement was less than that seen in the other studies (e.g., changes in BMI -4.09 kg/m² in Ozkan study; an open-label study). At the end of the study, weight increased above baseline in both groups, but those receiving orlistat gained less weight than

those receiving placebo (0.53 vs. 3.14 kg). A secondary analysis of the same data showed that early weight loss was a strong predictor of the 52-week favorable outcome in both groups.[43] However, subjects in the orlistat group were 2.4 times (95% CI: 1.34–4.46) more likely to experience a weight loss ≥5% after 12 weeks than those in the placebo group. In a 6-month study in 40 subjects, aged 14–18 years old with a BMI > 85th centile, no statistically significant reduction in BMI was observed between the orlistat and the placebo group.[41] Overall, however, the results of the clinical trials so far are in favor of orlistat with respect to changes in BMI although without a statistically significant improvement in lipid, insulin, and glucose profiles.

Metformin is another drug that is prescribed to obese children with a view to reducing their BMI. Metformin is commonly used in children over 10 years old with type 2 diabetes but is not FDA approved for obesity treatment. It reduces hepatic glucose production and intestinal glucose absorption and inhibits lipogenesis in addition to improving insulin sensitivity and the secretion of glucagon-like peptide.

At least 10 placebo-controlled have been conducted with metformin with a view to reducing obesity in children. The average dose of metformin was 1500 mg/day. Most of these trials were small, but four trials enrolled more than 100 patients. The duration of treatment was short (between 2 and 6 months) apart from one trial,[44] which studied 77 subjects, aged 13–18 years. BMI reduction ranged from −0.9 to −1.8 kg/m² compared with placebo. But metformin did not produce significant change in total fat mass, abdominal fat, or insulin. A metaanalysis of three randomized pediatric trials of metformin monotherapy in nondiabetic obese adolescents showed a small but not statistically significant change in BMI after 6 months (−0.17; CI: −0.62 to 0.28).

Another study conducted in 66 patients (aged 7–18 years; 29 prepubertal and 37 pubertal) showed that weight loss was modest but more pronounced in the metformin group (−4.9 ± 1.0 kg) than in the diet group (−1.7 ± 1.1 kg), whereas high sensitivity C-reactive protein and fibrinogen decreased more in the diet/exercise pubertal group. Baseline intrahepatic fat was high but decreased only in the diet/exercise pubertal group.[45]

Yanovski studied 100 severely obese and insulin-resistant children, aged 6–12 years old, randomized to either metformin (1000 mg) or placebo for 6 months.[46] Children in the metformin group had a statistically significant greater decreases in BMI (−0.11 SD score [95% CI −0.16 to −0.06]) than placebo (−0.04 [95% CI: −0.1 to 0.02]), while less weight gain was seen in the metformin group versus the placebo group (1.47 kg [−0.31 to 3.24] vs. 4.85 [2.84 to 6.85], respectively). Glucose and IR (HOMA) improved more in the metformin group [HOMA-IR index difference between metformin and placebo (−1.54 [95% CI: −2.65 to −0.44])].

The main adverse effects of metformin were transient diarrhea, abdominal discomfort, and nausea, which rarely led to withdrawal of patients. A small decrease in dose was shown to improve tolerability without affecting efficacy.

A systematic Cochrane review (2016) evaluated metformin (11 trials), sibutramine (6 trials), and orlistat (4 trials) and one trial combining metformin and fluoxetine. It showed that pharmacologic interventions usually have some positive effect on BMI, but nevertheless the reduction remains small. Trials were considered generally of low quality with high dropout rates. This Cochrane review confirmed previous findings and conclusions.

Glucagon-like peptide-1 receptor agonist (GLP-1) is one of the promising medications currently being evaluated in obese or overweight subjects because it can potentially reduce both metabolic risk and body weight. It reduces energy expenditure and appetite and slows down gastric emptying.[47–49] Two clinical trials have evaluated the effects in pediatric patients.[50,51] The pooled data treatment effects showed an average reduction in BMI at 3 months of −3.42 (96% CI −5.41 to −1.42%) compared with placebo. The most common adverse effect of GLP-1 was mild and transient nausea. However, these two trials were of short term (3 months) in a small number of patients (12 and 26, respectively), hence these results need to be interpreted with caution and need to be supported by long-term studies.

Recent US clinical practice guidelines recommend against using obesity medications in children and adolescents <16 years of age who are overweight and not obese, except in the context of clinical trials. They suggest that FDA-approved pharmacotherapy for obesity should be administered only after a concomitant lifestyle modification program of the highest intensity and only by clinicians who are experienced in the use of antiobesity agents. They suggest discontinuing medication and reevaluating the patient if the patient does not have a >4% BMI z-score reduction after 12-week treatment.[52]

Key Messages
- Orlistat is the only treatment approved for treating obesity in adolescents over the age of 12 years. There are no obesity drugs approved for younger children.
- Pharmacologic treatment should be restricted to at least severely obese children (BMI > 2.5 SD) with cardiovascular or liver comorbidities and be always combined with lifestyle modifications.
- Metformin has also been used for treating obesity in nondiabetic children and adolescents. However, it is not considered a weight-loss treatment.

- Both orlistat and metformin have shown a favorable but modest effect on BMI. The long-term effects are still unknown.
- In addition to a need for further data on the treatment of children with existing drugs, there is also a need for the development of more effective new drugs to treat obese children who have complications despite making lifestyle modifications.

Gastric Bypass

Surgical treatment is the only effective treatment in the long term when targeting the right population. Surgery has now become an option in morbidly obese adolescents after careful psychologic assessment. Different techniques have been used and have usually shown promising results.[53-55] Roux-en-Y gastric bypass laparoscopic is probably the most popular operation in obese adolescents because of encouraging long-term results and its reversibility. A 7-year follow-up study in a small group of patients (19 subjects) and 5-year follow-up in the Adolescent Morbid Obesity Surgery (AMOS) Swedish study (81 subjects) showed substantial weight loss and sustained improvement in metabolic risk factors as well as psychologic benefits. However there is still a need for randomized controlled trials to assess the long-term impact of surgery in adolescents.

This option can only be the last resort for a very small proportion of morbidly obese adolescents who have access to an experienced pediatric surgeon working in specialized centers capable of providing appropriate long-term follow-up.

Recent US endocrine guidelines recommend bariatric surgery in patients who have attained Tanner 4 or 5 pubertal development and final or near-final height, and in patients who have a BMI > 40 kg/m^2 or have a BMI of 35 kg/m^2 and significant comorbidities.

THE FUTURE

Tackling obesity is a "societal challenge, similar to climate change." All interventions that are addressed at the level of the individual are not sufficient and a whole system approach and review at national and international level should be considered.

There are a few new medications—administered alone or in combination—currently being approved (and/or investigated) in adults, e.g., lorcaserin,[56] combo naltrexone, and bupropion.[57] Some of these medications are likely to be evaluated in pediatric patients in the near future. It is now a regulatory obligation in the United States and the EU to assess new drugs in the pediatric population when their safety and efficacy have been shown in adults—and when they are likely to be of benefit to children. However, it should be emphasized again that only long-term placebo-controlled clinical trials in children and adolescents will determine the safety and efficacy of these new obesity drugs.

The future is likely to be based on a more targeted and individualized approach, which should involve better identification of the underlying factors, leading to being overweight and obese at different stages of growth and development—from in utero to adulthood. This comprises genetic screening, new pharmacologic treatments, and better policies to reduce the burden of obesity in the whole community not only at a local but also at an international level. While monogenic obesity will probably benefit most from future therapies (e.g., targeted gene therapies, recombinant leptin, MC4R agonists), the main effort should be focused on prevention with implementation of policies at local, national, and international levels[58]

REFERENCES

1. Ebbeling CB, Pawlak DB, Ludwig DS. Childhood obesity: public-health crisis, common sense cure. *Lancet.* 2002;360(9331):473–482. http://dx.doi.org/10.1016/S0140-6736(02)09678-2.
2. Atay Z, Bereket A. Current status on obesity in childhood and adolescence: prevalence, etiology, co-morbidities and management. *Obes Med.* 2016;3:1–9. http://dx.doi.org/10.1016/j.obmed.2016.05.005.
3. Gurnani M, Birken C, Hamilton J. Childhood obesity: causes, consequences, and management. *Pediatr Clin North Am.* 2015;62(4):821–840. http://dx.doi.org/10.1016/j.pcl.2015.04.001.
4. Viner RM, White B, Barrett T, et al. Assessment of childhood obesity in secondary care: OSCA consensus statement. *Arch Dis Child Educ Pract Ed.* 2012;97(3):98–105. http://dx.doi.org/10.1136/edpract-2011-301426.
5. Wright N, Wales J. Assessment and management of severely obese children and adolescents. *Arch Dis Child.* June 2016. http://dx.doi.org/10.1136/archdischild-2015-309103.
6. Haliloglu B, Bereket A. Hypothalamic obesity in children: pathophysiology to clinical management. *J Pediatr Endocrinol Metab.* 2015;28(5–6):503–513. http://dx.doi.org/10.1515/jpem-2014-0512.
7. Pluymen LPM, Smit HA, Wijga AH, Gehring U, De Jongste JC, Van Rossem L. Cesarean delivery, overweight throughout childhood, and blood pressure in adolescence. *J Pediatr.* 2016;179:111–117. http://dx.doi.org/10.1016/j.jpeds.2016.08.059. e3.
8. Kuhle S, Tong OS, Woolcott CG. Association between caesarean section and childhood obesity: a systematic review and meta-analysis. *Obes Rev.* 2015;16(4):295–303. http://dx.doi.org/10.1111/obr.12267.

9. Li HT, Zhou YB, Liu JM. The impact of cesarean section on offspring overweight and obesity: a systematic review and meta-analysis. *Int J Obes.* 2013;37(7):893–899. http://dx.doi.org/10.1038/ijo.2012.195.

10. Al Mamun A, Lawlor DA, Cramb S, O'Callaghan M, Williams G, Najman J. Do childhood sleeping problems predict obesity in young adulthood? Evidence from a prospective birth cohort study. *Am J Epidemiol.* 2007;166(12):1368–1373. http://dx.doi.org/10.1093/aje/kwm224.

11. Paul IM, Savage JS, Anzman SL, et al. Preventing obesity during infancy: a pilot study. *Obesity.* 2011;19(2):353–361. http://dx.doi.org/10.1038/oby.2010.182.

12. Alamian A, Wang L, Hall AM, Pitts M, Ikekwere J. Infant sleep problems and childhood overweight: effects of three definitions of sleep problems. *Prev Med Rep.* 2016;4:463–468. http://dx.doi.org/10.1016/j.pmedr.2016.08.017.

13. Al Mamun A, Lawlor DA, Alati R, O'Callaghan MJ, Williams GM, Najman JM. Does maternal smoking during pregnancy have a direct effect on future offspring obesity? Evidence from a prospective birth cohort study. *Am J Epidemiol.* 2006;164(4):317–325. http://dx.doi.org/10.1093/aje/kwj209.

14. Chiasson MA, Scheinmann R, Hartel D, et al. Predictors of obesity in a cohort of children enrolled in WIC as infants and retained to 3 years of age. *J Community Health.* 2016;41(1):127–133. http://dx.doi.org/10.1007/s10900-015-0077-2.

15. Lumeng JC, Somashekar D, Appugliese D, Kaciroti N, Corwyn RF, Bradley RH. Shorter sleep duration is associated with increased risk for being overweight at ages 9 to 12 years. *Pediatrics.* 2007;120(5):1020–1029. http://dx.doi.org/10.1542/peds.2006-3295.

16. Heerman WJ, Krishnaswami S, Barkin SL, McPheeters M. Adverse family experiences during childhood and adolescent obesity. *Obesity.* 2016;24(3):696–702. http://dx.doi.org/10.1002/oby.21413.

17. Sinha R, Fisch G, Teague B, et al. Prevalence of impaired glucose tolerance among children and adolescents with marked obesity. *N Engl J Med.* 2002;346(11):802–810. http://dx.doi.org/10.1056/NEJMoa012578.

18. Sperling MA. *Pediatric Endocrinology.* Elsevier Health Sciences; 2014:956–1014.

19. Juonala M, Magnussen CG, Berenson GS, et al. Childhood adiposity, adult adiposity, and cardiovascular risk factors. *N Engl J Med.* 2011;365(20):1876–1885. http://dx.doi.org/10.1056/NEJMoa1010112.

20. Simmonds M, Llewellyn A, Owen CG, Woolacott N. Predicting adult obesity from childhood obesity: a systematic review and meta-analysis. *Obes Rev.* 2016;17(2):95–107. http://dx.doi.org/10.1111/obr.12334.

21. Krassas GE, Tzotzas T. Do obese children become obese adults: childhood predictors of adult disease. *Pediatr Endocrinol Rev.* 2004;1(suppl 3):455–459.

22. Rogers I. The influence of birthweight and intrauterine environment on adiposity and fat distribution in later life. *Int J Obes.* 2003;27(7):755–777. http://dx.doi.org/10.1038/sj.ijo.0802316.

23. Kuh D, Hardy R, Chaturvedi N, Wadsworth MEJ. Birth weight, childhood growth and abdominal obesity in adult life. *Int J Obes Relat Metab Disord J Int Assoc Study Obes.* 2002;26(1):40–47. http://dx.doi.org/10.1038/sj.ijo.0801861.

24. Rolland-Cachera M-F, Deheeger M, Guilloud-Bataille M, Avons P, Patois E, Sempé M. Tracking the development of adiposity from one month of age to adulthood. *Ann Hum Biol.* 1987;14(3):219–229. http://dx.doi.org/10.1080/03014468700008991.

25. Papadimitriou A. Timing of adiposity rebound and prevalence of obesity. *J Pediatr.* 2015;167(2):498. http://dx.doi.org/10.1016/j.jpeds.2015.04.072.

26. Koyama S, Sairenchi T, Shimura N, Arisaka O. Association between timing of adiposity rebound and body weight gain during infancy. *J Pediatr.* 2015;166(2):309–312. http://dx.doi.org/10.1016/j.jpeds.2014.10.003.

27. Börnhorst C, Siani A, Tornaritis M, et al. Potential selection effects when estimating associations between the infancy peak or adiposity rebound and later body mass index in children. *Int J Obes.* November 2016. http://dx.doi.org/10.1038/ijo.2016.218.

28. Han JC, Lawlor DA, Kimm SYS. Childhood obesity – 2010: progress and challenges. *Lancet.* 2010;375(9727):1737–1748. http://dx.doi.org/10.1016/S0140-6736(10)60171-7.

29. Prince RL, Kuk JL, Ambler KA, Dhaliwal J, Ball GDC. Predictors of metabolically healthy obesity in children. *Diabetes Care.* 2014;37(5):1462–1468. http://dx.doi.org/10.2337/dc13-1697.

30. Arisaka O, Koyama S, Ichikawa G, Kariya K, Yoshida A, Shimura N. Pediatric obesity and adult metabolic syndrome. *J Pediatr.* 2014;164(6):1502. http://dx.doi.org/10.1016/j.jpeds.2014.02.050.

31. Manios Y, Birbilis M, Moschonis G, et al. Childhood obesity risk evaluation based on perinatal factors and family sociodemographic characteristics: CORE Index. *Eur J Pediatr.* 2013;172(4):551–555. http://dx.doi.org/10.1007/s00431-012-1918-y.

32. Helseth S, Haraldstad K, Christophersen K-A. A cross-sectional study of health related quality of life and body mass index in a Norwegian school sample (8–18 years): a comparison of child and parent perspectives. *Health Qual Life Outcomes.* 2015;13:47. http://dx.doi.org/10.1186/s12955-015-0239-z.

33. Robertson W, Murphy M, Johnson R. Evidence base for the prevention and management of child obesity. *Paediatr Child Health.* 2016;26(5):212–218. http://dx.doi.org/10.1016/j.paed.2015.12.009.

34. Oude Luttikhuis H, Baur L, Jansen H, et al. Cochrane review: interventions for treating obesity in children. *Evid Based Child Health Cochrane Rev J.* 2009;4(4):1571–1729. http://dx.doi.org/10.1002/ebch.462.

35. Monasta L, Batty GD, Macaluso A, et al. Interventions for the prevention of overweight and obesity in preschool children: a systematic review of randomized controlled trials. *Obes Rev.* 2011;12(5):e107–e118. http://dx.doi.org/10.1111/j.1467-789X.2010.00774.x.

36. Birch L, Perry R, Penfold C, Beynon R, Hamilton-Shield J. What change in body mass index is needed to improve metabolic health status in childhood obesity: protocol for a systematic review. *Syst Rev.* 2016;5:120. http://dx.doi.org/10.1186/s13643-016-0299-0.

37. Barlow SE. Expert committee recommendations regarding the prevention, assessment, and treatment of child and adolescent overweight and obesity: summary report. *Pediatrics.* 2007;120(suppl 4):S164–S192. http://dx.doi.org/10.1542/peds.2007-2329C.

38. McDuffie JR, Calis KA, Uwaifo GI, et al. Three-month tolerability of orlistat in adolescents with obesity-related comorbid conditions. *Obes Res.* 2002;10(7):642–650. http://dx.doi.org/10.1038/oby.2002.87.

39. McDuffie JR, Calis KA, Uwaifo GI, et al. Efficacy of orlistat as an adjunct to behavioral treatment in overweight African American and Caucasian adolescents with obesity-related co-morbid conditions. *J Pediatr Endocrinol Metab.* 2011;17(3):307–320. http://dx.doi.org/10.1515/JPEM.2004.17.3.307.

40. Ozkan B, Bereket A, Turan S, Keskin S. Addition of orlistat to conventional treatment in adolescents with severe obesity. *Eur J Pediatr.* 2004;163(12):738–741. http://dx.doi.org/10.1007/s00431-004-1534-6.

41. Chanoine J-P, Hampl S, Jensen C, Boldrin M, Hauptman J. Effect of orlistat on weight and body composition in obese adolescents: a randomized controlled trial. *JAMA.* 2005;293(23):2873–2883. http://dx.doi.org/10.1001/jama.293.23.2873.

42. Maahs D, de Serna DG, Kolotkin RL, et al. Randomized, double-blind, placebo-controlled trial of orlistat for weight loss in adolescents. *Endocr Pract.* 2006;12(1):18–28. http://dx.doi.org/10.4158/EP.12.1.18.

43. Chanoine J-P, Richard M. Early weight loss and outcome at one year in obese adolescents treated with orlistat or placebo. *Int J Pediatr Obes.* 2011;6(2):95–101. http://dx.doi.org/10.3109/17477166.2010.519387.

44. Wilson DM, Abrams SH, Aye T, et al. Metformin extended release treatment of adolescent obesity: a 48-week randomized, double-blind, placebo-controlled trial with 48-week follow-up. *Arch Pediatr Adolesc Med.* 2010;164(2):116–123. http://dx.doi.org/10.1001/archpediatrics.2009.264.

45. Mauras N, DelGiorno C, Hossain J, et al. Metformin use in children with obesity and normal glucose tolerance – effects on cardiovascular markers and intrahepatic fat. *J Pediatr Endocrinol Metab.* 2012;25(1–2):33–40. http://dx.doi.org/10.1515/jpem-2011-0450.

46. Yanovski JA, Krakoff J, Salaita CG, et al. Effects of metformin on body weight and body composition in obese insulin-resistant children. *Diabetes.* 2011;60(2):477–485. http://dx.doi.org/10.2337/db10-1185.

47. Edwards CMB, Stanley SA, Davis R, et al. Exendin-4 reduces fasting and postprandial glucose and decreases energy intake in healthy volunteers. *Am J Physiol Endocrinol Metab.* 2001;281(1):E155–E161.

48. Grill HJ, Hayes MR. The nucleus tractus solitarius: a portal for visceral afferent signal processing, energy status assessment and integration of their combined effects on food intake. *Int J Obes.* 2009;33(suppl 1):S11–S15. http://dx.doi.org/10.1038/ijo.2009.10.

49. Horowitz M, Flint A, Jones KL, et al. Effect of the once-daily human GLP-1 analogue liraglutide on appetite, energy intake, energy expenditure and gastric emptying in type 2 diabetes. *Diabetes Res Clin Pract.* 2012;97(2):258–266. http://dx.doi.org/10.1016/j.diabres.2012.02.016.

50. Kelly AS, Metzig AM, Rudser KD, et al. Exenatide as a weight-loss therapy in extreme pediatric obesity: a randomized, controlled pilot study. *Obes Silver Spring Md.* 2012;20(2):364–370. http://dx.doi.org/10.1038/oby.2011.337.

51. Kelly AS, Rudser KD, Nathan BM, et al. The effect of glucagon-like Peptide-1 receptor agonist therapy on body mass index in adolescents with severe obesity: a randomized, placebo-controlled, clinical trial. *JAMA Pediatr.* 2013;167(4):355–360. http://dx.doi.org/10.1001/jamapediatrics.2013.1045.

52. Styne DM, Arslanian SA, Connor EL, et al. Pediatric obesity-assessment, treatment, and prevention: an endocrine society clinical practice guideline. *J Clin Endocrinol Metab.* 2017;102(3):709–757. http://dx.doi.org/10.1210/jc.2016-2573.

53. Yitzhak A, Mizrahi S, Avinoach E. Laparoscopic gastric banding in adolescents. *Obes Surg.* 2006;16(10):1318–1322. http://dx.doi.org/10.1381/096089206778663823.

54. Inge T, Helmrath M, Vierra M. The Santoro III massive enterectomy: how can we justify the risks in obese adolescents? *Obes Surg.* 2010;20(12):1718–1719. http://dx.doi.org/10.1007/s11695-010-0291-z.

55. Vilallonga R, Himpens J, van de Vrande S. Long-term (7 years) follow-up of Roux-en-Y gastric bypass on obese adolescent patients (<18 years). *Obes Facts.* 2016;9(2):91–100. http://dx.doi.org/10.1159/000442758.

56. Smith SR, Weissman NJ, Anderson CM, et al. Multicenter, placebo-controlled trial of lorcaserin for weight management. *N Engl J Med.* 2010;363(3):245–256. http://dx.doi.org/10.1056/NEJMoa0909809.

57. Apovian CM, Aronne L, Rubino D, et al. A randomized, phase 3 trial of naltrexone SR/bupropion SR on weight and obesity-related risk factors (COR-II). *Obesity.* 2013;21(5):935–943. http://dx.doi.org/10.1002/oby.20309.

58. Nishtar S, Gluckman P, Armstrong T. Ending childhood obesity: a time for action. *Lancet Lond Engl.* 2016;387(10021):825–827. http://dx.doi.org/10.1016/S0140-6736(16)00140-9.

CHAPTER 16

Obesity and Depression

FLORIANA S. LUPPINO, MD, PHD • LEONORE M. de WIT, MSC, PHD

INTRODUCTION

It is often said that people with greater disposition are happier. We all have a picture of a voluptuous smiling Santa Claus as a shining example. Like this, there are various other examples of people who are more than happy with their larger size. However, obesity can also lead to unpleasant physical consequences and an internal struggle, possibly resulting in a negative impact on and contributing to someone's mental well-being.

Obesity and depression often co-occur and there is evidence for a bidirectional association between both diseases.[1] As from the 1980s, both obesity and depression have grown to be a major burden for public health and both diseases are associated with elevated morbidity and mortality.[2,3] Major depressive disorder (MDD) is ranked at number two on the list of burden of disease, globally. In low-income countries, it is at the eighth place, but at the first place in middle- and high-income countries. Soon, it will reach the first position globally, while ischemic heart disease, now at number four, will be third in rank.[4] The burden of disease, according to the WHO, is expressed as disability-adjusted life-years (DALYs) and is based on years lived in less than full health and years of life lost from premature death, in other words, "lost healthy life years."

Both depression and cardiovascular disease (CVD) are high in rank on the burden of disease list, but interestingly, among depressed individuals, there is a doubled risk for CVD.[5] Therefore, research has increasingly focused on etiologic factors, mechanisms of interaction, and pathways the two disorders might have in common.

Research indicates that both conditions are associated, and the association is probably mediated by the metabolic syndrome (MetSyn),[6] along with other closely related metabolic components. In particular, obesity is thought to be a key feature in this association.[7] Furthermore, both obesity and depression are associated with various chronic diseases, such as cancer, hypertension, diabetes mellitus, respiratory and ostheoarticular disease.[8,9] Therefore, gaining understanding on the mechanisms that explain the relation between obesity and depression is not only of great importance to public health but also could help to diminish the high costs involved in the healthcare sector.[10]

DEPRESSION
Epidemiology

Depression is one of the most common psychiatric disorders, along with anxiety, sleep disturbance, and alcohol abuse. Twenty percent of the population experiences a depressive disorder at some point in their life.[11] Moreover, the Global Burden of Disease 2000 estimates that 5.8% of men and 9.5% of women will experience a depressive episode in a 12-month period, depressive disorders are about twice as common among females and less common during childhood and adolescence, 2.5% and 8.0%, respectively.[12] Depression is often long-lasting with an average of 16 weeks and with a high relapse risk.[13] Among those who experience a first time episode of depression, 75% will have a subsequent period.[14] When individuals have multiple depressive episodes, the episodes tend to last longer, thus decreasing the prognostic outcomes. In other words, depression is a common condition, but with a high burden of disease, in need of adequate treatment to minimize the chance of unfavorable long-term outcomes.

Depressive Symptomatology Versus Diagnosis Depressive Disorder

Everyone experiences moments in life when they feel down or sad. Sometimes these feelings occur after experiencing a negative life event, such as a divorce or the loss of employment, and can be explained by the circumstances. And sometimes these feelings emerge without a direct cause. Regardless of their cause, these feelings are depressive symptoms. When mild or moderate in severity, they tend to disappear spontaneously after a few weeks. However, when the symptoms are persistent, more severe, and interfere with daily functioning, we might speak of a depressive disorder, in terms of a clinical diagnosis.

The presence of depressive symptoms should be distinguished from the presence of a Major depressive disorder (MDD) because the distinction is important, as the appropriate treatment is often different in both.

The diagnosis of an MDD, according to the golden standard, the Diagnostic and Statistical Manual of Mental Disorders (DSM) classification, is characterized by the presence of at least five of nine symptoms, for the duration of at least 2 weeks (Box 16.1). At least one of the symptoms is either (1) depressed mood or (2) loss of interest or pleasure, the so-called "main symptoms." The "accompanying symptoms" are unintentional changes in appetite and weight, sleep disturbances, psychomotor activity, fatigue, feelings of worthlessness thoughts of death and suicidal ideation. The symptoms can be present in different combinations.

Given the variety of possible combinations, the clinical heterogeneity within the diagnosis can be wide, as two patients who differ in all their symptoms may reach the same diagnosis of MDD nonetheless. For example, we have two patients, patient A and patient B. Patient A is a 43-year-old female, who for the last 2 months has been suffering from a depressed mood. She suffered from these complaints before, but to a lesser degree. In addition she suffers from a complete loss of appetite, causing her body weight to decrease from 60 to 56 kg, loss of energy, insomnia, and suicidal ideations. She is convinced that her death will free her loved ones, and these ideations are very vivid. Therefore she had repeatedly looked for opportunities to put an end to her life. She lost the motivation to undertake any daily activity, and her family, unlike previous times, is worried that she will, in fact, harm herself. The patient was hospitalized to protect her from a possible suicidal attempt and for pharmacologic treatment with an antidepressant (a tricyclic antidepressant, TCA) and an antipsychotic. Patient B is a 28-year-old male, who for the last 3 weeks is unable to experience pleasure in the things he used to enjoy, suffers from psychomotor agitation, experiences loss of energy, feels worthless, and feels unable to make even the simplest decisions. Although these complaints never completely fade, they are mostly present in the morning, while by the end of the day he feels better. Despite these complaints he manages to go to

> **BOX 16.1**
> Diagnostic Criteria of Major Depressive Disorder, According to the *DSM-V* Criteria. These Symptoms (At Least 5 of 9) Are Present for the Duration of At Least 2 Weeks. At Least One of the Symptoms Is Either (1) Depressed Mood or (2) Loss of Interest or Pleasure
>
> 1. **Depressed mood** most of the day, nearly every day, as indicated either by subjective report (e.g., feels sad or empty) or observation made by others (e.g., appears tearful).
>
> 2. Markedly diminished or **loss of interest or pleasure** in all, or almost all, activities most of the day, nearly every day (as indicated by either subjective account or observation made by others).
>
> 3. Significant weight loss when not dieting, or weight gain (e.g., a change of more than 5% of body weight in a month) or decrease or increase in appetite nearly every day.
>
> 4. Insomnia or hypersomnia nearly every day.
>
> 5. Psychomotor agitation or retardation nearly every day (observable by others, not merely subjective feelings of restlessness or being slowed down).
>
> 6. Fatigue or loss of energy nearly every day.
>
> 7. Feelings of worthlessness or excessive or inappropriate guilt (which may be delusional) nearly every day (not merely self-reproach or guilt about being sick).
>
> 8. Diminished ability to think or concentrate, or indecisiveness, nearly every day (either by subjective account or as observed by others).
>
> 9. Recurrent thoughts of death (not just fear of dying), recurrent suicidal ideation without a specific plan, or a suicide attempt or specific plan for committing suicide.

work. He fully remitted after ambulant treatment with a selective serotonin reuptake inhibitor (SSRI) and psychotherapy.

Both cases fulfill the *DSM-V* diagnostic criteria for MDD and show that disparities can be larger than similarities. They also show that, along with the heterogeneity of the diagnosis MDD, the treatment may vary accordingly. Because of this heterogeneity, recent research focuses on specific subtypes of depression (melancholic, atypical, combined, and unspecified). Atypical depression, according to the *DSM-V* classification, is characterized by positive mood reactions to some events, significant weight gain or increase in appetite, hypersomnia, heavy or leaden feelings in arms or legs, long-standing pattern of sensitivity to interpersonal rejection has found to be a strong predictor of obesity.[15]

Treatment of Depression

Depending on the level of functioning, the presence or absence of specific symptoms, and their severity, the chosen treatment may differ from patient to patient with respect to several aspects: the caregiver, the treatment setting, and the treatment itself. The treatment giver is the general practitioner (GP), a psychologist, or a psychiatrist. The treatment setting can be a primary care setting (ambulant treatment by a GP and/or psychologist), a secondary care setting (ambulant treatment by a psychologist and/or psychiatrist), or an inpatient setting where the patient is admitted in a mental healthcare institution and where a psychiatrist is the responsible caregiver. The therapy can consist of lifestyle adjustments (e.g., increase in physical activity, improvement of daily structure), psychotherapy, pharmacologic treatment, or a combination. In some cases, such as in therapy-resistant depression, electroconvulsive therapy is needed, which should be performed in a highly controlled inpatient environment. The pharmacologic treatment is by far the most used treatment form and includes several classes of medication. The most commonly used are SSRIs, selective serotonin and noradrenaline reuptake inhibitors, and TCAs. A meta-analysis by *Cuijpers* et al.[16] has shown that psychotherapy and pharmacotherapy are both equally effective, but when combined, the treatment is significantly more effective than pharmacotherapy alone. However, one should keep in mind that a certain level of cognitive functioning is needed for psychotherapy to be effective. In the most severe cases, such as inpatients, often suffering from severe concentration disturbances and apathy, improvement of the cognitive state has to be reached first, in most cases with pharmacologic treatment.

Etiologic Factors

Depression is one of the most studied psychologic disorders. This shows the complexity of the etiology of the disorder, involving genetic factors (e.g., a hereditable vulnerability for depressed mood), psychologic factors (e.g., self-esteem ergo personality), environmental factors (e.g., life events), social factors (e.g., marital and/or socioeconomic status), and hormonal changes. These factors can also have an impact on weight status and do even explain (in part) the interaction between depression and obesity.

OBESITY AND DEPRESSION

Obesity and Depression: A Confirmed Association

Numerous studies on the subject have been performed and pointed out a positive association between obesity and depression. Among these studies, also meta-analyses confirmed an association between both conditions. Since meta-analyses combine the results of several scientific studies, weighing the results of the individual studies according to the sample size, meta-analytic results have larger statistical power, and results are considered to be of greater value. There is also evidence that by treating one condition, the other will improve.[17]

A cross-sectional metaanalysis of 17 community-based studies,[18] including a total of more than 200,000 subjects, found a significant overall association between depression (i.e., depressive symptoms or depressive disorder according to the *DSM-IV* criteria) and obesity (i.e., a body mass index (BMI) $\geq 30\,\mathrm{kg/m^2}$), with and overall odds ratio (OR) of 1.26 (95% confidence interval [CI]: 1.17–1.36, $P < .001$). The association was also found in a longitudinal meta-analysis,[1] where 15 studies were analyzed, including approximately 55,000 subjects, that showed an even stronger and bidirectional association: the baseline population of obese nondepressed subjects had a 55% increased chance of developing depression. Vice versa, the baseline population of depressed but normal-weight subjects had a 58% increased chance of becoming obese over time ($\geq 10\,\mathrm{years}$).

Of all potential moderators (age, socioeconomic status), gender and severity of both depression and weight objectively play an important role. In line with the general prevalence rates, where females are more often affected by depression, it seems only logical that the association is strongest among females. Secondly, results indicate that the association is stronger in obese subjects (BMI $\geq 30\,\mathrm{kg/m^2}$) compared with overweight (BMI $25–29.99\,\mathrm{kg/m^2}$), as well in subjects with a depressive disorder compared with those with depressive symptoms ($P = 0.05$). This suggests a dose-response gradient. This "severity-gradient" of both conditions may even influence the distribution of the prevalence rates. In fact, in inpatient studies, where the MDD is considered to be more severe compared with MDD in outpatients, both genders are equally affected.[19]

As noted before, the presentation of MDD can be heterogeneous. Because appetite loss is one of the nine diagnostics criteria of depression, it seems paradoxical that MDD is associated with weight gain. However, studies that further investigate the different subtypes of depression increasingly show that especially the subtype of atypical depression is linked to obesity and disturbed lipid parameters, such as triglycerides and cholesterol levels.[20]

Mechanisms of Interaction

The evidence is convincing that there is indeed a causal relation between obesity and depression. There are several pathways (biologic, behavioral, psychologic, and pharmacologic) that may explain the relation between the two conditions, and they might even interact with each other.

The biologic pathways include several mechanisms that are considered to be involved, first, through activation of inflammatory pathways, often seen in case of weight gain.[21] Obesity might therefore be considered to be an inflammatory state, which in turn has repeatedly been associated with depression.[22] Second, hypothalamic-pituitary-adrenal axis (HPA axis) dysregulation, especially HPA axis hyperactivation, leading to hypercortisolism, is often seen in depression and thought to be induced by the depressive state (ergo stress) itself.[23] Hypercortisolism, which is considered to be one of the reliable findings in biologic psychiatry, is largely found in depression as a result of the experiences of psychologic stress and induces several metabolic changes, among which are disturbances in the fat metabolism. Third, a surplus of body adipose tissue in the body alters neuropeptide secretion levels, such as neuropeptide Y, and induces a state of hypercortisolism through the hypothalamus-sympathetic nervous system-adipose tissue innervation system.[24] Both neuropeptides and cortisol affect HPA axis functioning, in return affecting mood and thus leading to a depressed state.[25] Fourth, obesity is closely related to the onset of diabetes and increased insulin resistance.[26] Through its angiopathic characteristics, hyperglycemia could induce alterations in the brain[27] and increase the risk of depression.[28] And fifth is the activation of the autonomous nervous system:[29] the sympathetic nervous system, as part of the ANS, triggers intracellular signaling events that lead to lipolysis, thus changing the lipid levels and inducing body fat composition.[30]

Because in both Europe and the United States, thinness is considered a beauty ideal, because of a (perceived) lack of social acceptance and other sociocultural factors, overweight and obesity might induce psychologic distress, leading to increased body dissatisfaction and decreased self-esteem, both well-known risk factors for depression.[31] Disturbed eating patterns and eating disorders, as well as experiencing physical complaints as a direct consequence of obesity, are risk factors for depression as well.[32] Lack of social and physical activity,

a sedentary lifestyle, and a qualitatively poor diet are often seen in both obesity and depression. Research has shown that physical activity partially mediated the association between obesity and depression.[33]

Finally, the effects of psychotropic medication on metabolism should be kept in mind. Not only most TCAs but also some SSRIs and mirtazapine (tetracyclic antidepressant) are known to induce weight gain. Additionally, because of psychologic and or behavioral factors such as poor diet and lack of physical activity, the effects might synergize leading in long term to obesity (Fig. 16.1).[34]

PRELIMINARY CONCLUSIONS, CLINICAL IMPLICATIONS, AND FUTURE CONSIDERATIONS

In summary, depression is a common condition, with a lifetime prevalence of about 20%, that knows a less favorable outcome in case of frequent recurrence and longer-lasting episodes. The treatment differs from case to case, based on the presented symptomatology and its severity. The pharmacologic treatment, one of the most used treatment options, however effective, might affect one's metabolic state. Along with CVD, MDD reaches one of the top positions in the burden of disease list and often co-occur. Because metabolic disturbances, and obesity in special, seem to play a central role in the interactions between depression and CVD, the interaction of depression and obesity has been studied extensively as well.

Despite the brief overview given above, it seems clear that the association between depression and obesity is complex. First, the evidence shows a bidirectional relation between obesity and depression, with obesity causing depression after several years and vice versa. Second, the association between both conditions is not easily untangled because of the different mechanisms underlying the association, on the one hand, and the heterogeneity of depression itself. Despite the fact that there is evidence for several biologic, behavioral, psychologic, and pharmacologic factors influencing the association, the underlying mechanisms of interaction between obesity and depression need further examination. A deep understanding of these mechanisms might additionally give more treatment options. Furthermore, both conditions are a major burden for public health. Therefore unraveling the relation between obesity and depression is of important clinical relevance in terms of treatment and prevention. Because early detection and treatment of both conditions may help to prevent one another and therefore possibly even prevent secondary

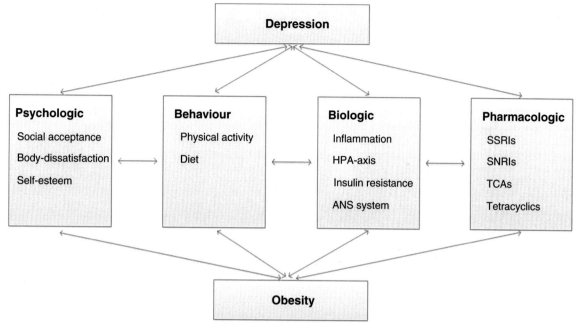

FIG. 16.1 Model of the different potential mechanisms of interaction in the association between depression and obesity. *ANS*, autonomous nervous system; *HPA*, hypothalamic-pituary-adrenal; *SNRI*, selective serotonin and noradrenalin reuptake inhibitors; *SSRI*, selective serotonin reuptake inhibitor; *TCA*, tricyclic antidepressant.

pathologies, understanding of the terms of interaction might also prevent unnecessary high costs in (mental) healthcare. This urges mental and somatic healthcare practitioners to collaborate closely with one another and thoroughly analyze and weight the different treatment options.

REFERENCES

1. Luppino FS, de Wit LM, Bouvy PF, et al. Overweight, obesity, and depression: a systematic review and meta-analysis of longitudinal studies. *Arch Gen Psychiatry.* 2010;67(3):220–229.
2. Cuijpers P, Vogelzangs N, Twisk J, Kleiboer A, Li J, Penninx BW. Comprehensive meta-analysis of excess mortality in depression in the general community versus patients with specific illnesses. *Am J Psychiatry.* 2014;171(4):453–462.
3. Vos T, Flaxman AD, Naghavi M, et al. Years lived with disability (YLDs) for 1160 sequelae of 289 diseases and injuries 1990–2010: a systematic analysis for the global burden of disease study 2010. *Lancet.* 2012;380(9859):2163–2196.
4. Mathers CD, Loncar D. Projections of global mortality and burden of disease from 2002 to 2030. *PLos Med.* 2006;3 (11):2011–2030.
5. Penninx BW, Beekman AT, Honig A, et al. Depression and cardiac mortality: results from a community-based longitudinal study. *Arch Gen Psychiatry.* 2001;58(3):221–227.
6. Bjorntorp P. Do stress reactions cause abdominal obesity and comorbidities? *Obes Rev.* 2001;2(2):73–86.
7. Despres JP, Lemieux I. Abdominal obesity and metabolic syndrome. *Nature.* 2006;444(7121):881–887.
8. Field AE, Coakley EH, Must A, et al. Impact of overweight on the risk of developing common chronic diseases during a 10-year period. *Arch Intern Med.* 2001;161(13):1581–1586.
9. Must A, McKeown NM. In: De Groot LJ, Chrousos G, Dungan K, et al., eds. *The Disease Burden Associated with Overweight and Obesity.* South Dartmouth, MA: Endotext; 2000.
10. Robinson RL, Grabner M, Palli SR, Faries D, Stephenson JJ. Covariates of depression and high utilizers of healthcare: impact on resource use and costs. *J Psychosom Res.* 2016;85:35–43.
11. de Graaf R, ten Have M, van Gool C, van Dorsselaer S. Prevalence of mental disorders and trends from 1996 to 2009. Results from The Netherlands mental health survey and incidence study-2. *Soc Psychiatry Psychiatr Epidemiol.* 2012;47(2):203–213.
12. Kessler RC, Avenevoli S, Costello EJ, et al. Prevalence, persistence, and sociodemographic correlates of DSM-IV

disorders in the national comorbidity survey replication adolescent supplement. *Arch Gen Psychiatry.* 2012;69(4): 372–380.

13. Kessler RC, Berglund P, Demler O, et al. The epidemiology of major depressive disorder: results from the national comorbidity survey replication (NCS-R). *JAMA.* 2003;289(23):3095–3105.

14. Kessing LV, Hansen MG, Andersen PK. Course of illness in depressive and bipolar disorders. Naturalistic study, 1994 1999. *Br J Psychiatry.* 2004;185:372 377.

15. Lasserre AM, Glaus J, Vandeleur CL, et al. Depression with atypical features and increase in obesity, body mass index, waist circumference, and fat mass: a prospective, population-based study. *JAMA Psychiatry.* 2014;71(8):880–888.

16. Cuijpers P, Berking M, Andersson G, Quigley L, Kleiboer A, Dobson KS. A meta-analysis of cognitive-behavioural therapy for adult depression, alone and in comparison with other treatments. *Can J Psychiatry.* 2013;58(7):376–385.

17. Lin CH, Chen CC, Wong J, McIntyre RS. Both body weight and BMI predicts improvement in symptom and functioning for patients with major depressive disorder. *J Affect Disord.* 2014;161:123–126.

18. de Wit L, Luppino F, van Straten A, Penninx B, Zitman F, Cuijpers P. Depression and obesity: a meta-analysis of community-based studies. *Psychiatry Res.* 2010;178(2):230–235.

19. Luppino FS, Bouvy PF, Giltay EJ, Penninx BW, Zitman FG. The metabolic syndrome and related characteristics in major depression: inpatients and outpatients compared: metabolic differences across treatment settings. *Gen Hosp Psychiatry.* 2014;36(5):509–515.

20. Lamers F, Vogelzangs N, Merikangas KR, de Jonge P, Beekman AT, Penninx BW. Evidence for a differential role of HPA-axis function, inflammation and metabolic syndrome in melancholic versus atypical depression. *Mol Psychiatry.* 2013;18(6):692–699.

21. Emery CF, Fondow MD, Schneider CM, et al. Gastric bypass surgery is associated with reduced inflammation and less depression: a preliminary investigation. *Obes Surg.* 2007;17(6):759–763.

22. Shoelson SE, Herrero L, Naaz A. Obesity, inflammation, and insulin resistance. *Gastroenterology.* 2007;132(6):2169–2180.

23. Belanoff JK, Kalehzan M, Sund B, Fleming Ficek SK, Schatzberg AF. Cortisol activity and cognitive changes in psychotic major depression. *Am J Psychiatry.* 2001;158(10):1612–1616.

24. Zhang W, Cline MA, Gilbert ER. Hypothalamus-adipose tissue crosstalk: neuropeptide Y and the regulation of energy metabolism. *Nutr Metab.* 2014;11.

25. Pasquali R, Vicennati V. Activity of the hypothalamic-pituitary-adrenal axis in different obesity phenotypes. *Int J Obes Relat Metab Disord.* 2000;24(suppl 2):S47–S49.

26. Holsboer F. The corticosteroid receptor hypothesis of depression. *Neuropsychopharmacology.* 2000;23(5):477–501.

27. Lee WJ, Lee YC, Ser KH, Chen JC, Chen SC. Improvement of insulin resistance after obesity surgery: a comparison of gastric banding and bypass procedures. *Obes Surg.* 2008;18(9):1119–1125.

28. Huber TJ, Issa K, Schik G, Wolf OT. The cortisol awakening response is blunted in psychotherapy inpatients suffering from depression. *Psychoneuroendocrinology.* 2006;31(7):900–904.

29. Peirce V, Carobbio S, Vidal-Puig A. The different shades of fat. *Nature.* 2014;510(7503):76–83.

30. Arnaldi G, Scandali VM, Trementino L, Cardinaletti M, Appolloni G, Boscaro M. Pathophysiology of dyslipidemia in Cushing's syndrome. *Neuroendocrinology.* 2010;92(suppl 1): 86–90.

31. Derenne JL, Beresin EV. Body image, media, and eating disorders. *Acad Psychiatry.* 2006;30(3):257–261.

32. Beesdo K, Jacobi F, Hoyer J, Low NC, Hofler M, Wittchen HU. Pain associated with specific anxiety and depressive disorders in a nationally representative population sample. *Soc Psychiatry Psychiatr Epidemiol.* 2010;45(1):89–104.

33. de Wit LM, Fokkema M, van Straten A, Lamers F, Cuijpers P, Penninx BW. Depressive and anxiety disorders and the association with obesity, physical, and social activities. *Depress Anxiety.* 2010;27(11):1057–1065.

34. McIntyre RS, Park KY, Law CW, et al. The association between conventional antidepressants and the metabolic syndrome: a review of the evidence and clinical implications. *CNS Drugs.* 2010;24(9):741–753.

CHAPTER 17

Visual Biases in Estimating Body Size

MARTIN J. TOVÉE, PHD • PIERS L. CORNELISSEN, MBBS, DPHIL

THE PROBLEM OF ESTIMATING BODY SIZE

There has been a steady rise in obesity levels in the developed world, which places significant pressure on public health resources.[1,2] A potential contributory factor to the rise in obesity is the failure of people to fully recognize their weight gain. If overweight individuals cannot accurately judge their weight and are unable to detect the fact that they are gaining weight, then their behavior will remain unchanged. Several studies suggest that overweight and obese people seem to underestimate their size and weight and may not be able to detect their weight gain.[3-9,35]

Of equal importance is the ability of healthcare professionals to detect obesity and weight change in their patients. For example, General Practitioners (GPs) are advised to screen and offer weight control to help overweight and obese patients, but this seems to happen comparatively rarely despite the fact that most people will see their GP at least once a year [35,41]. It is suggested that GPs underestimate the body mass index (BMI) of overweight and obese patients and therefore fail to either check their patient's weight or initiate a weight control discussion.[10]

A final important group of people who need to accurately estimate body size are the parents of school-aged children. Given the increasing levels of child obesity, it is important that their parents initiate changes in their child's diet and behaviors.[11,12] However, a significant proportion of parents underestimate their child's BMI and fail to undertake weight control measures.[13,14]

Thus, there is evidence from multiple sources that three important groups of people have difficulty in accurately assessing body mass. Why should this be? A number of basic perceptual biases make it a challenge to estimate body size, and the biases are particularly marked for overweight and obese bodies. In this chapter we will consider the three main visual biases that effect body judgments: contraction bias, adaptation, and Weber's law.

Contraction Bias

Previous studies suggest that we make judgments about complex stimuli, such as bodies, by reference to a template based on the average of all that class of stimuli

that we have seen—our "visual diet."[15,16] The visual bias in judging body size arises as a direct result of this way of estimating size. When one uses a standard reference or template for a particular kind of object (for example, a fence post) against which to estimate the size of other examples of that object, a form of visual bias called contraction bias occurs. The estimate is most accurate when a given object is of a similar size to the reference but becomes increasingly inaccurate as the magnitude of the difference between the reference and the object increases. When this happens, the observer estimates that the object is more similar in size to the reference than it actually is. As a result, an object smaller in size than the reference will be overestimated and an object larger will be underestimated. Thus, if we judge the size of a body by using a "reference body," which is based on an average of all the bodies we have seen in our life,[16] then individuals judging very thin bodies will overestimate the body size and individuals with very large bodies will underestimate the body size.[17,18] Thus, anyone trying to estimate the body size of an overweight or obese person will automatically tend to underestimate the body's size and judge it to be smaller than it is (see Fig. 17.1A).

Cornelissen et al.[18] suggest that the "reference" body people use for estimating women's body has a body weight of 70 kg. A value of 70 kg is the average body weight for adult women in the United Kingdom,[19] and its adoption as a reference value against which to judge other women's bodies would be consistent with people's visual diet shaping their reference body so that it reflects the population norm. As a result, contraction bias predicts that bodies below 70 kg will be increasingly overestimated and bodies above 70 kg will be increasingly underestimated, a result consistent with their findings. Based on the results reported by Cornelissen et al.,[18] contraction bias predicts that an observer who judges the weight of a 100-kg woman will underestimate her weight by approximately 10 kg.

Adaptation

The second visual bias also derives from the use of a reference standard to judge the body size. If someone

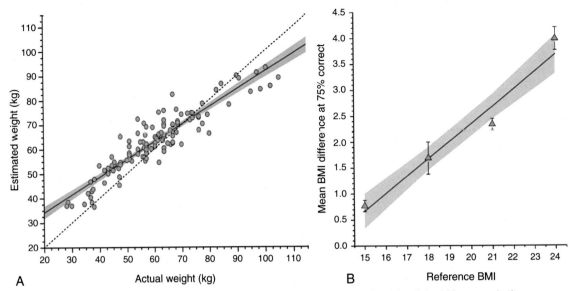

FIG. 17.1 (A) Scatterplot depicting the relationship between the actual weight of the 120 women in the images (kg) and the mean of the 29 female participants' estimations of their weight (one data point represents one image). The women in the images varied in weight from 28.2 to 104.9 kg. The *red line* represents the linear regression of estimated weight on actual weight and the *pink shaded region* its 95% confidence limits. The *dotted black line* represents the line of equality (which is where the observers' estimates should fall if they were perfectly accurate). **(B)** Plot of mean just noticeable difference (JND) as a function of the image body mass index (BMI) for the photos of real women. The *solid red line* represents the main effect of BMI on JND derived from a mixed model analysis, and the pink shading its 95% confidence band. The Weber fraction for this data is ~0.1. (Adapted from Cornelissen KK, Gledhill LJ, Cornelissen Piers L, Tovée MJ. Visual biases in judging body weight. *Brit J Health Psychol.* 2016;21:555–569, with permission.)

sees a large number of high BMI bodies, then their internal reference (what they perceive as a normal, representative body size) will change and be shifted toward a heavier body size (reflecting the higher proportion of heavier bodies making up their reference template). This is called visual adaptation. Just as faces are encoded in multiple independent dimensions, such as nose length or the distance between the eyes, bodies are also encoded in different feature dimensions.[15,20] Different features of body shape and composition (such as percentage body fat and muscle content) are encoded separately and can be independently adapted by visual experience.[21,37,38]

Therefore it is possible that the failure to recognize an overweight or obese body may be because the observer is comparing the body to their adapted reference body, which is much closer in size to the body being judged, as opposed to making a comparison against an absolute reference point that is not subject to adaptation.[6,7] The result of the adaptation is to shift what is regarded as a "normal" body size toward a bigger, heavier body, thus endorsing a heavier body

as an acceptable body size. The increasing number of people in our society who are overweight and obese means that our visual diet is increasingly filled with heavier bodies, which potentially has a positive feedback effect; more heavy people in the population means people's reference body is also bigger and heavier, which makes having a heavier body more acceptable.

The concept of what is a "normal" body can be artificially modified by a cognitive bias training program. For example, women with anorexia nervosa spend a great deal of time looking at low BMI bodies, including not only their own but also online as part of their obsession with the thin ideal,[22,23] and consider a much lower BMI to be normal.[17,24] This can be adjusted upward by a simple cognitive bias training program, which demonstrates the range of body sizes in the normal population and gives positive feedback on the point where the normal BMI lies.[25] A similar approach could be used to recalibrate the perception of a normal BMI in people who have a visual diet skewed toward higher BMI values.

However, this "visual diet" is not the only factor in judging what an acceptable body size is. For example, showing larger bodies in a positive light can increase the preference for larger bodies.[26] An example of this "visual valency" is the change in body preferences as people move between cultures. People living in rural KwaZulu-Natal in South Africa prefer a much larger BMI,[27] but people from KwaZulu-Natal moving to the United Kingdom shift their preferences toward a lower BMI. The average BMI of people in both regions is not significantly different; however, in KwaZulu-Natal a heavier body is associated with health and higher socioeconomic status, whereas in the United Kingdom the opposite is the case. Thus, one factor whether a particular body size is regarded as acceptable is the value placed on different body sizes by a particular culture or subculture. Therefore multiple factors can influence body preferences.

Weber's Law

Although contraction bias and adaptation could explain why people might underestimate overweight and obese bodies, there is another perceptual phenomenon described by Weber's law, which means it also gets progressively more difficult to detect an increase in body weight as we put weight on (see Fig. 17.1B). Weber's law states that the just noticeable difference (JND) between two stimuli will be a constant proportion of their size (the Weber fraction). This is calculated by the equation:

$$K = \Delta I / I$$

where I is the stimulus size, ΔI is the the minimum change in stimulus size required for it to be noticed, and K is the Weber fraction.

In practical terms this means that it is easier to notice, for example, a one-unit difference in BMI between two low BMI bodies than between two high BMI bodies. Over the full range of BMI, discriminating between higher BMI bodies requires progressively larger differences in BMI between stimuli. This means that as we get heavier it gets progressively harder to detect an increase in body mass. For example, for a height of 1.6 m, women with BMIs of ~22 (normal) and ~35 (obese) would just be able to detect increases in body weight of ~3 and ~5.5 kg, respectively.[18]

DISCUSSION

Thus a set of purely perceptual factors make it harder to detect both being obese and weight increase when obese, but this does not rule out more cognitive factors that are also playing an important role. Judging bodies has both perceptual and cognitive components.[39] The perceptual component is the ability to accurately estimate the shape and size of a body, and the cognitive component is how this estimation is interpreted. What is regarded as an acceptable body size or weight is influenced by cultural and media values; it is not just the sizes of the bodies we see every day in both real life and the media (visual diet), but also the positive or negative social values we put on them (visual valence) and the context in which we see them.[26-28,40] Additionally, the accuracy of the judgments may be modulated or influenced by the ethnic or social group of the observers and their own anthropometric or psychologic characteristics (e.g., Ref. 17,24,29).

Of course there are many potential cues to weight gain. For example, as you put on weight, your clothes become tighter and you can quantify any weight change by stepping on the bathroom scales. However, it is easy to rationalize tighter clothes (you can tell yourself that they have shrunk in the wash) and the bathroom scales themselves may be old and not very accurate (e.g., Ref. 30). Additionally, many people, particularly men (see e.g., Ref. 31), may not check their weight unless they had a reason to do so. If you look in the mirror and do not detect any weight change, then you will not have any reason to check your weight through standing on the scales.

The problems of detecting change in body size also represent a problem in people seeking to lose weight. Weber's law means that people who are overweight or obese have to lose a significantly larger amount of weight for it to be perceptible than someone of lower weight. As a result, they receive no positive visual feedback until they have lost a comparatively large amount of weight. This can be a problem because losing weight to improve their appearance is one of the reasons commonly given by overweight and obese people for undertaking weight control behaviors,[32-34] and if they cannot detect any change in appearance despite losing weight, it could undermine their resolve and reduce adherence and retention in weight-loss programs.

REFERENCES

1. Ogden CL, Carroll M, Curtin LR, McDowell MA, Tabak CJ, Flegal KM. Prevalence of overweight and obesity in the United States, 1999-2004. *JAMA.* 2006;295:1549–1555.
2. Swinburn BA, Sacks G, Hall KD, et al. The global obesity pandemic: shaped by global drivers and local environments. *Lancet.* 2011;378:804–814.

3. Kuchler F, Variyam JN. Mistakes were made: misperception as a barrier to reducing overweight. *Int J Obes.* 2003;27:856–886.

4. Kuskowska-Wolk A, Rössner S. The "true" prevalence of obesity: a comparison of objective weight and height measures versus self-reported and calibrated data. *Scand J Prim Health Care.* 1989;7:79–82.

5. Maximova K, McGrath JJ, Barnett T, O'Loughlin J, Paradis G, Lambert M. Do you see what I see? Weight status misperception and exposure to obesity among children and adolescents. *Int J Obes.* 2008;32:1008–1015.

6. Oldham M, Robinson E. Visual weight status misperceptions of men: why overweight can look like a healthy weight. *J Health Psychol.* 2015;20:1–10.

7. Robinson E, Kirkham TC. Is he a healthy weight? Exposure to obesity changes perception of the weight status of others. *Int J Obes.* 2013;38:663–667.

8. Truesdale K, Stevens J. Do the obese know they are obese? *N C Med J.* 2008;69:188–194.

9. Wetmore C, Modkdad AH. In denial: misperceptions of weight change among adults in the United States. *Prev Med.* 2012;56:93–100.

10. Robinson E, Parretti H, Aveyard P. Visual identification of obesity by healthcare professionals: an experimental study of trainee and qualified GPs. *Br J Gen Pract.* 2014;64:e703–e708.

11. Jackson-Leach R, Lobstein T. Estimated burden of paediatric obesity and co-morbidities in Europe. Part 1. The increase in the prevalence of child obesity in Europe is itself increasing. *Int J Pediatr Obes.* 2006;1:26–32.

12. Olds TIM, Maher C, Zumin SHI, et al. Evidence that the prevalence of childhood overweight is plateauing: data from nine countries. *Int J Pediatr Obes.* 2011;6:342–360.

13. Jones AR, Parkinson KN, Drewett RF, et al. Parental perceptions of weight status in children: the Gateshead Millennium Study. *Int J Obes.* 2011;35:953–962.

14. Duncan DT. Parental misperception of their child's weight status: clinical implications for obesity prevention and control. *Obesity.* 2011;19:2293.

15. Leopold DA, O'Toole AJ, Vetter T, Blanz V. Prototype-referenced shape encoding revealed by high-level aftereffects. *Nat Neurosci.* 2001;4:89–94.

16. Winkler C, Rhodes G. Perceptual adaptation affects attractiveness of female bodies. *Brit J Psychol.* 2005;96:141–154.

17. Cornelissen PL, Johns A, Tovée MJ. Body size over-estimation in women with anorexia nervosa is not qualitatively different from female controls. *Body Image.* 2013;10:103–111.

18. Cornelissen KK, Gledhill LJ, Cornelissen Piers L, Tovée MJ. Visual biases in judging body weight. *Brit J Health Psychol.* 2016;21:555–569.

19. *Health Survey for England.* Colchester, Essex, UK: National Centre for Social Research and University College London. Department of Epidemiology and Public Health. UK Data Archive; 2012.

20. Smith KL, Tovée MJ, Hancock PJB, Bateson M, Cox MAA, Cornelissen PL. An analysis of body shape attractiveness based on image statistics: evidence for a dissociation between expressions of preference and shape discrimination. *Vis Cogn.* 2007;15:927–953.

21. Rhodes G, Jeffery L, Boeing A, Calder A. Visual coding of human bodies: perceptual aftereffects reveal norm-based, opponent coding of body identity. *J Exp Psychol Hum Percept Perform.* 2013;39:313–317.

22. Norris ML, Boydell KM, Pinhas L, Katzman DK. Ana and the internet: a review of pro-anorexia websites. *Int J Eat Disord.* 2006;39:443–447.

23. Ransom DC, La Guardia JG, Woody EZ, Boyd JL. Interpersonal interactions on online forums addressing eating concerns. *Int J Eat Disord.* 2010;43:161–170.

24. Cornelissen KK, Bester A, Cairns P, Tovée MJ, Cornelissen PL. The influence of personal BMI on body size estimations and sensitivity to body size change in anorexia spectrum disorders. *Body Image.* 2015;13:75–85.

25. Gledhill LJ, Cornelissen KK, Cornelissen PL, Penton-Voak IP, Munafo MR, Tovée MJ. An interactive training program to treat body image disturbance. *Brit J Health Psychol.* 2017;22:60–76.

26. Boothroyd LG, Tovée MJ, Pollet TV. Visual diet versus associative learning as mechanisms of change in body size preferences. *PLoS One.* 2012;7:e48691. http://dx.doi.org/10.1371/journal.pone.0048691.

27. Tovée MJ, Swami V, Furnham A, Mangalparsad R. Changing perceptions of attractiveness as observers are exposed to a different culture. *Evol Hum Behav.* 2006;27:443–456.

28. Bateson M, Tovée MJ, George HR, Gouws A, Cornelissen PL. Humans are not fooled by size illusions in attractiveness judgements. *Evol Hum Behav.* 2014;35:133–139.

29. Robinson E, Hogenkamp PS. Visual perceptions of male obesity: a cross-cultural study examining male and female lay perceptions of obesity in Caucasian males. *BMC Public Health.* 2015;15:492.

30. Yorkin M, Spaccarotella K, Martin-Biggers J, Virginia Quick V, Byrd-Bredbenner C. Accuracy and consistency of weights provided by home bathroom scales. *BMC Public Health.* 2013;13:1194.

31. Striegel-Moore RH, Rosselli F, Perrin N, et al. Gender difference in the prevalence of eating disorder symptoms. *Int J Eat Disord.* 2009;42:471–474.

32. Clarke LH. Older women's perceptions of ideal body weights: the tensions between health and appearance motivations for weight loss. *Ageing Soc.* 2002;22:751–773.

33. Dixon JB, Dixon ME, O'Brien PE. Body image: appearance orientation and evaluation in the severely obese. Changes with weight loss. *Obes Surg.* 2002;12:65–71.

34. Hankey CR, Leslie WS, Lean MEJ. Why lose weight? Reasons for seeking weight loss by overweight but otherwise healthy men. *Int J Obes.* 2002;26:880–882.

35. Rahman M, Berenson AB. Self-Perception of Weight Gain Among Multiethnic Reproductive-Age Women. *Journal of Women's Health.* 2012;21:340–346.

36. NICE (National Institute for Health and Care Excellence). Obesity: guidance on the prevention, identification, assessment and management of overweight and obesity in adults and children. *Nice guidelines (CG43)*. 2006.

37. Brooks KR, Mond JM, Stevenson RJ, Stephen ID. Body Image Distortion and Exposure to Extreme Body Types: Contingent Adaptation and Cross Adaptation for Self and Other. *Front Neurosci*. 2016;10:334.

38. Sturman D, Stephen ID, Mond J, Stevenson RJ, Brooks KR. Independent Aftereffects of Fat and Muscle: implications for neural encoding, body space representation, and body image disturbance. *Sci Rep*. 2017;7:40392.

39. Cash TF, Deagle EA. The nature and extent of body-image disturbances in anorexia nervosa and bulimia nervosa: a meta-analysis. *Int J Eat Disord*. 1997;22:107–125.

40. Boothroyd LG, Jucker JL, Thornborrow T, et al. Television exposure predicts body size preferences in rural Nicaragua. *Brit J Psychol*. 2016;107:752–767.

41. NHS England. GP patient survey 2012/2013. Retrieved from http://www.england.nhs.uk/statistics/2013/06/13/2012-13-gp-patient-survey-aggregated-wave-1-and-2-results. 2013.

CHAPTER 18

Eating Disorders and Obesity

DR. ESTHER M. COHEN-TOVÉE, BA, MA, MPHIL

INTRODUCTION

Obesity is not classed as an eating disorder, but it does co-occur with some conditions that are classified as eating disorders, as well as with other mental health problems. It should be noted that there is significant challenge to the continued use in research and clinical practice of functional psychiatric diagnosis, due to concerns about validity, reliability, and utility, as described by, for example, Timini.[1] However, the categories in common current usage will be considered in this chapter because our current clinical evidence base relates largely to these (see Refs. 2,3 for a transdiagnostic approach to eating disorders). This chapter will give an overview of the links between obesity and eating disorders and will also note where obesity may arise as part of or in relation to another mental health problem. Psychological treatments for eating disorders that have relevance for obesity will also be described and their utility will be discussed.

Of all the eating disorders, obesity is most likely to be associated with binge eating disorder (BED), where the absence of behaviors aimed at compensating for the additional calories consumed (cf. bulimia nervosa below) leads inexorably to weight gain and sooner or later to obesity. The DSM-V definition of binge eating is "eating in a discrete period of time (for example, within any 2-hour period), an amount of food that is definitely larger than most people would eat in a similar period of time under similar circumstances," together with "a sense of lack of control over eating during the episode (for example, a feeling that one cannot stop eating or control what or how much one is eating)."[4]

For someone to receive a diagnosis of BED, binge eating will have occurred at least once a week for 3 months and will be associated with at least three of the following:

- eating much more rapidly than normal
- eating until feeling uncomfortably full
- eating large amounts of food when not feeling physically hungry
- eating alone because of feeling embarrassed by how much one is eating
- feeling disgusted with oneself, depressed, or very guilty afterward

People suffering from eating behavioral and psychological difficulties classified as bulimia nervosa (BN) are unlikely to gain so much weight as to reach a body mass index (BMI) of 30 or above, because of their compensatory behaviors such as purging after binge eating. However, some people develop BN when they are already close to or above the threshold for obesity; thus BN can be associated with obesity, and this complicates treatment (see below). Some people who meet diagnostic criteria for BN use methods of purging that are relatively ineffective as well as dangerous to their health (e.g., use of laxatives), and this group may also find that their BMI increases over time into the obese range. Similar patterns may develop in people with partial syndromes (previously described as EDNOS—Eating Disorder Not Otherwise Specified—DSM IV[5]). It is also possible to find a partial syndrome of anorexia nervosa in someone who is obese and is trying to lose weight by extreme dietary restriction.

PSYCHOLOGICAL AND PSYCHO-SOCIAL FACTORS IN DEVELOPING EATING DISORDERS AND OBESITY

A number of psychological and psycho-social factors have been shown to be related to the development of eating problems that lead to obesity. These include the following:

1. Stress and comfort eating as a coping strategy
2. Responsiveness to external cues (eating when appealing food is available whether or not one is hungry)
3. Consequences of excessive restraint over eating (biologic and psychological drives to overeat to compensate)
4. Body image disparagement—eating as a (counterproductive) coping strategy
5. Insufficient physical activity due to negative perceptions of oneself in relation to sport/exercise
6. Family attitudes toward food, eating, and dietary restraint
7. Social facilitation of overeating

BINGE EATING DISORDER

As noted above, BED has the greatest prevalence of obesity among many of the eating disorders, where 20%–30% of people with BED who request treatment are obese. BED has a point prevalence of 3.6% in people aged 16–90 in the United Kingdom, based on the results of a recent study in Southeast London.[6] In the United States, it affects 3.5% of adult females, 2% of adult males, and up to 1.6% of adolescents.[7] BED was recognized as a separate eating disorder comparatively recently (in 2013) and is similar to the more familiar disorder of BN, but crucially the compensatory behaviors following binge eating are largely or entirely absent. This is positive in that most of these compensatory behaviors are very bad for peoples' health (e.g., self-induced vomiting; abuse of laxatives, diuretics, or slimming tablets). However, it does mean that the additional calories consumed during binges inevitably lead to weight gain, and over a period of time individuals will become obese unless they are able to change their eating behaviors themselves or are willing to seek help.

BULIMIA NERVOSA

BN is most prevalent among young women and sometimes occurs following an episode of anorexia nervosa. It has been suggested that the different categorizations of eating disorders may actually be unhelpful and that what we are seeing is a continuum of eating disorders, along which people may move at different life stages and in relation not only to changing life circumstances but also changing biologic factors across the life span (see e.g., Fairburn's transdiagnostic model).[2] If someone develops BN following a partial recovery from anorexia nervosa, he/she is likely to be at a low or average body weight and BMI and although the binge–purge cycle leads to some variability in weight, this usually stays within the normal or underweight range. For some people, however, if the effects of purging are even less effective (purging is not as effective as people believe), or if their starting weight was quite high, they may develop obesity because the excess calories consumed during bingeing gradually cause weight gain.

ANOREXIA NERVOSA AND OBESITY

It may seem strange to include anorexia nervosa in this chapter. However, as mentioned above, it appears that eating disorders are on a continuum, and an individual may move along this continuum during his/her lifetime, presenting with a different constellation of difficulties at different times. Someone who has suffered with anorexia nervosa as a child, as a teenager, or in early adulthood may go on to have lifelong problems with eating and body image. If he/she develops obesity later in life, he/she may try to lose weight by extreme dietary restriction, and effectively develop all the features of anorexia, except for the low BMI, despite being obese.

PARTIAL SYNDROMES

The most widely prevalent eating disorders are partial syndromes, in which people display some but not all of the characteristics associated with an eating disorder and therefore do not fully meet the diagnostic criteria for the disorder. For example, someone who binge eats and does not use compensatory behaviors may not meet formal criteria for a diagnosis of BED if he/she binges less frequently than once a week over a 3-month period. However, he/she is still likely to become obese and may benefit from a psychological treatment very similar to that offered to someone with a diagnosis of BED.

OTHER MENTAL HEALTH PROBLEMS AND OBESITY

Depression may be accompanied by overeating or loss of appetite; the former may be associated with "comfort eating" and may lead to obesity, especially if the person was already overweight.

People with anxiety disorders and those who suffer from anxiety as well as another mental health problem may use eating to manage their anxiety.

The most significant problems, however, arise because weight gain can be a side effect of medication for a wide range of mental health problems, including depression, psychosis, and bipolar disorder.

TREATMENT FOR OBESITY WHERE IT IS PART OF AN EATING DISORDER

Psychological interventions for BN are well established with cognitive behavioral therapy (CBT) and interpersonal therapy, having similar outcomes at 9 months follow-up[8] and the transdiagnostic approach also showing good results,[3] and for most people the impact of ceasing both bingeing and compensatory behaviors on their weight is that it stabilizes within the pre-treatment range. For people whose BMI was 30 or above pre-treatment, additional interventions will be helpful once eating behaviors have been regularized (and any underlying issues addressed) to support gradual weight loss through a healthy eating and healthy lifestyle approach. However, this may be challenging as the studies of weight loss in BED show (see below).

BED can be successfully treated similar to BN[9]; however, the focus is on introducing regular eating patterns and addressing triggers for binge eating (biological, psychological, and social) because the compensatory behaviors are usually absent. Once eating has been regularized and exercise has been introduced, gradual weight loss should in theory follow; however, a review by Wilson et al.[10] concluded that although treatment response is good, significant weight loss does not occur. Behavioral weight loss programs such as the *LEARN Program for Weight Management*[11] have also been shown to be effective in treating BED symptoms but without achieving significant weight loss.[12]

For partial syndrome eating disorders, again the best course is to adapt the evidence-based psychological intervention for the full disorder, with additional work done to support gradual weight loss once the eating disorder symptoms are resolving. The shorter the duration of the problem, the more likely a good outcome can be achieved.

CLINICAL VIGNETTE

The following is based on amalgamation of a number of clinical examples and the names are not those of real individuals.

Ailsa was a single mother aged 27 with two young children aged 3 and 5. Her ex-partner Carl had sporadic contact with the children and would make derogatory comments about Ailsa's weight and body shape whenever he saw her. Ailsa had gained weight after her pregnancies, and after Carl left 2 years ago she began to diet, but this led to binge eating every night. Ailsa also started to binge when she felt lonely or anxious, and found that eating large amounts of "comfort" food helped her feel better. Before long, Ailsa's weight had increased into the obese range.

Ailsa's general practitioner noticed her weight gain and suggested a behavioral weight management program. However, Ailsa's self-esteem was low and she did not attend. She was then referred for CBT. Ailsa's therapist helped Ailsa make links between Carl's comments and the way she was putting herself down all the time. She also helped her consider that comfort eating was helpful only for a brief period and was

doing long-term damage to her health. Together they agreed on strategies to improve Ailsa's self-esteem and stop her internal self-critical thoughts. Triggers for binge eating were identified and Ailsa's therapist helped her to plan her day to minimize exposure to triggers and help her stick to a healthy eating plan. It was important for Ailsa to stand up to Carl and to seek support from friends and family. Ailsa managed to stop binge eating after a few weeks' of therapy, and her weight stabilized but did not go down. It was hard for Ailsa to stick with the healthy eating plan because she felt her children should be given treats such as crisps and biscuits, and it was then difficult for her to resist having some as well. With the help of a dietitian, healthy snacks were chosen that would be good for Ailsa and her children. Finally, Ailsa felt brave enough to start an exercise program, and this together with the healthy eating plan helped her start to lose weight in a sustainable way.

Further information, treatment advice, and self-help information are available at: http://eating-disorders.org.uk/information/compulsive-overeating-binge-eating-disorder/.

REFERENCES

1. Timimi S. No more psychiatric labels: why formal psychiatric diagnostic systems should be abolished. *Int J Clin Health Psychol.* 2014;14:208–215.
2. Fairburn CG, Cooper Z, Shafran R. Cognitive behavior therapy for eating disorders: a transdiagnostic theory and treatment. *Behav Res Ther.* 2003;41:509–528.
3. Fairburn CG, Bailey-Straebler S, Basden S, et al. A transdiagnostic comparison of enhanced cognitive behavior therapy (CBT-E) and interpersonal psychotherapy in the treatment of eating disorders. *Behav Res Ther.* 2015; 70:64–71.
4. American Psychiatric Association, APA. *Diagnostic and Statistical Manual of Mental Disorders* 5th ed. (DSM 5). Washington, DC: American Psychiatric Association; 2013.
5. American Psychiatric Association, APA. *Diagnostic and Statistical Manual of Mental Disorders* 4th ed. (DSM 4). Washington, DC: American Psychiatric Association; 1994.
6. Solmi F, Hotopf M, Hatch SL, Treasure J, Micali N. Eating disorders in a multi-ethnic inner-city UK sample: prevalence, comorbidity and service use. *Soc Psychiatry Psychiatr Epidemiol.* 2016;51:369.
7. Swanson SA, Crow SJ, Le Grange D, Swendsen J, Merikangas KR. Prevalence and correlates of eating disorders in adolescents. Results from the national comorbidity survey replication adolescent supplement. *Arch Gen Psychiatry.* 2011;68(7):714–723.

8. Agras WS, Walsh T, Fairburn CG, Wilson GT, Kraemer HC. A multicenter comparison of cognitive-behavioral therapy and interpersonal psychotherapy for bulimia nervosa. *Arch Gen Psychiatry*. 2000;57(5):459–466.

9. Agras WS, Telch CF, Arnow B, Eldredge K, Marnell M. One-year follow-up of cognitive-behavioral therapy for obese individuals with binge eating disorder. *J Consult Clin Psychol*. 1997;65(2):343–347.

10. Wilson GT, Grilo CM, Vitousek KM. Psychological treatment of eating disorders. *Am Psychol*. April 2007;62(3):199–216.

11. Brownell KD. *The LEARN Program for Weight Management*. vol. 2000. Dallas, TX: American Health; 2000.

12. Grilo CM, Masheb RM, Wilson GT, Gueorguieva R, White MA. Cognitive-behavioral therapy, behavioral weight loss, and sequential treatment for obese patients with binge eating disorder: a randomized controlled trial. *J Consult. Clin Psychol*. 2011;79(5):675–685.

CHAPTER 19

Motivational Interviewing and Mindfulness in Weight Management

LYNNE JOHNSTON, BA, MSC, PHD, CBT DIPLOMA, DCLIN PSYCH, AFBPSS •
CHARLOTTE HILTON, BSC, PHD • CLAIRE LANE, BA, PHD, DIPPSYCH,
DCLIN PSYCH

INTRODUCTION

A fundamental challenge within healthcare is adherence to lifestyle behavior change(s). Obesity is a consequence of dysregulation in *multiple* "lifestyle behaviors," which are often viewed in isolation. Typically, people struggle to sustain behavior changes across multiple health behaviors.[1] Many cooccurring factors impact on an individual's obesity; it is, therefore, essential to help patients understand their *own* maintaining behavioral patterns and the links between them.[2,3] Without this collaborative *process* taking place, there is a danger of falling into a "premature focus trap," i.e., prematurely focusing on a single "assumed" problematic behavior of importance.[4–6] Prematurely focusing on generic dietary and exercise-based "solutions" has arguably exacerbated the current obesity epidemic because the underlying complexities (for the individual) have not been adequately conceptualized. Understanding the "comaintaining impact" that various behavioral patterns have can help patients to decide which behaviors to change first and why (i.e., which will have the best impact on subsequent changes). Building this understanding is an essential first step. For a more comprehensive discussion of the role of collaborative and person-centered *formulation* within a weight management context, see Chapter 29. We fully acknowledge that wider social, cultural, and economic aspects need consideration and refer the reader to Chapter 29 for a fuller discussion of these issues.

A significant evidence base indicates that clinicians account for a substantial portion of outcome within treatment,[7] and one of the best predictors of patient outcome following an intervention is their assigned clinician. Clinicians directly impact on the patients' likelihood of engaging with treatment and in making changes. They can help their patients make changes or inadvertently *talk them out of it*. In this chapter, we consider the use of motivational interviewing (MI),

which was developed to address behavior change. We provide an overview of the key features of MI and some clinical examples of how it is being used within specialist weight management services (SWMSs). We conclude the chapter with a brief introduction to another approach (mindfulness) that has been gaining momentum within the academic literature and clinical practice. The critical consideration of either approach is not emphasizing *what* is done, but *how* it is done.

The primary purpose of this chapter is to provide an overview of MI within weight management specifically. We conceptualize obesity as a complex condition, often presenting alongside physical and psychological comorbidities (e.g., see Chapter 29 for an exploration of the importance of deconstructing obesity). As mentioned previously, from a behavior change perspective, it is important to recognize that obesity is usually best conceptualized as a consequence of <u>multiple</u> underlying behaviors that are dysregulated (i.e., sleep, activity, eating patterns). It is from this position that we demonstrate how MI can assist with the assessment and treatment of obesity. The secondary purpose of this chapter is to acknowledge the growing interest in mindfulness, highlight how mindfulness has been used within a weight management context, and signpost the reader to relevant literature.

DECONSTRUCTING OBESITY BEHAVIORS

When practitioners conceptualize obesity as a consequence of multiple behaviors, they can start unpacking, with the patient, the various behaviors that may have *caused* (proximal and distal factors) and are *maintaining* the obesity. In psychology, we call this process "formulation" and we aim to do this in a collaborative way with patients.[8,9] Within MI, when we think about *formulation*, we are engaging in a process of *focusing*.[6] As an example, we have listed in Table 19.1 lifestyle behaviors that may have an impact on an individual's weight

TABLE 19.1		
Examples of Some Specific Behaviors That Can Have an Impact on an Individual's Weight		
Broad Area	**Health-Enhancing Behaviors to Increase**	**Problematic Health Behaviors to Reduce**

Dietary	• Planning and prioritization of own needs to ensure:
	  • regular eating patterns
	  • regular intake of water
	  • type of food: nonprocessed
	  • correct combination of food groups (e.g., protein, fruit, vegetables, carbohydrates, dairy)
		• Portion sizes (reduce)
		• Food groups (trans fats and sugars)
		• Type of food: processed fast-foods
		• Takeaway food
		• Eating patterns: long gaps
		• Food/alcohol as a coping strategy (emotional regulation)
		• Fizzy sugary drinks

Activity	• Structured "exercise" • Everyday movement: integrating activity within the daily routines (i.e., active transport) • Type of activity • Intensity and duration	• Sedentary behaviors (work, home); how long, how often • Depression symptoms (i.e., avoidance cycles and rumination) • Social phobia/anxiety symptoms (i.e., avoidance cycles associated with fear of social ridicule)
Sleep	• Regular sleep routine • Wearing a mask (CPAP) for effective treatment of sleep apnea • Sleep hygiene interventions (i.e., routines around sleep wake cycles, no distractions in the room)	Not wearing the sleep mask (CPAP) for sleep apnea Phone/laptop use in bed TV/radio on as "background noise"—all night
Substance misuse		Alcohol misuse (excess, dependency, emotional regulation) Drugs (prescribed or illegal) Food (binge eating disorder [BED]; bulimia nervosa [BN])

CPAP, continuous positive airway pressure.

(this is not exhaustive). For some lifestyle behaviors, the aim will be to *reduce* a problematic or harmful behavior (e.g., overeating); for others, it will be to start or increase a health-enhancing behavior (e.g., physical activity). When psychologists work with patients to explore the impact of these behaviors on each other (i.e., formulation of the comaintaining systems), it becomes obvious which behaviors to start to change first and why (e.g., increase planning, to reduce gaps between meals, to minimize overeating/binge eating episodes on high fat/sugar foods).

Formulation as a "process," as well as an "outcome" (usually in diagrammatic and/or narrative form), helps to avoid the premature focus trap. Crucially, all of the following examples could be occurring within the same individual. MI as an approach can be extremely helpful in working with the person to help him/her to resolve his/her ambivalence for change and to build and strengthen his/her own internal motivation for change.

WHAT IS MOTIVATIONAL INTERVIEWING?

MI is a behavior change counseling method that originated from the field of addictions in the early 1980s.[10]

A central tenet is that it is a person/patient-centered approach that builds on the relational components of Carl Rogers. Rogers believed in the human capacity to exercise free choice and to change via a process of *self-actualization*. Rogerian principles of acceptance and empathic understanding underpin the relational aspects of MI.[7,11] Yet, MI has a directional aspect (i.e., to guide the person toward change). One of the key aims of MI is to help an individual to resolve their feelings of ambivalence regarding a change in behavior,[5] attitude, or belief.[6] The originators have defined the approach as "a collaborative conversation style for strengthening a person's own motivation and commitment to change."[6(p12)] A "grounded" definition (from an Alaskan elder reflecting after an MI workshop) states: "MI with someone is like entering their home. One should enter with respect, interest and kindness, affirm what is good, and refrain from providing unsolicited advice and rearranging their furniture" (*Personal Communication*: Steve Berg-Smith, 2014).

The origins of MI are explained by William Miller,[10] where he describes how he was encouraged to explicitly articulate the implicit therapeutic decision-making processes that he had learned from his patients. He worked with a group of young Norwegian psychologists (in Bergen, in 1982) and used role-play methods to demonstrate his approach. His Norwegian supervisees asked him to explicate his internal thought processes by asking questions such as "Why did you say *that?*" "Why didn't you push harder at that point?" and "Why did you do this instead of that?"[10(p153)] Over the next few years the face validity of this method became increasingly appealing to clinicians. One UK-based clinician, struck by the concepts and methods that Miller articulated, was Stephen Rollnick. After a chance meeting in Australia, in the mid-1980s, Miller and Rollnick decided to put their ideas together into a book.[4]

There are now over 3000 articles and book chapters and several books written on MI. We refer the interested reader to an extensive bibliography at http://motivational interviewing.org/motivational-interviewing-resources.[12]

Within the current context, MI has been shown to increase physical activity among low-income communities in the United Kingdom[13] and significantly increased readiness to change and confidence in ability to control binge eating.[14] A randomized controlled trial (RCT) comprising 51 postoperative bariatric patients has indicated that MI improves perceived readiness, confidence, and self-efficacy for change. Participants also reported improvements in binge eating symptomatology and some measures of dietary adherence across a 12-week follow-up period.[15]

Spirit of Motivational Interviewing

Central to MI, and underpinning the approach, is the notion of the MI "spirit," which refers to the overall style of the consultation. In her explanation of what defines the spirit, Moyers[7] emphasizes the core elements of the relationship as being (1) collaboration (equal partnership), (2) support of autonomy (emphasizing choice and control), (3) evoking rather than installing, and (4) accurate empathy.[7(p359)] She notes an increased emphasis (in recent years) to the role of compassion and acceptance, the later additions being an implicit aspect when working in the best interests of the patient. For example, imagine the qualities needed in a person to enable us to feel safe enough to disclose to them a deeply held personal secret. Imagine that the secret may cause us significant levels of embarrassment, guilt, anger, and fear and that we may be afraid of being judged unfavorably. It is likely that the qualities that we imagine in the hypothetical person (i.e., that we wish to make the disclosure to) are consistent with the qualities associated with the spirit of MI.

A common metaphor is that the MI spirit is much like dancing (moving together) rather than wrestling (pushing against) with a patient. MI spirit embodies the interpersonal processes underpinning the approach (i.e., it is the way in which it is done that is fundamental). The spirit of MI is directly associated with the therapeutic alliance[16] and subsequent favorable patient outcomes (e.g., improved eating behaviors and life quality).[7,17] Such is the importance of MI Spirit that a consultation without it is considered MI inconsistent. Furthermore, an overreliance on the skills and strategies, at the expense of spirit, runs the risk of the therapeutic relationship being fractured and the behavior change process being thwarted. The emphasis here is on the way in which the practitioner engages with the patient (i.e., warm, collaborative, respectful, compassionate, evoking, affirming, empathetic, and honoring of the other person's autonomy, wisdom, and worth) rather than the provision of standardized ingredients as one may find when following a recipe or set of uniform content (i.e., as in a behavior change taxonomy) of what "should" be said or done. The MI spirit is the embodiment of *process* and is about the therapeutic ethos: "MI is done for and with a person"[6(p15)] it is not done on them or to them. Central to MI, and fundamental to the spirit, is a practitioner's ability to relinquish the role of "expert" and instead enhance, empathically, the patient's autonomy in the decisional and treatment planning process.[7]

Low levels of the interpersonal factors that reflect MI spirit during a consultation have consistently been shown to be linked to poor outcomes.[18] Specifically, practitioner empathy predicts increased retention and positive behavioral changes across a wide range of patients and settings.[19] Such is the importance of the spirit of an MI consultation that there is an increasing awareness of the value of assessing these processes adequately so that a better understanding of their role in interpreting treatment outcomes can be established.[18] Consequently, there needs to be a greater emphasis on training and supporting clinicians to develop the skills associated with MI spirit.[7] The way a specific treatment approach is delivered (process) is more important, if not more so, than the treatment content. Separating content (what) and process (how) is analogous to considering whether it is the ingredients (what) or method or chef (how and who) that determine the quality of the meal. A disproportional focus on MI clinical trials, which exclusively address content (what) and observed outcomes, rather than the all-important interpersonal processes that impacted on these outcomes, runs the risk of MI itself falling foul of its own *premature focus trap*.[20] Consequently, it is the spirit of MI that arguably best reflects the primary and reoccurring focus of this chapter—that it is not purely *what specifically* is done but *how* (i.e., *when, why, where*, and in what way within the interpersonal dynamic [between two people or in a group]) that is critical to supporting people through change.

Ambivalence

It is not uncommon that people feel *in two minds* about changing behaviors, and it is this ambivalence that is central to MI practice. People's attitudes/beliefs and desires do not always reflect their behavior (i.e., eating high-fat/high-sugar foods and engaging in little physical activity despite wanting to lose weight). This incongruence between attitudes and behavior was coined as "cognitive dissonance."[21] An MI approach aims to help a person to resolve his/her ambivalence and strengthen the congruence between a patient's values (e.g., healthy weight, independence in older age, not being a burden on family members) and the behaviors that are consistent with such values. An MI approach aims to achieve this through the implementation of a variety of strategies

that are explored collaboratively with the patient. For example, an MI approach seeks to increase the patient's intrinsic (or internally driven) motivation and help him/her to identify his/her own reasons for change rather than those that may be assumed and imposed on him/her by an "expert practitioner" (i.e., as a medical model may do). An MI approach embraces feelings of ambivalence that are commonly experienced by patients by allowing for a full exploration of the pros and cons of the behavior under consideration for change. This can be achieved through the skillful use of a strategy called the "decisional balance."[22] The perceived discrepancy between the current behavior (e.g., lack of regulation in eating behaviors, binge/overeating episodes) and future value-consistent or value-driven goals (e.g., healthy weight, absence of chronic health problems) often serves as a powerful motivator for change and thereby helps to resolve ambivalence. Box 19.1 provides a schematic summary of a typical decisional balance matrix completed by a patient within an SWMS.

BOX 19.1
Example of a Decisional Balance Matrix Exploring the Pros and Cons of Regular Healthy Eating

PROS OF INCREASED LEVELS OF REGULATION AROUND EATING BEHAVIORS
- I would like to have better control over my blood sugar levels
- I might be less likely to get to a point of starvation and then reach for crisps and chocolates
- I might be able to have more control over my eating and have less of a tendency to overeat
- I would be less likely to engage in secret binges
- I need to reduce my feelings of guilt and shame about binge eating and overeating
- I may learn to notice when I am actually hungry
- I would start to learn to eat in public without feeling such shame/guilt
- I could potentially lose weight and feel healthier
- It might increase my metabolic rate if I stop putting my body into starvation mode
- I could save some money
- I would really like to reduce the risk of health consequences such as diabetes
- I would love to feel more comfortable eating in front of friends and family again and finally eliminate my "dirty little secret"
- My moods might improve because I had thought the triggers were actually bad moods rather than physical hunger, but now I'm realizing that it is my hunger levels that are the problem and that's caused by the gaps
- If my moods improve, my relationship with my partner may also improve

CONS OF INCREASED LEVELS OF REGULATION AROUND EATING BEHAVIORS
- I will need to plan more
- It will take a lot of effort
- I will need to involve other people to remind me and they might not "get it"; they may see me eating and make comments like "no wonder you're fat" or "should you be eating that"
- I might have to say "no" more often to other people to prioritize my own needs and that feels uncomfortable
- It feels like yet another thing I have to think about
- What if I fail?
- What if I gain more weight?
- What if it just makes me even more hungry and I turn into a grazer
- What if other people see me as being selfish

BOX 19.1
Example of a Decisional Balance Matrix Exploring the Pros and Cons of Regular Healthy Eating—cont'd

PROS OF NOT EATING REGULARLY
- I don't have to think about it
- It's easy
- I can carry on doing what I have already done around my eating without thinking about stuff
- I've been doing this all my life; I'm not sure I can change
- I enjoy the binges when they are happening; it's the feeling afterward I hate
- I look forward to my dinners more when I feel like I have not eaten anything for a while
- I enjoy the feeling of being really, really hungry
- I can save taking the risk of failure
- I'm not setting myself up to be disappointed
- I can eat what I want and when I want and don't have to think, plan or discuss it with other people
- I don't risk the chance of other people ridiculing me

CONS OF NOT EATING REGULARLY
- Nothing changes and I would feel terrible
- I would still feel really disappointed in myself
- My weight will probably continue to increase and I really need to stop gaining weight
- I would be more at risk of health problems as I get older
- I'm setting a really bad example to my kids and that makes me really want to change. My daughter has started to skip breakfast and I don't think she is using her dinner money for food at school
- I'm spending quite a bit of money each week on junk foods' like chocolate and crisps; I would like to reduce that and spend it on my kids
- Sometimes I feel so tired I can't be bothered cooking and that makes me feel really guilty
- My tiredness and low moods are getting worse
- I'm storing up fat (and health problems) for the future
- My blood sugar is all over the place and I know that increases my risk of diabetes. My mum had diabetes and she lost the feeling in her feet- that really terrifies me and I don't want that to happen to me
- I know I am doing myself harm and that's always at the back of my mind. I need to change that
- My body is going into starvation mode everyday which is not good
- I think it is having an impact on my sleep because I'm eating junk food late at night and I don't want that
- It makes me feel really bad about myself after I have done it and on some occasions I actually make myself sick to feel better. But that only happens occasionally…

Related to ambivalence is a patient's readiness to change. MI considers that perceived readiness is often assessed via a combination of how <u>important</u> the changes in behavior are to the patient and how <u>confident</u> they are to undertake such changes. These scaling questions also serve an additional purpose and are capable of eliciting language from the patient which reflects varying levels of commitment to change (change talk). This is addressed in detail later. However, in the context of scaling questions, a practitioner may respond to the value given by the patient by inquiring why a lower number was not provided and/or what would have to happen or change for the patient to increase his/her value in response to each of the scaling questions. The intention of doing so is to invite the patient to justify his/her perceived importance and confidence to change and thereby elicit change talk (i.e., language in favor of changing a specific behavior).[23] Box 19.2 provides some practical examples of

questions a clinician may ask to establish a patient's perceived readiness to change and to evoke change talk.

Resistance and Discord
Earlier conceptions of MI referred to the notion of "patient resistance" to change,[5] and this is still prevalent in mainstream healthcare practice.[24] More recently MI has rejected this term because it erroneously suggests that the problems encountered in the change process reside solely in the patient rather than being a consequence of the interpersonal exchange between patient and clinician. Consequently, "resistance" is now considered a consequence of a rupture or breakdown in the therapeutic alliance and referred to as discord.[6] Common examples include patients' need to defend themselves and signals that the practitioner is perceived as an adversary rather than an advocate (e.g., interrupting, disengagement), as well as the clinician's own mood or approach (e.g., tired, stressed, or distracted).[6]

BOX 19.2
Scaling Questions to Help Assess Patient
Readiness and Elicit Change Talk

ASSESSING IMPORTANCE

Practitioner: "On a scale of 1–10, with 1 being not at all important and 10 being extremely important, how important is it for you to eat more regularly?"

ASSESSING CONFIDENCE

Practitioner: "On a scale of 1–10, with 1 being not at all confident and 10 being extremely confident; how confident are you that you can eat more regularly?"

Generally, the greater a person's perceived importance and confidence, the higher his/her perceived readiness to change will be[6]

EXAMPLE FOLLOW-UP QUESTIONS TO ELICIT CHANGE TALK

Practitioner: "You've rated the importance of regular eating as 5, why not a lower number such as 2 or 3, for example?"
    And/or
Practitioner: "You've rated your confidence to eat more regularly as 3. What would have to happen for you to rate your confidence higher such as 4 or 5, for example?"

Box 19.3 presents a sample dialogue between a patient and clinician with examples of discord language. For added context, examples of sustain talk (patient language that favors maintaining current [unhealthy] behaviors) are also provided (sustain talk is addressed further in the next subsection). The context of the example dialogue is that the patient and clinician are discussing the implementation of the change plan. The patient has not managed to maintain the implementation of their plan because of attending a wedding, which caused a break in the routine. Eating patterns became erratic because of long car journeys, lack of control over when and what they ate, and increased alcohol consumption.

Sustain Talk and Change Talk

Sustain talk and *change talk* result from the interpersonal interaction between patient and practitioner. Sustain talk refers to patient language that favors maintaining current (unhealthy) behaviors, whereas change talk reflects speech that supports the change process and movement toward particular valued-goals. Sustain talk and change talk are important to MI because they demonstrate an individual's level of interest and motivation to engage in the change process. Change

BOX 19.3
Example Dialogue to Show Discord (and Sustain Talk)

Practitioner: "So tell me, how have you been getting on with your change plan?"
    Patient: "Well if I'm honest, it's been quite difficult this week. You see, I attended my sister's wedding last weekend and that kind of derailed things a bit."
    Practitioner: "Derailed things? In what way? What went wrong?"
    Patient: "Well, we had a really long car journey to get there and I wasn't driving so didn't have control over when we stopped for breaks. I couldn't find any healthy food at the service station. So I ended up getting a burger, fries, and fizzy drink cause I was starving. That was the start of things going wrong and it just spiraled from there really…."
    Practitioner: "That's really disappointing; sounds like you just failed at the first hurdle" because of a lack of willpower (*note that the practitioner's intention may have been to provide a complex reflection although this is a poor example and is likely to be perceived as confrontational and judging/blaming). This can be exacerbated further by a confrontational tone/body language and demonstrates how the practitioner's approach may contribute to discord.*
    Patient: "No, not really, it wasn't my fault. Things were out of my control" (*discord: feeling blamed*).

Practitioner: "OK so that was the journey. But why didn't you stick to the change plan at the wedding?"
    Patient: "Well it was a wedding (a celebration) so of course there was lots of unhealthy food and alcohol available. Like I said, it's a celebration so I wasn't going to be miserable when everyone else was enjoying themselves. Why should I have to deprive myself? It's not as if my sister gets married every week" (*discord: justifying/ sustain talk*).
    Practitioner: "But if you do go ahead and have the gastric bypass this type of behavior is just not an option. Have you *actually* thought through the implications of what weight loss surgery is all about? This is life-changing surgery and you CANNOT eat and drink like everyone else—wedding or no wedding!"
    Patient: "Well I just thought I'll have a final *blow out* before the surgery. It was my sister's wedding after all. I don't socialize very often so it's not that bad" (*discord: minimizing/sustain talk*).
    Practitioner: "Yes, but you do socialize with food/ drinks being a key focus and…"
    Patient: (interrupts) "No, no I don't, I don't think you really understand what it's like for me" (*discord: interrupting/rupture in the therapeutic alliance*).

BOX 19.4
Different Types of Change Talk and Example Keywords to Listen for

Desire	Want to, like to, love to, prefer to, wish
Ability	Able, can, confident, have done before, could, might, possible, probably
Reasons	Specific arguments for change (e.g., Why do it? Why is this important? What would be good about it? Why now?)
Need	Have to, need to, got to
Commitment	I will, I'm doing X, I guarantee

talk serves as a powerful motivator because it is generated by the patient (rather than the practitioner) and demonstrates their own *desires, abilities, reasons and needs for change*. These forms of change talk are usually coupled with *commitment, activation* and *taking steps* subtypes and referred to by the acronym DARN-CAT.[25] Examples of the different types of change talk (DARN) and associated keywords to listen for in relation to each are shown in Box 19.4.

Box 19.5 revisits the decisional balance matrix cited earlier (Box 19.1) with the change talk and sustain talk differentiated by quadrant (i.e., the two diagonals). The different types of change talk are also included and the keywords or phrases to listen out for are shown in **bold**.

BOX 19.5
Example of a Decisional Balance Matrix Exploring the Pros and Cons of Regular Healthy Eating with *Change Talk* **and** *Sustain Talk* **Statements Added and Types of Change Talk Highlighted in** **Bold**

PROS OF INCREASED LEVELS OF REGULATION AROUND EATING BEHAVIORS
Change Talk Statements and Type (DARN-C)
Keywords in **bold** to show the type of change talk evoked

- I would **like** to have better control over my blood sugar levels (Desire)
- I **might be less likely** to get to a point of starvation and then reach for crisps and chocolates (Ability)
- I might be **able** to have more control over my eating and have less of a tendency to overeat (Ability)
- I **would** be less likely to engage in secret binges (Ability/Reason)
- I **need** to reduce my feelings of guilt and shame about binge eating and overeating (Need)
- I **may** learn to notice when I am actually hungry (Ability/Reason)
- I **would** start to learn to eat in public without feeling such shame/guilt (Ability/Reason)
- I **could** potentially lose weight and feel healthier (Ability)
- It **might** increase my metabolic rate if I stop putting my body into starvation mode (Ability/Reason)
- I **could** save some money (Ability/Reason)
- I would really **like** to reduce the risk of health consequences such as diabetes (Desire)
- I would **love** to feel more comfortable eating in front of friends and family again and finally **eliminate my "dirty little secret"** (Desire/Reason)
- My moods **might** improve because I had thought the triggers were actually bad moods rather than physical hunger but now I'm realizing that it is my **hunger levels that are the problem** and that's caused by the gaps (Ability/Reason)
- If my moods improve, **my relationship** with my partner may also improve (Reason)

CONS OF INCREASED LEVELS OF REGULATION AROUND EATING BEHAVIORS
Sustain Talk Statements

- I will need to plan more
- It will take a lot of effort
- I will need to involve other people to remind me and they might not "get it"; they may see me eating and make comments such as "no wonder you're fat" or "should you be eating that"
- I might have to say "no" more often to other people to prioritize my own needs and that feels uncomfortable
- It feels like yet another thing I have to think about
- What if I fail?
- What if I gain more weight?
- What if it just makes me even more hungry and I turn into a grazer?
- What if other people see me as being selfish?

BOX 19.5

Example of a Decisional Balance Matrix Exploring the Pros and Cons of Regular Healthy Eating with *Change Talk* and *Sustain Talk* Statements Added and Types of Change Talk Highlighted in **Bold**—cont'd

Pros of Not Eating Regularly (Sustain Talk Statements)

- I don't have to think about it
- It's easy
- I can carry on doing what I have already done around my eating without thinking about stuff
- I've been doing this all my life; I'm not sure I can change
- I enjoy the binges when they are happening; it's the feeling afterward I hate
- I look forward to my dinners more when I feel like I have not eaten anything for a while
- I enjoy the feeling of being really, really hungry
- I can save taking the risk of failure
- I'm not setting myself up to be disappointed
- I can eat what I want and when I want and don't have to think, plan, or discuss it with other people
- I don't risk the chance of other people ridiculing me

Cons of Not Eating Regularly
Change Talk Statements and Type (DARN-C)
Keywords in **bold** to show the type of Change Talk evoked

- Nothing changes and I would feel terrible (Reason)
- I would still feel really disappointed in myself (Reason)
- My weight will probably continue to increase and I really **need** to stop gaining weight (Need)
- I'm would be more at risk of health problems as I get older (Reason)
- I'm setting a really bad example to my kids and that makes me really **want** to change. My daughter has started to skip breakfast and I don't think she is using her dinner money for food at school (Desire/Reason)
- I'm **spending quite a bit of money** each week on junk foods such as chocolate and crisps; I would **like** to reduce that and spend it on my kids (Reason/Desire)
- Sometimes I feel so tired I can't be bothered cooking and that **makes me feel really guilty** (Reason)
- **My tiredness and low moods are getting worse** (Reason)
- I'm storing up fat (and health problems) for the future (Reason)
- My blood sugar is all over the place and I know that increases my **risk of diabetes**. My mum had diabetes and she lost the feeling in her feet- that really **terrifies me** and I don't **want** that to happen to me (Reason/Desire).
- I know **I am doing myself harm** and that's always at the back of my mind. I **need** to change that. (Reason/Need)
- My **body is going into starvation mode** everyday, which is not good (Reason)
- I think it is **having an impact on my sleep** because I'm eating junk food late at night and I don't **want** that (Reason/Desire)
- It **makes me feel really bad about myself** after I have done it and on some occasions I actually make myself sick to feel better. But that only happens occasionally... (Reason)

Open questions, Affirmations, Reflective Listening, and Summaries—The Microskills of Motivational Interviewing

Central to an MI-consistent conversation are the microskills used in MI. These microskills comprise open questions, affirmations, reflective listening, and summaries (OARS).[5,6] Open questions refer to questions that do not invite a brief response (e.g., "in what way has your binge eating been a problem to you?" rather than "do you want to stop binge eating?"). Affirmations are considered as statements of appreciation—typically that reflect the clinician's genuine observation of the patient's strengths (e.g., "you're a very determined person"). Reflective listening is fundamental to MI and is a key way in which to communicate empathetic understanding to a patient. The deeper the reflection (i.e., complex reflections that tap into meaning and emotion), the more empathetic it is likely to be.

On a basic level a reflective listening statement is simply a way of checking that what the clinician heard was what was actually meant by the patient. For example, a patient may say "I think I eat too much take-out food" and the practitioner may respond with a simple reflection of "you believe that your consumption of take-out food is excessive" to invite elaboration and/or to prompt some exploration of what is meant by "too much" (i.e., frequency, volume, type of processed components of take-out food, etc.) by the patient. However, overuse of simple reflections can damage the therapeutic relationship, challenge the expression of empathy, and stifle attempts to explore the underlying emotion and meaning behind what is communicated by the patient.

A skillful practitioner will integrate some simple reflections but will usually employ a greater number of complex reflections into a consultation. This avoids the risk of repeating back (parrot fashion) everything that the patient has said. Complex reflections may be usefully considered as a hypothesis test. The practitioner may attempt to tap into the underlying meaning or the emotion behind the patient's words or they offer an educated guess at what was actually meant by a patient's statement (e.g., "you're aware that it's become a habit and it's starting to have an impact on your health; that's concerning you"; or, a more tentative reflection would be: "you wonder if the amount of take-out food you are consuming is excessive and if it might be impacting negatively on your health"). A reflective listening statement is more powerful than a reflective question and often helps the conversation to develop to a deeper level and for the patient to gain new/or greater understanding of the underlying issues. Good quality reflective statements tend to evoke further elaboration and help the patient to feel understood. This contributes to building and maintaining empathy because complex reflections help both the patient and clinician to gain a deeper understanding of the emotion and meaning behind what is said. As an overall strategy, reflective listening is perhaps best understood as both a method of checking interpretation and also as a means to deepen the therapeutic alliance. Miller and Rollnick[6] emphasize that clinicians are unlikely to do harm with good quality reflective listening; it is a fundamental and basic (yet not simple) skill within an MI practitioner's toolbox.

> **BOX 19.6**
> **Example of a Summary**
>
> On the one hand, you want to lose weight because you are worried about the impact on your health, specifically your diabetes, back/knee pain, and blood pressure. Yet you describe a pattern of eating that has developed over a number of years where you are having long gaps in between meals, especially during the day, and then overeating from approximately 6 p.m. onward. This is really frustrating for you. You describe a tendency to binge on chocolate around 10.30 p.m. when your partner goes to bed. This leaves you feeling guilty and angry because you know this is having a direct impact on your weight; it can feel like you're *cutting off your nose to spite your face*" You want to change but you're not sure where to start. You have gone through an endless cycle of *yo-yo dieting* for years and that has been feeling really overwhelming. You feel like the binges give you a "cuddle from the inside" but at the same time you know they sabotage your weight loss attempts. It has been a long and isolating journey for you and it now feels like weight loss surgery is your last and only hope.

Summaries tend to be useful in gathering up the content and/or process of what has been said. They can be useful at the end of specific segments or after the use of a specific strategy. They are helpful in checking understanding or at times when a change of direction may be required. It can often be helpful to summarize both sides of a person's ambivalence via a "double-sided" reflective summary. Reflective summaries are a useful way to demonstrate that the clinician has been listening carefully to what has been said and can convey empathy and understanding in the same way that a reflective statement can. Again, a summary that captures the meaning and emotion behind the patient's words is likely to be more powerful than a simple description of what has been said. Summaries serve as a useful opportunity for the clinician to summariz both change talk and sustain talk. Adding structure to a summary by way of identifying links between key issues can be a helpful way of "containing" information that patients may feel is somewhat overwhelming to them. Acknowledging this can be helpful to a client (see Box 19.6).

Summaries may also appear throughout the consultation. For example, in the form of a collecting summary "what else?" generates the opportunity for the patient and clinician to collaboratively explore all the factors that may be helping or hindering the change process more thoroughly than without this invitation.

An interesting use of a summary can be to ask the patient what he/she feels the key themes are to summarize from a consultation. This can be a useful way for the clinician to check the aspects of the consult that have stood out for the patient. Asking a patient to summarize a specific strategy such as a decisional balance regarding the costs and benefits of changing or not changing may also help a clinician to hear where the priorities are, in what order, where the emotion is, and why.

Using Elaboration, Affirmations, Reflections, Summaries to Respond to Change Talk

A skillful practitioner will seek to elicit and explore change talk and sustain talk within the context of a strong therapeutic alliance (i.e., maintaining MI spirit). Careful use of specific strategies (e.g., follow-up questions to scaling question responses) may be used to evoke change talk from the patient and can guide the discussion toward the patient's values and how a change in behavior may be more in line with such values (or how their current behaviors are inconsistent). The elicitation of sustain talk is considered as a consequence of the interpersonal interaction. When change talk does occur, it is important that practitioners respond in a manner that is likely to reinforce and strengthen the patient's intentions and behavior and therefore MI-consistent responses to change talk include *elaboration, affirmations, reflections, summaries* (EARS). The acronym EARS is often used to describe these responses to change talk. Box 19.7 provides an example of one change talk statement generated from Box 19.1 (e.g., I would like to have better control over my blood sugar levels) and then outlines some potential responses that the clinician may offer in line with EARS.

BOX 19.7
Example of Possible Responses to Strengthen and Reinforce Change Talk Using EARS (Elaboration, Affirmations, Reflections, Summaries)

CHANGE TALK STATEMENT: "I WOULD LIKE TO HAVE BETTER CONTROL OVER MY BLOOD SUGAR LEVELS (DESIRE)"
- Possible elaboration questions:
  - **"Because...?"** (A simple way of asking why via an incomplete sentence to tap into meaning.)
  - **"Tell me more about that?"** (A fairly standard elaboration response.)
  - "Why do you **think** regular eating would improve your control over blood sugar levels?" (This type of question allows the clinician to explore the client's understanding but also emphasizes personal control by asking for the client's thoughts not what they have heard from others.)
  - "What would it **mean** for you, if you were able to achieve better control over your blood sugar levels?" (This type of question will help the clinician to start to tap into the underlying meaning for the client; this will often lead onto values/life goals.)
  - "What might be the **benefits** of better control over your blood sugar levels?" (This type of question will tap into the **pros of change** specifically but crucially eliciting the patient's understanding of the benefits.)
  - "What **concerns** you have about your current control over your blood sugar levels." (This type of question will tap into the **cons of the no-change** position or status quo specifically; crucially eliciting the patient's understanding of the benefits.)

- "Why would that be?" (This type of question again taps into the client's understanding of the issues and from their own perspective, again emphasizing personal control.)
- "In what way?" (A fairly standard elaboration response and another way of asking "why" without asking directly.)
- "How would you **feel** if you were able to gain better control over your blood sugar levels? (and why?)" (This type of question will help the clinician to start to tap into the benefits and underlying emotion associated with positive change; this will often lead onto discussion of meaning, which in turn can link into a deeper level of discussion around values/life goals.)
- "What do you make of that?" (This is a type of analyzing and synthesizing question, which again taps into the patient's understanding and can start to draw out the broader meaning/implications for change but importantly from the clients perspective.)

CHANGE TALK STATEMENT: "I WOULD LIKE TO HAVE BETTER CONTROL OVER MY BLOOD SUGAR LEVELS (DESIRE)"
- Possible affirmations:
  - "That's great."
  - "It's good that you know what you want to change and why."
  - "You're a very determined person."
  - "You have a good level of insight."

BOX 19.7

Example of Possible Responses to Strengthen and Reinforce Change Talk Using EARS (Elaboration, Affirmations, Reflections, Summaries)—cont'd

CHANGE TALK STATEMENT: "I WOULD LIKE TO HAVE BETTER CONTROL OVER MY BLOOD SUGAR LEVELS (DESIRE)"

- Possible reflective listening responses:
  - "It feels like this is something that you have been thinking about for a while." (This type of reflection should generate a bit more elaboration from the client.)
  - "This is a bit of a concern to you and you're wondering if it is something you might be ready to address." (By paradoxically deemphasizing the importance "bit of a concern," it put the onus on the client to come back and say "actually it is more than a bit of a concern"; the second part of this reflective listening statement allows the ambivalence to be heard by the client. Again, this should lead to further elaboration.)
  - "Your blood sugar control is important to you and you want to get this in hand to avoid longer-term health problems." (This type of reflection is adding some extra meaning back to the client. They have not quite said this so the meaning is inferred.)
  - "You're worried about this but at the same time you're not quite sure if you are ready to change things." (This is a reflection with emotion added but also captures the person's ambivalence about change. If accurate this will strengthen rapport. If it is inaccurate they client will clarify the inaccuracy.)
  - "On the one hand, you want better control over your blood sugar levels but, on the other, you're not convinced you will be able to implement the regular eating patterns to the extent that it would make a lasting difference." (Again, this reflects the ambivalence between the desired outcome and the effort required to achieve this. By reflecting the ambivalence back to the client it avoids the temptation for the clinician to move into "fixing mode" referred to as the righting reflex.)

CHANGE TALK STATEMENT: "I WOULD LIKE TO HAVE BETTER CONTROL OVER MY BLOOD SUGAR LEVELS (DESIRE)"

- Possible summary:
  - This will depend on what else has been elicited and how the dialogue unfolds. However, it will generally include the key themes or examples of change talk statements generated; for example:
  - "You want to get better control over your blood sugar levels. One way that you have been trying to do this is to reduce the long gaps, and also to eat the types of foods that the dietitian has been recommending. One way that you have been monitoring the gaps, as well as the types of foods you are eating, has been to complete the self-monitoring sheets. This was a real struggle initially because you were frightened of family members finding the sheets and judging you. However, you are now getting into the habit of filling them out and you're recognizing when and why the gaps are occurring. You're seeing consistent links between the long gaps and specific episodes of binge eating on high-fat/high-sugar food groups. This is often worse toward the end of the day and especially on days where you have skipped lunch or eaten a less balanced lunch."
  - It can be helpful to add structure to a summary, especially when clients are feeling overwhelmed or do not initially see the links between themes, difficulties, or behaviors (e.g., "You talked about three key issues in relation to gaining better control: First…; Second…; Third").
  - An alternative is to ask the client to offer the summary. This can be helpful to listen to in terms of the order in which the client presents the information back. What is the first thing they mention? What did they miss out? Where did they express most emotion and why?
  - A summary can also be used when you want to shift focus or change direction. This can be helpful at the end of specific strategies such as a decisional balance; two futures; readiness, importance; or confidence ruler.

FOUR PROCESSES IN MOTIVATIONAL INTERVIEWING: APPLICATION TO WEIGHT MANAGEMENT

The conceptual development of MI has evolved and the most recent schematic representation is termed the "four processes model."[6] The model comprises engaging, focusing, evoking, and planning and specific details of the "what," "how," and "when" of each phase are presented below. Fig. 19.1 presents a visual representation of the four process model. It is important to understand that because each process is added to the consult, the preceding ones must be maintained, otherwise the structure of the consult will collapse.

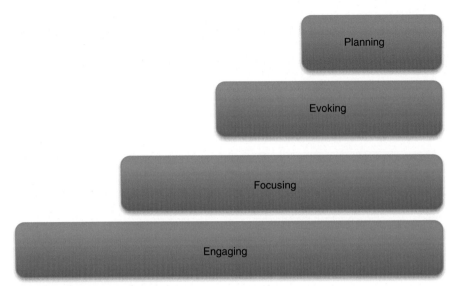

FIG. 19.1 Interdependent four processes of motivational interviewing.

Engaging

The predominant focus of MI is to engage the patient in a collaborative working relationship and create the relational foundation.[6] Although the process of engaging is conceptualized as the first of the four processes, it is essential to view engagement as a critical component of the complete therapeutic journey. Without engagement there is no journey. Useful strategies to help enhance engagement may include "a typical day/week" whereby the patient is invited to describe, in more depth, the impact of factors that may contribute to the maintenance of weight gain behaviors and the associated comorbidities (e.g., poor sleep patterns, patterns of behavioral avoidance, long gaps between meals, triggers for episodes of overeating or binge eating).

We have written previously about the reciprocal links between obesity and depression[26-28] and refer the interested reader to Chapter 16 for a recent review. Although this focuses on one specific mental health comorbidity (depression), the range of biopsychosocial factors associated with obesity and a range of comorbid conditions (see Fig. 19.2) exemplifies the need to engage and fully explore contributing underlying and comaintaining factors for, and between, multiple comorbidities. Exploring the links in this way avoids the premature focus on factors that the clinician may assume are most important to the patient.[5]

Engagement also avoids assuming that the patient is ready, willing, and able to engage in a specific behavior change process and knows what is required to make and maintain the changes identified. A strong focus on engagement as a therapeutic process reduces the likelihood that the clinician will provide unsolicited information regarding standardized "solutions" that could damage the all-important therapeutic alliance. A clinician's fundamental desire to want to "fix" or provide "solutions" and improve a patient's circumstances is referred to as the "righting reflex."[5] The process of engaging helps clinicians to be aware of an inherent desire to fix (often via one-dimensional premature information provision or solutionism). An MI-consistent approach avoids this and instead allows for the emergence of the patients story with respect to their weight-gain journey and, in addition to building trust and rapport, generates a favorable position from which to focus on those behaviors that are most likely to facilitate change.

Focusing

We have outlined earlier in this chapter (and in Chapter 29), the complex nature of the psychology of obesity. We argue that behavioral factors associated with weight gain are multifaceted and best represented and understood as a biopsychosocial construction.[29] Our approach to the assessment and treatment of obesity reflects this complexity. With specific focus on MI, the process of focusing facilitates the collaborative strategic

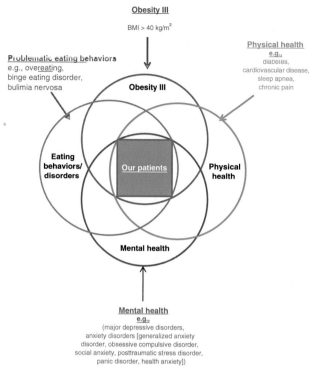

FIG. 19.2 Common comorbid-presenting difficulties within specialist weight management services.

discussion (between patient and clinician) to establish where the most significant behavioral impact(s) on health improvements are likely to be made. Without this focusing process there is a genuine risk that the patient and clinician will engage well but without any clear direction or strategic focus of where the journey is going and what the specific goals may be. For this reason, focusing has been previously described as "an ongoing process of seeking and maintaining direction."[6(p94)] Within MI the directional components of focusing are toward change and in helping an individual to resolve their internal ambivalence. Skilled use (by the clinician) of the microskills (OARS and EARS) described earlier are integral to the way in which this is done.

Arguably, one of the most powerful therapeutic experiences for patients when undertaking the focusing process is the shift from a predominant focus on weight as an outcome to a more dynamic and inclusive exploration of the behavioral factors that have contributed to this outcome. Clinically, our patients report this to be a novel and extremely valuable experience because it helps them to begin to understand <u>why</u> their previous attempts to weight management (e.g., commercial weight loss and exercise programs) have failed (i.e., a premature focus on a simplified one size fits all

solution).[28] By engaging in a focusing process, contributions to perpetual feelings of failure, inadequacy, and low self-worth that often result from unsuccessful weight loss attempts can be avoided (see Fig. 29.3, Chapter 29).

Fig. 19.3 provides an illustrated example of how common factors important to a patient's weight loss journey may be <u>initially</u> mapped out between patient and practitioner and explored. Mapping things out in this way helps to identify and mutually agree how to focus the consultation. Crucially, there are likely to be connections/relationships between the factors identified and written into the map. The clinician and patient will usually work together to unpack these links. Blank circles are provided to add additional factors of importance as they arise.

Such is the importance of a collaborative approach between the patient and clinician in exploring and identifying the most appropriate focus for treatment/therapy, that the similarities between the focusing phase of MI and a formulation approach[8,9] has been suggested previously.[26,27] Within the context of weight management and weight loss surgery, we provide a detailed account of the utility of a five P's formulation framework[30] in Chapter 29 of this book. Sufficient

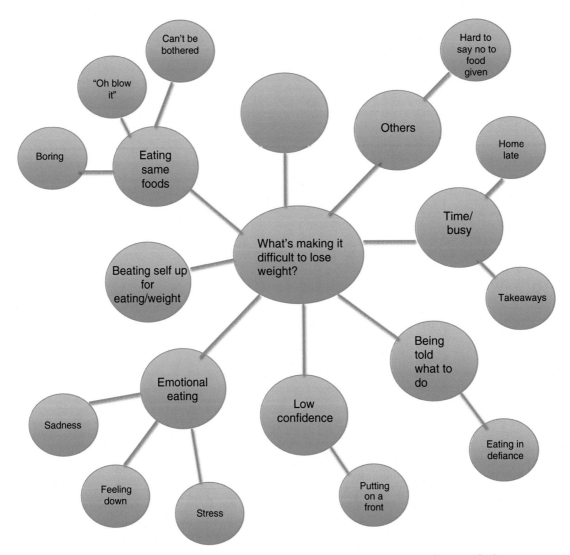

FIG. 19.3 Sample focusing map used in a specialist weight management service consultation.

engagement and focusing with the patient means that both parties are clear about where the journey is heading; this provides the directional platform for change whereby the third MI-process, evoking, is particularly helpful.

Evoking

Exploring the potential discrepancy between current behaviors (e.g., those that contribute to weight gain) and the person's broader goals and values (e.g., healthy aging [not being a burden on family; maintaining independence in late life]) serves as a useful strategy to elicit change talk. A critical consideration, perhaps not just

with respect to the evoking phase of MI, but to the very nature of conversations about change behavior, is that a person's own faith and hope and/or belief in his/her ability to change serve as a powerful motivator. Arguably, this is something that we have more commonly come to identify as self-efficacy.[31]

The primary purpose of evoking is for the clinician to elicit change talk from the patient and then to respond in a way that reinforces or strengthens this (using EARS; see Box 19.7). People tend to feel a greater commitment to what they hear themselves saying,[6] and for this reason, it is important that the clinician continues to resist their "righting reflex" and instead construct

> ### BOX 19.8
> Example of a dialogue which will either elicit *Change Talk* or *Sustain Talk* depending on the way the follow-up question is asked
>
> **EXAMPLE 1: ELICITATION OF CHANGE TALK (UNDERLINED)**
>
> *Practitioner 1*: "On a scale of 1–10, how ready are you to eat breakfast every morning, where 1 is not at all ready and 10 is extremely ready?"
>
> *Patient*: "I would say that I am around 5 out of 10."
>
> *Practitioner 1*: "Why a 5 and not a 1 or a 2?"
>
> *Patient*: Because I know that I should do it. I've been to the dietetic classes and they have talked to me about metabolism and why having breakfast "switches this on." I guess if I had my breakfast, I wouldn't feel so hungry by 10 a.m.; that's when I start to eat the wrong stuff (e.g., fried breakfast at the work's canteen) and I end up just picking all day from there.
>
> **EXAMPLE 2: ELICITATION OF SUSTAIN TALK (UNDERLINED)**
>
> *Practitioner 2*: On a scale of 1–10, how ready are you to eat breakfast every morning, where 1 is not at all ready and 10 is extremely ready?
>
> *Patient*: I would say that I am around 5 out of 10.
>
> *Practitioner 2*: Why a 5 and not a 9 or a 10?
>
> *Patient*: Because I don't have time. It's just such a manic rush in our house first thing. By the time I get up, get them ready for school, do their packed lunches, and walk the dog, I have literally got time to shower and get dressed before I have to leave. I don't even have time to dry my hair....

This patient has previously skipped breakfast in favor of an unhealthy breakfast later in the morning and/or snacking during the morning. Practitioner 1 evokes change talk (underlined); whereas Practitioner 2 evokes sustain talk (underlined). The difference in both examples is simply in the wording of the follow-up question from the practitioner.

Another strategy to elicit change talk involves inviting the patient to reflect on times before the problem emerged and to compare this with the current situation. In this strategy ("looking back"), a clinician may ask, "What was it like for you before you gained weight?" A patient may respond that they were: "More sociable, more active; or that their self-confidence was higher." This highlights the discrepancy between how things may have been better previously compared with the current situation, which can enhance a person's belief in the possibility of their health improving again (e.g., when they can identify the behavioral comaintaining processes that keep the current situation going; see Fig. 29.3, Chapter 29).

Similarly, a strategy named "looking forward" invites the person to consider how their life may be different, if changes were made and improvements occurred with respect to the problems that they are currently experiencing (e.g., decreased weight and improved health outcomes such as increased mobility). A clinician may use the same strategy, in a slightly different way to explore how a patient would feel if no changes or improvements were made when they look ahead. The use of both strategies (i.e., looking at the benefits of future change, as well as the negatives of a future with no changes) has been coined "two possible futures." Looking at both sides of the future in this way elicits change talk across the diagonal's outlines in Box 19.5. A skillful practitioner will then use EARS (see Box 19.7) in response and can chose to direct the consultation toward only the change talk or to more fully explore both change talk and sustain talk. The clinician's role of enhancing the patient's perceived self-efficacy through the use of the microskills (e.g., OARS and EARS) and additional strategies described here serves to build the foundation for the last of the four processes: collaborative planning for change.

Planning

It is striking to consider that helping a person to plan change is something that, in less person-centered and MI-consistent healthcare settings, is almost always prematurely introduced by the clinician. Yet, we see here how much collaborative work has to be undertaken first. This is akin to a joint process of detective work

questions that are designed to elicit change talk[27(p60)] or to elicit both sides of the patient's ambivalence (i.e., change and sustain talk) and help them to understand how this may be incompatible with values and life goals.

Although the use of carefully constructed open questions comprise one way to elicit change talk,[6,27] there are a number of specific strategies that may be specifically used for this aim. For example, the importance and confidence scaling questions referred to earlier have the capacity to generate either *change talk* or *sustain talk* from the values given depending on how the clinician responds via a simple follow-up question: "Why X and not a lower number?" (evokes change talk) versus "Why X and not a higher number?" (evoke sustain talk). The example dialogue in Box 19.8 below highlights this subtle difference with a specific example of a patient trying to eat a breakfast in the morning.

between the patient and clinician, to establish whether the person wants to be there; if they have someone who they are willing and able to work with, who they feel comfortable to be honest and disclose things to (e.g., binge eating); if they have a clear focus and direction for change; and if they are at a point where they are actually ready, willing, and able to move toward a planning stage for change (i.e., they have resolved their long-term ambivalence and linked this discrepancy to important life values/goals). If a person *is* ready, then the collaborative process of planning helps to shift the focus of the consultation from the *why* of change, to the *how to go about it*. The volume, strength, and type of change talk that is heard usually provides a good indicator as to whether a person is ready to move toward planning. For example, the type of change talk may start to move toward more commitment language involving more concrete examples of action-oriented or doing words or imagined scenarios. As mentioned earlier, recapitulating (summarizing) the change talk that has been heard sets the scene well for moving into planning. However, if uncertain, a clinician may simply ask the patient a question that indicates a movement into action planning. An example may be: "Would it be OK if we considered how you might start to incorporate meal planning into your daily routine?" or "if we were to discuss how you might go about being more regulated around your eating behaviors, would that be getting ahead of things?"

Additional strategies to check that it is appropriate to move toward developing a change plan is to ask a "key question" such as "What are you thinking about in terms of how you <u>could</u> better manage your weight at this point?" or "What options are you considering, as a first step, in making a change to your eating patterns?" It is important during this transitional phase from the *why* to the *how* not to rush things. Indeed, this is an important consideration throughout. Remembering to "sit back" and allowing the patient adequate time can help to avoid the temptation to "fill the silence" with further questions (or even worse, unsolicited solutions). An MI-consistent consultation may create the first opportunity for someone to reflect meaningfully on the complexity of all that contributes to his/her weight, wellness, and illness and as such the clinician's ability to sit with and tolerate the uncertainty of not knowing or rushing a plan can often be a powerful experience for a patient. There is a serious risk that the righting reflex can raise its ugly head at this point and it is crucial that the clinician remains patient and stays in evoke mode.

Throughout this chapter we have consistently referred to the importance of *how* things are said or the

way in which things are done. This is equally, if not more important, than what is said or done. Collaboratively developing a change plan with a patient is no exception and builds on the same skills used during the preceding three phases of MI and underpinned by MI Spirit. In general terms, the clearer (and more specific) the goal, the better the clarity and focus of the planning will be. Weight management and obesity is a complex condition. How well the clinician had identified with the patient (engagement) and what behavior is likely to yield the most benefit (focusing) will impact upon the clarity and focus of planning. Additionally, it may be easier to identify progress against short-, medium-, and longer-term goals when they are broken down into process (how) and outcome (what) goals, and when they are much more specific.

During the planning process, the strength of change talk is an important consideration. For example, "I will do" is a much stronger indication of intention than "I might do." Clinicians can better help their patients to develop their own change plan in an MI-consistent way by eliciting and strengthening a person's intentions to implement the emerging plan. One such approach is to elicit "implementation intentions"[32] that comprise (1) a specific plan of action and (2) a statement of intent to do it. This strategy is also useful when identifying what smaller steps might constitute contributing to a much larger long-term goal (i.e., smaller process goals then leading to a larger outcome goal). For example, I will walk to the shops twice this week (on Monday afternoon at 2 p.m. and Friday morning at 9.30 a.m.) may reflect a smaller component of the longer-term goal of wanting to be more physically active. Similar to exploring both the perceived pros and cons of behavior change, within the planning process, a clinician may invite the patient to consider any reluctance or concerns they have about the change plan and this generates the opportunity to again adopt a collaborative approach to problem solving anything that is anticipated to hinder the change process. Box 19.9 offers an overview of what a typical change plan might look like within the context of weight management.

RECOMMENDATIONS FOR TRAINING

Introductory training in MI varies in duration. Typically, a 3-day course with follow-up supervision tailored around eight stages of learning[33] may be a starting point for grounding in the approach. To develop proficiency, attendance at more advanced workshops and ongoing supervision are recommended alongside the assessment of practitioner skills via audiovisual

BOX 19.9
Change Plan Worksheet Example

THE CHANGE I WANT TO MAKE:

1. Reducing gaps between meals

THE MOST IMPORTANT REASONS WHY I WANT TO MAKE THESE CHANGES ARE:

1. To increase my Metabolic Rate
2. To help regulate my blood sugar levels
3. To help to regulate my mood
4. To improve my energy levels

THE STEPS I PLAN TO TAKE FOR THE CHANGES ARE:

1. To have breakfast each morning
2. To take regular snacks to work for morning and afternoon (e.g., fruit, nuts, yogurts, crackers)
3. To make a packed lunch for work every night before bed
4. To do my shopping weekly to ensure always plenty of healthy options available
5. To make sure I don't go longer than 3–4 h between food intake

THE WAYS OTHER PEOPLE CAN HELP ME ARE:

1. My partner can encourage me to eat breakfast
2. My work colleagues can encourage me to have healthy snacks
3. My computer/watch/phone can alert me for regular snack times
4. My boss to allow me to have a regular lunch break away from my desk

I WILL KNOW THAT MY PLAN IS WORKING IF:

1. I am eating regularly
2. My mood improves
3. I feel less tired

SOME THINGS THAT COULD INTERFERE WITH MY PLAN ARE:

1. Busy work schedule
2. Not going shopping regularly enough
3. Not taking snacks into work
4. Being on holiday
5. Colleagues' birthday—chocolate temptations!
6. Being off sick from work
7. Weekends

WHAT I WILL DO IF THE PLAN IS NOT WORKING:

1. Review plan with the specialist weight management services
2. Review plan with partner/colleague/friend/family/employer

feedback. However, it should be stressed that, as with the implementation of <u>any</u> therapeutic skill, attendance at a single MI workshop alone is highly unlikely to result in the level of skill development required for effective clinical practice. The Health Foundation[34] has explored the evidence base for the most effective ways to train practitioners in MI. Their report suggests that effective training techniques should adopt a workshop <u>and</u> coaching model to enhance **skill** development rather than simply **knowledge** development. Furthermore, that training should include workshops not self-guided study; practice sessions and role plays; ongoing supervision; various engagement techniques; application to real behaviors; and practice with others (i.e., trainees, actors/simulated patients). In summarizing the factors that makes for successful training in MI, the Health Foundation suggests that training is most effective when: it begins early in an individual's career; it explores the spirit of MI and not simply the technical skills or specific strategies; ample opportunity for practice, feedback, and ongoing development is included; and ongoing supervision is provided.

The use of the Motivational Interviewing Treatment Integrity Scale (MITI)[35] is often recommended to offer a transparent approach to coding and coaching and to aid skill implementation and development. Practitioners interested in developing proficiency in the clinical application of MI do so by attending appropriate training and engaging in opportunities to assess skills via ongoing coaching, critical self-reflection, audio-video analysis of mock (and where ethically viable) real-life consultations, and assessment via appropriate coding tools such as the MITI[35] or the Motivational Interviewing Skills Code.[36]

Arguably, the use of such scales in isolation is somewhat reductionist in that they do not fully capture the complexity of the interpersonal and dynamic processes involved in a therapeutic clinical interaction. In our own clinical supervision, we use detailed feedback involving video/audio analysis of real-life practice with more extensive clinically focused coding systems (e.g., those that incorporate both qualitative and quantitative feedback on practice; and tools that explore the interpersonal dynamic rather than simply a coding framework that focuses on one half of the dancing partnership [i.e., the practitioner]). We have recently suggested that the use of Computer Assisted Qualitative Data Analysis Systems (CAQDAS) such as QSR-NVivo (http://www.qsrinternational.com/what-is-nvivo)[37] offer much potential to aid the process of clinical skill development[38] within MI. CAQDAS systems offer a much greater degree of transparency[39] in the analysis of complex data. Developments in such software allow a greater level of precision in analysis by facilitating direct coding from video and audio data.

Appropriate training, skill development, and assessment impact on all-important treatment fidelity (i.e., is what a practitioner claiming to demonstrate, an accurate reflection of the [MI] method). This is particularly important with respect to investigations of the impact and efficacy of MI as a valuable assessment and treatment method. Inaccurate and poor quality representations of MI within research settings and clinical trials result in a poor understanding of the utility of the approach.

SUMMARY

The integration of MI within a weight management setting has the capacity to help address collaboratively (between patient and practitioner) the complexity of obesity and avoid a premature and inappropriate focus on simplistic weight loss methods. We have demonstrated how the four processes (engaging, focusing, evoking, and planning) and the use of specific microskills in MI (open questions, affirmations, reflective listening, and summaries: OARS) and strategies (e.g., decisional balance; two futures; scaling questions; looking back/forward) provide a practical and evidence-based approach to structuring therapeutic conversations with patients. Central to the MI approach is an emphasis on the spirit. Crucially, this reflects the interpersonal processes needed to build trust, empathy, and rapport (to enhance the therapeutic relationship). It is not only *what* is done but also *how* it is done that is critical to supporting people through the change process. This is also true of mindfulness-based approaches within weight management, which we turn to next to briefly introduce the reader to an additional approach which is gaining momentum.

MINDFULNESS IN WEIGHT MANAGEMENT

There has been an increased interest in mindfulness-based interventions (MBIs) within clinical health psychology generally[40,41] and within the context of weight management interventions specifically.[42,43] We acknowledge this interest in the utility of mindfulness approaches; however, we do not intend to provide a full exploration and critique of such interventions here. Rather, we highlight key features with respect to weight management and signpost to relevant further reading.

Mindfulness is not a new approach. Although the origins of mindfulness are more spiritual than clinical,

it is increasingly being promoted as a valuable clinical approach.[44] Various approaches to mindfulness have appeared in the clinical literature[45] although a common theme is the importance of paying attention in a particular way, purposefully and nonjudgmentally, to the present moment.[46] An example of mindful eating, therefore, refers to engaging with heightened awareness during eating. Patients may be encouraged to pay close attention to the processes involved in eating slowly and consider in detail the taste, what thoughts they have while chewing, the sensation of swallowing, and feelings of satiety, for example. An example mindful eating script can be found at http://hfhc.ext.wvu.edu/r/download/114469.[47]

The discrepancy of how things are and how a person would like them to be is something that is shared with MI. Mindfulness conceptualizes this observation as an opportunity for individuals to identify and alter behaviors that may contribute to undesirable outcomes (e.g., weight gain).[48] To this end, mindfulness-based cognitive therapy (MBCT)[48] has been introduced into the clinical arena as a viable treatment option for depression, anxiety, and social functioning.[49]

The evidence for the utility of MBIs for behaviors associated with weight management is unclear. Kearney et al.[50] revealed that participation in a 4-month mindfulness program had no impact on emotional or uncontrolled eating. Similarly, Miller, et al.[51] compared a mindful eating to a diabetes self-management intervention among adults with type 2 diabetes and found no significant differences in treatment outcomes over a 3-month period. A mindful restaurant eating intervention was shown to be effective in promoting weight management in perimenopausal women.[43] However, this study suffered similar limitations to those aforementioned in that the study period was only 6 months.

With respect to physical activity, an exploratory randomized controlled trial (RCT) revealed that neither an MBI nor one designed to increase implementation intentions impacted on physical activity, BMI, or body composition compared with controls.[52] However, it is reasonable to suggest that similar to MI, mindfulness is a skill that requires commitment and practice to develop proficiency and the 5 minutes daily over a 6-month period that were required for the study design may not have been sufficient to yield a significant impact on the physiological outcome variables. An exploratory RCT of a mindfulness-based weight loss intervention for women showed at 6 months significantly greater increases in physical activity compared with controls ($P < .05$) but no significant differences in weight loss or mental health. Although interestingly, reductions in

BMI were mediated primarily by reductions in binge eating. A recent systematic review that assessed the impact of mindfulness on binge eating, emotional eating, and/or weight change revealed that mindfulness decreases binge eating and emotional eating, but that evidence for its effect on weight was unclear.[53] A further systematic review and metaanalysis indicated that there were medium to large effect sizes of mindfulness interventions on binge eating although there was high statistical heterogeneity among the studies.[54]

Reviews of the effectiveness of MBIs for obesity-related eating behaviors[55,56] have provided support and a recent RCT that assessed the use of mindfulness to manage weight post–bariatric surgery revealed that mindfulness reduced emotional eating up to 6 months but not weight.[57] However, because of the breadth of what is considered a mindfulness-based approach (e.g., from yoga to MBCT), it is difficult to establish what approach or combination may be the most effective. Furthermore, the RCT is favored as the approach to exploring the application of mindfulness to behaviors related to weight management. However, this approach may be limited because it lacks the ability to be able to assess the process-related factors associated with the quality and impact of mindfulness studies. Unlike qualitative approaches, there is no scope to understand participant experiences of how often they practiced mindfulness during the study period and what their experiences of it as an intervention actually were. Evidence of the value of assessing MBI's qualitatively can be seen in allied health-related research such as the experiences of breast cancer patients.[58] However, similar research relevant to weight management has been slow to respond.

Therefore, once again, the notion of *how* we do things is relevant for MBIs and practice too. For example, it has been suggested that the most important consideration for clinicians who want to implement mindfulness approaches is their own meditation experience.[59] In this respect, considerations of treatment fidelity are also highly relevant to mindfulness-based practice and the assessment of their utility within weight management services. Indeed, Dimidjian and Segal[60] have called for a greater attention to promoting an integrated approach to core research questions, enhanced methodological quality of individual studies, and increased logical links among stages of clinical translation to increase the potential of MBIs to impact positively for individuals and communities. Given that the current evidence for MBIs would seem to suggest that they are effective in helping to manage some of the behaviors associated with weight gain (e.g., binge eating, emotional eating),[52,53,56] it is reasonable to suggest that

MBIs have the capacity to influence weight loss. However, as we have seen, weight management is a complex area that is highly subjective and the very nature of attempting to standardize interventions in an effort to establish what works for whom, when, and under what conditions may be counterproductive. Understanding the utility and impact of MBIs for weight management is in its relative infancy. However, what is clear currently is that empathy and compassion both for self (as the practitioner) and the patients with whom we work are vital components of healthcare[61] and this is a shared concept with both MI and mindfulness.

CONCLUSIONS AND RECOMMENDATIONS

Weight management is complex and therefore this is best addressed via methods that have the capacity to address this complexity. An outcome (or medical-model) only focus is limited in its ability to explore all the behaviors that contribute to a person's ability to manage their weight and is typically prematurely focused on weight loss. MI adopts a person-centered approach to supporting people through their weight loss journey. Relinquishing the clinician role as expert, avoiding the righting reflex and instead integrating the four processes (engaging, focusing, evoking, and planning) and the microskills of MI (open questions, affirmations, reflective listening and summaries: OARS) alongside additional strategies, is much more suited to addressing the broad range of behaviors associated with weight management.

There is a growing interest in the use of mindfulness and MBIs within a weight management context although current research would suggest that the impact of such approaches on weight loss is limited. However, there are some indications that MBIs have the capacity to impact on some of the behaviors associated with weight gain (e.g., binge eating, emotional eating), and therefore, future research may help to inform the utility of MBIs in weight management further.

Something that is central to both MI and mindfulness is the importance of process-related factors (i.e., an emphasis on not only what is done but how it is done). For MI this consideration reflects MI spirit, which is central to the expression of empathy and the development of the therapeutic relationship. For mindfulness, the variance in what is considered mindful practice is problematic, at least from the perspective of gaining a clearer understanding of what works for whom (and under what conditions). However, this variance may also reflect the subjective nature of what approach may have the most impact for someone with complex weight-related issues.

For example, yoga may be sufficient to help one person adjust his/her weight-related behaviors, whereas for another MBCT may be better suited.

"One size does not fit all" and therefore a formulation-based individualized intervention is needed within specialist services. Arguably, MI as an approach is very well suited to compliment this approach. The concept of MI can be learned reasonably quickly. However, becoming a skillful MI practitioner is something that develops with practice, ongoing coaching, and supervision. There has been an increased recognition and focus, in recent years, on the importance of the relationship in MI (with an emphasis on interpersonal processes)[7] as with any interpersonal approach, it is the therapeutic alliance which is crucial.

REFERENCES

1. Naar-King S, Earnshaw P, Breckon J. Toward a universal maintenance intervention: integrating cognitive behavioral treatment with motivational interviewing for maintenance of behavior change. *J Cogn Psychother*. 2013;27(2):126–137. http://dx.doi.org/10.1891/0889-8391.27.2.126.
2. Hutchison A, Johnston L. Exploring the potential of case formulation within exercise psychology. *J Clin Sport Psychol*. 2013;7(1):60–76. http://dx.doi.org/10.1123/jcsp.7.1.60.
3. Johnston LH, Hutchison AJ. Influencing health behaviour: applying theory to practice. In: Scott A, Gidlow C, eds. *Clinical Exercise Science*. 2015. London: Routledge; 2016:224–246.
4. Miller WR, Rollnick S. *Motivational Interviewing: Preparing People to Change Addictive Behavior*. London: Guilford Press; 1991.
5. Miller W, Rollnick S. *Motivational Interviewing: Preparing People for Change*. 2nd ed. London: Guilford Press; 2002.
6. Miller W, Rollnick S. *Motivational Interviewing*. 3rd ed. New York, NY: Guilford Press; 2013.
7. Moyers T. The relationship in motivational interviewing. *Psychotherapy*. 2014;51(3):358–363. http://dx.doi.org/10.1037/a0036910.
8. Johnstone L, Dallos R. Introduction to formulation. In: Johnstone L, Dallos R, eds. *Formulation in Psychology and Psychotherapy*. London: Routledge; 2006:1–16.
9. Johnstone L, Dallos R. *Formulation in Psychology and Psychotherapy*. 2nd ed. London: Routledge; 2013.
10. Miller W. Motivational interviewing with problem drinkers. *Behav Psychother*. 1983;11(02):147–172. http://dx.doi.org/10.1017/s0141347300006583.
11. Rogers C. *A Way of Being*. 1st ed. Boston: Houghton Mifflin; 1980.
12. Motivational Interviewing Network Trainers (MINT). Motivational Interviewing Resources. Available at: http://motivationalinterviewing.org/motivational-interviewing-resources. Accessed January 25th, 2017.
13. Hardcastle S, Blake N, Hagger M. The effectiveness of a motivational interviewing primary-care based intervention on physical activity and predictors of change in a disadvantaged community. *J Behav Med*. 2012;35(3):318–333. http://dx.doi.org/10.1007/s10865-012-9417-1.
14. Vella-Zarb R, Mills J, Westra H, Carter J, Keating L. A randomized controlled trial of motivational interviewing+self-help versus psychoeducation+self-help for binge eating. *Int J Eat Disord*. 2014;48(3):328–332. http://dx.doi.org/10.1002/eat.22242.
15. David L, Sockalingam S, Wnuk S, Cassin S. A pilot randomized controlled trial examining the feasibility, acceptability, and efficacy of adapted motivational interviewing for post-operative bariatric surgery patients. *Eat Behav*. 2016;22:87–92. http://dx.doi.org/10.1016/j.eatbeh.2016.03.030.
16. Norcross J. *Psychotherapy Relationships that Work*. 2nd ed. New York: Oxford University Press; 2011.
17. Moyers T, Houck J. Combining motivational interviewing with cognitive-behavioral treatments for substance abuse: lessons from the COMBINE research project. *Cogn Behav Pract*. 2011;18(1):38–45. http://dx.doi.org/10.1016/j.cbpra.2009.09.005.
18. Miller W, Moyers T. The forest and the trees: relational and specific factors in addiction treatment. *Addiction*. 2014;110(3):401–413. http://dx.doi.org/10.1111/add.12693.
19. Moyers T, Miller W. Is low therapist empathy toxic? *Psychol Addict Behav*. 2013;27(3):878–884. http://dx.doi.org/10.1037/a0030274.
20. Hilton C, Lane C, Johnston L. Has motivational interviewing fallen into its own premature focus trap? *Int J Adv Couns*. 2016;38(2):145–158. http://dx.doi.org/10.1007/s10447-016-9262-y.
21. Festinger L. *A Theory of Cognitive Dissonance*. 1st ed. Evanston, Ill. [u.a.]: Row, Peterson; 1957.
22. Miller W, Rose G. Motivational interviewing, decisional balance: contrasting responses to client ambivalence. *Behav Cogn Psychother*. 2013;43(02):129–141. http://dx.doi.org/10.1017/s1352465813000878.
23. Glynn L, Moyers T. Chasing change talk: the clinician's role in evoking client language about change. *J Subst Abuse Treat*. 2010;39(1):65–70. http://dx.doi.org/10.1016/j.jsat.2010.03.012.
24. Barton J, Dew K, Dowell A, et al. Patient resistance as a resource: candidate obstacles in diabetes consultations. *Sociol Health Illn*. 2016;38(7):1151–1166. http://dx.doi.org/10.1111/1467-9566.12447.
25. Amrhein P, Miller W, Yahne C, Palmer M, Fulcher L. Client commitment language during motivational interviewing predicts drug use outcomes. *J Consult Clin Psychol*. 2003;71(5):862–878. http://dx.doi.org/10.1037/0022-006x.71.5.862.
26. Watt A, Johnston LH, Wells T. Sticky plasters and septic wounds: one dietitian's journey in weight management (Part 1). *Complete Nutr*. 2016;16(1):60–62.

27. Watt A, Johnston LH, Wells T. Sticky plasters and septic wounds: one dietitian's journey in weight management (Part 2). *Complete Nutr.* 2016;16(2):60–62.

28. Watt A, Johnston LH, Wells T. One size does not fit all: using a formulation approach within specialist weight management services. *Diet Today.* 2016.

29. Andrasik F, Goodie J, Peterson A. Biopsychosocial assessment. In: *Clinical Health Psychology.* 1st ed. London: Guilford Press; 2015.

30. Dudley R, Kuyken W. Formulation in cognitive behavioural therapy: There is nothing either good or bad, but thinking makes it so. In: Johnstone L, Dallos R, eds. *Formulation in Psychology and Psychotherapy.* London: Routledge; 2006:17–46.

31. Bandura A. *Social Learning Theory.* 1st ed. Englewood Cliffs, NJ: Prentice Hall; 1977.

32. Rise J, Thompson M, Verplanken B. Measuring implementation intentions in the context of the theory of planned behavior. *Scand J Psychol.* 2003;44(2):87–95. http://dx.doi.org/10.1111/1467-9450.00325.

33. Miller W, Moyers T. Eight stages in learning motivational interviewing. *J Teach Addict.* 2006;5(1):3–17. http://dx.doi.org/10.1300/j188v05n01_02.

34. The Health Foundation. *Research Scan: Training Professionals in Motivational Interviewing.* London: The Health Foundation; 2011.

35. Moyers TB, Manuel JK, Ernst D. *Motivational Interviewing Treatment Integrity Coding Manual 4.0.* Unpubl Manual; 2014.

36. Miller WR, Moyers TB, Ernst D, Amrhein P. Manual for the Motivational Interviewing Skills Code: Version 2.1. Available at: http://casaa.unm.edu/download/misc.pdf. Accessed January 25, 2017.

37. QSR International. What is NVIVO? http://www.qsrinternational.com/what-is-nvivo. Accessed January 25, 2017.

38. Johnston L, McMaster F, Hilton C. *How Can QSR NVivo Software Help People Reflect on Their Clinical Practice and Supervision? Motivational Interviewing Network of Trainers International Conference and Annual Training of New Trainers (TNT).* Berlin, Germany; 2015.

39. Bringer J, Johnston L, Brackenridge C. Maximizing transparency in a doctoral thesis 1: the complexities of writing about the use of QSR*NVIVO within a grounded theory study. *Qual Res.* 2004;4(2):247–265. http://dx.doi.org/10.1177/1468794104044434.

40. Loucks E, Britton W, Howe C, Eaton C, Buka S. Positive associations of dispositional mindfulness with cardiovascular health: the new England family study. *Int J Behav Med.* 2014;22(4):540–550. http://dx.doi.org/10.1007/s12529-014-9448-9.

41. Roberts K, Danoff-Burg S. Mindfulness and health behaviors: is paying attention good for you? *J Am Coll Health.* 2010;59(3):165–173. http://dx.doi.org/10.1080/07448481.2010.484452.

42. Mantzios M, Giannou K. Group vs. Single mindfulness meditation: exploring avoidance, impulsivity, and weight management in two separate mindfulness meditation settings. *Appl Psychol Health Well-Being.* 2014;6(2):173–191. http://dx.doi.org/10.1111/aphw.12023.

43. Timmerman G, Brown A. The effect of a mindful restaurant eating intervention on weight management in women. *J Nutr Educ Behav.* 2012;44(1):22–28. http://dx.doi.org/10.1016/j.jneb.2011.03.143.

44. Carmody J. Evolving conceptions of mindfulness in clinical settings. *J Cogn Psychother.* 2009;23(3):270–280. http://dx.doi.org/10.1891/0889-8391.23.3.270.

45. Langer E, Moldoveanu M. The construct of mindfulness. *J Soc Issues.* 2000;56(1):1–9. http://dx.doi.org/10.1111/0022-4537.00148.

46. Kabat-Zinn J. *Wherever You Go, There You Are.* 1st ed. New York: Hyperion; 1994.

47. West Virginia University. Eating One Raisin: A First Taste of Mindfulness. http://hfhc.ext.wvu.edu/r/download/114469. Accessed January 25th 2017.

48. Segal Z, Williams J, Teasdale J. *Mindfulness-based Cognitive Therapy for Depression.* 2nd ed. New York: Guilford Press; 2013.

49. Askey-Jones R, Flanagan E. Mindfulness-based cognitive therapy in clinical practice. *Ment Health Pract.* 2016;19(5):28–35. http://dx.doi.org/10.7748/mhp.19.5.28.s19.

50. Kearney D, Milton M, Malte C, McDermott K, Martinez M, Simpson T. Participation in mindfulness-based stress reduction is not associated with reductions in emotional eating or uncontrolled eating. *Nutr Res.* 2012;32(6):413–420. http://dx.doi.org/10.1016/j.nutres.2012.05.008.

51. Miller C, Kristeller J, Headings A, Nagaraja H. Comparison of a mindful eating intervention to a diabetes self-management intervention among adults with type 2 diabetes. *Health Educ Behav.* 2014;41(2):145–154. http://dx.doi.org/10.1177/1090198113493092.

52. Cleobury L, Tapper K. Exploratory randomised controlled trial of a mindfulness and implementation intention intervention to target physical activity and BMI. *Appetite.* 2012;59(2):623. http://dx.doi.org/10.1016/j.appet.2012.05.051.

53. Katterman S, Kleinman B, Hood M, Nackers L, Corsica J. Mindfulness meditation as an intervention for binge eating, emotional eating, and weight loss: a systematic review. *Eat Behav.* 2014;15(2):197–204. http://dx.doi.org/10.1016/j.eatbeh.2014.01.005.

54. Godfrey K, Gallo L, Afari N. Mindfulness-based interventions for binge eating: a systematic review and meta-analysis. *J Behav Med.* 2014;38(2):348–362. http://dx.doi.org/10.1007/s10865-014-9610-5.

55. Godsey J. The role of mindfulness based interventions in the treatment of obesity and eating disorders: an integrative review. *Complement Ther Med.* 2013;21(4):430–439. http://dx.doi.org/10.1016/j.ctim.2013.06.003.

56. O'Reilly G, Cook L, Spruijt-Metz D, Black D. Mindfulness-based interventions for obesity-related eating behaviours: a literature review. *Obes Rev.* 2014;15(6):453–461. http://dx.doi.org/10.1111/obr.12156.

57. Chacko S, Yeh G, Davis R, Wee C. A mindfulness-based intervention to control weight after bariatric surgery: preliminary results from a randomized controlled pilot trial. *Complement Ther Med*. 2016;28:13–21. http://dx.doi.org/10.1016/j.ctim.2016.07.001.

58. Schellekens M, Jansen E, Willemse H, van Laarhoven H, Prins J, Speckens A. A qualitative study on mindfulness-based stress reduction for breast cancer patients: how women experience participating with fellow patients. *Support Care Cancer*. 2015;24(4):1813–1820. http://dx.doi.org/10.1007/s00520-015-2954-8.

59. Caldwell K, Baime M, Wolever R. Mindfulness based approaches to obesity and weight loss maintenance. *J Ment Health Couns*. 2012;34(3):269–282. http://dx.doi.org/10.17744/mehc.34.3.t016616717774643.

60. Dimidjian Segal Z. Prospects for a clinical science of mindfulness-based intervention. *Am Psychol*. 2015;70(7):593–620. http://dx.doi.org/10.1037/a0039589.

61. Raab K. Mindfulness, self-compassion, and empathy among health care professionals: a review of the literature. *J Health Care Chaplain*. 2014;20(3):95–108. http://dx.doi.org/10.1080/08854726.2014.913876.

CHAPTER 20

The Role of Physical Activity and Exercise in Managing Obesity and Achieving Weight Loss

DR. MATTHEW D. CAMPBELL, PHD, ACSM CEP, BSC •
DR. ZOE H. RUTHERFORD, PHD, MSC, BSC

INTRODUCTION

Our curiosity, individually and as a society, is a continuous and unrelenting driver in the search of a magical weight loss quick fix. Ask almost anyone and he/she will tell you that it is certainly not exercise, however. Even in those individuals who value exercise and understand its associated benefits, many view exercise as daunting and as a long, slow, arduous slog. Unsurprisingly, a common question often encountered within a clinical setting is how much exercise is needed to lose weight and keep the weight off and what type of exercise will achieve this most effectively. The answer is not always obvious or, indeed, consistent. The sheer abundance of easily accessible information at the hands of the public is simply overwhelming and, to the scientific and medical community, of alarming concern. The vast majority of advice served to us online or through media outlets is out of control; information is often oversimplified and overextrapolated at best and is inaccurate, unsubstantiated, and of conflicting opinion at worst.

A logical place to start is to define what is meant by *exercise*. Is exercise the same as being physically active? Are we physically active if we exercise but spend large periods of the day sedentary? How much, and how much of what, yields the greatest weight loss success? And, how does this affect our health in a wider context? The aim of this chapter is to offer some clarity when considering these questions through a review of the available scientific evidence regarding exercise-based weight loss interventions.

EXERCISE, PHYSICAL ACTIVITY, PHYSICAL INACTIVITY, AND SEDENTARINESS

Exercise and physical activity, and physical inactivity and sedentariness, respectively, are often thought of as synonymously interchangeable—but they are not necessarily. *Physical activity* can be thought of as any form of bodily movement that results in increasing energy expenditure above resting levels. Energy expenditure is a continuous variable ranging from low to high and is the product, and interaction, of the intensity, duration, and frequency of activity.[1,2] It is important to acknowledge that everyone performs some degree of physical activity, but the amount largely differs from person to person, as well as within a given person, and that this is subject to personal choice and the demands of everyday life. The term *exercise* is often confused with *physical activity*,[3] and this is understandable because both involve bodily movement that expends energy in relation to intensity, frequency, and duration. However, exercise differs in that it is planned, structured, repetitive, and purposive and is simply a component of physical activity.[1,3] Exercise itself can be subdivided into classifications largely including aerobic exercise, high-intensity intermittent exercise, and resistance exercise. A comprehensive overview of exercise modality is beyond the scope of this chapter, but interested readers are directed to the American College of Sports Medicine Exercise Testing and Prescription Guidelines.[4]

Conversely, physical inactivity is the opposite, whereby time is spent in a resting state (sitting, sleeping). In this respect, sedentariness is a component of physical inactivity characterized by prolonged periods during waking hours spent at low levels of energy expenditure, such as prolonged sitting at home, at work, or in transport, but not sleep.[5] Activities that propagate sedentariness, such as television viewing, are termed sedentary behaviors.

AEROBIC EXERCISE

Aerobic exercise involves the continuous and rhythmic use of large muscle groups,[4] such as walking, jogging, cycling, and swimming. In practical terms, this means sustaining a self-perceived moderate-to-vigorous exercise intensity for a prolonged period. Current guidance stipulates that people with obesity should engage in aerobic exercise 5–7 days/week, with each session lasting 45–60 min[4,6] such that the amount of exercise undertaken within in a week totals a minimum of 150 min.[7] This recommendation serves as the minimum amount of exercise needed to maintain health, not weight loss however. Those individuals seeking to lose weight or prevent weight regain over the long term are advised to increase exercise duration to 200–300 min/week.[6,8,9] For most individuals, this equates to expending over 2000 kcal/week (or over 400 kcal/session). To put this into perspective, most individuals would need to walk or jog 1 mile to expend 100 calories, which is the same as one slice of bread or four heaped tablespoons of sugar. Based on this guidance, it is clear that a substantial amount of aerobic exercise is needed for people with obesity to lose weight or maintain weight loss in those who have successfully lost weight. However, weight loss resulting from aerobic exercise is highly variable due, at least in part, to individual differences in total energy expenditure for a set amount of given exercise and subsequent compensatory changes in dietary caloric intake.[10]

In studies evaluating weight change in response to aerobic exercise prescription consistent with current guidance, most demonstrate only modest weight loss and some demonstrate no weight loss at all.[11–14] For example, in the Inflammation and Exercise (INFLAME) study[11] (n = 129), 4 months of aerobic exercise training resulted in only minimal weight loss (~0.4 kg), which was no different to a nonexercise control group. In line with this investigation, the Dose Response to Exercise in Women (DREW) study[12] assessed weight loss in response to performing aerobic exercise consistent with public health recommendations in postmenopausal women (n = 464) over a 6-month duration. Despite achieving adherence rates, the researchers observed no significant changes in weight (~–2.2 kg). Interestingly, in this study the authors found that weight loss

remained minimal even when aerobic exercise was performed at 150% of public health recommendations (~–0.6 kg). The Targeted Risk Reduction Intervention through Defined Exercise (STRRIDE) study[13] (n = 84) investigated the interaction between exercise amount and intensity, assessing 6 months of exercise training at (1) a low amount at a moderate intensity, (2) a low amount at a vigorous intensity, or (3) a high amount at a vigorous intensity. Irrelevant of the exercise intensity, weight loss was the lowest with the least amount of exercise performed (moderate intensity ~–0.6 kg vs. vigorous intensity ~–0.2 kg), and although weight loss was greater when increasing exercise amount, the total weight lost was still minimal (~–1.5 kg). In a cohort of people with type 2 diabetes, the Diabetes Aerobic and Resistance Exercise (DARE) study[14] (n = 251) observed statistically significant weight loss after 22 weeks of aerobic training compared with a nonexercise control group, although the amount of weight lost was once again minimal (~0.74 kg).

It is important to note that the aforementioned studies represent the strongest research design to evaluate changes in weight from aerobic exercise training because they have a large sample size of people who are overweight or obese at baseline, feature supervised exercise training sessions to ensure high rates of compliance, report strong adherence rates, include a control group for comparing changes in weight, and controlled confounding factors, such as complementary dietary interventions. Overall, people who are overweight or obese seeking to lose weight through aerobic exercise alone (i.e., without a complementary dietary intervention such as caloric restriction) can expect to experience weight loss in a range of no weight loss to ~2 kg (0%–3% loss in body weight) when adhering to a training program consistent with current guidelines. With this in mind, clinicians should caution their patients, and practitioners should make clear to their clients, that the chances of substantial weight loss are unlikely at these exercise training levels without caloric restriction.[7] An important limitation of the present data in this area is that sufficiently robust long-term (>1 year) and time-course studies are not currently available.

Within the literature, some studies implementing supervised aerobic exercise training do demonstrate significant weight reduction in the absence of caloric restriction.[7,15,16] However, these interventions have prescribed exercise at levels that far exceed the minimum amount of exercise recommended according to public health guidance.[7] In one study, an 8% reduction in body weight was achieved in people with obesity after only 12 weeks of aerobic exercise training without altering dietary habits.[15] The exercise prescription in this study translated to an energy expenditure of ~700 kcal/session; for an individual weighing ~90 kg this is equivalent to cycling leisurely for ~2 h or, in food terms, the same calories contained in a cheeseburger and medium portion of fries. In a different study,[15] overweight (body mass index [BMI] >27 kg m²) premenopausal women followed 14 weeks of aerobic exercise training with an energy expenditure of 500 kcal/session, and this resulted in a 6.8% reduction in weight. In addition, in an investigation by Donnelly and colleagues[7] a 5.3% reduction in weight was observed in overweight men after 16 weeks of aerobic exercise training expending ~2000 kcal/week—which, in terms of recommended calorie intake for an average women, is equivalent to abstaining from food for a whole day. Notably, in this study, women participating in the exercise intervention did not have a significant reduction in weight (~−0.7 kg), although, any prospective weight gain was prevented whereas this was not in a nonexercise control group (~+2.9 kg). In light of the above, it is possible to achieve clinically significant weight loss with aerobic exercise training in the absence of caloric restriction, but exercise training volume must be substantially greater than levels currently recommended, and the results are likely to be variable. For the general population and the average person with obesity, such training volumes are unlikely to be practical or sustainable.

HIGH-INTENSITY INTERMITTENT-BASED EXERCISE

High-intensity intermittent exercise—which is often termed interval or HIIT training—involves performing repeated bouts of exercise at an intense effort interspersed by low-intensity exercise or periods of rest with varied recovery times. The exercise periods may range from 5 s to 8 min long with recovery periods varying in length and with total exercise duration lasting between 20 and 60 min.[4]

The most obvious advantage of high-intensity exercise is the shorter time frame needed to expend an appropriate amount of energy.[17] This is an important consideration because when energy expenditure is matched, the reduction in weight is the same as when exercising for 300 min/week at a moderate intensity or 200 min/week at a vigorous intensity.[18] Interestingly, Ross and colleagues[18] observed differential changes in body fat distribution, following a high-intensity versus aerobic-based exercise training program. Following 24 weeks of a high-intensity exercise program,

abdominal obesity was reduced by ~4.6 cm (range −6.2 to 3.0 cm) compared with a reduction of ~3.6 cm (range −5.1 to 2.2 cm) following an aerobic training program of equivalent length. Considering that a reduction in abdominal girth of ~5 cm is associated with 9% lower mortality risk,[19] this finding is all the more clinically relevant. In addition, increasing exercise intensity may provide additional health benefits beyond increased energy expenditure.[18,20,21]

RESISTANCE EXERCISE

Resistance training is primarily designed to improve muscle fitness by exercising a muscle or a muscle group against external resistance (such as free weights, weight machines, body weight, elastic tubing, medicine balls, or even common household products). The caveat with resistance exercise is that it is important to ensure maintenance of correct technique to minimize injury, which, for most nonexercising individuals, requires proper tuition and supervision. Guidelines for undertaking resistance exercise differ depending on whether hypertrophy, muscular strength, power, and endurance are the targeted outcomes.[4] Resistance exercise should form an important part of any exercise training program because it is associated with many exercise-specific health benefits, such as the prevention of sarcopenia and preservation of bone mineral density, both of which are associated with aging and inactivity.[22,23] However, resistance exercise is often overlooked from a weight management perspective. Overall, little evidence exists, demonstrating that resistance exercise training alone promotes weight loss. In one study conducted by Church and colleagues,[24] 9 months of resistance exercise training did not result in a significant change in weight compared with a nonexercise control group, and this seems to be a consistent finding within the literature.[14,25] Although resistance exercise may not improve weight loss per se, resistance training does contribute to the reduction of body fat[7] and increases lean body mass.[26] Thus, people with obesity performing resistance exercise may not see significant reductions in weight, whereas they can expect improvements in body composition.

COMBINED AEROBIC AND RESISTANCE EXERCISE

There are very few randomized controlled trials (RCTs) investigating whether combining aerobic and resistance exercise training leads to greater weight loss compared with aerobic or resistance exercise training alone. Of the available evidence, however, it would seem that weight loss following participation in a combined aerobic and resistance exercise training program results in similar reductions to performing aerobic exercise training alone.[14,24] With this said, combining aerobic and resistance exercise training may result in enhanced effects for other health indicators. For example, looking at the HART-D[14,24] and DARE[15] trials, data would suggest that the combined effects of resistance and aerobic exercise training in people with type 2 diabetes promote greater changes in glycemic control compared with those performing aerobic exercise alone.

PHYSICAL INACTIVITY AND SEDENTARY TIME: WHY IS BEING ACTIVE IMPORTANT BEYOND WEIGHT LOSS?

Sedentary Behavior and Physical Inactivity

A goal of obesity management is to recommend safe, sustainable, and science-based behaviors to the public. Recommending exercise or general improvements in physical activity levels at lower intensities, if demonstrated to be effective, hold great promise because these may provide a more achievable and realistic solution for the vast majority of the unfit, inactive population if the perceived exertion is low enough. Indeed, it is important that we consider nonfatiguing and safe types of physical activity in the lower end of the physical activity continuum, because the proportion of the population that require sedentary interventions have the greatest health concerns. With this in mind, the biggest question still requiring unanswered is what behaviors are most effective and practical to prescribe.

Historically, the approach taken has been to emphasize moderate-to-vigorous exercise.[27,28] However, the effect of "too much sitting" is not the same as not performing enough exercise.[29-32] There has been a rapid emergence in research, indicating that sedentary behavior is associated with disease risk, independent of exercise levels.[29-36] Data indicates that, even in individuals who exercise twice the recommended 150 min/week level, sedentary time (expressed as either total time spent sitting or total daily nonexercise activity) are similar to those who almost never exercise.[37] Long periods of inactivity are typical in modern-day lifestyles. Indeed, when accumulating time spent sitting at work and at home, it is not unreasonable to suggest that many of us spend ~10 h/day spent inactive. In fact, recent studies indicate that most people sit more than half of every day or between 50% and 75% of the waking day.[37] From a weight management perspective, total sitting time across the life span appears to be associated with abnormal glucose and lipid metabolism, diabetes,[38-42]

metabolic syndrome,[43-52] and overall cardiometabolic risk[53-55] and all-cause mortality[54,56,57] independent of BMI and whether one participates in moderate-to-vigorous exercise or not. Therefore, although it is plausible that sedentary behavior promotes excess body fat and this in turn contributes to disease risk, epidemiologic data also elude to a need to consider additional, more distinct, mechanisms beyond body fat and BMI. This is likely because the physiologic processes mediating the effects of sedentary behavior on health operate via acute and transient metabolic processes, which are not on the same time scale in which changes in body composition take to occur.[58-61]

A large proportion of research investigates the dual effect of sitting down for long periods (to watch TV for example) combined with feeding (i.e., eating snacks or meals).[62] From a practical and ecological perspective, this direction of research is helpful because this is largely representative of modern-day living. It is certainly plausible to hypothesize that eating during prolonged periods spent sedentary is detrimental to health, such as unhealthy postprandial responses.[57,63-65] This is highly relevant considering that people with obesity typical display poor postprandial responses, including elevated 2-h glucose,[53] prolonged and exaggerated lipemia,[53,54] fasting insulin,[55] and lower high-density lipoprotein (HDL) cholesterol.[53] Bearing in mind that people with obesity are placed at a substantially increased risk of developing type 2 diabetes and metabolic syndrome, it is possible that this risk is likely augmented by successive acute episodes of disturbed postprandial metabolism that are perpetually manifested by prolonged periods spent inactive. Fundamental to this concept is that muscle cells constantly sense and respond to their environment. Thus, ensuring regular stimulation through increasing physical activity over the whole day is important. This means that metabolically important muscle tissue is potentially responsive to *total* time spent active, not just time spent performing isolated bouts of exercise. In support of this, inactivity invokes molecular processes notably through a rise in the expression and repression of specific genes.[66] Hence, evidence suggests that the detrimental effects of prolonged inactivity may not be completely counteracted by isolated moderate-to-vigorous exercise. This implies that there is value in interrupting sedentariness with light-intensity activities, such as standing or walking, at least in physically inactive subjects.[60,67]

Accumulating evidence from large observational studies have indicated that breaking up long periods spent sedentary may improve cardiometabolic risk[68-70] and reduce mortality from all causes[71] independent of the amount of moderate-to-vigorous exercise performed.[52] Unsurprisingly, this has provoked the inclusion of recommendations around reducing sedentary behavior, specifically stating that long periods of sitting should be interrupted regularly with physical activity[72,73] and office-working adults should aim to increase their standing and light-intensity activity to between 2 and 4 h/day.[74] From a weight management perspective, studies have demonstrated that interrupting sedentary time is related to a lower waist circumference[53,63,68,69] and BMI.[68] However, it is important to stress that some of the most robust evidence available suggests that it is not necessarily how sedentary time is accumulated, but that it is total time spent being sedentary that carries the largest risk; total sedentary time is significantly related to metabolic syndrome,[52] glucose tolerance and postprandial handling,[53,63,68,69,75] and inflammation,[69,76] with most of these risk factors remaining significant even when total time spent sedentary is adjusted for breaks[52,68] and waist circumference or BMI.[53,63,75,76]

Studies that compare a single day of sitting are insightful because the time is short enough to identify some of the more potent responses that are obviously independent of changes in body composition.[58–61] In one tightly controlled laboratory-based study, participants were exposed to a nonsedentary condition consisting of a large duration of intermittent low-intensity physical activity to counterbalance sitting time throughout ~66% of the waking day. Such activities in this condition were diverse and designed to mimic many of the typical activities of daily living, such as dishwashing, folding clothes, and putting away groceries. This corresponded to an estimated energy expenditure of ~44 kcal/h greater than in a sedentary control condition. This intensity of physical activity is relatively light and is below the range described as "health promoting" in physical activity guidelines; yet, the authors observed a 39% reduction in insulin-stimulated glucose uptake (tracer-determined plasma glucose uptake per unit of insulin) after a night of rest and before getting out of bed.[59] In a second study[59] the effect of acute and intermittent walking was assessed at two different intensities during the postprandial period in overweight and/or obese middle-aged adults.[59] An insightful and novel finding of that study was that, despite a twofold difference in walking speeds (2.0 vs. 3.6–4.0 mph), glucose and insulin responses through the postprandial period were essentially identical, suggesting that the metabolic benefits of this range of intermittent activity are independent of intensity. It remains to be seen if an even lower intensity activity that could be sustained for

longer and integrated into a large part of the day to displace more sedentary time would be more potent. This is important because many overweight and unfit individuals may find walking ~4 mph in bouts lasting only 2 min difficult. In addition, regardless of fitness and weight, it may not be practical for many people to alter the workplace or other domains to replace many hours of sedentary time with moderate or vigorous activity. Even in people who can exercise for an hour per day, Duvivier et al.[60] reported that replacing sedentary time with a large amount of nonexercise physical activity was more effective than exercise in reducing plasma triglyceride, non-HDL cholesterol, and postprandial insulin. Interestingly, in support of Stephens et al.,[59] the authors concluded that duration was *more* important than intensity because the caloric expenditure of exercise versus nonexercise activity was matched.[60]

The currently available prospective experimental studies do advocate that breaking up sitting time and replacing it with light-intensity ambulatory physical activity and standing may be a stimulus sufficient enough to induce acute favorable changes in the postprandial metabolic parameters, at least in physically inactive people and in those with type 2 diabetes. Despite convincing evidence of the positive effects of replacing prolonged sitting with light-intensity physical activity in physically inactive subjects, a higher intensity or volume seems to be more effective in rendering such positive outcomes in young habitually, physically active subjects.[71] Breaking up sitting time fundamentally implies interrupting prolonged periods spent sitting in environments such as the work place (i.e., desk-bound office work) or home (i.e., during TV watching). Therefore it is of the upmost importance that strategies for "breaking up sitting" are both feasible, that is, capable of interrupting prolonged sitting without disturbing or impairing attention to task, and effective in improving cardiometabolic parameters. In this context, a recent review by Torbeyns et al.[77] reported that active workstations (such as standing or treadmill workstations) seemed to positively affect important health parameters while not affecting work efficiency. Therefore, this may be regarded as a feasible and effective vehicle to reduce sitting time in the work place; however, this body of evidence is not without methodological limitations that affect their direct translation to real life.[78] Moreover, such recommendations should be made with the individual patient in mind as some individuals may be unable to tolerate periods of standing.

In clinical practice, it is difficult to motivate some individuals to perform aerobic exercise training at a sufficient level to achieve significant weight loss.

Indeed, many individuals find the prospect of radically changing their lifestyle to incorporate exercise training daunting or even unrealistic. A tool often used by clinicians and exercise practitioners is to concentrate on decreasing the time spent sedentary through increasing daily physical activity levels rather than the promotion of exercise sessions. An easy, inexpensive, and accessible tool for monitoring physical activity habits and prescribing physical activity modification is the use of pedometers. Pedometers are devices that count the number of steps that an individual accumulates through the day.[79] The current consensus states that obtaining less than 5000 steps per day is indicative of sedentary behavior, whereas greater than 10,000 steps suggest a more active lifestyle. Pedometer-based interventions where sedentary participants increase physical activity to 10,000 steps or 2000–4000 above baseline levels have shown some positive effects for weight loss; in general, however, weight loss tends to be very modest (2 kg).[79] Richardson et al.[80] performed a meta-analysis on pedometer-based interventions without caloric restriction (median duration 16 weeks) and observed that the pooled estimated change in weight was ~−1.3 kg. Therefore, although decreasing total sedentary behavior through increasing step count may provide some, albeit little, weight loss, little empirical evidence exists that a pedometer-based program alone without caloric restriction can promote clinically significant weight loss.

Traditionally, the management of energy balance has been achieved through an increase in physical activities to enhance energy expenditure, which is mostly accompanied by dietary restriction. However, it is suggested that daily activities may not only affect an individual's energy expenditure but also play a role in the control of appetite and energy intake. Evidence has shown that physical activity,[81-83] sedentary behaviors, and sleeping duration[22,32] can also affect energy consumption at all ages.

TV viewing is currently one of the main sedentary pastimes at all ages, and many publications have underlined its association with overweight and obesity.[84] Although this association has been attributed to the low energy expenditure it requires, it has been reported that watching TV is also associated with increased meal frequency and food consumption,[85-91] regardless of appetite sensations.[92,93] Children and adolescents have been shown to consume a substantial proportion of their daily energy while watching TV,[86,94,95] and also that food choice is altered in which energy dense and palatable food items are self-selected, whereas fruit and vegetables are neglected.[88,90,96-98]

Although watching TV remains the preferred leisure-time activity of most children and adolescents, the interest and practice of video games has been growing recently in youth.[99] More than 50% of children report eating while playing computer or video games.[100] This contemporary trend has been related to the progression of overweight and obesity[101-104] and has been primarily attributed to decreased energy expenditure with seated video-gaming.[105] However, the practice of computer-related activities promotes overconsumption of food in adolescents[106] and adults.[106,107] However, not all video games involve sedentary sitting patterns. Active video games (involving large body movements) are popular and may result in increased energy expenditure, which may offset increases in energy intake.[108-111] Indeed, the energy expenditure of active gaming has been found to be up to two to three times the energy expended during seated television viewing[112,113] and even higher than walking at 1.5 mph while watching TV. However, increases in energy expenditure from active video games are unlikely to produce any weight loss due to possible compensations in food intake and/or compensatory activity adjustments.[110,114-116]

A plethora of studies have been conducted examining the appetite, appetite-regulatory hormone, and energy intake responses to acute and chronic exercise.[117] Current evidence suggests that increasing energy expenditure during short-term exercise training days elicit partial compensations in energy intake.[7,118-131] Furthermore, a recent systematic review concluded that longer-term exercise training studies (>2 weeks to 18 months) typically observe no change in energy intake across the training intervention;[132] however, it is important to note that the available literature is prone to a number of methodological shortcomings (unsupervised exercise, self-reported energy intake), which makes it difficult to interpret the findings with confidence. In one study directly comparing isoenergetic 3-day energy deficits imposed by either diet or exercise, it was reported that dietary restriction stimulated a compensatory increase in ad libitum energy intake, which was not observed in response to exercise.[133] This supports the findings from acute studies demonstrating rapid compensatory changes (appetite, appetite-regulatory hormones, energy intake) in response to diet, but not to exercise-induced energy deficits.[134,135] These findings suggest that dietary restriction may represent a greater challenge to appetite regulation and energy balance than exercise, highlighting the importance of exercise to facilitate weight management/loss.[9,117]

DIET VERSUS EXERCISE-INDUCED WEIGHT LOSS

Ross and colleagues[15] exposed 52 men to one of four conditions for 3 months: (1) diet-induced weight loss, (2) exercise-induced weight loss, (3) exercise without weight loss, or (4) a control group. Both the diet-induced and exercise-induced weight loss groups lost approximately 7 kg of weight (~8% weight reduction). In addition, both groups demonstrated a significant reduction in total fat mass and visceral fat and an increase in glucose disposal. Interestingly, however, a greater reduction in total fat mass was evident under the exercise-induced weight loss group compared with the diet-induced weight loss group. Furthermore, improvements in cardiorespiratory fitness and visceral fat were observed in both exercise groups with or without weight loss, whereas this was not observed in the diet-induced weight loss group.

These observations by Ross and colleagues[136] further highlight that exercise training confers important health benefits to people with obesity even when weight loss is not achieved. Despite the possibility of improving cardiovascular risk factors through dieting alone, exercise training should be encouraged with a focus on improving cardiorespiratory fitness, which is independently associated with the risk of cardiovascular disease, type 2 diabetes, and overall mortality.

EXERCISE TRAINING COUPLED WITH CALORIC RESTRICTION

It is well recognized that for those wishing to achieve significant weight loss, caloric restriction is likely to yield greater results than exercise alone.[137] However, the literature is less clear whether weight loss from caloric restriction is enhanced by adding exercise training or increasing overall physical activity levels. In a metaanalysis of weight loss interventions, Miller and colleagues[137] determined that the rate of weight loss was similar following caloric restriction alone (~0.98 kg/week) or following caloric restriction combined with exercise training (~1.0 kg/week). However, it is important to note that the weight loss achieved in this study exceeds by far that of exercise training alone (~0.2 kg/week). Therefore, it is not unreasonable to conclude that the majority of weight loss, resulting from combined exercise and caloric restriction interventions, is largely attributed to the contribution of caloric restriction. As discussed previously, however, exercise and physical activity play important roles in overall weight maintenance and also cardiovascular fitness[138]—which improves in direct response to aerobic

exercise training[136] but not with caloric restriction alone. Although caloric restriction may have a more profound and consistent effect on weight loss compared with exercise training, the importance of the latter should not be undervalued and form an important part of a weight-loss program.[15,137]

As previously established, the dose response effect of exercise-induced weight loss is not clear. However, this is not the case when exercise is coupled with caloric restriction.[139] Jakicic and colleagues[139] observed a dose response between long-term weight loss and the amount of self-reported weekly exercise over an 18-month period. Those individuals who exercised greater than 200 min/week lost considerably more weight compared with those who exercised between 150 and 199 min/week and those who failed to achieve more than 150 min/week (~−13.1 kg vs. ~−8.5 kg vs. ~−3.5 kg, respectively). This was supported by findings in a different study by Jakicic et al.,[139] investigating a weight loss intervention that is composed of both caloric restriction and exercise training in women. Following 12 months of caloric restriction coupled with exercise training, the women in the study exercising more than 200 min/week (13.6%) achieved a significantly greater proportion of weight loss compared with those exercising at 150–199 min/week (9.5%), and greater still than those exercising for 150 min/week (4.7%). Lastly, Anderson et al.[140] evaluated the effect of a low-fat, low-calorie diet (1200 kcal/day) in combination with either structured aerobic exercise training or lifestyle activity (increasing physical activity to recommended levels), and both groups lost approximately ~8 kg of weight following 16 weeks of the program. On follow-up 1 year after the intervention, those who were most active were reported to have lost additional weight (~−1.9 kg), whereas a substantial amount of weight was regained in those who were reported to be least active (~+4.9 kg). These findings illustrate that exercise has an important role not only in weight loss, when coupled with dietary modification, but also in longer-term weight management following successful weight loss.

DIFFERENCES IN EXERCISE-INDUCED WEIGHT LOSS RESPONSE BETWEEN SEXES

The efficacy of exercise as a successful strategy for weight management varies markedly between individuals.[141] Interestingly, it has been suggested that sex may be a primary factor that affects the ability of structured exercise to promote weight loss and/or facilitate weight management.[142] In general, studies have demonstrated that men experience greater weight loss than women in response to a supervised program of exercise when exercise is prescribed at a similar duration and relative intensity across the sexes.[122,123,143,144] However, in many studies, the exercise-induced energy expenditure was substantially greater in men than women, and when energy expenditure is matched, weight loss is similar between sexes.[125,126,145] A common finding in the literature is the degree of individual variation in the weight loss response to exercise training in both sexes.[125,126,141,146–148] It has been suggested that individual differences in compensatory behavior, which negate the exercise-induced energy deficit, may be responsible for the variability.[141] Specifically, evidence of increased hunger and energy intake have been reported in individuals who experience a lower-than-expected weight loss after a period of exercise training.[141,147,148] For a more comprehensive review of this literature the reader is directed to an excellent article by Thackray and colleagues,[117] which discusses the interaction of exercise, appetite, and sex in weight management.

EXERCISE AND PHYSICAL ACTIVITY INTERVENTIONS TARGETED AT OBESE CHILDREN AND YOUTH

Childhood obesity is a known independent risk factor for obesity in adulthood. Moreover, problems in endocrine and cardiovascular functioning, as well as mental health concerns, are prevalent in children and adolescents with obesity,[149] which often persist into adulthood.[150] In short, being obese in childhood is an important early risk factor for adult morbidity and mortality.[150,151]

When data are pooled, childhood exercise interventions are associated with a statistically significant reduction in BMI compared with nonexercise control conditions.[152] However, the magnitude of BMI change following exercise interventions is unlikely to achieve a level to be considered as clinically significant.[153] With this said, the level of change required to achieve population-wide public health significance for obesity prevention among nonobese children is not entirely known.[152]

Interestingly, when assessing the pooled effects of different types of intervention studies (i.e., sedentary behavior vs. sedentary behavior + physical activity vs. sedentary behavior + physical activity + diet) separately, none has demonstrated a significant effect in BMI reduction, and multicomponent studies (i.e., sedentary behavior + physical activity or sedentary behavior + physical activity + diet) were no more effective in

BMI reduction than interventions aimed at tackling sedentary behavior alone[152,154]; however, this is not always shown especially when multicomponent interventions include counseling and/or medication.[155]

From a practical perspective, it may be that alerting one behavior is easier to accomplish than altering two or more behaviors at the same time for children. In fact, most multiple health behavior change interventions in children failed to achieve significant changes, and the successful ones were all found in adults.[156] However, it is important to note that in the meta-analysis conducted by Liao et al.,[152] the effect of the interventions on targeted behavior change (i.e., sedentary behavior, physical activity, dietary intake) was not evaluated. Therefore, it is not clear whether the BMI reduction in multicomponent interventions was a result of a decrease in sedentary behavior, an increase in physical activity, an improvement in diet, or any combination thereof. In addition, the analysis included both prevention studies (interventions that targeted the general population) and treatment studies (interventions that were exclusively for overweight and obese children), which may have attenuated the observed effect of BMI reduction as the effect size is generally higher in treatment studies.[114,155,157]

Interestingly, studies in which the intervention has been prescribed in clinic include multicomponent interventions. Often in clinical practice, there is emphasis on the provision of all available evidence-based strategies for BMI reduction to patients, but this does not necessarily consider how pragmatic this may be within the limited contact time available. Bearing this in mind, clinical health practitioners might want to consider focusing solely on one behavior change component to reduce BMI for pediatric patients.

A limitation of the majority of evidence available is a failure to report socioeconomic status and ethnicity, and almost all studies have been conducted in North America and Europe. Childhood obesity is a global problem and the prevalence rate is increasing in developing countries and cultures.[158,159] Children's lifestyles are different across countries and cultures, and therefore lifestyle interventions, such as sedentary behavior interventions, to prevent childhood obesity may not be generalizable and universally effective. In addition, it is important to consider that an important part of any child's weight management should be the inclusion of a structured and supported parent/family behavior change component as a child is unlikely to be able to directly modify his/her own lifestyle individually.

THE WIDER BENEFITS OF PHYSICAL ACTIVITY

Regardless of the amount of weight loss, clinicians should emphasize that numerous health benefits occur in the absence of weight loss and that maintenance of an active lifestyle will reduce the risk of future weight gain.[7,160] Clinical trials of exercise training that report no weight loss or modest weight loss (<5 kg) still report numerous health benefits for overweight and obese adults with risk factors for disease. These benefits include improvements in cardiorespiratory fitness,[12,161] glucose control,[14,24] endothelial function,[162,163] lipoprotein particle size,[13] and HDL;[164] reduction in visceral fat and fat distribution;[165–169] and improvement in the quality of life.[170,171] This is true whether regular aerobic exercise is performed or general physical activity levels are increased through, for example, step counting.[172]

For overweight and obese individuals, the benefits of weight loss are clear and consistent. However, in individuals with established cardiovascular disease, the clinical impact of weight loss may not be as clear. Recent data suggest that, in individuals with cardiovascular disease, higher BMI levels are associated with better survival rates compared with those with lower levels.[173] This phenomenon has been termed the "obesity paradox" and has been shown in a variety of cardiovascular conditions, including heart failure, hypertension, and coronary heart disease.[173] Much of these data are epidemiologic in nature, therefore reverse causation may be an important factor. More research is needed to determine the extent to which the relationships are explained by the obesity paradox and whether actively losing weight or weight maintenance is protective against mortality-specific populations. Many studies that show weight loss with physical activity as a component have shown improvements in cardiovascular disease risk factors,[22] reduced progression to type 2 diabetes,[174] and lower mortality.[136] Importantly, higher cardiorespiratory fitness levels appear to be protective against mortality in all BMI categories[175] and alter the relationship of the obesity paradox. Thus the current evidence suggests that overweight/obese individuals should still participate in exercise training but focus on moderate weight loss objectives. However, further investigation of the obesity paradox is certainly warranted.

COMMUNITY-BASED ADULT WEIGHT MANAGEMENT

Although the literature presented thus far has examined the dose-response relationship between exercise and weight loss in a controlled environment or research design through clinical trials, the tools available to clinicians, such as general practitioners (GPs), in the "real world" require further inspection in terms of what works. Many GPs will prescribe their patients with an evidence-based weight loss intervention in line with the Exercise is Medicine model[176] that takes place in the community through a variety of locations (e.g., leisure centers, community centers, sporting locations) and delivered by different providers (e.g., health trainers, exercise professionals, football in the community). Interventions are usually based on reducing weight for general health or to improve health markers associated with metabolic disease risk.

Evidence-based guidance for weight loss provision in the United Kingdom outline that interventions should include a combination of physical activity and dietary change and that they are part of a program of behavior change.[177] Typically these interventions consist of dietary education, goal setting, peer-support and exercise instruction, and additional low-cost/free physical activity/exercise opportunities (instructed and noninstructed sessions, such as gym memberships, swimming, and walking). One of the key performance indicators of such interventions is that participants should lose 5% of their starting weight over the normal duration of the intervention (10–12 weeks[178]).

Although there has been a large increase in research examining the efficacy of community-based behavior change weight management interventions in adults over the last 10 years, there remains a limited critical mass in terms of the quality of these studies when reporting external validity of the different components, which makes it difficult to generalize their results.[179] This is largely because of the "real-world" settings that these interventions take place, which means that RCTs are not appropriate and research, therefore, tends to be quasiexperimental. The lack of process information and additional measures of body fatness and distribution (waist circumference), fitness, and health (BP, lipid, and glucose profiles) also means that it is difficult to interpret the reason for some of the smaller reductions in weight loss that are typically observed.[180]

For example, in a randomized control study of overweight (BMI >27 kg m²) Taiwanese adults with metabolic syndrome, a community-based exercise intervention consisted of one 40-min instructor led aerobic session per week, which was supplemented by an additional five 40-min aerobic or walking-based sessions.[181] Participants in the intervention group were supported by volunteers who were trained in delivering health messages and who sent reminders via text messages or phone calls (vs. control group who had access to exercise but no support). After 6 months and with 97% compliance, the weight loss of the intervention group reduced their body weight by 1.1 kg ($P<.000$) (vs. −0.65 kg in the control group). Within the intervention group, this minimal change in weight was accompanied, however, by a reduction in waist circumference of 3.63 cm and favorable changes in systolic blood pressure (SBP), diastolic blood pressure (DBP), and HDL, which are all markers for cardiometabolic health.

In a pragmatic RCT, Hunt and colleagues[182] examined a weight loss and healthy living program for overweight and obese men delivered by Scottish Premier League football clubs (FFIT). Seven hundred forty-seven men aged between 35 and 65 years were randomized to receive the FFIT intervention or comparator (1:1), stratified by club. FFIT was delivered free of charge to participants by trained community coaching staff employed by clubs. Sessions took place every week for 12 weeks at the club's home stadium, and each 90-min session combined advice on healthy diet with physical activity. As men became fitter, the balance of classroom and physical activity sessions changed to focus on physical activity and the shorter classroom sessions focused on revision. After the 12-week program 47% of men significantly reduced their weight by 5% (vs. −7%) and 37% (vs. −11%) of men were able to have achieved this at 12-month follow-up. Similar quasiexperimental studies have found comparable reductions in body weight as well as waist circumference and fitness (6-min walk) in the short term (12 weeks) in both men (−4.96 kg, −6.29 cm, 70.22 m; $P<.05$) and women (−4.26 kg, −5.90 cm, 35.29 m; $P<.05$).

As with the clinical-based trials, it is important that practitioners do not rely solely on weight loss as a marker for health in community interventions, because the benefits of increased fitness and waist circumference, in particular, may be a stronger predictor of improvements in cardiometabolic health. This is especially important for delivery staff to recognize that modest reductions in weight, despite an increase in physical activity and modification in diet, may demotivate individuals when a goal setting approach is used, and additional measures of body fatness and fitness may help them to stay motivated and change behavior long term.

SUMMARY

It must be recognized that recommendations should be used in the context of an individual's needs, goals, and initial abilities. In this regard, a sliding scale as to the amount of time allotted and intensity of effort should be carefully gauged for weight loss or weight

maintenance. The important factor is to design a program for the individual to provide achievable and sustainable weight loss and/or management and to ensure adherence to a physically active lifestyle to profit from the vast array of health benefits but at a lower risk of dropout. With this in mind, permanent lifestyle change should be emphasized rather than the adoption of exercise or physical activity alone.

REFERENCES

1. Caspersen CJ, Powell KE, Christenson GM. Physical activity, exercise, and physical fitness: definitions and distinctions for health-related research. *Public Health Rep.* 1985;100(2):126.
2. Taylor HL, Jacobs DR, Schucker B, Knudsen J, Leon AS, Debacker G. A questionnaire for the assessment of leisure time physical activities. *J Chronic Dis.* 1978;31(12):741–755.
3. Taylor HL. Physical activity: is it still a risk factor? *Prev Med.* 1983;12(1):20–24.
4. Medicine ACoS. *ACSM's Guidelines for Exercise Testing and Prescription.* Lippincott Williams & Wilkins; 2013.
5. Owen N, Leslie E, Salmon J, Fotheringham MJ. Environmental determinants of physical activity and sedentary behavior. *Exerc Sport Sci Rev.* 2000;28(4):153–158.
6. McQueen MA. Exercise aspects of obesity treatment. *Ochsner J.* 2009;9(3):140–143.
7. Donnelly J, Blair S, Jakicic J, Manore M, Rankin J, Smith B. Appropriate physical activity intervention strategies for weight loss and prevention of weight regain for adults. (41:459, 2009) *Med Sci Sports Exerc.* 2009;41(7):1532.
8. Jakicic JM, Clark K, Coleman E, et al. American College of Sports Medicine Position Stand. Appropriate intervention strategies for weight loss and prevention of weight regain for adults. *Med Sci Sports Exerc.* 2001;33(12):2145–2156.
9. Donnelly JE, Blair SN, Jakicic JM, Manore MM, Rankin JW, Smith BK. American College of Sports Medicine Position Stand. Appropriate physical activity intervention strategies for weight loss and prevention of weight regain for adults. *Med Sci Sports Exerc.* 2009;41(2):459–471.
10. Thomas D, Bouchard C, Church T, et al. Why do individuals not lose more weight from an exercise intervention at a defined dose? An energy balance analysis. *Obes Rev.* 2012;13(10):835–847.
11. Church TS, Earnest CP, Thompson AM, et al. Exercise without weight loss does not reduce C-reactive protein: the INFLAME study. *Med Sci Sports Exerc.* 2010;42(4):708.
12. Church TS, Earnest CP, Skinner JS, Blair SN. Effects of different doses of physical activity on cardiorespiratory fitness among sedentary, overweight or obese postmenopausal women with elevated blood pressure: a randomized controlled trial. *JAMA.* 2007;297(19):2081–2091.

13. Kraus WE, Houmard JA, Duscha BD, et al. Effects of the amount and intensity of exercise on plasma lipoproteins. *N Engl J Med.* 2002;347(19):1483–1492.

14. Sigal RJ, Kenny GP, Boulé NG, et al. Effects of aerobic training, resistance training, or both on glycemic control in type 2 diabetes: a randomized trial. *Ann Intern Med.* 2007;147(6):357–369.

15. Ross R, Dagnone D, Jones PJ, et al. Reduction in obesity and related comorbid conditions after diet-induced weight loss or exercise-induced weight loss in men: a randomized, controlled trial. *Ann Intern Med.* 2000;133(2):92–103.

16. Ross R, Janssen I, Dawson J, et al. Exercise-induced reduction in obesity and insulin resistance in women: a randomized controlled trial. *Obes Res.* 2004;12(5):789–798.

17. Committee PAGA. *Physical Activity Guidelines Advisory Committee Report.* Washington, DC: US Department of Health and Human Services; 2008.

18. Ross R, Hudson R, Stotz PJ, Lam M. Effects of exercise amount and intensity on abdominal obesity and glucose tolerance in obese adults: a randomized trial. *Ann Intern Med.* 2015;162(5):325–334.

19. Berentzen TL, Jakobsen MU, Halkjaer J, Tjønneland A, Overvad K, Sørensen TI. Changes in waist circumference and mortality in middle-aged men and women. *PLoS One.* 2010;5(9):e13097.

20. Gillen JB, Gibala MJ. Is high-intensity interval training a time-efficient exercise strategy to improve health and fitness? *Appl Physiol Nutr Metab.* 2013;39(3):409–412.

21. Weston KS, Wisløff U, Coombes JS. High-intensity interval training in patients with lifestyle-induced cardiometabolic disease: a systematic review and meta-analysis. *Br J Sports Med.* 2014;48(16):1227–1234.

22. Haskell WL, Lee I-M, Pate RR, et al. Physical activity and public health: updated recommendation for adults from the American College of Sports Medicine and the American Heart Association. *Circulation.* 2007;116(9):1081.

23. Winett RA, Carpinelli RN. Potential health-related benefits of resistance training. *Prev Med.* 2001;33(5):503–513.

24. Church TS, Blair SN, Cocreham S, et al. Effects of aerobic and resistance training on hemoglobin A1c levels in patients with type 2 diabetes: a randomized controlled trial. *JAMA.* 2010;304(20):2253–2262.

25. Bateman LA, Slentz CA, Willis LH, et al. Comparison of aerobic versus resistance exercise training effects on metabolic syndrome (from the studies of a targeted risk reduction intervention through defined exercise-STRRIDE-AT/RT). *Am J Cardiol.* 2011;108(6):838–844.

26. McGuigan MR, Tatasciore M, Newton RU, Pettigrew S. Eight weeks of resistance training can significantly alter body composition in children who are overweight or obese. *J Strength & Cond Res.* 2009;23(1):80–85.

27. Colberg SR, Sigal RJ, Fernhall B, et al. Exercise and type 2 diabetes the American College of Sports Medicine and the American Diabetes Association: joint position statement. *Diabetes Care.* 2010;33(12):e147–e167.

28. Health UDo, Services H, Health UDo, Services H. *Physical Activity Guidelines for Americans;* 2008.

29. Hamilton MT, Hamilton DG, Zderic TW. Exercise physiology versus inactivity physiology: an essential concept for understanding lipoprotein lipase regulation. *Exerc Sport Sci Rev.* 2004;32(4):161.

30. Hamilton MT, Healy GN, Dunstan DW, Zderic TW, Owen N. Too little exercise and too much sitting: inactivity physiology and the need for new recommendations on sedentary behavior. *Curr Cardiovasc Risk Rep.* 2008;2(4):292–298.

31. Hamilton M, Owen N. *Sedentary Behavior and Inactivity Physiology. Physical Activity and Health.* 2nd ed. Champaign, Illinois: Human Kinetics; 2012:59–61.

32. Hamilton MT, Hamilton DG, Zderic TW. Role of low energy expenditure and sitting in obesity, metabolic syndrome, type 2 diabetes, and cardiovascular disease. *Diabetes.* 2007;56(11):2655–2667.

33. Edwardson CL, Gorely T, Davies MJ, et al. Association of sedentary behaviour with metabolic syndrome: a meta-analysis. *PLoS One.* 2012;7(4):e34916.

34. Saunders TJ, Larouche R, Colley RC, Tremblay MS. Acute sedentary behaviour and markers of cardiometabolic risk: a systematic review of intervention studies. *J Nutr Metab.* 2012;2012.

35. Thorp AA, Owen N, Neuhaus M, Dunstan DW. Sedentary behaviors and subsequent health outcomes in adults: a systematic review of longitudinal studies, 1996–2011. *Am J Prev Med.* 2011;41(2):207–215.

36. Wilmot EG, Edwardson CL, Achana FA, et al. Sedentary time in adults and the association with diabetes, cardiovascular disease and death: systematic review and meta-analysis. *Diabetologia.* 2012;55:2895–2905.

37. Craft LL, Zderic TW, Gapstur SM, et al. Evidence that women meeting physical activity guidelines do not sit less: an observational inclinometry study. *Int J Behav Nutr Phys Act.* 2012;9(1):1.

38. Kriska A, Delahanty L, Edelstein S, et al. Sedentary behavior and physical activity in youth with recent onset of type 2 diabetes. *Pediatrics.* 2013;131(3):e850–e856.

39. George ES, Rosenkranz RR, Kolt GS. Chronic disease and sitting time in middle-aged Australian males: findings from the 45 and up Study. *Int J Behav Nutr Phys Act.* 2013;10(1):1.

40. Hu FB, Leitzmann MF, Stampfer MJ, Colditz GA, Willett WC, Rimm EB. Physical activity and television watching in relation to risk for type 2 diabetes mellitus in men. *Arch Intern Med.* 2001;161(12):1542–1548.

41. Krishnan S, Rosenberg L, Palmer JR. Physical activity and television watching in relation to risk of type 2 diabetes the black Women's health study. *Am J Epidemiol.* 2009;169(4):428–434.

42. Tonstad S, Butler T, Yan R, Fraser GE. Type of vegetarian diet, body weight, and prevalence of type 2 diabetes. *Diabetes Care.* 2009;32(5):791–796.

43. Bertrais S, Beyeme-Ondoua JP, Czernichow S, Galan P, Hercberg S, Oppert JM. Sedentary behaviors, physical activity, and metabolic syndrome in middle-aged French subjects. *Obes Res.* 2005;13(5):936–944.

44. Dunstan D, Salmon J, Owen N, et al. Associations of TV viewing and physical activity with the metabolic syndrome in Australian adults. *Diabetologia*. 2005;48(11):2254–2261.

45. Ford ES, Kohl HW, Mokdad AH, Ajani UA. Sedentary behavior, physical activity, and the metabolic syndrome among US adults. *Obes Res*. 2005;13(3):608–614.

46. Gao X, Nelson ME, Tucker KL. Television viewing is associated with prevalence of metabolic syndrome in Hispanic elders. *Diabetes Care*. 2007;30(3):694–700.

47. Li C-L, Lin J-D, Lee S-J, Tseng R-F. Associations between the metabolic syndrome and its components, watching television and physical activity. *Public Health*. 2007;121(2):83–91.

48. Chang P-C, Li T-C, Wu M-T, et al. Association between television viewing and the risk of metabolic syndrome in a community-based population. *BMC Public Health*. 2008;8(1):1.

49. Chen X, Pang Z, Li K. Dietary fat, sedentary behaviors and the prevalence of the metabolic syndrome among Qingdao adults. *Nutr Metab Cardiovasc Dis*. 2009;19(1):27–34.

50. Sisson SB, Camhi SM, Church TS, et al. Leisure time sedentary behavior, occupational/domestic physical activity, and metabolic syndrome in US men and women. *Metab Syndr Relat Disord*. 2009;7(6):529–536.

51. Trinh OT, Nguyen ND, Phongsavon P, Dibley MJ, Bauman AE. Metabolic risk profiles and associated risk factors among Vietnamese adults in Ho Chi Minh City. *Metab Syndr Relat Disord*. 2010;8(1):69–78.

52. Bankoski A, Harris TB, McClain JJ, et al. Sedentary activity associated with metabolic syndrome independent of physical activity. *Diabetes Care*. 2011;34(2):497–503.

53. Henson J, Yates T, Biddle SJ, et al. Associations of objectively measured sedentary behaviour and physical activity with markers of cardiometabolic health. *Diabetologia*. 2013;56(5):1012–1020.

54. Wijndaele K, Orrow G, Ekelund U, et al. Increasing objectively measured sedentary time increases clustered cardiometabolic risk: a 6 year analysis of the ProActive study. *Diabetologia*. 2014;57(2):305–312.

55. Ekelund U, Griffin SJ, Wareham NJ. Physical activity and metabolic risk in individuals with a family history of type 2 diabetes. *Diabetes Care*. 2007;30(2):337–342.

56. Koster A, Caserotti P, Patel KV, et al. Association of sedentary time with mortality independent of moderate to vigorous physical activity. *PLoS One*. 2012;7(6):e37696.

57. Matthews CE, George SM, Moore SC, et al. Amount of time spent in sedentary behaviors and cause-specific mortality in US adults. *Am J Clin Nutr*. 2012;95(2):437–445.

58. Dunstan DW, Kingwell BA, Larsen R, et al. Breaking up prolonged sitting reduces postprandial glucose and insulin responses. *Diabetes Care*. 2012;35(5):976–983.

59. Stephens BR, Granados K, Zderic TW, Hamilton MT, Braun B. Effects of 1 day of inactivity on insulin action in healthy men and women: interaction with energy intake. *Metabolism*. 2011;60(7):941–949.

60. Duvivier BM, Schaper NC, Bremers MA, et al. Minimal intensity physical activity (standing and walking) of longer duration improves insulin action and plasma lipids more than shorter periods of moderate to vigorous exercise (cycling) in sedentary subjects when energy expenditure is comparable. *PLoS One*. 2013;8(2):e55542.

61. Manohar C, Levine JA, Nandy DK, et al. The effect of walking on postprandial glycemic excursion in patients with type 1 diabetes and healthy people. *Diabetes Care*. 2012;35(12):2493–2499.

62. Van Uffelen JG, Wong J, Chau JY, et al. Occupational sitting and health risks: a systematic review. *Am J Prev Med*. 2010;39(4):379–388.

63. Cooper A, Sebire S, Montgomery A, et al. Sedentary time, breaks in sedentary time and metabolic variables in people with newly diagnosed type 2 diabetes. *Diabetologia*. 2012;55(3):589–599.

64. Balkau B, Mhamdi L, Oppert J-M, et al. Physical activity and insulin sensitivity the RISC study. *Diabetes*. 2008;57(10):2613–2618.

65. Lahjibi E, Heude B, Dekker J, et al. Impact of objectively measured sedentary behaviour on changes in insulin resistance and secretion over 3 years in the RISC study: interaction with weight gain. *Diabetes Metab*. 2013;39(3):217–225.

66. Bey L, Akunuri N, Zhao P, Hoffman EP, Hamilton DG, Hamilton MT. Patterns of global gene expression in rat skeletal muscle during unloading and low-intensity ambulatory activity. *Physiol Genomics*. 2003;13(2):157–167.

67. Peddie MC, Bone JL, Rehrer NJ, Skeaff CM, Gray AR, Perry TL. Breaking prolonged sitting reduces postprandial glycemia in healthy, normal-weight adults: a randomized crossover trial. *Am J Clin Nutr*. 2013;98(2):358–366.

68. Healy GN, Dunstan DW, Salmon J, et al. Breaks in sedentary time beneficial associations with metabolic risk. *Diabetes Care*. 2008;31(4):661–666.

69. Healy GN, Matthews CE, Dunstan DW, Winkler EA, Owen N. Sedentary time and cardio-metabolic biomarkers in US adults: NHANES 2003–06. *Eur Heart J*. 2011:ehq451.

70. Saunders TJ, Chaput J-P, Goldfield GS, et al. Prolonged sitting and markers of cardiometabolic disease risk in children and youth: a randomized crossover study. *Metabolism*. 2013;62(10):1423–1428.

71. Katzmarzyk PT. Standing and mortality in a prospective cohort of Canadian adults. *Med Sci Sports Exerc*. 2014;46(5):940–946.

72. Brown WJ, Bauman AE, Bull FC, Burton NW. *Development of Evidence-based Physical Activity Recommendations for Adults (18–64 Years): Report Prepared for the Australian Government Department of Health*; August 2012. 2013.

73. Bull F, Biddle S, Buchner D, Ferguson R, Foster C, Fox K. *Physical Activity Guidelines in the UK: Review and Recommendations*. School of Sport, Exercise and Health Sciences, Loughborough University; 2010.

74. Buckley JP, Hedge A, Yates T, et al. The sedentary office: a growing case for change towards better health and productivity. Expert statement commissioned by Public Health England and the Active Working Community Interest Company. *Br J Sports Med*. 2015. http://dx.doi.org/10.1136/bjsports-2015-094618.

75. Healy GN, Dunstan DW, Salmon J, et al. Objectively measured light-intensity physical activity is independently associated with 2-h plasma glucose. *Diabetes Care*. 2007;30(6):1384–1389.

76. Henson J, Yates T, Edwardson CL, et al. Sedentary time and markers of chronic low-grade inflammation in a high risk population. *PLoS One*. 2013;8(10):e78350.

77. Torbeyns T, Bailey S, Bos I, Meeusen R. Active workstations to fight sedentary behaviour. *Sports Med*. 2014;44(9):1261–1273.

78. Benatti FB, Ried-Larsen M. The effects of breaking up prolonged sitting time: a review of experimental studies. *Med Sci Sports Exerc*. 2015;47(10):2053–2061.

79. Tudor-Locke C, Bassett Jr DR. How many steps/day are enough? *Sports Med*. 2004;34(1):1–8.

80. Richardson CR, Newton TL, Abraham JJ, Sen A, Jimbo M, Swartz AM. A meta-analysis of pedometer-based walking interventions and weight loss. *Ann Fam Med*. 2008;6(1):69–77.

81. Blundell JE, Stubbs RJ, Hughes DA, Whybrow S, King NA. Cross talk between physical activity and appetite control: does physical activity stimulate appetite? *Proc Nutr Soc*. 2003;62(03):651–661.

82. Martins C, Morgan L, Truby H. A review of the effects of exercise on appetite regulation: an obesity perspective. *Int J Obes*. 2008;32(9):1337–1347.

83. Thivel D, Blundell JE, Duché P, Morio B. Acute exercise and subsequent nutritional adaptations. *Sports Med*. 2012;42(7):607–613.

84. Swinburn B, Shelly A. Effects of TV time and other sedentary pursuits. *Int J Obes*. 2008;32:S132–S136.

85. Sonneville KR, Gortmaker SL. Total energy intake, adolescent discretionary behaviors and the energy gap. *Int J Obes*. 2008;32:S19–S27.

86. Matheson DM, Killen JD, Wang Y, Varady A, Robinson TN. Children's food consumption during television viewing. *Am J Clin Nutr*. 2004;79(6):1088–1094.

87. Stroebele N, de Castro JM. Television viewing is associated with an increase in meal frequency in humans. *Appetite*. 2004;42(1):111–113.

88. Coon KA, Goldberg J, Rogers BL, Tucker KL. Relationships between use of television during meals and children's food consumption patterns. *Pediatrics*. 2001;107(1):e7.

89. Crespo CJ, Smit E, Troiano RP, Bartlett SJ, Macera CA, Andersen RE. Television watching, energy intake, and obesity in US children: results from the third National Health and Nutrition Examination Survey, 1988–1994. *Am J Dis Child*. 2001;155(3):360–365.

90. French SA, Story M, Neumark-Sztainer D, Fulkerson JA, Hannan P. Fast food restaurant use among adolescents: associations with nutrient intake, food choices and behavioral and psychosocial variables. *Int J Obes Relat Metab Disord*. 2001;25(12).

91. Mcnutt SW, Hu Y, Schreiber GB, Crawford PB, Obarzanek E, Mellin L. A longitudinal study of the dietary practices of black and white girls 9 and 10 years old at enrollment: the NHLBI Growth and Health Study. *J Adolesc Health*. 1997;20(1):27–37.

92. Bellisle F, Dalix A, Slama G. Non food-related environmental stimuli induce increased meal intake in healthy women: comparison of television viewing versus listening to a recorded story in laboratory settings. *Appetite*. 2004;43(2):175–180.

93. Temple JL, Giacomelli AM, Kent KM, Roemmich JN, Epstein LH. Television watching increases motivated responding for food and energy intake in children. *Am J Clin Nutr*. 2007;85(2):355–361.

94. Gore SA, Foster JA, DiLillo VG, Kirk K, West DS. Television viewing and snacking. *Eat Behav*. 2003;4(4):399–405.

95. Van den Bulck J, Van Mierlo J. Energy intake associated with television viewing in adolescents, a cross sectional study. *Appetite*. 2004;43(2):181–184.

96. Blass EM, Anderson DR, Kirkorian HL, Pempek TA, Price I, Koleini MF. On the road to obesity: television viewing increases intake of high-density foods. *Physiol Behav*. 2006;88(4):597–604.

97. Francis LA, Lee Y, Birch LL. Parental weight status and girls' television viewing, snacking, and body mass indexes. *Obes Res*. 2003;11(1):143–151.

98. Rey-López JP, Ruiz JR, Ortega FB, et al. Reliability and validity of a screen time-based sedentary behaviour questionnaire for adolescents: the HELENA study. *Eur J Public Health*. 2012;22(3):373–377.

99. Christakis DA, Ebel BE, Rivara FP, Zimmerman FJ. Television, video, and computer game usage in children under 11 years of age. *J Pediatr*. 2004;145(5):652–656.

100. Moag-Stahlberg A, Miles A, Marcello M. What kids say they do and what parents think kids are doing: the ADAF/knowledge networks 2003 family nutrition and physical activity study. *J Acad Nutr Diet*. 2003;103(11):1541.

101. Schneider M, Dunton GF, Cooper DM. Media use and obesity in adolescent females. *Obesity*. 2007;15(9):2328–2335.

102. Ray M, Jat KR. Effect of electronic media on children. *Indian Pediatr*. 2010;47(7):561–568.

103. Carvalhal MM, Padez MC, Moreira PA, Rosado VM. Overweight and obesity related to activities in Portuguese children, 7–9 years. *Eur J Public Health*. 2007;17(1):42–46.

104. Stettler N, Signer TM, Suter PM. Electronic games and environmental factors associated with childhood obesity in Switzerland. *Obes Res*. 2004;12(6):896–903.

105. Janz KF, Mahoney LT. Maturation, gender, and video game playing are related to physical activity intensity in adolescents: the Muscatine study. *Pediatr Exerc Sci*. 1997;9:353–363.

106. Chaput J-P, Visby T, Nyby S, et al. Video game playing increases food intake in adolescents: a randomized crossover study. *Am J Clin Nutr.* 2011;93(6):1196–1203.

107. Chaput J-P, Drapeau V, Poirier P, Teasdale N, Tremblay A. Glycemic instability and spontaneous energy intake: association with knowledge-based work. *Psychosom Med.* 2008;70(7):797–804.

108. Mathieu M-E, Kakinami L. Active video games could be the solution to the increased energy intake reported with sedentary video games. *Am J Clin Nutr.* 2011;94(4):1150–1151.

109. Graves L, Stratton G, Ridgers ND, Cable NT. Energy expenditure in adolescents playing new generation computer games. *Br J Sports Med.* 2008;42(7):592–594.

110. Peng W, Lin J-H, Crouse J. Is playing exergames really exercising? A meta-analysis of energy expenditure in active video games. *Cyberpsychol Behav Soc Netw.* 2011;14(11):681–688.

111. Barnett A, Cerin E, Baranowski T. Active video games for youth: a systematic review. *J Phys Act Health.* 2011.

112. Graf DL, Pratt LV, Hester CN, Short KR. Playing active video games increases energy expenditure in children. *Pediatrics.* 2009;124(2):534–540.

113. Lanningham-Foster L, Foster RC, McCrady SK, Jensen TB, Mitre N, Levine JA. Activity-promoting video games and increased energy expenditure. *J Pediatr.* 2009;154(6):819–823.

114. Maddison R, Foley L, Mhurchu CN, et al. Effects of active video games on body composition: a randomized controlled trial. *Am J Clin Nutr.* 2011;94(1):156–163.

115. Lyons EJ, Tate DF, Ward DS, Wang X. Energy intake and expenditure during sedentary screen time and motion-controlled video gaming. *Am J Clin Nutr.* 2012;96(2):234–239.

116. Mellecker RR, Lanningham-Foster L, Levine JA, McManus AM. Energy intake during activity enhanced video game play. *Appetite.* 2010;55(2):343–347.

117. Thackray AE, Deighton K, King JA, Stensel DJ. Exercise, appetite and weight control: are there differences between men and women? *Nutrients.* 2016;8(9):583.

118. Whybrow S, Hughes DA, Ritz P, et al. The effect of an incremental increase in exercise on appetite, eating behaviour and energy balance in lean men and women feeding ad libitum. *Br J Nutr.* 2008;100(05):1109–1115.

119. Staten MA. The effect of exercise on food intake in men and women. *Am J Clin Nutr.* 1991;53(1):27–31.

120. Stubbs RJ, Sepp A, Hughes DA, et al. The effect of graded levels of exercise on energy intake and balance in free-living men, consuming their normal diet. *Eur J Clin Nutr.* 2002;56:129–140.

121. Farah N, Malkova D, Gill J. Effects of exercise on postprandial responses to ad libitum feeding in overweight men. *Med Sci Sports Exerc.* 2010;42(11):2015–2022.

122. Westerterp KR, Meijer GA, Janssen EM, Saris WH, Ten Hoor F. Long-term effect of physical activity on energy balance and body composition. *Br J Nutr.* 1992;68(01):21–30.

123. Donnelly JE, Hill JO, Jacobsen DJ, et al. Effects of a 16-month randomized controlled exercise trial on body weight and composition in young, overweight men and women: the midwest exercise trial. *Arch Intern Med.* 2003;163(11):1343–1350.

124. Irving BA, Weltman J, Patrie JT, et al. Effects of exercise training intensity on nocturnal growth hormone secretion in obese adults with the metabolic syndrome. *J Clin Endocrinol Metab.* 2009;94(6):1979–1986.

125. Caudwell P, Gibbons C, Hopkins M, King NA, Finlayson G, Blundell JE. No sex difference in body fat in response to supervised and measured exercise. *Med Sci Sports Exerc.* 2013;45(2):351–358.

126. Donnelly JE, Honas JJ, Smith BK, et al. Aerobic exercise alone results in clinically significant weight loss for men and women: midwest exercise trial 2. *Obesity.* 2013;21(3):E219–E228.

127. Wade GN, Jones JE. Neuroendocrinology of nutritional infertility. *Am J Physiol Regul Integr Comp Physiol.* 2004;287(6):R1277–R1296.

128. Hagobian TA, Braun B. Physical activity and hormonal regulation of appetite: sex differences and weight control. *Exerc Sport Sci Rev.* 2010;38(1):25–30.

129. Lieberman DE. Is exercise really medicine? An evolutionary perspective. *Curr Sports Med Rep.* 2015;14(4):313–319.

130. Hagobian TA, Sharoff CG, Stephens BR, et al. Effects of exercise on energy-regulating hormones and appetite in men and women. *Am J Physiol Regul Integr Comp Physiol.* 2009;296(2):R233–R242.

131. Hagobian TA, Yamashiro M, Hinkel-Lipsker J, Streder K, Evero N, Hackney T. Effects of acute exercise on appetite hormones and ad libitum energy intake in men and women. *Appl Physiol Nutr Metab.* 2012;38(999):66–72.

132. Donnelly JE, Herrmann SD, Lambourne K, Szabo AN, Honas JJ, Washburn RA. Does increased exercise or physical activity alter ad-libitum daily energy intake or macronutrient composition in healthy adults? A systematic review. *PLoS One.* 2014;9(1):e83498.

133. Cameron JD, Goldfield GS, Riou M-È, Finlayson GS, Blundell JE, Doucet É. Energy depletion by diet or aerobic exercise alone: impact of energy deficit modality on appetite parameters. *Am J Clin Nutr.* 2016;103(4):1008–1016.

134. King JA, Wasse LK, Ewens J, et al. Differential acylated ghrelin, peptide YY3-36, appetite, and food intake responses to equivalent energy deficits created by exercise and food restriction. *J Clin Endocrinol Metab.* 2011;96(4):1114–1121.

135. Alajmi N, Deighton K, King JA, et al. Appetite and energy intake responses to acute energy deficits in females versus males. *Med Sci Sports Exerc.* 2016;48(3):412–420.

136. Swift DL, Lavie CJ, Johannsen NM, et al. Physical activity, cardiorespiratory fitness, and exercise training in primary and secondary coronary prevention. *Circ J.* 2013;77(2):281–292.

137. Miller WC, Koceja D, Hamilton E. A meta-analysis of the past 25 years of weight loss research using diet, exercise or diet plus exercise intervention. *Int J Obes.* 1997;21(10):941–947.

138. Redman LM, Heilbronn LK, Martin CK, Alfonso A, Smith SR, Ravussin E. Effect of calorie restriction with or without exercise on body composition and fat distribution. *J Clin Endocrinol Metab.* 2007;92(3):865–872.

139. Jakicic JM, Winters C, Lang W, Wing RR. Effects of intermittent exercise and use of home exercise equipment on adherence, weight loss, and fitness in overweight women: a randomized trial. *JAMA.* 1999;282(16):1554–1560.

140. Andersen RE, Wadden TA, Bartlett SJ, Zemel B, Verde TJ, Franckowiak SC. Effects of lifestyle activity vs structured aerobic exercise in obese women: a randomized trial. *JAMA.* 1999;281(4):335–340.

141. King NA, Hopkins M, Caudwell P, Stubbs R, Blundell JE. Individual variability following 12 weeks of supervised exercise: identification and characterization of compensation for exercise-induced weight loss. *Int J Obes.* 2008;32(1):177–184.

142. Donnelly JE, Smith BK. Is exercise effective for weight loss with ad libitum diet? Energy balance, compensation, and gender differences. *Exerc Sport Sci Rev.* 2005;33(4):169–174.

143. Despres J, Bouchard C, Savard R, Tremblay A, Marcotte M, Theriault G. The effect of a 20-week endurance training program on adipose-tissue morphology and lipolysis in men and women. *Metabolism.* 1984;33(3):235–239.

144. Potteiger JA, Jacobsen DJ, Donnelly JE, Hill JO. Glucose and insulin responses following 16 months of exercise training in overweight adults: the midwest exercise trial. *Metabolism.* 2003;52(9):1175–1181.

145. Martins C, Kulseng B, King N, Holst JJ, Blundell J. The effects of exercise-induced weight loss on appetite-related peptides and motivation to eat. *J Clin Endocrinol Metab.* 2010;95(4):1609–1616.

146. Barwell ND, Malkova D, Leggate M, Gill JM. Individual responsiveness to exercise-induced fat loss is associated with change in resting substrate utilization. *Metabolism.* 2009;58(9):1320–1328.

147. Caudwell P, Hopkins M, King NA, Stubbs RJ, Blundell JE. Exercise alone is not enough: weight loss also needs a healthy (mediterranean) diet? *Public Health Nutr.* 2009;12(9A):1663–1666.

148. King NA, Caudwell PP, Hopkins M, Stubbs JR, Naslund E, Blundell JE. Dual-process action of exercise on appetite control: increase in orexigenic drive but improvement in meal-induced satiety. *Am J Clin Nutr.* 2009;90(4):921–927.

149. Krebs NF, Jacobson MS, Nutrition AAoPCo. Prevention of pediatric overweight and obesity. *Pediatrics.* 2003;112(2):424.

150. Freedman DS, Dietz WH, Srinivasan SR, Berenson GS. The relation of overweight to cardiovascular risk factors among children and adolescents: the Bogalusa Heart Study. *Pediatrics.* 1999;103(6):1175–1182.

151. Must A, Strauss RS. Risks and consequences of childhood and adolescent obesity. *Int J Obes Relat Metab Disord.* 1999:23.

152. Liao Y, Liao J, Durand CP, Dunton GF. Which type of sedentary behaviour intervention is more effective at reducing body mass index in children? A meta-analytic review. *Obes Rev.* 2014;15(3):159–168.

153. Ford AL, Hunt LP, Cooper A, Shield JP. What reduction in BMI SDS is required in obese adolescents to improve body composition and cardiometabolic health? *Arch Dis Child.* 2010;95(4):256–261.

154. van Grieken A, Ezendam NP, Paulis WD, van der Wouden JC, Raat H. Primary prevention of overweight in children and adolescents: a meta-analysis of the effectiveness of interventions aiming to decrease sedentary behaviour. *Int J Behav Nutr Phys Act.* 2012;9(1):1.

155. Seo D-C, Sa J. A meta-analysis of obesity interventions among US minority children. *J Adolesc Health.* 2010;46(4):309–323.

156. Prochaska JJ, Spring B, Nigg CR. Multiple health behavior change research: an introduction and overview. *Prev Med.* 2008;46(3):181–188.

157. Saelens BE, Sallis JF, Wilfley DE, Patrick K, Cella JA, Buchta R. Behavioral weight control for overweight adolescents initiated in primary care. *Obes Res.* 2002;10(1):22–32.

158. James PT, Leach R, Kalamara E, Shayeghi M. The worldwide obesity epidemic. *Obes Res.* 2001;9(S11):S228–S233.

159. Gupta N, Goel K, Shah P, Misra A. Childhood obesity in developing countries: epidemiology, determinants, and prevention. *Endocr Rev.* 2012;33(1):48–70.

160. Fogelholm M, Kukkonen-Harjula K. Does physical activity prevent weight gain–a systematic review. *Obes Rev.* 2000;1(2):95–111.

161. Johannsen NM, Swift DL, Lavie CJ, Earnest CP, Blair SN, Church TS. Categorical analysis of the impact of aerobic and resistance exercise training, alone and in combination, on cardiorespiratory fitness levels in patients with type 2 diabetes. *Diabetes Care.* 2013;36(10):3305–3312.

162. Swift DL, Earnest CP, Blair SN, Church TS. The effect of different doses of aerobic exercise training on endothelial function in postmenopausal women with elevated blood pressure: results from the DREW study. *Br J Sports Med.* 2012;46(10):753–758.

163. Sixt S, Rastan A, Desch S, et al. Exercise training but not rosiglitazone improves endothelial function in prediabetic patients with coronary disease. *Eur J Cardiovasc Prev Rehabil.* 2008;15(4):473–478.

164. Kodama S, Tanaka S, Saito K, et al. Effect of aerobic exercise training on serum levels of high-density lipoprotein cholesterol: a meta-analysis. *Arch Intern Med.* 2007;167(10):999–1008.

165. Kim M-K, Tomita T, Kim M-J, Sasai H, Maeda S, Tanaka K. Aerobic exercise training reduces epicardial fat in obese men. *J Appl Physiol.* 2009;106(1):5–11.

166. Thomas EL, Brynes AE, McCarthy J, et al. Preferential loss of visceral fat following aerobic exercise, measured by magnetic resonance imaging. *Lipids.* 2000;35(7):769–776.

167. Lee S, Kuk JL, Davidson LE, et al. Exercise without weight loss is an effective strategy for obesity reduction in obese individuals with and without Type 2 diabetes. *J Appl Physiol.* 2005;99(3):1220–1225.

168. Giannopoulou I, Ploutz-Snyder L, Carhart R, et al. Exercise is required for visceral fat loss in postmenopausal women with type 2 diabetes. *J Clin Endocrinol Metab.* 2005;90(3):1511–1518.

169. Mourier A, Gautier J-F, De Kerviler E, et al. Mobilization of visceral adipose tissue related to the improvement in insulin sensitivity in response to physical training in NIDDM: effects of branched-chain amino acid supplements. *Diabetes Care.* 1997;20(3):385–391.

170. Myers VH, McVay MA, Brashear MM, et al. Exercise training and quality of life in individuals with type 2 diabetes. *Diabetes Care.* 2013;36(7):1884–1890.

171. Martin CK, Church TS, Thompson AM, Earnest CP, Blair SN. Exercise dose and quality of life: a randomized controlled trial. *Arch Intern Med.* 2009;169(3):269–278.

172. Bravata DM, Smith-Spangler C, Sundaram V, et al. Using pedometers to increase physical activity and improve health: a systematic review. *JAMA.* 2007;298(19):2296–2304.

173. Lavie CJ, Milani RV, Ventura HO. Obesity and cardiovascular disease: risk factor, paradox, and impact of weight loss. *J Am Coll Cardiol.* 2009;53(21):1925–1932.

174. Group DPPR. Reduction in the incidence of type 2 diabetes with lifestyle intervention or metformin. *N Engl J Med.* 2002;2002(346):393–403.

175. McAuley PA, Kokkinos PF, Oliveira RB, Emerson BT, Myers JN. Obesity paradox and cardiorespiratory fitness in 12,417 male veterans aged 40 to 70 years. *Mayo Clin Proc.* 2010.

176. Lobelo F, Stoutenberg M, Hutber A. The exercise is medicine global health initiative: a 2014 update. *Br J Sports Med.* 2014. http://dx.doi.org/10.1136/bjsports-2013-093080.

177. NICE CfPHEa, Care NCCfP. Obesity: the prevention, identification, assessment and management of overweight and obesity in adults and children; 2006.

178. NICE. *Weight Management: Lifestyle Services for Overweight or Obese Adults.* London: National Institute for Health and Care Excellence; 2014.

179. Partridge S, Juan SH, McGeechan K, Bauman A, Allman-Farinelli M. Poor quality of external validity reporting limits generalizability of overweight and/or obesity lifestyle prevention interventions in young adults: a systematic review. *Obes Rev.* 2015;16(1):13–31.

180. Rutherford Z, Gough B, Seymour-Smith S, et al. 'Motivate': the effect of a football in the community delivered weight loss programme on over 35-year old men and women's cardiovascular risk factors. *Soccer Soc.* 2014;15(6):951–969.

181. Chang SH, Chen MC, Chien NH, Lin HF. Effectiveness of community-based exercise intervention programme in obese adults with metabolic syndrome. *J Clin Nurs.* 2016;25(17–18):2579–2589.

182. Hunt K, Wyke S, Gray CM, et al. A gender-sensitised weight loss and healthy living programme for overweight and obese men delivered by Scottish Premier League football clubs (FFIT): a pragmatic randomised controlled trial. *Lancet.* 2014;383(9924):1211–1221.

CHAPTER 21

Weight Management Programs

PAMELA DYSON, PHD, RD

ABBREVIATIONS

ACA Affordable Care Act
BBC British Broadcasting Corporation
BT Behavioral therapy
CAMWEL Camden Weight Loss program
CVD Cardiovascular disease
DEHKO Development Program for the Prevention and Care of Diabetes in Finland
DPP Diabetes Prevention Program
DPS Diabetes Prevention Study
GCWMS Glasgow and Clyde Weight Management Service
GI Glycemic index
JC Jenny Craig
kcal Kilocalorie
LDL Low-density lipoprotein

MJ Megajoule
NDPP National Diabetes Prevention Program
NHS National Health Service
NHS DPP NHS Diabetes Prevention Program
NICE National Institute for Health and Care Excellence
NWCR National Weight Control Registry
RC Rosemary Conley
RCT Randomized controlled trial
SW Slimming World
TOPS Take Off Pounds Sensibly
UK United Kingdom
US United States
WATCH Worcester Area Trial for Counseling in Hyperlipidemia
WW WeightWatchers

INTRODUCTION

Globally, many countries, including the United States, the United Kingdom, Australia, China, and India, have formulated guidelines for the management of obesity.[1–5] Structured lifestyle programs, incorporating dietary advice, physical activity, and behavioral interventions, are generally recommended as the first-line strategy for weight loss, because simply giving people advice alone or a printed leaflet to lose weight is largely ineffective.[6] Traditionally, many weight management interventions involve one-to-one counseling and support, and it is widely recognized that interventions targeting individuals are expensive, are labor-intensive, and may not result in meaningful weight loss and that group-based structured interventions are more effective.[7]

In primary care, where the majority of weight management takes place, it has been established that counseling alone for weight loss is largely ineffective, but there is evidence that multicomponent interventions integrating diet, physical activity, and behavioral strategies can improve outcomes.[8] Many weight management programs incorporating these strategies have been developed over the years, and these programs are offered by both commercial providers and the health sector to groups and to individuals.

COMPONENTS OF WEIGHT MANAGEMENT PROGRAMS

Commercial Programs

Commercial weight loss group programs are probably the best known and most widely used and provide a variety of strategies for weight loss, although relatively few have robust evidence of efficacy. Table 21.1 shows the characteristics of commercial groups[9–13] with published studies of efficacy. The majority of commercial programs offer energy-restricted dietary interventions with an emphasis on foods seen as healthful, including fruit, vegetables, lean meat and poultry, seafood, eggs, low- or nonfat dairy, and wholegrain cereals. Energy-dense foods high in fat and sugar are restricted or substituted with reduced-energy versions. Physical activity is promoted and most programs recommend aiming for the internationally recognized standard of 150 min of moderate to vigorous physical activity per week (or 30 min/day on 5 days per week)[14].

Behavioral therapy (BT) increases weight loss when compared with diet and physical activity interventions alone[15] and is commonly incorporated into commercial weight loss programs. BT includes three specific characteristics: goal setting, process orientation, and focusing on small, manageable changes. The behavioral

TABLE 21.1
Characteristics of Commercial Weight Management Groups With Published Efficacy

Programme	Description	Dietary Intervention	Physical Activity Intervention	Behavioral Intervention	Frequency and Length of Contact
WeightWatchers[9]	Available as: 1. Weekly support groups led by trained consultants who have lost weight with optional eSource online support 2. WeightWatchers online 3. WeightWatchers at home (postal support)	Energy restriction achieved by ProPoints Switch, consisting of ProPoints Plan and/or Filling and Healthy Plan. Individual daily allowance of points allocated. Foods high in lean protein and dietary fiber are lower in points; members are encouraged to use points on these foods rather than energy-dense foods higher in sugar and fat	Daily physical activity is promoted, with the use of an activity monitor. Extra points can be earned through increased physical activity	Based on the transtheoretical model of behavior change using goal setting, action plans, self-monitoring, and progress evaluation	Initial group lasts 60–70 min. Weekly groups last 30–40 min
Slimming World[10]	Available as: 1. Weekly support groups led by trained consultants with online dietary support 2. Online diet plan and support	Energy restriction achieved by Food Optimising using Extra Easy or Extra Easy SP. Designed to be permissive rather than restrictive and emphasizes fruit, vegetables, lean meat and poultry, fish, and low-fat dairy produce	Physical activity encouraged by the use of Body Magic designed to increase daily activity to a goal of 150 min/week of moderate to vigorous activity using bronze, silver, gold, and platinum awards	Based on transactional analysis, motivational interviewing, and compassionate mind theory. Groups avoid criticism, control, or judgment and use self-monitoring, cost-benefit analysis, visualization, and flexible restraint	Weekly groups lasting 1–1.5 h
Rosemary Conley[11]	Available as: 1. Weekly support and exercise classes led by trained consultants 2. Online plan and support	Low-fat (any food containing <5% fat), low-GI, high-fiber diet. Begins with a Fat Attack Fortnight with energy restricted to 1200 kcal/day	Physical activity is a core component, most classes include 45-min supervised exercise session. 30 min/day of moderate to vigorous activity recommended	Based on social cognitive theory and self-efficacy with reasoned action and planned behavior. Group support and role modelling through visualization are offered	Weekly groups lasting 1–2 h
Jenny Craig[12]	Meal replacement system where the majority of food is provided	Low-fat diet with three prepared meals and one snack provided daily, along with added fruit, vegetables, unsaturated fats, and nonfat dairy products	Exercise goals of 30 min of moderate to vigorous physical activity on ≥5 days/week	Uses goal setting and self-monitoring	Weekly one-to-one counseling visits or telephone contact
Nutrisystems[13]	Meal replacement system with prepackaged foods provided	Energy-restricted diet providing 1250 kcal/day for women and 1550 kcal/day for men. High-fiber, low-GI diet with lean protein supplemented by fruit and vegetables	Three 10-min sessions of exercise recommended daily	Uses self-monitoring	One-to-one counseling with online community forum

GI, glycemic index.

strategies used in commercial programs are varied, but they are usually underpinned by recognized theoretic principles and include components such as self-monitoring, stimulus control, slower eating, health education, problem-solving, and social support.[16]

The advantages of commercial programs include wide availability, and many of the more established programs have evidence of efficacy. The disadvantage of most commercial programs is the cost, although many programs are now available on prescription through the NHS in the United Kingdom. In the United States, the 2010 Affordable Care Act provided new incentives for states to cover obesity screening and counseling, and this is likely to result in increased referrals to commercial weight management programs.[17]

Programs Delivered by the Health Sector

Most experts now recognize that obesity management is a complex issue, and treatment is not the sole responsibility of the physician, although primary care is often the first port of call for advice about weight management.[18] In the United Kingdom, for example, the National Institute for Health and Care Excellence recommends an integrated approach for the prevention and management of obesity with a systems-wide strategy involving health workers, public health services, and local communities. This approach includes referrals by health professionals to lifestyle weight management programs for both adults and children.[19,20]

In response to these demands, health services in countries including the United Kingdom, the United States, Finland, and Australia have developed structured lifestyle programs for weight management. Many of these programs, e.g., the Diabetes Prevention Program (DPP) in the United States[21] and the Diabetes Prevention Study in Finland,[22] were high-intensity research programs delivered in academic units by a multidisciplinary team, and their translation to usual practice has been questioned because they have limited availability, affordability, and acceptability.[23] However, these trials have contributed to the development of effective components for weight management programs and have shaped interventions offered by many health services.[24,25]

Dietary advice formulated from these academic studies includes the following recommendations:

- Energy restriction/portion-controlled diet providing 1200–1800 kcal/day (5.0–7.5 MJ) designed to promote 5%–10% weight loss
- Total fat intake ≤30% total energy
- Saturated fat intake ≤10% total energy
- Dietary fiber intake ≥15 g/1000 kcal (4.2 MJ)

Guidelines for physical activity are formulated in either daily (30 min/day) or weekly (150 min/week) amounts in line with internationally agreed recommendations.[14] Behavioral interventions underpin the majority of weight management programs offered by the health sector and commonly include social support, self-monitoring, and intensive personalized support.

There are many examples of weight management programs offered by the health sector in primary care,[26–34] and the characteristics of those with published evidence of efficacy are shown in Table 21.2.

EFFICACY OF WEIGHT MANAGEMENT PROGRAMS
Body Weight

Evidence from randomized controlled trials (RCTs) demonstrates that multicomponent weight management programs are effective in promoting weight loss (Table 21.3). Commercial programs show mean weight losses of 3.5–7.9 kg, with more modest weight losses of 1.6–5.1 kg seen with programs delivered by the health sector. There are few head-to-head trials assessing the most effective program for weight loss, but one RCT in the United Kingdom, which compared three commercial programs (WW, SW, and RC) with three NHS programs (Size Down, a nurse-led, and a pharmacist-led intervention), reported that all programs resulted in significant weight loss at 12 weeks (1.37–4.43 kg), but only the commercial programs achieved significantly greater weight loss (mean difference 2.3 kg) at 1-year follow-up.[32] The results from this RCT suggested that WW was the most effective intervention, and this was supported by a further study of an NHS primary care slimming on referral scheme comparing RC, SW, and WW, which reported that those attending WW lost more weight (mean difference 1.15 kg).[38] A more recent trial, designed to assess noninferiority of the three programs commonly used in the United Kingdom (an NHS program, RC, and SW), compared with WW failed to show significant differences at 1-year follow-up and concluded that differences between commercial programs were small and of minor clinical importance.[37] The British Broadcasting Corporation "diet trials" also reported significant weight loss over 6 months with no differences between WW, RC, Slim-Fast, and the Atkins diet,[48] and a 1-year study in the United States comparing WW, the Ornish diet, the Zone diet, and the Atkins diet stated that there were no significant differences in weight loss between diets.[49] In summary, it appears that commercial programs are slightly more effective for weight loss than those offered by the health sector, but there appears to be little or no difference between commercial programs.

TABLE 21.2
Characteristics of Weight Management Groups Delivered by the Health Sector With Published Efficacy

Program	Description	Dietary Intervention	Physical activity Intervention	Behavioral Intervention	Frequency and Length of Contact
UNITED STATES					
Think Health![26]	Group-based program adapted from the DPP, focused on African-American and Hispanic adults and delivered by primary care workers	Energy restriction of 1200–1800 kcal/day and fat restriction of 30–40 g/day aiming for weight loss of 5%–10%	Increased physical activity aiming for 150 min/week	Behavioral counseling including goal setting, self-monitoring, addressing negative thoughts, stimulus control, stress management, and social cues	Monthly groups over 1–2 years
POWER-UP[27]	Study comparing usual care, brief lifestyle counseling, and enhanced lifestyle counseling in overweight, hypertensive subjects	"Balanced diet" providing 1200–1800 kcal/day. Energy derived from macronutrients: 15%–20% from protein, 20%–35% from fat, 45%–65% energy from carbohydrate. Enhanced group also offered sibutramine, orlistat, and meal replacements	Gradual increase in physical activity to 180 min/week, monitored by pedometer	Lifestyle coaching offered to brief and enhanced groups only, together with self-monitoring	3-monthly visits for usual care group and monthly visits for brief and enhanced groups over 12 months follow-up
Davis Martin et al.[28]	Study comparing usual care to culturally sensitive tailored interventions in African-American women	Healthier food choices and meal preparation tips	Tailored physical activity recommendations based on current activity levels	Based on social cognitive theory and the trans-theoretical model including self-efficacy, social support, self-reinforcement, goal setting, stimulus control, and contingency planning	Monthly visits lasting 15 min each over 6 months follow-up in the intervention group
Worcester Area Trial for Counseling in Hyperlipidemia (WATCH)[29]	Study comparing usual care, nutrition counseling service, and nutrition counseling service with office support in hyperlipidemic subjects	Low-fat diet based on recommendations from the National Cholesterol Education Program using Dietary Risk Assessment	None	Assessment of resources for change using strengths and barriers, developing plan for change and goal setting	According to need, follow-up over 12 months

UNITED KINGDOM

Program	Delivery	Diet	Physical activity	Behavioral approach	Sessions
Glasgow and Clyde Weight Management Service (GCWMS)[30]	Community-based program delivered by dietitians with psychological support	600 kcal deficit diet with recommended portions from the five food groups, aiming for weight loss of ≥5 kg	Increased physical activity	Cognitive behavioral approaches including goal setting, self-monitoring, cognitive restructuring, and relapse prevention	Nine fortnightly sessions over 16 weeks
Camden Weight Loss (CAMWEL) program[31]	Individualized weight management program	Healthy eating and portion control	Incorporating physical activity into daily life	Social cognitive theory, goal setting, systems thinking, treatment adherence, and behavior change techniques	Fourteen 30-min sessions over 36 weeks
NHS Size Down[32]	Group-based program run in community centers by support workers trained by dietitians	Healthy eating based on the Eatwell Plate	Gradual increase in daily physical activity	Based on the transtheoretical model of behavior change and including goal setting, stages of change, and self-monitoring	Weekly 2-h sessions over 6 weeks
Counterweight[33]	Group-based structured model for weight management in primary care, delivered by practice nurses	Healthy eating based on the Balance of Good Health aiming for weight loss of 5%–10%	Gradual increase in daily physical activity aiming for 30 min/day on most days of the week	Based on the transtheoretical model of behavior change and including goal setting, self-monitoring, stimulus control, and relapse management	Six 1-h group sessions over 3 months

AUSTRALIA

Program	Delivery	Diet	Physical activity	Behavioral approach	Sessions
Weigh Forward[34]	Group or individual sessions delivered by practice nurses	Reducing energy intake	Increasing energy expenditure	Behavioral strategies including readiness to change and goal setting	Fortnightly meetings for 12 weeks

TABLE 21.3
Comparative Weight Losses Between Different Weight Management Programs

Program	Number of Studies	Number of Individuals Receiving Named Intervention	Mean Length of Follow-up (weeks)	Mean Weight Loss (kg)
COMMERCIAL PROGRAMS				
WeightWatchers[17,23,35–38]	12	3352	37.2	4.3
Slimming World[32,37,38]	3	1521	38.7	4.4
Rosemary Conley[32,37,38]	3	1034	38.7	3.5
Jenny Craig[39–41]	3	360	60.0	7.9
Nutrisystems[42–44]	3	111	16.0	7.1
PROGRAMS DELIVERED BY HEALTH SERVICES				
Think Health![45]	1	124	52	1.6
POWER-UP[27]	1	260	104	3.7
Davis Martin et al.[28]	1	71	24	2.0
WATCH[29]	1	315	52	2.3
Glasgow and Clyde Weight Management Service (GCWMS)[30]	1	2976	Completion of Phase 1, defined as attending four or more sessions	Not reported Among 809 completers, 35.5% lost ≥5 kg
Camden Weight Loss (CAMWEL) program[31]	1	191	52	2.39
NHS Size Down[32]	1	100	52	2.37
Counterweight[46,47]	2	8134 825	52 104	3.0[46], 3.7[47]
Weigh Forward[34]	1	258	24	5.1

Cardiovascular Risk Reduction

Modest weight losses of 5%–10% are associated with significant improvements in cardiovascular disease (CVD) risk factors including blood pressure and lipid concentrations.[50,51] The majority of RCTs of weight management programs do not report CVD endpoints such as myocardial infarction or stroke, and the data for surrogate endpoints such as blood pressure and lipid concentrations are limited. In addition, very few trials of weight management programs have investigated long-term (1 year or more) CVD risk factor outcomes, with the majority reporting changes at 3 and 6 months. A systematic review and metaanalysis of the effects of commercial programs on CVD risk factors in studies lasting at least 12 months reported that the current evidence available for these programs do not demonstrate clear benefits for CVD risk factor reduction,[52] and that head-to-head comparisons fail to demonstrate superiority for any named program.[53] However, conclusions

were limited by the lack of studies, high attrition rates, and the fact that the majority of participants did not have underlying CVD or CVD risk factors with both blood pressure and lipid concentrations relatively well controlled at baseline.

The majority of weight management programs in the health sector have not reported CVD outcomes.[26,28,30,32–34] Three programs have evaluated effects of interventions on CVD risk factors and most report small differences of limited clinical significance. The CAMWEL (Camden Weight Loss) program in the United Kingdom reported blood pressure only and found no difference between the intervention and control group,[31] and two studies in the United States both reported some benefit in the enhanced intervention group. The POWER-UP study showed reductions in blood pressure and improvements in lipid concentrations in all groups and this appeared to be related to weight loss, but the differences were only statistically significant for triglyceride and low-density lipoprotein (LDL) concentrations.[27] The WATCH (Worcester Area Trial for Counseling in Hyperlipidemia) study also reported significant improvements in LDL and total cholesterol in the enhanced lifestyle intervention group, but the change was not statistically significant compared with standard treatment.[29] Overall, data are lacking for CVD risk factor reduction in weight management programs delivered by health services.

Diabetes Prevention

Obesity accounts for 80%–85% of the risk of type 2 diabetes and, as the strongest modifiable risk factor, is the main focus for prevention.[54] There is robust evidence from academic RCTs showing that lifestyle interventions as part of a structured program reduce progression to diabetes in high-risk populations by 50%.[55] Many countries, including Australia, Finland (DEHKO), the United States (NDPP), and the United Kingdom (NHS DPP), have attempted to apply diabetes prevention at the population level using structured weight management programs designed for individuals at high risk.[56–59] However, the translation of efficacy from RCT to real-world conditions tends to dilute effectiveness, because more wide-spread programs need to address issues such as infrastructure for program delivery, the intensity of the intervention, staffing, resources, and sustainability.[59] This has been demonstrated in the United States, with the adaptation of the DPP into the National Diabetes Prevention Program (NDPP). The original DPP was a high-intensity lifestyle program where individuals were offered one-to-one lifestyle coaching by trained nutritionists, exercise physiologists, or behavioral psychologists at weekly intervals for 16 weeks and subsequent monthly group and individual sessions. The NDPP offers diverse group programs in community settings, with weekly meetings over 4–12 months delivered by a variety of personnel including health workers (usually nurses and/or dietitians and nutritionists), peer educators, and lay leaders.[60] These differences in intensity and delivery translate to differences in efficacy assessed by weight loss; in the DPP, mean weight losses over the first year were 7%[21] compared with 4% in community programs based on DPP,[60] although both results were probably clinically significant.

COST-EFFECTIVENESS OF WEIGHT MANAGEMENT PROGRAMS

There is limited evidence for the cost-effectiveness of weight management programs, although a systematic review has suggested that they are cost-effective.[61] An international study that evaluated referral to a commercial weight management program against standard care provided by general practitioners reported that the commercial group was a highly cost-effective strategy for weight management[62] and for those at risk of weight-related comorbidities.[63] A head-to-head analysis comparing WW, JC, VTrim (a lifestyle program) and three pharmaceutical products suggested that the only cost-effective lifestyle program was WW.[64]

LIMITATIONS OF WEIGHT MANAGEMENT PROGRAMS

Sustainability

Cynicism is often expressed about the sustainability of weight management generally over the long-term, and this also applies to multicomponent programs, where it has been reported that weight changes were small and weight regain was common.[61] Combining behavioral interventions with diet and physical activity in structured programs demonstrate small but significant effects on maintenance of weight loss at 2-year's follow-up,[65] but trials rarely last beyond 2 years, and it is challenging to draw conclusions about sustainability of weight loss from RCTs lasting less than 6 months. Audit data can provide some indication of long-term weight loss maintenance, and an analysis of participants attending WW reported that members achieved an initial mean weight loss of 12.2 kg, but that average weight regain at 5-year's follow-up was 7.4 kg, indicating an overall loss from baseline of 4.8 kg.[66] SW have reported data at 12 months follow-up in 45,395 people who completed at least 75% of sessions, and weight losses were reported as 12.7 kg, with no difference between men and women.[67] However, attrition rates were not reported in either of these audits, and data were presented for completers only. Data at 7-year's follow-up are available from the Take Pound Off Sensibly program, a nonprofit peer-led group intervention in the United States, and show that mean weight losses in 2289 individuals was 8.3 kg, although attrition rates were extremely high at 94%.[68]

Attrition

Attrition rates in weight loss interventions are notoriously high and range from 10%–80%.[69] Studies using commercial weight loss programs have reported attrition rates between 40% and 60% over ≥12-month's follow-up,[70] and similar rates have been reported for community programs offered by health services.[46]

Applicability

The majority of those who use weight management programs for weight loss in the United Kingdom are white, middle-aged, and female, and concern has been expressed about inequalities in access and provision of interventions for all who would benefit from weight loss.[71] A study of the uptake of weight management programs in primary care in the United Kingdom identified that males, younger people, and those from more deprived areas were less likely to participate in a weight loss trial,[72] leading to speculation that tailored interventions should be designed specifically for men,[73] adapted for different ethnic groups[26,28,74] and for deprived populations.[71]

SUMMARY AND RECOMMENDATIONS

Integrated weight management programs incorporating diet, physical activity, and behavioral strategies are effective in achieving clinically meaningful weight losses of approximately 2–8 kg, although there is less evidence for efficacy for reducing the risk of obesity-related comorbidities. Commercial weight management programs are more successful for weight loss than those offered by the health sector or nonprofit organizations, with no strong evidence of superiority of a specific named program. Referral to these programs should be offered as an option for first-line treatment of obesity.

REFERENCES

1. Garvey WT, Mechanick JI, Brett EM, et al. American Association of Clinical Endocrinologists and American College of Endocrinology comprehensive clinical practice guidelines for medical care of patients with obesity. Executive summary. *Endocr Pract.* 2016;22(7):842–884.
2. National Institute for Health and Care Excellence. *Obesity: Identification, Assessment and Management.* London: NICE CG189; 2014.
3. National Health and Medical Research Council. *Clinical Practice Guidelines for the Management of Overweight and Obesity in Adults, Adolescents and Children in Australia.* Melbourne: National Health and Medical Research Council; 2013.
4. Chen C, Lu FC, Department of Disease Control Ministry of Health, PR China. The guidelines for prevention and control of overweight and obesity in Chinese adults. *Biomed Environ Sci.* 2004;17(suppl 1):1–36.
5. Misra A, Chowbey P, Makkar B, et al. Consensus statement for diagnosis of obesity, abdominal obesity and the metabolic syndrome for Asian Indians and recommendations for physical activity, medical and surgical management. *J Assoc Physicians India.* 2009;57:163–170.
6. Franz MJ, VanWormer JJ, Crain AL, et al. Weight-loss outcomes: a systematic review and meta-analysis of weight-loss clinical trials with a minimum 1-year follow-up. *J Am Diet Assoc.* 2007;107(10):1755–1767.
7. Paul-Ebhohimhen V, Avenell A. A systematic review of the effectiveness of group versus individual treatments for obesity. *Obes Facts.* 2009;2(1):17–24.
8. Johns DJ, Hartmann-Boyce J, Jebb SA, Aveyard P, Behavioural Weight Management Review Group. Diet or exercise interventions vs combined behavioral weight management programs: a systematic review and meta-analysis of direct comparisons. *J Acad Nutr Diet.* 2014;114(10):1557–1568.
9. WeightWatchers. https://www.weightwatchers.com.
10. Slimming World. https://www.slimmingworld.co.uk.
11. Conley R. https://www.rosemaryconley.com.
12. Craig J. https://www.jennycraig.com.
13. Nutrisystem. https://www.nutrisystem.com.
14. World Health Organisation. *Global Recommendations on Physical Activity for Health.* Geneva Switzerland: WHO; 2010.
15. Wadden TA, Webb VL, Moran CH, Bailer BA. Lifestyle modification for obesity: new developments in diet, physical activity, and behavior therapy. *Circulation.* 2012;125(9):1157–1170.
16. Jacob JJ, Isaac R. Behavioural therapy for the management of obesity. *Indian J Endocrinol Metab.* 2012;16(1):28–32.
17. Gudzune KA, Doshi RS, Mehta AK, et al. Efficacy of commercial weight-loss programs: an updated systematic review. *Ann Intern Med.* 2015;162(7):501–512.
18. Kirk SF, Penney TL. The role of health systems in obesity management and prevention: problems and paradigm shifts. *Curr Obes Rep.* 2013;2(4):315–319.
19. National Institute for Health and Care Excellence. *Weight Management: Lifestyle Services for Overweight or Obese Adults [PH53].* London, UK: NICE; 2014.
20. National Institute for Health and Care Excellence. *Weight Management: Lifestyle Services for Overweight or Obese Children and Young People [PH47].* London, UK: NICE; 2014.
21. Knowler WC, Barrett-Connor E, Fowler SE, et al. Reduction in the incidence of type 2 diabetes with lifestyle intervention or metformin. *N Engl J Med.* 2002;346(6):393–403.
22. Tuomilehto J, Lindstrom J, Eriksson JG, et al. Prevention of type 2 diabetes mellitus by changes in lifestyle among subjects with impaired glucose tolerance. *N Engl J Med.* 2001;344(18):1343–1350.
23. O'Neil PM, Miller-Kovach K, Tuerk PW, et al. Randomized controlled trial of a nationally available weight control program tailored for adults with type 2 diabetes. *Obesity (Silver Spring).* 2016;24(11):2269–2277.
24. Ryan DH, Espeland MA, Foster GD, et al. Look AHEAD (Action for Health in Diabetes): design and methods for a clinical trial of weight loss for the prevention of cardiovascular disease in type 2 diabetes. *Control Clin Trials.* 2003;24(5):610–628.

25. Lindström J, Peltonen M, Tuomilehto J. Lifestyle strategies for weight control: experience from the Finnish Diabetes Prevention Study. *Proc Nutr Soc.* 2005;64(1):81–88.

26. Kumanyika S, Fassbender J, Phipps E, et al. Design, recruitment and start up of a primary care weight loss trial targeting African American and Hispanic adults. *Contemp Clin Trials.* 2011;32(2):215–224.

27. Wadden TA, Volger S, Sarwer DB, et al. A two-year randomized trial of obesity treatment in primary care practice. *N Engl J Med.* 2011;365:1969–1979.

28. Davis Martin PD, Rhode PC, Dutton GR, Redmann SM, Ryan DH, Brantley PJ. A primary care weight management intervention for low-income African-American women. *Obesity.* 2006;14:1412–1420.

29. Ockene IS, Hebert JR, Ockene JK, et al. Effect of physician-delivered nutrition counseling training and an office-support program on saturated fat intake, weight, and serum lipid measurements in a hyperlipidemic population: Worcester Area Trial for Counseling in Hyperlipidemia (WATCH). *Arch Intern Med.* 1999;159:725–731.

30. Morrison DS, Boyle S, Morrison C, Allardice G, Greenlaw N, Forde L. Evaluation of the first phase of a specialist weight management programme in the UK National Health Service: prospective cohort study. *Public Health Nutr.* 2012;15(1):28–38.

31. Nanchahal K, Power T, Holdsworth E, et al. A pragmatic randomised controlled trial in primary care of the Camden Weight Loss (CAMWEL) programme. *BMJ Open.* 2012;2:e000793.

32. Jolly K, Daley A, Adab P, et al. A randomised controlled trial to compare a range of commercial or primary care led weight reduction programmes with a minimal intervention control for weight loss in obesity: the lighten up trial. *BMC Public Health.* 2010;10:439.

33. The Counterweight Project Team. A new evidence-based model for weight management in primary care: the counterweight programme. *J Hum Nutr Diet.* 2004;17:191–208.

34. Hemmes RA, Adam N, Dixon JB. Weigh forward: a clinical audit of weight management in Australian general practice. *Clin Obes.* June 2016;6(3):202–209.

35. Baetge C, Earnest CP, Lockard B, et al. Efficacy of a randomized trial examining commercial weight loss programs and exercise on metabolic syndrome in overweight and obese women. *Appl Physiol Nutr Metab.* 2017:1–12.

36. Jakicic JM, Rogers RJ, Kovacs SJ, et al. A commercial program is effective for weight loss and improving health-related outcomes in adults. *Med Sci Sports Exerc.* 2016;48(5 suppl 1):1083–1084.

37. Madigan CD, Daley AJ, Lewis AL, Jolly K, Aveyard P. Which weight-loss programmes are as effective as weight watchers?: non-inferiority analysis. *Br J Gen Pract.* 2014;64(620):e128–e136.

38. Dixon KJ, Shcherba S, Kipping RR. Weight loss from three commercial providers of NHS primary care slimming on referral in North Somerset: service evaluation. *J Public Health (Oxf).* 2012;34(4):555–561.

39. Rock CL, Flatt SW, Pakiz B, et al. Weight loss, glycemic control, and cardiovascular disease risk factors in response to differential diet composition in a weight loss program in type 2 diabetes: a randomized controlled trial. *Diabetes Care.* 2014;37(6):1573–1580.

40. Rock CL, Flatt SW, Sherwood NE, Karanja N, Pakiz B, Thomson CA. Effect of a free prepared meal and incentivized weight loss program on weight loss and weight loss maintenance in obesity and overweight women: a randomized controlled trial. *JAMA.* 2010;304(16):1803–1811.

41. Rock CL, Pakiz B, Flatt SW, Quintana EL. Randomized trial of a multifaceted commercial weight loss program. *Obesity (Silver Spring).* 2007;15(4):939–949.

42. Foster GD, Wadden TA, Lagrotte CA, et al. A randomized comparison of a commercially available portion-controlled weight-loss intervention with a diabetes self-management education program. *Nutr Diabetes.* 2013;3:e63.

43. Figueroa A, Vicil F, Sanchez-Gomes MA, et al. Effects of diet and/or low-intensity resistance exercise training on arterial stiffness, adiposity, and lean mass in obese postmenopausal women. *Am J Hypertens.* 2013;26(3):416–423.

44. Foster GD, Borradaile KE, Vander Veur SS, et al. The effects of a commercially available weight loss program among obese patients with type 2 diabetes: a randomized study. *Postgrad Med.* 2009;121(5):113–118.

45. Kumanyika SK, Fassbender JE, Sarwer DB, et al. One-year results of the Think Health! study of weight management in primary care practices. *Obesity (Silver Spring).* 2012;20(6):1249–1257.

46. Counterweight Project Team. Evaluation of the Counterweight Programme for obesity management in primary care: a starting point for continuous improvement. *Br J Gen Pract.* 2008;58(553):548–554.

47. Counterweight Project Team. The implementation of the counterweight programme in Scotland, UK. *Fam Pract.* 2012;29(suppl 1):i139–i144.

48. Truby H, Baic S, deLooy A, et al. Randomised controlled trial of four commercial weight loss programmes in the UK: initial findings from the BBC "diet trials". *BMJ.* 2006;332(7553):1309–1314.

49. Dansinger ML, Gleason JA, Griffith JL, Selker HP, Schaefer EJ. Comparison of the Atkins, Ornish, Weight Watchers, and Zone diets for weight loss and heart disease risk reduction: a randomized trial. *JAMA.* 2005;293(1):43–53.

50. Van Gaal LF, Mertens IL, Ballaux D. What is the relationship between risk factor reduction and degree of weight loss? *Eur Heart J Suppl.* 2005;7:L21–L26.

51. Wing RR, Lang W, Wadden TA, et al. Benefits of modest weight loss in improving cardiovascular risk factors in overweight and obese individuals with type 2 diabetes. *Diabetes Care.* 2011;34(7):1481–1486.

52. Mehta AK, Doshi RS, Chaudhry ZW, et al. Benefits of commercial weight-loss programs on blood pressure and lipids: a systematic review. *Prev Med.* 2016;90:86–99.

53. Vakil RM, Doshi RS, Mehta AK, et al. Direct comparisons of commercial weight-loss programs on weight, waist circumference, and blood pressure: a systematic review. *BMC Public Health.* 2016;16:460.

54. Hauner H. Obesity and diabetes. In: Holt RIG, Cockram CS, Flyvbjerg A, Goldstein BJ, eds. *Textbook of Diabetes.* 4th ed. Oxford: Wiley-Blackwell; 2010.

55. Gillies CL, Abrams KR, Lambert PC, et al. Pharmacological and lifestyle interventions to prevent or delay type 2 diabetes in people with impaired glucose tolerance: systematic review and meta-analysis. *BMJ.* 2007;334:299.

56. Australian diabetes prevention programmes. Available at: https://www.diabetesaustralia.com.au/prevention. Accessed 10 January 2017.

57. Finnish Diabetes Association. *Programme for the Prevention of Type 2 Diabetes in Finland 2003–2010.* Tampere, Finland: FDA; 2003.

58. Mitchell NS, Prochazka AV, Glasgow RE. Time to RE-AIM: why community weight loss programs should be included in academic obesity research. *Prev Chronic Dis.* 2016;13:E37.

59. NHS England Diabetes Prevention Programme. Available at: https://www.england.nhs.uk/ourwork/qual-clin-lead/diabetes-prevention/. Accessed 10 January 2017.

60. Ali MK, Echouffo-Tcheugui J, Williamson DF. How effective were lifestyle interventions in real-world settings that were modeled on the diabetes prevention program? *Health Aff (Millwood).* 2012;31(1):67–75.

61. Loveman E, Frampton GK, Shepherd J, et al. The clinical effectiveness and cost-effectiveness of long-term weight management schemes for adults: a systematic review. *Health Technol Assess.* 2011;15(2):1–182.

62. Fuller NR, Colagiuri S, Schofield D, et al. A within-trial cost-effectiveness analysis of primary care referral to a commercial provider for weight loss treatment, relative to standard care–an international randomised controlled trial. *Int J Obes (Lond).* 2013;37(6):828–834.

63. Fuller NR, Carter H, Schofield D, et al. Cost effectiveness of primary care referral to a commercial provider for weight loss treatment, relative to standard care: a modelled lifetime analysis. *Int J Obes (Lond).* August 2014;38(8):1104–1109.

64. Finkelstein EA, Kruger E. Meta- and cost-effectiveness analysis of commercial weight loss strategies. *Obesity (Silver Spring).* 2014;22(9):1942–1951.

65. Dombrowski SU, Knittle K, Avenell A, Araújo-Soares V, Sniehotta FF. Long term maintenance of weight loss with non-surgical interventions in obese adults: systematic review and meta-analyses of randomised controlled trials. *BMJ.* 2014;348:g2646.

66. Lowe MR, Miller-Kovach K, Phelan S. Weight-loss maintenance in overweight individuals one to five years following successful completion of a commercial weight loss program. *Int J Obes Relat Metab Disord.* 2001;25(3): 325–331.

67. Lavin JH, Pallister C, Morris L, Horgan G, Stubbs J. 12 month weight outcomes in 45,395 high-engagers with the Slimming World weight management programme. *Obes Facts.* 2013;6:189.

68. Mitchell NS, Polsky S, Catenacci VA, Furniss AL, Prochazka AV. Up to 7 years of sustained weight loss for weight-loss program completers. *Am J Prev Med.* 2015;49(2): 248–258.

69. Moroshko I, Brennan L, O'Brien P. Predictors of dropout in weight loss interventions: a systematic review of the literature. *Obes Rev.* 2011;12(11):912–934.

70. Dyson P. Commercial weight loss programmes: are they effective for people with type 2 diabetes?. *Pract Diabetes.* 2015;32(4):137–141a.

71. Relton C, Li J, Strong M, et al. Deprivation, clubs and drugs: results of a UK regional population-based cross-sectional study of weight management strategies. *BMC Public Health.* 2014;14:444.

72. Ahern AL, Aveyard P, Boyland EJ, Halford JC, Jebb SA, WRAP trial team. Inequalities in the uptake of weight management interventions in a pragmatic trial: an observational study in primary care. *Br J Gen Pract.* 2016;66(645):e258–e263.

73. Robertson C, Avenell A, Boachie C, et al. Should weight loss and maintenance programmes be designed differently for men? A systematic review of long-term randomised controlled trials presenting data for men and women: the ROMEO project. *Obes Res Clin Pract.* 2016;10(1):70–84.

74. Fitzgibbon ML, Stolley M, Schiffer L, et al. Obesity reduction black intervention trial (ORBIT): design and baseline characteristics. *J Womens Health (Larchmt).* 2008;17(7):1099–1110.

CHAPTER 22

Breakfast for the Prevention and Treatment of Obesity

JAVIER T. GONZALEZ, PHD

INTRODUCTION

Breakfast has no universally common definition and has been defined in a number of ways, including: the first meal of the day; eaten before or at the start of daily activities; within 2 h of waking; or within a specific time frame, such as between 0600 and 1000 h[1]; an energy content of at least 20% of daily energy needs,[2] or in some self-report studies, the definition is left to the participant's discretion.[3,4] A recent definition that attempted to logically consider potential limitations of others is "the first meal consumed within 2 h after the longest sleep in any 24 h period, thus normally also reflecting the longest daily duration spent in the fasted-state and the only time most humans are genuinely post-absorptive".[5]

Guidelines from public health authorities[6–8] and charities[9] recommend regular consumption of breakfast to assist with weight loss/maintenance. Moreover, some even specify the type of foods to consume, such as "unsweetened wholegrain cereals or bread, lower fat milk and a portion of fruit".[6] These guidelines appear to be followed by most people in the United Kingdom and United States, because ~80% of people report regularly consuming breakfast,[1,10] and the most common form of breakfast is cereal and milk based.[1]

EPIDEMIOLOGICAL LINKS BETWEEN BREAKFAST HABITS AND OBESITY

There is a wealth of observational evidence on links between breakfast and obesity. At least 58 observational studies (with 88 independent groups) spanning the globe have been published on the relationship between breakfast consumption and obesity, with evidence from over 30 countries and 5 continents.[11] A cumulative meta-analysis of these data supports public health guidelines that regular breakfast consumption is associated with a lower risk of obesity. Specifically, the odds ratio of obesity with regularly skipping breakfast was reported to be 1.55 (95% confidence interval [CI]: 1.46–1.65, $P = 10^{-42}$). This impressive P value

represents exceptionally strong evidence of an association. Interestingly, there was sufficient evidence for most people to be confident of an association (e.g., $P < .001$) before the year 2000; yet, there is continuing observational data being published, confirming this association across various populations.[11] However, a correlation is not evidence of cause and effect, a concept that should always be carefully considered, particularly in nutrition research where randomized controlled trials can reveal effects that directly oppose observational-based hypotheses.[12] Moreover, the relationship between breakfast and obesity could still be spurious or an artifact of publication bias.[11] Randomized control trials allow for more certainty of cause and effect between diet and health outcomes and thus will inform the majority of this chapter.

BREAKFAST FOR THE PREVENTION OF OBESITY

Because obesity is a consequence of a sustained positive energy balance, and breakfast habits relate to body mass index even within the non-obese range, then if breakfast habits causally affect obesity risk, studying energy balance components in non-obese individuals can reveal the potential mechanisms by which breakfast consumption may influence obesity risk. For example, it is commonly reported by laypersons that skipping breakfast increases food intake for the rest of the day (i.e., energy intake compensation). For this to reduce body mass then energy intake compensation must surpass the energy contained in breakfast and also be sustained over time. Moreover, the potential for breakfast to modulate components of energy expenditure should also be considered alongside energy intake, because increased energy intake could be surpassed by larger increases in expenditure.

By definition, lean and obese individuals within the same environment have different energy balance regulation. Therefore, the effect of regular breakfast consumption on energy balance could differ between obese versus lean individuals, and thus guidelines may need to be tailored for prevention versus treatment of obesity. Accordingly, lean individuals will be considered first (prevention), before examining the causal role of breakfast on energy balance in obese individuals (treatment).

Energy Balance

Acute responses

The acute (within-day) energy balance responses to breakfast in lean adults have been explored in relatively few trials. Although studies have determined energy intake, fewer determined both energy intake and expenditure in tandem. It is commonly assumed that breakfast skipping results in overconsumption later in the day, resulting in a positive energy balance and, over time, weight gain. However, the balance of evidence does not support this. The majority of studies report either no difference[13–15] or a marginal increase[13,16–19] in energy intake at subsequent meals (e.g., lunch or lunch + dinner). Importantly, the increase in energy intake is almost always insufficient to account for the energy intake that is missed with breakfast skipping[20] (Fig. 22.1A).

Breakfast is occasionally deemed by laypersons to "kick-start your metabolism." Consumption of any food increases energy expenditure above fasting, known as the thermic effect of feeding (TEF). TEF is a result of the digestion, absorption, and metabolism of nutrients and is proportional to the energy consumed and dependent on the nutrient composition of foods. For example, based on biochemistry, the TEF of protein,

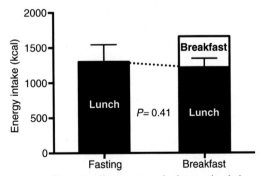

FIG. 22.1 Energy intake across a single morning in lean individuals who either remained fasted until ~1100h or consumed breakfast at ~0800h in a laboratory environment. Data are means ± 95% confidence interval. (Adapted from Gonzalez JT, Veasey RC, Rumbold PL, Stevenson EJ. Breakfast and exercise contingently affect postprandial metabolism and energy balance in physically active males. *Br J Nutr.* 2013;110(4):721–732, with permission.)

alcohol (ethanol), carbohydrate, and fat ingestion is expected to be ~23%, ~12%–27% (depending on the pathway utilized), ~6%, and ~3%, respectively.[21,22] This increase in energy expenditure is therefore modest and insufficient to offset the energy consumed at breakfast (Fig. 22.1A and B).

Studies that determined energy expenditure alongside energy intake have typically reported a more positive (less negative) energy balance with breakfast consumption[14] (Fig. 22.1). However, it should be noted that all within-day studies of energy balance have been performed in a laboratory environment and therefore any influence of breakfast consumption on energy balance behaviors, such as spontaneous physical activity energy expenditure (PAEE), may not be detectable.

Chronic responses

Acute studies have typically been confined to a laboratory environment, whereas longer-term experiments have explored more of the free-living energy balance response to breakfast consumption or omission. Combining laboratory studies with free-living observations permits a better understanding of the influence of breakfast on each individual component of energy expenditure. For example, the measurement of resting metabolic rate and/or postprandial thermogenesis requires tightly controlled conditions, and thus their measurement is most accurately performed in a laboratory environment. In contrast, for a measure of PAEE to be reflective of habitual patterns, its measurement requires free-living conditions to permit interaction with the environment.

Resting metabolic rate and postprandial thermogenesis appear to be largely unaffected by regular breakfast consumption,[23,24] and thus the focus on breakfast and PAEE is growing. Few randomized controlled trials on breakfast consumption have accurately determined PAEE despite this being the most dynamic component of energy expenditure.[25] Some have attempted to use heart rate alone[26] or pedometer scores alone[26,27] to assess PAEE in response to 7 days of breakfast consumption versus omission. These studies demonstrated that morning heart rate was higher when breakfast was consumed compared with that when breakfast was skipped,[26] although this did not translate into a higher daily heart rate, nor a higher daily pedometer score.[26,27] A more sensitive method of measuring PAEE under free-living conditions is to combine heart rate with accelerometry and branched-equation modeling.[28] This method has been shown to be accurate when compared with doubly labeled water[29] and has the added benefit of providing information on the intensity and temporal nature of PAEE.

A recent study employing combined heart rate and accelerometry provided the first causal evidence that breakfast consumption increases daily PAEE compared with extended morning fasting. Participants who were randomized to consume breakfast each day for 6 weeks (≥700 kcal of energy prior to 1100 h and ≥350 kcal of which was consumed within 2 h of waking) were 442 kcal/day (95% CI: 34, 851 kcal/day) more physically active than those randomized to breakfast omission (water only from waking until midday; Fig. 22.2).[23] This difference in daily PAEE was mostly driven by a higher morning PAEE and in light intensity PAEE (such as fidgeting and walking). The magnitude of this increase in PAEE is likely to be important from a public health standpoint, as this is broadly equivalent to the energy expenditure of government physical activity guidelines[30] and raises the question whether breakfast consumption assists in adherence to physical activity guidelines.

Chronic effects of breakfast consumption on energy intake in lean individuals, however, are less clear. Some have demonstrated that 2 weeks of breakfast omission increases energy intake (~91 kcal/day) compared with breakfast consumption,[24] whereas others have demonstrated that breakfast omission leads to a lower daily energy intake (~539 kcal/day) over 6 weeks (albeit also with a lower energy expenditure; Fig. 22.2).[23] Notwithstanding the issue that these studies were reliant on self-reported energy intake, the discordant results may be explained by experimental design, whereby the omission of breakfast results in a higher energy intake when the breakfast energy replaced later in the day,[24] as opposed to allowing all energy intake postmidday to vary,[23] thus requiring greater compensation of energy intake to surpass the energy skipped prior to midday. The overall energy balance response in the only study of this kind to report both energy intake and energy expenditure would indicate that, in lean adults, breakfast consumption would result in either little change or, if anything, a more positive (or less negative) energy balance compared with breakfast omission.[23]

Body Mass and Adiposity
Given the energy balance response in lean individuals indicates that higher energy expenditure with breakfast

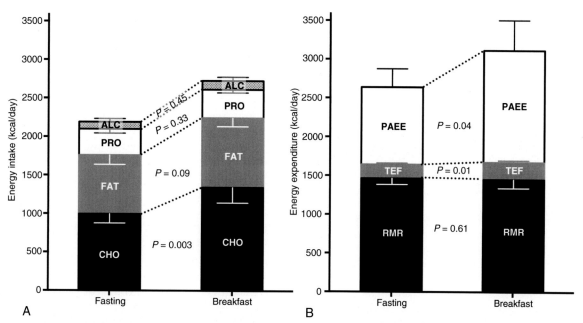

FIG. 22.2 Energy intake **(A)** and energy expenditure **(B)** in lean individuals randomized to either remain fasting until midday or consume breakfast before 1100 h each day for 6 weeks. *ALC*, alcohol; *CHO*, carbohydrate; *PAEE*, physical activity energy expenditure; *PRO*, protein; *RMR*, resting metabolic rate; *TEF*, thermic effect of feeding. Data are means ± 95% confidence interval. (Adapted from Betts JA, Richardson JD, Chowdhury EA, Holman GD, Tsintzas K, Thompson D. The causal role of breakfast in energy balance and health: a randomized controlled trial in lean adults. *Am J Clin Nutr.* 2014;100(2):539–547, with permission.)

consumption is countered (and may be surpassed) by higher energy intake, the net effect on energy balance is negligible.[23] Consistent with this, changes in body mass were unaffected by 6 weeks of breakfast consumption. Moreover, the change in fat mass was also unaffected by breakfast consumption (~0.21 kg in both groups).[23] Therefore, the current evidence does not support a causal role of breakfast consumption in the prevention of obesity.

Metabolic Health
Metabolic health is most often defined by the ability to maintain blood glucose, cholesterol and triglyceride concentrations within appropriate ranges. Exaggerated postprandial glucose or triglyceride concentrations are associated with mortality and morbidity.[31] Even in populations considered healthy (fasting and 2-h postprandial glucose <6.1 and <7.8 mmol/L, respectively), those with higher postprandial glucose concentrations relative to fasting have a ~10%–20% increased risk of heart disease or stroke.[32] Accordingly, the effects of regular breakfast consumption on blood glucose and lipid concentrations have important implications for health guidelines in both obese and nonobese individuals.

Acute responses
Because the most common breakfasts consumed in economically developed countries are high in carbohydrates, the initial response to breakfast consumption is an immediate rise in blood glucose concentrations. In healthy individuals, this rise is relatively transient, returning to baseline within 2 h.[14,17] More interestingly, the glycemic response to a subsequent meal appears to be influenced by prior breakfast consumption, whereby the ingestion of breakfast reduces postprandial glucose excursions to subsequent meals,[14,16,17] also known as "the second-meal effect."[33] The reduction in postprandial glycemia is also sometimes accompanied by a reduction in insulinemia,[14,17] suggestive of improved insulin sensitivity. The second-meal effect is apparent with both high-carbohydrate and high-protein breakfasts,[14,34] but not with high-fat breakfasts, whereby a tendency for an *increased* glycemic response to lunch has been observed.[35] Plasma triglycerides, however, do not display a second-meal effect, and in fact, the postprandial triglyceride response to lunch is greater after breakfast versus extended morning fasting.[36]

Chronic responses
Causal evidence on the effects of regular breakfast consumption on metabolic health in lean individuals is somewhat discordant and may depend on the breakfast size/composition. Two weeks of regular consumption of modest (~162 kcal), fiber-rich (7 g fiber) breakfast (consumed prior to 0800 h daily) has been shown to reduce total cholesterol concentrations compared with consumption of the same foodstuffs between 1200 and 1330 h daily.[24] This reduction was driven by a decrease in LDL cholesterol concentrations. In contrast, 6 weeks regular consumption of a larger (>700 kcal) breakfast did not result in any differences in fasting plasma cholesterol or triglyceride concentrations, compared with extended morning fasting.[23] Furthermore, other markers of metabolic health were also unaffected by breakfast consumption in both these studies, such as fasting plasma glucose, insulin, interleukin-6, and C-reactive protein concentrations.[23,24]

Aspects of metabolic health that may be improved by regular breakfast consumption are glucose control and/or peripheral insulin sensitivity. It has been shown that regular breakfast consumption for 6 weeks reduces interstitial glucose variability in the afternoon and evening, compared with extended morning fasting[23]. With regard to insulin sensitivity, fasting measures of plasma insulin and glucose provide a greater representation of hepatic insulin sensitivity, whereas postprandial measures are more heavily influenced by peripheral insulin sensitivity. Postprandial markers of insulin sensitivity (e.g., plasma insulin concentrations) have been shown to improve (i.e., lower insulin concentrations) with breakfast consumption by some,[24] and although others have not observed this at the whole-body level,[23] adipose tissue-specific indices of insulin sensitivity have been observed to improve with breakfast consumption.[23] It should be borne in mind, however, that adipose tissue is quantitatively a minor site of postprandial glucose disposal, and therefore until muscle-specific measures and/or hyperinsulinemic-euglycemic clamp studies are performed, the causal role of breakfast consumption on insulin sensitivity will remain unclear.

BREAKFAST FOR THE TREATMENT OF OBESITY
Energy Balance
Acute responses
There is currently an almost complete absence of evidence pertaining to the acute effects of breakfast consumption on energy balance components in obese individuals. One of the only studies to have investigated this to date found that, when obese individuals consumed a carbohydrate-rich breakfast containing ~521 kcal, their energy intake at an ad libitum lunch provided 3 h after breakfast was 817 ± 325 kcal. When breakfast was omitted, energy intake at lunch was not

different from the breakfast trial (869 ± 354 kcal). Accordingly, when the energy intake from breakfast was taken into account, then total energy intake was ~469 kcal higher with breakfast consumption versus omission. This response is, therefore, similar to that seen in lean individuals (Fig. 22.1), although, if anything, lean individuals have been observed to compensate in response to breakfast by reducing lunch energy intake (albeit insufficiently),[17] whereas obese individuals under similar experimental conditions do not compensate for breakfast with subsequent lunch intake.[15]

One study combined measures of energy intake with energy expenditure in response to breakfast consumption in overweight individuals. When a standardized lunch was provided and dinner and subsequent snacks were consumed ad libitum, breakfast consumption (~498 kcal) resulted in a higher carbohydrate and protein—but not fat—intake over a 24-h period, compared with breakfast omission.[19] Energy intake was 2344 kcal (interquartile range: 1913, 2777 kcal) when breakfast was omitted and 2516 kcal (interquartile range: 2363, 3324 kcal) when breakfast was consumed, and therefore any changes in energy intake with dinner and snack intake were insufficient to compensate for breakfast energy intake. The difference in energy expenditure pre-lunch, with breakfast omission (365 kcal, 95% CI: 342, 388 kcal) compared with breakfast consumption (411, 95% CI: 388, 434 kcal), was modest and predictable based on TEF. Consequently, after consumption of a standardized lunch, there was no difference in energy expenditure between breakfast consumption versus breakfast omission.[19] Lean and overweight/obese individuals therefore appear to respond broadly similarly in an acute laboratory setting to breakfast consumption, compared with extended morning fasting, whereby the energy intake at breakfast is not fully compensated for at the next available feeding opportunity. Similarly, breakfast consumption increases energy expenditure (TEF) in both lean and overweight individuals, but this effect is small and is only ever a fraction of the energy ingested in a meal.

Chronic responses

The lack of sufficient compensation in acute energy intake with breakfast consumption appears to be mitigated over a 6-week period in obese individuals, whereby people randomized to consume breakfast (≥700 kcal before 1100 h daily) report an energy intake that does not substantially differ from those randomized to skip breakfast (Fig. 22.3A; i.e., compensation with energy intake).

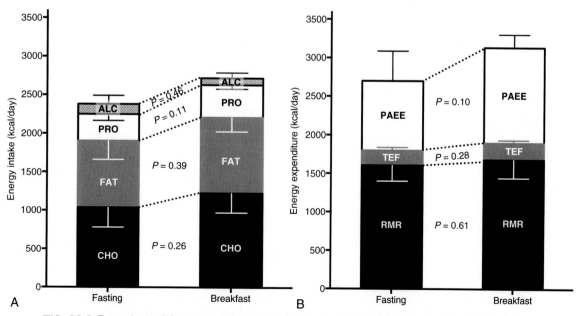

FIG. 22.3 Energy intake **(A)** and energy expenditure **(B)** in obese individuals randomized to either remain fasting until midday or consume breakfast before 1100 h each day for 6 weeks. *ALC*, alcohol; *CHO*, carbohydrate; *PAEE*, physical activity energy expenditure; *PRO*, protein; *RMR*, resting metabolic rate; *TEF*, thermic effect of feeding. Data are means ± 95% confidence interval. (Adapted from Chowdhury EA, Richardson JD, Tsintzas K, Thompson D, Betts JA. Effect of extended morning fasting upon ad libitum lunch intake and associated metabolic and hormonal responses in obese adults. *Int J Obes.* 2016;40(2):305–311, with permission.)

Energy expenditure appeared to respond in a similar direction to that seen in lean individuals, albeit with less magnitude. For example, resting metabolic rate was unaltered by breakfast consumption versus omission, as was postprandial thermogenesis. A higher PAEE prior to midday was observed with breakfast consumption compared with fasting (~188 kcal), but this effect was not seen across the entire day (Fig. 22.3B). Daily PAEE may not respond as robustly to breakfast consumption in obese individuals due to a "floor effect" whereby in lean individuals, removal of breakfast lowers daily PAEE, whereas obese individuals have a lower baseline PAEE, and thus less of a decrease in PAEE with breakfast omission.

Body Mass and Adiposity

The compensation in energy intake seen with breakfast consumption in obese individuals appears to translate into body mass because there is no detectable difference in body mass with consumption of a large breakfast (≥700 kcal) when compared with extended morning fasting (1.0 kg, 95% CI: 0.2, 1.7 kg, compared with 0.2 kg, 95% CI: −0.5, 1.0 kg, respectively).[37] Similarly, dual-energy x-ray absorptiometry-derived adipose tissue mass did not respond differently to breakfast consumption compared with fasting.[37] In contrast, consumption of a modest (~350 kcal) breakfast, as either cornflakes or oat porridge over 4 weeks, prevents the decrease in body mass seen with extended morning fasting in overweight individuals.[38] However, neither of these tightly controlled studies provide support for the efficacy of breakfast consumption for the treatment of obesity (or overweight).

Although tightly controlled trials are of use in determining efficacy and proof-of-principle, there is also a benefit of conducting trials employing more ecological validity. In this regard, it is of benefit to governments and public health authorities to know whether *the recommendation* to eat breakfast has effectiveness for weight loss. In the largest study of this kind to date, 309 overweight or obese participants were randomized to one of three groups for a 16-week intervention: control, breakfast, or no-breakfast groups. The control group received a handout providing generic dietary advice that did not specifically refer to breakfast. The breakfast group received generic advice plus a handout that instructed participants to consume breakfast prior to 1000 h daily and provided some suggestions of healthy breakfasts. The no-breakfast group received the generic advice plus a handout that instructed participants to not consume any foods or energy-containing beverages until 1100 h each day. Over the 16 weeks, all groups lost weight (~0.7 kg), but the advice to either consume or not to consume breakfast did not affect weight loss compared with the control group. Therefore, the current evidence base does not support the guidance to regularly consume breakfast for the treatment of obesity. Breakfast habits appear to have a little, if any, causal role in net weight loss and guidelines should focus on other strategies that assist with the maintenance of a negative energy balance.

Metabolic Health

Acute responses

The second-meal effect is also present in obese (or overweight) individuals, whereby consumption of a carbohydrate-rich breakfast results in a lower plasma glucose response to lunch.[15,19] Post-lunch plasma insulin concentrations are also sometimes,[15] but not always,[19] lower when a breakfast has previously been consumed, suggesting that insulin sensitivity may be acutely improved with breakfast consumption. The exaggerated triglyceride response to lunch when breakfast has been consumed is also seen in overweight individuals.[19] The acute metabolic responses to breakfast consumption therefore seem to be similar between both lean and obese individuals, whereby a carbohydrate-rich breakfast improves glucose control but raises triglyceride concentrations at the next meal.

Chronic responses

The chronic metabolic response to breakfast consumption in obese individuals may also depend on the size of breakfast. Consumption of a moderately sized breakfast (~350 kcal), either cornflakes or oat porridge, in overweight individuals prevents the increase in total cholesterol concentrations seen when breakfast is omitted for 4 weeks.[38] This response, however, was not observed when obese individuals consumed a larger (≥700 kcal) carbohydrate-rich breakfast over 6 weeks.[37] Furthermore, consistent evidence indicates that in overweight and obese individuals, breakfast consumption does not influence fasting concentrations of HDL cholesterol, LDL cholesterol, glucose, insulin, or triglycerides[37,38], at least in a relatively short time frame. Further markers of cardiovascular disease risk, such as interleukin-6 and C-reactive protein, also do not appear to be influenced by 6 weeks of breakfast consumption.[37]

Similarly to lean individuals, the one aspect of metabolic health that does appear to be improved by regular breakfast consumption in obese individuals is peripheral insulin sensitivity. The evidence for this comes from the insulin response to an oral glucose tolerance test, which showed a decline with 6 weeks of regular breakfast consumption relative to extended morning fasting.[37] Nonetheless, the similar limitation of a lack of gold-standard measures of peripheral insulin sensitivity means further research is required to confirm this potential health effect of regular breakfast consumption. Therefore, early evidence indicates that regular breakfast consumption may reduce total cholesterol concentrations (when the breakfast is modestly sized) and increase peripheral insulin sensitivity in overweight/obese individuals, but other markers of metabolic health appear to be unaffected.

INTERACTIONS BETWEEN BREAKFAST AND OTHER GUIDELINES FOR PREVENTION OF OBESITY

In addition to regular breakfast consumption, public health guidelines make numerous other recommendations for the prevention of obesity and their potential interaction with breakfast consumption warrants attention. The key guideline that could most readily interact with breakfast consumption is the recommendation to be more physically active to avoid a low energy expenditure.[6] This is encouraged to take place as either active travel (cycling or walking to work or school), partaking in sport, or exercise and increasing activity as part of daily routines (taking the stairs instead of the lift).

Although breakfast consumption may facilitate light intensity physical activity, particularly in the morning, and thus potentially assist in raising energy expenditure, this may not necessarily be the case when a bout of exercise or activity is imposed, such as with an active commute to work. In this scenario, the effect of breakfast on physical activity may be prohibited because the activity bout is dictated by other factors. Furthermore, exercise is known to influence appetite, and thus the subsequent energy balance response to the breakfast-exercise interaction is of interest. In this regard, there is little long-term data on this, but acute studies suggest that omitting breakfast prior to exercise reduces total energy intake, and thus energy balance up to 24 h,[14,18,39] warranting longer-term studies.

PERSPECTIVES ON THE FUTURE

The evidence base for breakfast and energy balance is still relatively small, and therefore the causal evidence to draw on is primarily studies of high-carbohydrate breakfasts. It therefore remains to be seen whether some of the potential benefits of breakfast consumption on energy expenditure can be maintained with other types of breakfasts, through stronger suppression of appetite and energy intake to achieve a negative (or less positive) energy balance. Potential candidates to explore in this regard are breakfasts rich in protein and calcium[40,41] and the role of caffeine in stimulating physical activity.[42]

With the recent increases in the prevalence and accessibility of wearable monitors, the ability to measure energy balance components, and even interstitial glucose concentrations, under free-living conditions is improving. With the use of these technologies, researchers can begin to explore the role of breakfast consumption in the prevention and treatment of obesity. The first randomized controlled trial to explore the role of breakfast consumption on energy balance components suggests that when lean people regularly consume a large, carbohydrate-rich breakfast over a 6-week period, then daily PAEE is increased relative to extended morning fasting. The increase in daily PAEE is driven by higher levels of light-to-moderate intensity physical activities in the morning. However, breakfast consumption of this type in lean people also leads to a higher daily energy intake, and thus the net effect on energy balance and body weight is negligible. These differences between breakfast consumption and omission appear to be much less prevalent in obese individuals, whereby energy intake is not substantially altered, nor is total PAEE. Nonetheless, breakfast consumption does still increase morning PAEE in obese individuals. Although it appears that breakfast consumption plays a little, if any, causal role in net energy balance and thus body weight changes, a higher energy turnover is likely to have positive effects on health, as indicated by potential improvements in peripheral insulin sensitivity with regular breakfast consumption.

REFERENCES

1. Gibson SA, Gunn P. What's for breakfast? Nutritional implications of breakfast habits: insights from the NDNS dietary records. *Nutr Bull.* 2011;36(1):78–86.
2. Timlin MT, Pereira MA. Breakfast frequency and quality in the etiology of adult obesity and chronic diseases. *Nutr Rev.* 2007;65(6 Pt 1):268–281.
3. Deshmukh-Taskar PR, Radcliffe JD, Liu Y, Nicklas TA. Do breakfast skipping and breakfast type affect energy intake, nutrient intake, nutrient adequacy, and diet quality in young adults? NHANES 1999–2002. *J Am Coll Nutr.* 2010;29(4):407–418.

4. Deshmukh-Taskar PR, Nicklas TA, O'Neil CE, Keast DR, Radcliffe JD, Cho S. The relationship of breakfast skipping and type of breakfast consumption with nutrient intake and weight status in children and adolescents: the National Health and Nutrition Examination Survey 1999–2006. *J Am Diet Assoc.* 2010;110(6):869–878.

5. Betts JA, Chowdhury EA, Gonzalez JT, Richardson JD, Tsintzas K, Thompson D. Is breakfast the most important meal of the day? *Proc Nutr Soc.* 2016:1–11.

6. NICE. Preventing excess weight gain (NICE guideline 7). In: *Agency HD.* London, 2015.

7. Zeratsky K. Why Does Eating a Healthy Breakfast Help Control Weight? http://www.mayoclinic.org/food-and-nutrition/expert-answers/FAQ-20058449.

8. SurgeonGeneral.gov. *The Surgeon General's Call to Action to Prevent and Decrease Overweight and Obesity: Overwegith in Children and Adolescents;* 2001. http://www.surgeongeneral.gov/library/calls/obesity/fact_adolescents.html.

9. Foundation BH. Facts not Fads – Your Simple Guide to Healthy weight loss, vol. M22015:36–37.

10. Wyatt HR, Grunwald GK, Mosca CL, Klem ML, Wing RR, Hill JO. Long-term weight loss and breakfast in subjects in the national weight control registry. *Obes Res.* 2002;10(2):78–82.

11. Brown AW, Bohan Brown MM, Allison DB. Belief beyond the evidence: using the proposed effect of breakfast on obesity to show 2 practices that distort scientific evidence. *Am J Clin Nutr.* 2013;98(5):1298–1308.

12. The effect of vitamin E and beta carotene on the incidence of lung cancer and other cancers in male smokers. The Alpha-Tocopherol, Beta Carotene Cancer Prevention Study Group. *N Engl J Med.* 1994;330(15):1029–1035.

13. Levitsky DA, Pacanowski CR. Effect of skipping breakfast on subsequent energy intake. *Physiol Behav.* 2013;119:9–16.

14. Gonzalez JT, Veasey RC, Rumbold PL, Stevenson EJ. Breakfast and exercise contingently affect postprandial metabolism and energy balance in physically active males. *Br J Nutr.* 2013;110(4):721–732.

15. Chowdhury EA, Richardson JD, Tsintzas K, Thompson D, Betts JA. Effect of extended morning fasting upon ad libitum lunch intake and associated metabolic and hormonal responses in obese adults. *Int J Obes.* 2016;40(2):305–311.

16. Astbury NM, Taylor MA, Macdonald IA. Breakfast consumption affects appetite, energy intake, and the metabolic and endocrine responses to foods consumed later in the day in male habitual breakfast eaters. *J Nutr.* 2011;141(7):1381–1389.

17. Chowdhury EA, Richardson JD, Tsintzas K, Thompson D, Betts JA. Carbohydrate-rich breakfast attenuates glycaemic, insulinaemic and ghrelin response to ad libitum lunch relative to morning fasting in lean adults. *Br J Nutr.* 2015:1–10.

18. Clayton DJ, Barutcu A, Machin C, Stensel DJ, James LJ. Effect of breakfast omission on energy intake and evening exercise performance. *Med Sci Sports Exerc.* 2015;47(12):2645–2652.

19. Thomas EA, Higgins J, Bessesen DH, McNair B, Cornier MA. Usual breakfast eating habits affect response to breakfast skipping in overweight women. *Obes (Silver Spring).* 2015;23(4):750–759.

20. Clayton DJ, James LJ. The effect of breakfast on appetite regulation, energy balance and exercise performance. *Proc Nutr Soc.* 2016;75(3):319–327.

21. Flatt JP. The biochemistry of energy expenditure. In: Bray GA, ed. *Recent Advances in Obesity Research.* London, United Kingdom: Newman Publishing; 1978:211–228.

22. Schutz Y. Role of substrate utilization and thermogenesis on body-weight control with particular reference to alcohol. *Proc Nutr Soc.* 2000;59(4):511–517.

23. Betts JA, Richardson JD, Chowdhury EA, Holman GD, Tsintzas K, Thompson D. The causal role of breakfast in energy balance and health: a randomized controlled trial in lean adults. *Am J Clin Nutr.* 2014;100(2):539–547.

24. Farshchi HR, Taylor MA, Macdonald IA. Deleterious effects of omitting breakfast on insulin sensitivity and fasting lipid profiles in healthy lean women. *Am J Clin Nutr.* 2005;81(2):388–396.

25. Thompson D, Batterham AM, Markovitch D, Dixon NC, Lund AJ, Walhin JP. Confusion and conflict in assessing the physical activity status of middle-aged men. *PLoS One.* 2009;4(2):e4337.

26. Halsey LG, Huber JW, Low T, Ibeawuchi C, Woodruff P, Reeves S. Does consuming breakfast influence activity levels? An experiment into the effect of breakfast consumption on eating habits and energy expenditure. *Public Health Nutr.* 2012;15(2):238–245.

27. Reeves S, Huber JW, Halsey LG, Villegas-Montes M, Elgumati J, Smith T. A cross-over experiment to investigate possible mechanisms for lower BMIs in people who habitually eat breakfast. *Eur J Clin Nutr.* 2015;69(5):632–637.

28. Thompson D, Batterham AM, Bock S, Robson C, Stokes K. Assessment of low-to-moderate intensity physical activity thermogenesis in young adults using synchronized heart rate and accelerometry with branched-equation modeling. *J Nutr.* 2006;136(4):1037–1042.

29. Silva AM, Santos DA, Matias CN, et al. Accuracy of a combined heart rate and motion sensor for assessing energy expenditure in free-living adults during a double-blind crossover caffeine trial using doubly labeled water as the reference method. *Eur J Clin Nutr.* 2015;69(1):20–27.

30. Bull FCatEWG. Physical activity guidelines in the U.K.: review and recommendations. In: *Health Do.* 2010.

31. Nordestgaard BG, Benn M, Schnohr P, Tybjaerg-Hansen A. Nonfasting triglycerides and risk of myocardial infarction, ischemic heart disease, and death in men and women. *JAMA.* 2007;298(3):299–308.

32. Ning F, Zhang L, Dekker JM, et al. Development of coronary heart disease and ischemic stroke in relation to fasting and 2-hour plasma glucose levels in the normal range. *Cardiovasc Diabetol.* 2012;11:76.

33. Gonzalez JT. Paradoxical second-meal phenomenon in the acute post-exercise period. *Nutrition.* 2014;30(9):961–967.

34. Chen MJ, Jovanovic A, Taylor R. Utilizing the second-meal effect in type 2 diabetes: practical use of a soya-yogurt snack. *Diabetes Care.* 2010;33(12):2552–2554.

35. Frape DL, Williams NR, Scriven AJ, Palmer CR, O'Sullivan K, Fletcher RJ. Diurnal trends in responses of blood plasma concentrations of glucose, insulin, and C-peptide following high- and low-fat meals and their relation to fat metabolism in healthy middle-aged volunteers. *Br J Nutr.* 1997;77(4):523–535.

36. Allerton DM, Campbell MD, Gonzalez JT, Rumbold PL, West DJ, Stevenson EJ. Co-ingestion of whey protein with a carbohydrate-rich breakfast does not affect glycemia, insulinemia or subjective appetite following a subsequent meal in healthy males. *Nutrients.* 2016;8(3).

37. Chowdhury EA, Richardson JD, Holman GD, Tsintzas K, Thompson D, Betts JA. The causal role of breakfast in energy balance and health: a randomized controlled trial in obese adults. *Am J Clin Nutr.* 2016;103(3):747–756.

38. Geliebter A, Astbury NM, Aviram-Friedman R, Yahav E, Hashim S. Skipping breakfast leads to weight loss but also elevated cholesterol compared with consuming daily breakfasts of oat porridge or frosted cornflakes in overweight individuals: a randomised controlled trial. *J Nutr Sci.* 2014;3:e56.

39. Bachman JL, Deitrick RW, Hillman AR. Exercising in the fasted state reduced 24-hour energy intake in active male adults. *J Nutr Metab.* 2016;2016:1984198.

40. Gonzalez JT, Green BP, Brown MA, Rumbold PL, Turner LA, Stevenson EJ. Calcium ingestion suppresses appetite and produces acute overcompensation of energy intake independent of protein in healthy adults. *J Nutr.* 2015;145(3):476–482.

41. Gonzalez JT, Stevenson EJ. Calcium co-ingestion augments postprandial glucose-dependent insulinotropic peptide1-42, glucagon-like peptide-1 and insulin concentrations in humans. *Eur J Nutr.* 2014;53(2):375–385.

42. Schubert MM, Hall S, Leveritt M, Grant G, Sabapathy S, Desbrow B. Caffeine consumption around an exercise bout: effects on energy expenditure, energy intake, and exercise enjoyment. *J Appl Physiol (1985).* 2014;117(7):745–754.

CHAPTER 23

Overview of a Range of Diets in Obesity Management

HELEN LONG, BSc (HONS) • GRACE STONEBANKS, BSc (HONS)

INTRODUCTION

Despite rates of obesity increasing globally, access to dietary advice has never been easier. There is a direct relationship between a negative balance of energy intake and energy requirements to the rate of weight loss. Most diets achieve this through the restriction of one or more macronutrients (carbohydrate, fat, and protein). This chapter aims to review a range of popular macronutrient-restrictive diets currently available in obesity management and evaluate the evidence of their success in weight reduction and sustainability. Fad diets (diets involving unusual eating patterns or combinations of food) have a very limited evidence base and their reputability usually comes from a celebrity endorsement. These will not be reviewed in this chapter because of insufficient supporting research and these diets are usually unsustainable long term.

Diets can be split into two categories:
1. Very-low-calorie diets (VLCD)—less than 800 kcal/day
2. Conventional diets—over 800 kcal/day

CONVENTIONAL DIETS

Low-Carbohydrate Diet

Low- and very-low-carbohydrate diets provide 60–130 g/day and 0–60 g/day, respectively. Popular diets based on this model include the Atkins, South Beach, and Dukan.

Typically, low-carbohydrate diets are low in fibre in the UK, thiamine, folate, potassium, calcium, magnesium, iron, and vitamins A, E, and B_6.

Overall, restricting carbohydrates has been shown to be effective for stimulating weight loss up to 6 months, more so than low-fat diets. However, this was not sustained at 12 months.[1] Early weight loss can be attributed to fluid loss and glycogenolysis. In a recent study, it was also shown that low-carbohydrate diets can cause cognitive deficits because of a lack of energy from blood glucose, which is normally produced in the breakdown of carbohydrates. In addition, a study showed low-carbohydrate diets to affect myocardial energy substrates

and insulin signaling both of which play a role in the protection of ischemic myocardium. Low-carbohydrate diets led to an increase in 3-hydroxybutyrate and lower circulating insulin, resulting in impaired ventricular performance, along with lower myocardial glycogen stores and glycogen utilization.[2] Low-carbohydrate diets have also been shown to prolong the QT interval in an ECG, which is of clinical importance because of an increased risk for ventricular dysrhythmia and sudden death.[3]

Low-Fat Diets

Fat-focused diets can encompass a restriction of specific types of fat or of fats overall.

A reduction in total dietary fat to 30% or less of daily energy intake is recommended in almost all dietary guidelines. This equates to approximately 30 g of fat per 1000 calories consumed. Some fat-focused diets advise not necessarily a restriction of fat intake but an adjustment of the ratios of different types of fat consumed. For example, Mediterranean diet, this encourages the consumption of monounsaturated, as opposed to saturated fats, which are found in red meats and dairy. Long-term studies have shown that low-fat diets can result in weight loss and be sustained over a number of years and can have cardiovascular health benefits.[4,5] Fat-soluble vitamins A, E, D, and K and essential fatty acids n-3 and n-6 are involved in immune response, vision, bone density, blood clotting, and skin health. Therefore, some fat needs to be incorporated into the diet to avoid deficiencies in the aforementioned vitamins/fatty acids.

High-Protein Diets

High-protein diets promote the increased consumption of energy intake from protein sources and are usually coupled with a decreased consumption of carbohydrates.

They can also include aspects of fat restriction and/or modification. Protein in large amounts can cause the body to excrete inflated amounts of calcium via the urine, which can lead to bone loss and the formation of

---

BOX 23.1
Current Portion Size Recommendations for the United Kingdom

What is a portion: Carbohydrate
1 medium slice of bread
Pasta (boiled) 2–3 tablespoons
Rice (boiled) 2–3 tablespoons
2 egg-sized new potatoes (boiled)
1 medium baked potato (with skin)
Porridge oats: 3 tablespoons
Breakfast cereal: 3 tablespoons
What is a portion: Protein
Cooked meat 60–90 g
Cooked white fish, oily and canned fish 140 g
2 medium eggs
Beans and pulses 150 g
Soya/tofu 100 g
Nuts/peanut butter 30 g
What is a portion: Fruit and vegetables
All fresh, frozen and tinned 80 g
Dried fruit 30 g
What is a portion: Fats
Butter or spread 5 g
Oil 3 g
What is a portion: Dairy
Milk/milk alternative 200 mL
Yoghurt 125 g
Hard cheese 30 g

Data from British Dietetic Association. Food Fact Sheet: Portion Sizes. Available at: https://www.bda.uk.com/foodfacts/portionsizesfoodfactsheet.pdf; 2016.

BOX 23.2
Handy Guides to Portion Sizes

Carbohydrates: fist sized
Beans, pulses, soya, and tofu: 4 tablespoons
Meat and fish: Palm of your hand
Vegetables/salad: 2 handfuls
Fruit: cupped handful
Top of your thumb: oil or fat
Cheese: matchbox size
Milk: Third of a pint

Data from British Dietetic Association. Food Fact Sheet: Diabetes – Type 2. Available at: https://www.bda.uk.com/foodfacts/diabetestype2.pdf; 2015.

---

kidney stones.[6] A dietary intake that is very low in carbohydrate can also lead to the development of ketosis, a process where the body uses its fat stores for energy because it is unable to mobilize glucose because of reduced insulin production. A common misconception about carbohydrates is that they can attribute to weight gain. However, at 3.45 kcal/g, they have the lowest calorie load of all the macronutrients, with protein and fat providing 4 and 9 kcal/g respectively.

Proteins are associated with early satiety, which in turn can encourage weight loss[7]; however, short-terms side effects often cited include constipation, fatigue, halitosis, headaches, thirst, polyuria, and nausea.

Very-Low-Calorie Diets
VLCD are perhaps the most controversial of the various dietary treatments available for use in the management of obesity.[8] They should not generally be considered as a first-line weight loss intervention. Circumstances where it would be indicated is in individuals with a BMI >30 kg/m^2 [9] who require rapid weight loss, for example, before surgery.

PORTION CONTROL
Over the last 1000 years the portion size of main courses has increased by 69% and plate size by 66%.[10] An increase in meal portions has not been shown to correlate with an increased feeling of satiety.[11] Large quantities of any food group can have a detrimental effect on health. The current portion size recommendations for the United Kingdom are shown in Box 23.1.

A practical guide to portion sizes is shown in Box 23.2.

CONCLUSION
Overall, no conventional diet is preferable for guaranteed long-term sustainable weight loss. The most important factor in successful weight loss is choosing an eating pattern that is achievable for the individual and continuing to adjust macronutrient intake to continue the weight loss momentum. Long-term weight maintenance is often the most difficult part of weight loss and ensuring nutritional adequacy is essential. Therefore a macronutrient balanced approach is generally recommended.

REFERENCES

1. Nordman AJ, Nordam A, Briel M, et al. Effects of low-carbohydrate vs low-fat diets on weight loss and cardiovascular risk factors: a meta-analysis of randomized control trials. *Arch Intern Med.* 2006;166:285–293.

2. Wang P, Tate JM, Lloyd SG. Low carbohydrate diet decreases myocardial insulin signalling and increased susceptibility to myocardial ischemia. *Life Sci.* 2008;83:836–844.

3. Crowe TC. Safety of low-carbohydrate diets. *Obes Rev.* 2005;6:235–245.

4. Howard BV, Manson JE, Stefanick ML, et al. Low fat dietary pattern and weight change over 7 years: the women's health initiative dietary modification trial. *JAMA.* 2006;295(1):39–49.

5. Fung TT, van Dam RM, Hankinson SE, et al. Low carbohydrate diets and all-cause and cause-specific mortality: 2 cohort studies. *Ann Intern Med.* 2010;153(5):289–298.

6. Prentice A, Schoenmakers I, Laskey MA, et al. Nutrition and bone growth and development. *Proc Nutr Soc.* 2006;65:348–360.

7. Foster GD, Wyatt HR, Hill JO, et al. A randomized trial of a low carbohydrate diet for obesity. *N Engl J Med.* 2003;348(21):2082–2090.

8. DOMUK: Position Statement on Very Low Energy Diets in the Management of Obesity. Dieticians in Obesity Management 2007. Available at: http://domuk.org/wpcontent/uploads/2007/02/very-low-energy-diets.pdf.

9. Pearson D, Grace C. Treatment options: the evidence for what works. In: *Weight Management Practitioners Guide.* West Sussex: Wiley-Blackwell; 2012:27.

10. Wansink B, Wansink CS. The largest last supper: depictions of foods portions and plate size increased over the millennium. *Int J Obes.* 2010;34:943–944.

11. Ello-Martin JA, Ledikwe JH, Rolls BJ. The influence of food portion size and energy density on energy intake: implementations for weight management. *Am Soc Clin Nutr.* 2005;82(1):2365–2415.

12. British Dietetic Association. *Food Fact Sheet: Portion Sizes;* 2016. Available at: https://www.bda.uk.com/foodfacts/portionsizesfoodfactsheet.pdf.

13. British Dietetic Association. *Food Fact Sheet: Diabetes – Type 2;* 2015. Available at: https://www.bda.uk.com/foodfacts/diabetestype2.pdf.

CHAPTER 24

New Approach to Type 2 Diabetes Reversal in Obesity: Acute Calorie Restriction

SARAH STEVEN, MBCHB (HONS), MRCP, PHD

OBESITY, EXCESS INTRAORGAN FAT AND RISK OF TYPE 2 DIABETES

Type 2 diabetes is characterized by two pathophysiologic defects: insulin resistance and reduced insulin secretory capacity.[1] Insulin resistance usually precedes a diagnosis of type 2 diabetes by many years; however, this defect is insufficient on its own to cause blood glucose levels to rise.[2] The ability to maintain normal glucose tolerance in insulin resistant individuals is determined by the ability of the pancreatic β cells to acutely increase insulin secretion. Although type 2 diabetes has been viewed as a chronic, progressive condition, whereby inexorable decline in insulin secretion inevitably results in insulin dependence, it is now established that type 2 diabetes is clearly reversible following bariatric surgery[3] or very low–calorie diet (VLCD).[4]

Obesity is a major predictor of the risk of type 2 diabetes; compared with those of healthy weight, there is a seven times greater risk of diabetes in obese individuals and a threefold increased risk in those who are overweight.[5] However, only about 30% of people with a body mass index (BMI) of more than 40 kg/m² develop diabetes.[6] This may be, in part, because of the fact that BMI does not reflect body composition, particularly fat mass and distribution, which seems to be an important determinant of the metabolic sequelae of obesity. Although insulin resistance is common in people with type 2 diabetes and is exacerbated by obesity, individuals with normal weight can develop type 2 diabetes if their β cell function is sufficiently compromised. In the entire UK Prospective Diabetes Study cohort of individuals with type 2 diabetes (1977–1991), the BMI curve has only a slight right skew, demonstrating that the majority of these individuals had a BMI of less than 30 kg/m² (see Fig. 24.1). There is clearly a balance between insulin resistance and insulin secretory capacity regardless of body weight. The concept of a personal fat threshold has recently been described

and hypothesized that each individual will only experience the metabolically deleterious effects of intraorgan fat accumulation when this exceeds a level of tolerability specific to that individual and unrelated to body weight or BMI.[7] There are likely to be individual susceptibility factors that determine the development of the metabolic consequences of obesity. One example is the PNPLA3 genotype that results in high liver fat levels, but with individuals seemingly relatively protected from insulin resistance.[8] The responsible G allele of PNPLA3 is believed to code for a lipase that is ineffective in triglyceride hydrolysis. In individuals homozygous for the mutation, it appears that fat metabolites

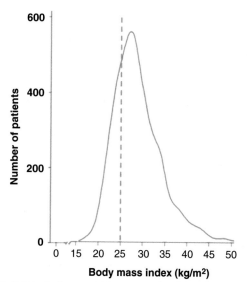

FIG. 24.1 Body mass index curve of UKPDS population. (From Taylor R, Holman RR. Normal weight individuals who develop type 2 diabetes: the personal fat threshold. *Clin Sci (Lond)*. 2015;128:405–410 © the Biochemical Society, with permission.)

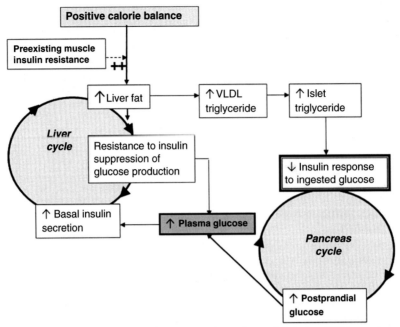

FIG. 24.2 The twin-cycle hypothesis regarding the etiology of type 2 diabetes. *VLDL*, very low–density lipoprotein. (From Taylor R. Pathogenesis of Type 2 diabetes: Tracing the reverse route from cure to cause. *Diabetologia*. 2008;51:1781–1789 © Springer, with permission.)

that are deleterious to the insulin signaling pathway, such as diacylglycerol and ceramides, are sequestered as inert triglyceride.

There is compelling data linking excess liver fat to impaired hepatic insulin sensitivity. More than 90% of obese patients with type 2 diabetes have nonalcoholic fatty liver disease (NAFLD).[9] NAFLD can progress to nonalcoholic steatohepatitis and cirrhosis. It is now the commonest cause of liver disease in the developed world,[10] and is thought to be the reason for 15%–20% of all liver transplants. Excess liver fat seems to precede a diagnosis of type 2 diabetes,[11] as does an increase in alanine transaminase.[12] Hepatic steatosis correlates with the failure of insulin to suppress hepatic glucose production,[13] which is the major determinant of fasting blood glucose levels (see Fig. 24.2). An environment of hyperglycemia and hyperinsulinemia, such as seen in the early stages of type 2 diabetes, promotes hepatic de novo lipogenesis. Newly synthesized triglyceride in the liver can be oxidized, exported as very low–density lipoprotein (VLDL), or stored as hepatic fat.[14] Because transport of fatty acid into mitochondria for oxidation is inhibited by the malonyl-CoA produced during de novo lipogenesis, newly synthesized triglyceride is preferentially directed toward storage or export. A bidirectional relationship

between excess calorie intake and liver fat accumulation has been demonstrated. Overfeeding obese individuals by 1000 kcal/day for 3 weeks results in 2% weight gain and 27% increase in hepatic fat content,[15] whereas, during calorie restriction, it appears that intrahepatic fat stores are mobilized rapidly and before visceral or subcutaneous fat stores are affected.[4,16]

Data regarding the relevance of pancreatic steatosis in the pathophysiology of type 2 diabetes are more limited, and this may be, in part, due to the limitations of imaging techniques to precisely measure pancreas fat content. The pancreas moves with respiration and β cells (which comprise only about 1% of the pancreatic mass) cannot be distinguished from acinar cells and intrapancreatic adipocytes. Postmortem studies have demonstrated a relationship between BMI and pancreatic fat content but not diabetes status.[17,18] However, these studies are limited by small numbers, the fact that postmortem pancreatic tissue undergoes autolysis by lipases and that some fat is removed during histologic processing. Clinical studies of acute calorie restriction in type 2 diabetes have demonstrated a fall in pancreatic fat levels alongside recovery of insulin secretion.[4] Recent data show that weight loss achieved by bariatric surgery decreases excess pancreatic fat specifically in type 2 diabetes and is not just weight related.[19] In these clinical studies, a considerable overlap in pancreas fat levels between individuals with type 2 diabetes and those with normal glucose tolerance has been demonstrated, again suggesting individual susceptibility to the deleterious effects of excess fat.

OVERVIEW OF THE USE OF VERY LOW–CALORIE DIET IN TYPE 2 DIABETES

The benefits of significant weight loss achieved through an intensive lifestyle intervention on glycemic control in type 2 diabetes have been recognized for decades.[20–22] A low-calorie diet for 7 weeks with 8 kg weight loss lowered the fasting plasma glucose level significantly, increased whole body insulin sensitivity, and resulted in a marked increase in the suppression of hepatic glucose production alongside an 81% reduction in hepatic fat content.[23]

VLCDs have been used since the 1970s to promote rapid weight loss and consequent improvement in glucose tolerance. They are defined as a calorie intake of <800 kcal/day. Initially, there were safety concerns following episodes of sudden death during extreme VLCD in the 1970s. However, this appeared to be related to the cardiac effects of protein-calorie malnutrition, and with modern nutritionally balanced VLCDs, which use high-quality proteins, these concerns are no longer warranted.[24] Common minor adverse effects associated with VLCD, which include cold intolerance, dry skin, hair loss, constipation, headaches, fatigue, and dizziness, are generally self-limiting and transient. Other potential effects are gallstones, increased serum uric acid levels, precipitation of gout, and reduced bone mineral density. There is a specific advantage of VLCD over a low-calorie diet (800–1200 kcal/day) in the time taken to achieve significant weight loss. It is also worth acknowledging the motivating effect of rapid weight loss and rapid improvement in blood glucose levels during a VLCD, the convenience of meal replacement, and the potential beneficial effects of mild ketosis, which may act as an appetite suppressant.

Two systematic reviews of studies using VLCDs in people with type 2 diabetes demonstrated consistent effects on glucose levels and cardiovascular risk factors, high tolerability, and good safety outcomes.[25,26] The use of VLCD has recently become part of national guidance regarding obesity management in specific clinical scenarios. The recommendation by National Institute for Clinical Excellence (NICE) is that VLCD should not be used routinely when BMI is > 30 kg/m² but rather reserved for a multicomponent weight management strategy for people who are obese and who have a clinically assessed need to lose weight rapidly.[27] The use of a VLCD is not part of the current NICE type 2 diabetes guidelines. The National Obesity Forum considers that a VLCD may be suitable for weight loss for anyone with a BMI above 30 kg/m² and under medical supervision and for overweight patients with a BMI below 30 kg/m² who have type 2 diabetes or other comorbidities.[28]

METABOLIC CHANGES DURING DIABETES REVERSAL USING VERY LOW–CALORIE DIET

Insights into the mechanisms determining the rapid improvement in blood glucose levels during VLCD were gained in a study using an 8-week VLCD in individuals with short-duration type 2 diabetes using gold standard tests of β cell function and insulin sensitivity. In all 11 participants, with a mean BMI of 33.6 ± 1.2 kg/m², fasting plasma glucose had normalized within 7 days of VLCD. Alongside this, hepatic insulin sensitivity normalized and there was a 30% reduction in liver fat content as measured using the three-point Dixon magnetic resonance method (see Fig. 24.3).[4] By the end of the 8-week VLCD, there was restoration of first-phase insulin secretion alongside a reduction in pancreatic fat content ($8.0 \pm 1.6\%$ to $6.2 \pm 1.1\%$).

Using the same 8-week VLCD protocol, a group of 29 individuals with type 2 diabetes of variable duration (0.5–23 years) underwent a VLCD and then a 6-month weight maintenance phase.[29] Weight decreased from 98.0 ± 2.6 kg to 83.8 ± 2.4 kg and remained stable for the subsequent 6-month period (84.7 ± 2.5 kg). The pathophysiologic changes following the VLCD were improved first-phase insulin secretion, decreased pancreatic fat content, decreased hepatic fat content, improved hepatic insulin sensitivity, and decreased hepatic VLDL$_1$-triglyceride production. After the VLCD, 41% of the group achieved a fasting plasma glucose level in the nondiabetic range (<7 mmol/L) and 45% at the end of the 6-month weight maintenance period. After the VLCD, hepatic fat content normalized in those who achieved a nondiabetic fasting glucose levels (12.8 ± 2.7 to $2.2 \pm 0.2\%$) and those who did not (8.2 ± 1.1 to $2.2 \pm 0.1\%$). There was no reaccumulation of hepatic fat during the weight maintenance period. In addition, the beneficial effects on serum triglycerides, total cholesterol, non–high-density lipoprotein cholesterol, and VLDL$_1$ mass were sustained with weight maintenance. There was a clinically significant and sustained improvement in both systolic and diastolic blood pressure.

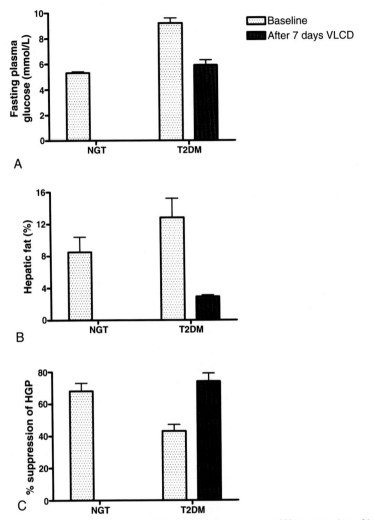

FIG. 24.3 **(A)** Fasting plasma glucose levels, **(B)** hepatic fat content and **(C)** suppression of hepatic glucose production (HGP) by insulin at baseline in individuals with type 2 diabetes mellitus (T2DM) and normal glucose tolerant (NGT) controls and in those with T2DM after 7 days of very low–calorie diet (VLCD). (Adapted from Lim EL, Hollingsworth KG, Aribisala BS, et al. Reversal of type 2 diabetes: normalisation of beta cell function in association with decreased pancreas and liver triacylglycerol. *Diabetologia*. 2011;54:2506–2514 © Springer, with permission.)

The beneficial effect on glucose control during VLCD seems to be accounted for by improvements in both insulin secretion and insulin sensitivity. However, the metabolic effects of caloric restriction per se may be, at least in part, independent of body weight reduction. Although weight is noted to improve gradually during a VLCD, the majority of the reduction in glucose levels consistently occurs within the first 10 days of dieting.[4,20,30] This relationship, between calorie intake and blood glucose levels, is bidirectional; glucose levels increase rapidly after resumption of normal eating after a VLCD, despite no initial weight regain.

LIMITATIONS TO REVERSAL OF TYPE 2 DIABETES

Following bariatric surgery, reversal of diabetes is thought to depend on the degree of achieved weight loss, subsequent weight regain, duration of diabetes, pre-surgery diabetes treatment requirements, preoperative

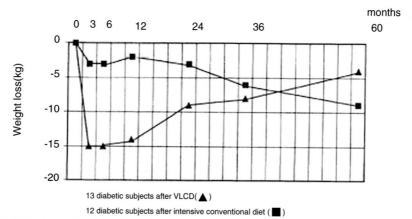

FIG. 24.4 Weight loss after intensive self-selected diet treatments: very low–calorie diet (VLCD) (*triangles*) and conventional diet (*squares*). (From Paisey RB, Frost J, Harvey P, et al. Five year results of a prospective very low calorie diet or conventional weight loss programme in type 2 diabetes. *J Human Nutr Diet*. 2002;15:121–127 © John Wiley and Sons, with permission.)

HbA1c, and choice of bariatric procedure.[31] After bariatric surgery, it is has been noted that in individuals who do not achieve diabetes reversal in the early postoperative period, there is a gradual improvement over time in parallel with weight loss.[32] It is hypothesized that early reversal of diabetes after surgery is determined by the potential for recovery of insulin secretory capacity, whereas later improvement of glucose control is determined by improved insulin sensitivity achieved through substantial weight loss.[33] A retrospective study demonstrated that a diabetes duration of more than 10 years was associated with lower diabetes reversal rates following Roux-en-Y gastric bypass surgery (42% vs. 68%).[34] Using a VLCD, a similar effect of diabetes duration on reversibility was noted; however, reversal of long-duration diabetes, even at a duration of 15 years, has been demonstrated, but is less likely to be achieved than in short-duration disease.[35] Diabetes duration may just represent a surrogate and insensitive marker for decreased insulin secretory capacity as opposed to being a factor that limits diabetes reversibility per se. Liver fat levels fall in both long- and short-duration diabetes. The clinical characteristics associated with a glucose response to a VLCD are younger age, shorter diabetes duration, better baseline glycemic control, and less requirement for diabetes therapies. However, the critical factors in determining those who achieve a fasting plasma glucose level less than 7 mmol/L following a VLCD seem to relate to insulin secretion. Those who respond to the VLCD differed from those who did not in terms of having higher baseline plasma insulin levels, a degree of β cell response to intravenous glucose

at baseline and recovery of acute insulin secretory capacity to nondiabetic levels after the VLCD. Nonresponders appeared to have a state of relative insulin deficiency, lower serum insulin levels, diminished first-phase insulin response, and lower maximal insulin secretory capacity, as well as higher baseline fasting β-hydroxybutyrate and nonesterified fatty acid levels. Baseline insulin secretory capacity and the recovery of this following VLCD to nondiabetic levels seem to be key to achieving diabetes reversal. The constancy of the arginine-induced insulin response implies persistence of the insulin secretory mechanism in reversible type 2 diabetes despite loss of glucose responsiveness. This is consistent with the concept that type 2 diabetes may be a condition of β cell dedifferentiation rather than β cell loss.[36] Even if blood glucose levels do not normalize, a major benefit in cardiovascular risk is anticipated given the improvement in blood pressure and blood lipids. Even if the effects are not maintained in the long term, the legacy effect that a period of normoglycemia confers is likely to give substantial benefits in decreasing the risk of complications.

WEIGHT MAINTENANCE FOLLOWING A VERY LOW–CALORIE DIET

A major concern regarding the use of VLCD is the high rate of weight recidivism after relaxation of calorie restriction (see Fig. 24.4).[37]

It is thought that only 20% of individuals manage to lose 10% body weight and maintain this for at least 1 year.[38] It has been proposed that this may be due to

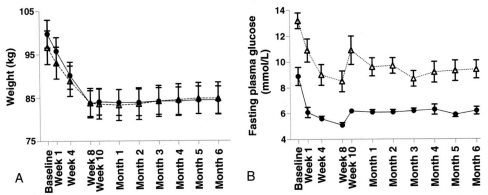

FIG. 24.5 **(A)** Weight and **(B)** fasting plasma glucose levels during an 8-week very low–calorie diet (VLCD), followed by 2 weeks of return to isocaloric diet, then 6 months of weight maintenance in individuals with type 2 diabetes. Responders (*circles*) achieved a fasting plasma glucose level of <7 mmol/L after the VLCD and nonresponders (*triangles*) did not. (Adapted from Steven S, Hollingsworth KG, Al-Mrabeh A, et al. Very Low-Calorie Diet and 6 Months of Weight Stability in Type 2 Diabetes: Pathophysiological Changes in Responders and Nonresponders. *Diabetes Care.* 2016;39:808–815 © American Diabetes Association, with permission.)

compensatory homeostatic changes during weight loss achieved during a VLCD such as increased hunger, increased circulating ghrelin, and reduced circulating GLP-1 and PYY. The durability of the beneficial effects of a VLCD after return to normal eating is crucial in determining the utility of this intervention in clinical practice. Case reports do suggest the potential for durability of the beneficial effects of a VLCD for up to 3 years.[39] Key to long-term maintenance of weight loss is the concept that returning to "normal eating" does not mean returning to previous calorie intake. Rather it means a major change to habitual eating patterns, to adjust to a dietary intake that is isocaloric with the new body weight. A VLCD should incorporate behavior modification elements to focus on the development of healthy, sustainable eating habits and encouragement of increased physical activity levels. These issues were not addressed in early studies on follow-up after VLCD. In a recent study, participants had been counseled in advance of the need to become used to eating approximately one-third less than previously.[29] During the 6-month weight maintenance phase, participants were supported by a structured individualized program with monthly reviews, based on goal setting, action planning, and barrier identification. The primary goal of this phase was to prevent weight regain by individualized dietary advice guided by weight trajectory. Physical activity was encouraged, but food behaviors were the priority. In this study, weight loss was maintained at 6 months following the VLCD, as was the improvement in fasting plasma glucose (see Fig. 24.5). There is potential that the newer glucose lowering agents

that augment weight loss, such as GLP-1 agonists, DPPIV inhibitors, and SGLT2 inhibitors, might enhance both the effects of a VLCD and the maintenance of weight loss in the longer term, and this possibility remains to be studied.

Although the main advantage of bariatric surgery over VLCD is thought to be long-term maintenance of weight loss, even following gastric bypass surgery, there is weight regain and diminution of diabetes reversal rates after 15 years.[40] Following bariatric surgery, changes in incretin hormone secretion, such as increased postprandial GLP-1 and PYY secretion and decreased ghrelin, are likely to reduce appetite and induce taste changes.[41]

COMPARISON OF EFFECTS OF VERY LOW–CALORIE DIET AND BARIATRIC SURGERY

It has been recognized since the 1950s that negative calorie balance, particularly acute and significant calorie restriction, rather than weight loss per se, has a profound role in regulating glucose metabolism. These first observations were made by bariatric surgeons observing individuals who did not proceed to the Greenville Bypass, but followed the same diet as those who did. These individuals achieved rapid improvement in blood glucose levels, similar to those individuals who underwent bypass surgery.[42] Bariatric surgery is currently the most effective treatment for reversal of type 2 diabetes.[43] Similar weight loss, approximately 14% of body weight, is achieved by 8 weeks of VLCD compared to 8 weeks after gastric bypass surgery.[44] The mechanisms determining normalization of glucose levels following bariatric surgery have been hypothesized to relate to alterations in incretin hormones following manipulation of gastrointestinal system.[45] However, the evidence for this being a primary mechanism is lacking. An alternative hypothesis to explain the profound change in metabolism following bariatric surgery relates to the obligate calorie restriction enforced by the surgery. A recent study compared the immediate metabolic responses 7 days after bariatric surgery with that after 7 days of a VLCD in individuals with type 2 diabetes and found that, despite greater weight loss after surgery, the improvement in fasting plasma glucose was modest and not significantly greater than 7 days after VLCD.[44] In addition, the increased meal-stimulated GLP-1, noted only in the surgery group, was not accompanied by any additional benefits over the diet group. This study used a semisolid 100 kcal meal for measurement of incretin hormone and insulin secretion rather than a standard 75-g oral glucose tolerance test. The latter would be highly nonphysiologic in individuals following gastric bypass surgery. Finally, some clinical studies have even shown superiority of acute calorie restriction over bariatric surgery on achieved glucose levels.[46,47]

Practical Aspects of This Approach

Knowledge that type 2 diabetes is a potentially reversible metabolic syndrome is helpful to individuals at diagnosis. Rather than a chronic progressive disease with a requirement for the sequential addition of therapies over time and the inevitable development of multisystem complications, type 2 diabetes should be tackled proactively from diagnosis, with targeted strategies to help achieve significant weight loss implemented at diagnosis. The intense interest, from individuals with type 2 diabetes and health care professionals, following publication of clinical studies on the use of VLCD in type 2 diabetes suggests that this could be a useful therapeutic intervention.[48] The remarkably low dropout rate during VLCD studies is encouraging; however, it must be acknowledged that these studies were performed in selected and highly motivated individuals.[49] In general, a systematic review of VLCD in individuals with diabetes has shown high tolerability and good safety outcomes.[25] Key practical aspects are the need to review antidiabetic agents prior to starting a VLCD to minimize hypoglycemia, to monitor blood pressure throughout with reduction in antihypertensives as necessary, and to make a dietary and physical activity plan for long-term weight maintenance (see Box 24.1). Weight regain can be avoided when reintroduction

BOX 24.1
Considerations When Using a Very Low–Calorie Diet (VLCD) in Type 2 Diabetes

1. Exclude alternative diagnoses than type 2 diabetes, such as MODY or LADA.
2. Review medications; stop those associated with hypoglycemia if possible.
3. Set a weight loss target—consider body weight loss of 15%–20%.
4. Forward plan ongoing calorie restriction/physical activity for long-term weight maintenance.
5. Consider microvascular complications—regular retinal screening if significant retinopathy.
6. Advise patients to ensure good hydration is maintained throughout VLCD.
7. Monitor blood pressure during VLCD and consider reduction in antihypertensives.

of food after a VLCD is done in a planned manner, with definitive prescription of food type and amount, emphasizing continuing high vegetable intake and adding in foods up to the specified restricted daily calorie intake. The critical factor determining the outcome after VLCD appears to be insulin secretory capacity at baseline and the extent of recovery of this following VLCD. It is hypothesized that there is a required minimum number of β cells retaining the capacity to redifferentiate and hence allow regain of function. Even in individuals who do not achieve normalization of glucose levels, it is likely that the benefits of significant weight loss to blood pressure and lipids are likely to confer long-term benefits in terms of cardiovascular risk. In addition, weight loss achieved through lifestyle modification[50] and bariatric surgery[51] has been shown to result in improvement in the histological features of nonalcoholic steatohepatitis, a precursor to the development of cirrhosis. A community-based study (DiRECT: Diabetes REmission Clinical Trial) is now underway of individuals with type 2 diabetes randomized to a low-calorie diet with structured individualized weight maintenance or to best possible guideline-based care. This will help determine the practical application of this approach in larger, primary care populations.[52]

CONCLUSIONS

Type 2 diabetes mellitus can now be understood to be a metabolic syndrome that is potentially reversible by substantial weight loss achieved through VLCD. The extent of weight loss required to reverse type 2 diabetes is greater than that conventionally advised, with recent studies suggesting a target of approximately 15 kg. A distinction can therefore be made between weight loss that improves glycemic control, but leaves blood glucose levels abnormal, and weight loss sufficient to normalize glucose metabolism. Not all individuals with type 2 diabetes will be willing to make the changes necessary, but for those who do, metabolic health may be regained and sustained in just under one-half. Weight loss achieved using a VLCD can be maintained by following a structured, individualized weight maintenance program, and in doing so, improvements in glucose control, blood pressure, lipid profiles and liver fat content can also be maintained. These observations carry profound implications for the health of individuals, management of type 2 diabetes, and for the economics of future diabetes care within the National Health Service (NHS).

REFERENCES

1. Ferrannini E, Natali A, Muscelli E, et al. Natural history and physiological determinants of changes in glucose tolerance in a non-diabetic population: the RISC Study. *Diabetologia.* 2011;54:1507–1516.
2. Taylor R. Insulin resistance and type 2 diabetes. *Diabetes.* 2012;61:778–779.
3. Buchwald H, Avidor Y, Braunwald E, et al. Bariatric surgery: a systematic review and meta-analysis. *JAMA.* 2004;292:1724–1737.
4. Lim EL, Hollingsworth KG, Aribisala BS, Chen MJ, Mathers JC, Taylor R. Reversal of type 2 diabetes: normalisation of beta cell function in association with decreased pancreas and liver triacylglycerol. *Diabetologia.* 2011;54:2506–2514.
5. Abdullah A, Peeters A, de Courten M, Stoelwinder J. The magnitude of association between overweight and obesity and the risk of diabetes: a meta-analysis of prospective cohort studies. *Diabetes Res Clin Pract.* 2010;89:309–319.
6. Gregg EW, Cheng YJ, Narayan KM, Thompson TJ, Williamson DF. The relative contributions of different levels of overweight and obesity to the increased prevalence of diabetes in the United States: 1976–2004. *Prev Med.* 2007;45:348–352.
7. Taylor R, Holman RR. Normal weight individuals who develop type 2 diabetes: the personal fat threshold. *Clin Sci (Lond).* 2015;128:405–410.
8. Kantartzis K, Peter A, Machicao F, et al. Dissociation between fatty liver and insulin resistance in humans carrying a variant of the patatin-like phospholipase 3 gene. *Diabetes.* 2009;58:2616–2623.
9. Tolman KG, Fonseca V, Dalpiaz A, Tan MH. Spectrum of liver disease in type 2 diabetes and management of patients with diabetes and liver disease. *Diabetes Care.* 2007;30:734–743.
10. de Alwis NMW, Day CP. Non-alcoholic fatty liver disease: the mist gradually clears. *J Hepatol.* 2008;48:S104–S112.
11. Shibata M, Kihara Y, Taguchi M, Tashiro M, Otsuki M. Nonalcoholic fatty liver disease is a risk factor for type 2 diabetes in middle-aged Japanese men. *Diabetes Care.* 2007;30:2940–2944.
12. Sattar N, McConnachie A, Ford I, et al. Serial metabolic measurements and conversion to type 2 diabetes in the west of Scotland coronary prevention study: specific elevations in alanine aminotransferase and triglycerides suggest hepatic fat accumulation as a potential contributing factor. *Diabetes.* 2007;56:984–991.
13. Seppala-Lindroos A, Vehkavaara S, Hakkinen A, et al. Fat accumulation in the liver is associated with defects in insulin suppression of glucose production and serum free fatty acids independent of obesity in normal men. *J Clin Endocrinol Metab.* 2002;87:3023–3028.
14. Adiels M, Olofsson S-O, Taskinen M-R, Boren J. Overproduction of very low density lipoproteins is the hallmark of the dyslipidaemia in the metabolic syndrome. *Arterioscler Thromb Vasc Biol.* 2008;28:1225–1236.
15. Sevastianova K, Santos A, Kotronen A, et al. Effect of short-term carbohydrate overfeeding and long-term weight loss on liver fat in overweight humans. *Am J Clin Nutr.* 2010;96:727–734.
16. Taylor R. Pathogenesis of Type 2 diabetes: tracing the reverse route from cure to cause. *Diabetologia.* 2008;51:1781–1789.
17. Saisho Y, Butler AE, Meier JJ, et al. Pancreas volumes in humans from birth to age one hundred taking into account sex, obesity, and presence of type-2 diabetes. *Clin Anat.* 2007;20:933–942.
18. Clark A, Wells CA, Buley ID, et al. Islet amyloid, increased A-cells, reduced B-cells and exocrine fibrosis: quantitative changes in the pancreas in type 2 diabetes. *Diabetes Res.* 1998;9:151–159.
19. Steven S, Hollingsworth KG, Small PK, et al. Weight loss decreases excess pancreatic triacylglycerol specifically in type 2 diabetes. *Diabetes Care.* 2016;39:158–165.
20. Henry RR, Schaeffer L, Olefsky JM. Glycaemic effects of intensive caloric restriction and isocaloric refeeding in non-insulin dependent diabetes mellitus. *J Clin Endocrinol Metab.* 1985;61:917–925.
21. Pi-Sunyer X, Blackburn G, Brancati FL, et al. Reduction in weight and cardiovascular disease risk factors in individuals with type 2 diabetes: one-year results of the look AHEAD trial. *Diabetes Care.* 2007;30:1374–1383.
22. Gregg EW, Chen H, Wagenknecht LE, et al. Association of an intensive lifestyle intervention with remission of type 2 diabetes. *JAMA.* 2012;308:2489–2496.
23. Petersen K, Dufour S, Befroy D, Lehrke M, Hendler R, Shulman G. Reversal of nonalcoholic hepatic steatosis, hepatic insulin resistance, and hyperglycemia by moderate weight reduction in patients with type 2 diabetes. *Diabetes.* 2005;54:603–608.
24. Basciani S, Costantini D, Contini S, et al. Safety and efficacy of a multiphase dietetic protocol with meal replacements including a step with very low calorie diet. *Endocrine.* 2015;48:863–870.

25. Sellahewa L, Khan C, Lakkunarajah S, Idris I. A systematic review of evidence on the use of very low calorie diets in people with diabetes. *Curr Diabetes Rev.* 2015; [Epub ahead of print].

26. Leslie WS, Taylor R, Harris L, Lean MEJ. Weight losses with low-energy formula diets in obese patients with and without type 2 diabetes: systematic review and meta-analysis. *Int J Obes.* 2016:1–6.

27. NICE. *Obesity: Identification, Assessment and Management of Overweight and Obesity in Children, Young People and Adults.* Available at: https://www.nice.org.uk/guidance/cg189; 2014.

28. *Position Statement on the Application of Very Low Energy Diets in Achieving Weight Loss in the Management of Obesity.* Available at: http://www.nationalobesityforum.org.uk/images/stories/_Final_version_NOF_consensus_statement_VLEDs.pdf; July 2010.

29. Steven S, Hollingsworth KG, Al-Mrabeh A, et al. Very low-calorie diet and 6 months of weight stability in type 2 diabetes: pathophysiological changes in responders and nonresponders. *Diabetes Care.* 2016;39:808–815.

30. Anderson J, Kendall C, Jenkins D. Importance of weight management in type 2 diabetes: review with meta-analysis of clinical studies. *J Am Coll Nutr.* 2003;22:331–339.

31. Hayes M, Hunt L, Foo J, Tychinskaya Y, Stubbs RA. Model for predicting the resolution of type 2 diabetes in severely obese subjects following Roux-en Y gastric bypass surgery. *Obes Surg.* 2011;21:910–916.

32. Kashyap S, Louis E, Kirwan J. Weight loss as a cure for type 2 diabetes? Fact or fantasy. *Expert Rev Endocrinol Metab.* 2011;6:557–561.

33. Dixon J, Zimmet P, Alberti K, Rubino F. Bariatric surgery: an IDF statement for obese type 2 diabetes. *Diabet Med.* 2011;28:628–642.

34. Hall TC, Pellen MGC, Sedman PC, Jain PK. Preoperative factors predicting remission of type 2 diabetes mellitus after Roux-en-Y gastric bypass surgery for obesity. *Obes Surg.* 2010;20:1245–1250.

35. Steven S, Taylor R. Restoring normoglycaemia by use of a very low calorie diet in long- and short-duration type 2 diabetes. *Diabet Med.* 2015;32:1149–1155.

36. White M, Shaw JAM, Taylor R. Type 2 diabetes: the pathologic basis of reversible β-cell dysfunction MG. *Diabetes Care.* 2016;39:2080–2088.

37. Paisey RB, Frost J, Harvey P, et al. Five year results of a prospective very low calorie diet or conventional weight loss programme in type 2 diabetes. *J Hum Nutr Diet.* 2002;15:121–127.

38. Wing RR, Hill JO. Successful weight loss maintenance. *Annu Rev Nutr.* 2001;21:323–341.

39. Peters C, Steven S, Taylor R. Reversal of type 2 diabetes by weight loss despite presence of macro- and microvascular complications. In: Draznin B, Wang CL, Rubin D, eds. *Diabetes Case Studies.* Alexandria, VA: American Diabetes Association; 2015:271–274.

40. Sjostrom L, Peltonen M, Jacobson P, et al. Association of bariatric surgery with long-term remission of type 2 diabetes and with microvascular and macrovascular complications. *JAMA.* 2014;311:2297–2304.

41. Batterham RL, Cummings DE. Mechanisms of diabetes improvement following bariatric/metabolic surgery. *Diabetes Care.* 2016;39:893–901.

42. Pories W, Swanson M, MacDonald K, et al. Who would have thought it? An operation proves to be the most effective therapy for adult-onset diabetes mellitus. *Ann Surg.* 1995;222:339–352.

43. Schauer PR, Kashyap SR, Wolski K, et al. Bariatric surgery versus intensive medical therapy in obese patients with diabetes. *N Engl J Med.* 2012;366:1567–1576.

44. Steven S, Hollingsworth KG, Small PK, et al. Calorie restriction and not glucagon-like peptide-1 explains the acute improvement in glucose control after gastric bypass in Type 2 diabetes. *Diabet Med.* 2016;33:1723–1731.

45. Knop FK. Resolution of type 2 diabetes following gastric bypass surgery: involvement of gut-derived glucagon and glucagonotropic signalling? *Diabetologia.* 2009;52:2270–2276.

46. Isbell J, Tamboli R, Hansen E, et al. The importance of caloric restriction in the early improvement in insulin sensitivity after Roux-en-Y gastric bypass surgery. *Diabetes Care.* 2010;33:1438–1442.

47. Lingvay I, Guth E, Islam A, Livingston E. Rapid improvement in diabetes after gastric bypass surgery: is it the diet or surgery. *Diabetes Care.* 2013;36:2741–2747.

48. Steven S, Lim EL, Taylor R. Population response to information on reversibility of Type 2 diabetes. *Diabet Med.* 2013;30:e135–e138.

49. Rehackova L, Arnott B, Araujo-Soares V, Adamson AA, Taylor R, Sniehotta FF. Efficacy and acceptability of very low energy diets in overweight and obese people with type 2 diabetes mellitus: a systematic review with meta-analysis. *Diabet Med.* 2016;33:580–589.

50. Vilar-Gomez E, Martinez-Perez Y, Calzadilla-Bertot L, et al. Weight loss through lifestyle modification significantly reduces features of nonalcoholic steatohepatitis. *Gastroenterology.* 2015;149:367–378.

51. Lassailly G, Caiazzo R, Buob D, et al. Bariatric surgery reduces features of nonalcoholic steatohepatitis in morbidly obese patients. *Gastroenterology.* 2015;149:379–388.

52. Leslie WS, Ford I, Sattar N, et al. The diabetes remission clinical trial (DiRECT): protocol for a cluster randomised trial. *BMC Fam Pract.* 2016;17:20.

CHAPTER 25

Historical Drug Therapies in Obesity

AYAT BASHIR, MBBS • JOLANTA U. WEAVER, MRCP, FRCP, PHD, CTLHE

INTRODUCTION

The increasing prevalence of obesity has led to progress toward pharmacologic and nonpharmacologic approaches for weight loss. Within the last 60 years, treatments for weight loss have changed throughout these times. From the advent of thyroid extract to amphetamine use, the fenfluramine era, and more recently sibutramine and rimonabant, several drug therapies have existed to tackle the global obesity epidemic. However, knowledge and understanding has advanced over the years leading to withdrawal of several key past pharmacologic players in different countries. This has mainly been due to further understanding of implications of mechanism of action to side effect profile of such medications. The aim of this chapter is thus to review historical drug therapies used in the management of obesity and to establish lessons learnt from their development and use.

LAXATIVES

The 2nd century AD welcomed the development of therapies to treat obesity in which Greek physicians prescribed laxatives and purgatives.[1] However, patients developed several medical complications particularly from chronic use. Chronic diarrhea results in metabolic disturbances, including hypokalemia and related metabolic alkalosis. Concomitant purging by vomiting exacerbates this effect.[2] Bowel dysfunction has also been reported with prolonged laxatives in addition to chronic kidney disease and subsequent renal failure.[2,3] This was hastily recognized as a harmful method of treatment. Unfortunately, laxative abuse exists to date, in particular, among patients with anorexia nervosa and bulimia.[2]

THYROID HORMONE

The preparation of thyroid hormone in the late 19th century has been argued to be the beginning of pharmacotherapy for obesity management.[4] The prescription of thyroid hormone extract, which was already in use among patients with hypothyroidism, became popular primarily because of its thermogenic properties. An increased metabolic rate was observed in patients and the hormone was used to induce weight loss[5] (Fig. 25.1). However, the main consequence of increasing metabolic rate was the loss of lean tissue rather than fat, and it has been shown that a loss of lean tissue leads to increased mortality.[5] The additional adverse effects also included loss of mineral bone density leading to osteoporosis.[6] As thyroid hormone also causes cardiac muscle hypertrophy, this leads to an increase in cardiac workload,[7] a complication already existing as a consequence of obesity. Thyroid hormones also influence multiple aspects of lipid, carbohydrate, and protein metabolism, and the ultimate effects of hyperthyroidism were observed in patients taking this as weight loss therapy.[7] Thus, it was considered appropriate that this form of therapy was no longer used to manage obesity.

However, over the 15 years, thyroid hormone analogues have been developed. They aim to uncouple beneficial effects from deleterious effects.[8] Selective thyroid hormone mimetics have shown to promote fat loss in animal models; these effects can be separated from harmful effects on heart and muscle.[9] However, in short clinical trials of low-dose agents, such as thyroid hormone receptor β-specific agonist (GC-1), weight loss was not reported and it was noted that GC-1 is less effective in promoting weight loss despite stimulating basal metabolic rate.[8] Thus studies on thyroid hormone mimetics are still at their infancy, and as yet limitations exist in the translation of these drugs from animal to human models regarding their pharmacologic efficacy and toxicity.[10]

DINITROPHENOL

2-4-Dinitrophenol (DNP) was one of the first antiobesity therapy used in the 1930s.[11] Its effect was first noticed among factory workers who were exposed to this and lost weight. It was shown to cause weight loss

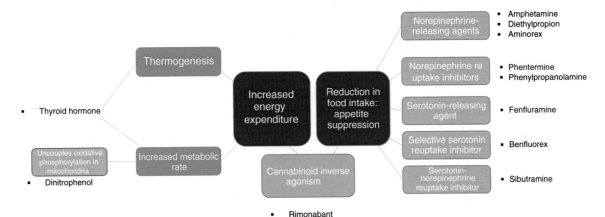

FIG. 25.1 **Anti-Obesity Drugs: Mechanism of Action.** The mechanism of action of historical drug therapies in obesity. Early drug therapies focused on increased energy expenditure through thermogenesis and increasing the basal metabolic rate. Therapies include the use of thyroid hormone extract and dinitrophenol. Later therapies aimed to focus on appetite suppression through development of drugs acting on monoamine neurotransmitters, such as norepinephrine, serotonin, and dopamine. This included amphetamines, phentermine, and fenfluramine. More recently, agents, such as rimonabant, acting on the endocannabinoid system have been developed.

by uncoupling oxidative phosphorylation, leading to a heightened metabolic rate and increased fat metabolism.[11] The rapid consumption of calories was thought to occur because of the shift in the proton electrochemical gradient, which results in potential energy dissipating as heat, instead of being converted to ATP.[12] This mechanism of action also leads to an accumulation of pyruvate and lactic acids. Unlike thyroid hormone, which was used for weight loss, it did not impact on nitrogen excretion and thus was postulated to cause fat rather than lean muscle mass loss.[13] The resultant excess heat production led to uncontrolled hyperthermia following failed mechanisms of thermoregulatory homeostasis, which results in significant morbidity and mortality.[11] Within a few years of its use, several adverse effects including toxic hyperthermia, hepatotoxicity, formation of cataracts, and few cases of agranulocytosis were reported.[14] Because of the severe adverse effects of this drug, it was banned in 1938. However, at present DNP is marketed on the Internet without regulation, in particular to the bodybuilding population attempting to lose weight. To address the growing use, the Food Standards Agency issued warning in 2011 that this product is "not fit for human consumption" given short- and long-term effects.[15]

agents targeting the central biogenic amine system. Amphetamine-based compounds are often referred to as sympathomimetics, i.e., their effects mimic certain effects of stimulating the sympathetic nervous system, e.g., increased heart rate, increased blood pressure.[16] Weight reduction through a reduction in food intake and a decrease in appetite was observed because of the action of amphetamines on hypothalamic receptors.[17] They lead to the release of norepinephrine and, to a lesser extent, dopamine and serotonin, increasing the CNS activity and resting energy expenditure.[17]

Benzedrine (amphetamine sulfate) was among the first amphetamines to be used for the management of obesity.[18] During clinical testing, increased energy, alertness, and weight loss were reported; however, more notably, evidence of abuse and addiction was observed.[16] Despite this, "rainbow pills" were prescribed on a widely basis.[19] They consisted of nonstandard combination of amphetamine, thyroid hormone, and diuretics for weight loss and β-blockers and benzodiazepines to manage side effects.[19] Understandably, there was a high tendency for drug toxicity, including hyperthyroidism, digitalis toxicity, hypokalemia,[19] and they were subsequently withdrawn.

AMPHETAMINES AND RAINBOW PILLS

Introduction of the amphetamines, compounds that are known for their central nervous system (CNS)-stimulant properties, led to the advent of antiobesity

AMPHETAMINE ANALOGUES

To reduce the addictive potential of the amphetamine–based antiobesity drugs, analogues were developed with varying dopamine and serotonin receptor specificities.

This included drugs such as phentermine, phenylpropanolamine, and diethylpropion.

Phentermine

In 1959, phentermine was developed predominantly for short-term use and it is one of the oldest pharmacologic agents approved by the United States Food and Drug Administration (FDA) for weight loss.[20] Its mechanism of action is thought to be characterized by appetite suppression through norepinephrine release and to a lesser extent through dopamine and serotonin release.[21] Therefore, it was thought that is had a lower potential for addiction than other amphetamine–based therapies. This was demonstrated in an intervention trial in which withdrawing phentermine from patients accustomed to long–term use for weight loss did not lead to drug cravings.[22]

In relation to side effect profile and efficacy, only a few randomized controlled trials exist with only a short-term duration of therapy reported. A metaanalysis of six short-term studies of phentermine showed that, among completers, transient symptoms of CNS stimulation, such as insomnia, irritability, and anxiety, were more common in patients receiving either continuous (24%) or intermittent (27%) therapy than in those receiving placebo (8%).[23]

In 2000, the European Medicines Agency advised withdrawal of phentermine due to an unfavorable risk-to-benefit ration; however, in 2003 a successful legal challenge in the European courts by a UK manufacturer of phentermine led to its reinstatement. Therefore, in several countries including the United States, it is used for a short period of time to promote weight loss, if exercise and calorie reduction are not sufficient, and in addition to exercise and calorie reduction.

Phenylpropanolamine

Phenylpropanolamine has a structure and function similar to amphetamine. It is primarily a selective agonist at the α-adrenergic receptor as well as a catecholamine reuptake inhibitor.[16] It also exerts its action at the β-receptor and CNS. Its anorectic effects are thought to be due to CNS stimulation. It was shown to be an independent risk factor for hemorrhagic stroke in women among its association with other adverse effects, including cardiovascular toxicity and headaches in a case-controlled study.[24]

DIETHYLPROPION

Diethylpropion is a phenylethylamine ring compound with minor sympathomimetic properties.[25] It increases the release of noradrenaline in the synaptic cleft of the hypothalamic neurons, thus stimulating noradrenergic receptors and inhibiting hunger.[26] It is thought to have less stimulant effects than amphetamine. A randomized double-blind placebo-controlled study of the long-term efficacy of diethylpropion focused on cardiovascular and psychiatric safety aspects.[27] The study included 69 obese healthy adults and the mean weight loss within 12 months was 10.6%.[27] Dry mouth and insomnia were the most common adverse events observed.[27] The study had several limitations, including the fact it was conducted on a small scale, participants were predominantly of women, and it has been carried out at one only center. Therefore, these results cannot be extrapolated to men, older patients, or patients with comorbidities.

AMINOREX

Aminorex fumarate (2-amino-5-phenyl-oxazoline) is similar to epinephrine and amphetamine in chemical structure,[28] and its toxic effects have been attributed predominantly to the release of catecholamines and norepinephrine. In 1965, aminorex became available in Switzerland, Austria, and Germany. However, the incidence of primary pulmonary hypertension (PPH) in these three countries increased between 1965 and 1972.[29] Symptoms including dyspnea on exertion, syncope, and chest pain (symptoms of PPH) lagged 6–12 months after starting the drug.[28] It was withdrawn from the market in 1968. The experience with aminorex in obesity pharmacotherapy brought to light the potential association of obesity drugs with PPH and also the importance of assessing the long-term impact of a drug on discontinuation.

FENFLURAMINE AND DEXFENFLURAMINE

Fenfluramine causes the feeling of fullness and reduced appetite.[30] It disrupts vesicular storage of the neurotransmitter, causing the release of serotonin in addition to reversing serotonin transporter function.[31] The combination of fenfluramine and phentermine (Fen-Phen) induced weight loss in a study carried out in 1992.[32] However by 1997, it was discovered that right-sided and left-sided valvular regurgitation was associated with fenfluramine. These results were soon generalized to fenfluramine's stereoisomer dexfenfluramine. Increased rates of pulmonary hypertension were observed in both medications and they were withdrawn from the market in 1997.[33]

BENFLUOREX

Benfluorex is a selective serotonin reuptake inhibitor, which is related to fenfluramine. It was thought to have lipid-lowering and anorectic actions.[34] Because of reports of pulmonary artery hypertension and valvular abnormalities, this drug was withdrawn from the market.[35] It was postulated that the development of valvular regurgitation was due to the action of one of its metabolites, norfenfluramine, on the 5-HT2B receptor expressed on heart valves.[34] A large multinational randomized prospective trial in patients with type 2 diabetes reported a threefold increase in the incidence of echocardiographic evidence of valvular regurgitation with benfluorex compared with the insulin-sensitizing drug pioglitazone.[35]

SIBUTRAMINE

Sibutramine, a selective serotonin and norepinephrine reuptake inhibitor was approved by FDA regulators in 1997. Clinical trials demonstrated that sibutramine induced weight loss and improved lipid profile and glucose tolerance, but it also increased blood pressure and pulse rate.[36] In 2010 the Sibutramine Cardiovascular Outcomes Trial (SCOUT), a randomized cardiovascular outcomes study in patients with cardiovascular disease, diabetes mellitus, or both, found that sibutramine caused a greater rate of cardiovascular events.[37] The benefit-risk profile of sibutramine was considered unfavorable by the FDA given the uncertainties surrounding the cardiovascular implications of the drug; therefore this drug was voluntarily withdrawn from the market.[38]

RIMONABANT

The development of rimonabant introduced a new mechanism of action in the battle against obesity, cannabinoid inverse agonism.[39] Clinical trials showed weight loss and improvement in metabolic parameters, but they also showed depression and anxiety.[39] Rimonabant for Prevention of Cardiovascular Events (CRESCENDO), a long-term cardiovascular outcomes trial, was terminated after revealing an increased rate of serious psychiatric side effects including suicide at mean follow-up of 14 months.[40] Rimonabant was eventually withdrawn from the European market in 2009.[25]

CONCLUSION

There is no doubt that historical discoveries and trials have assisted in the development of antiobesity medications and our understanding of therapeutic targets. We have learnt from the past decades the importance of recognizing the complex mechanisms that lead to weight gain and establishing the counterregulatory hormonal, metabolic, and neurochemical pathways involved. We have also learnt the chronicity of the disease in itself poses difficulties when developing safe therapies and also the importance of recognizing associated comorbidities. As this cohort of patients are often considered high risk, history has demonstrated the significance of acquiring cardiovascular and neurocognitive safety data and postmarketing surveillance. Research should focus on understanding the potential for adverse effects, not just the primary therapeutic aim. In recent years there have been advances in the development of animal models that may facilitate a greater understanding of the pathogenesis and pathophysiology of cardiovascular adverse effects. This may assist in developing safer and more tolerated therapies. However, ultimately given the significant number of withdrawn therapies historically, it is important to recognize that long-term research and development needs to be conducted in this field.

REFERENCES

1. Christopoulou-Aletra H, Papavramidou N. Methods used by the hippocratic physicians for weight reduction. *World J Surg.* 2004;28(5):513–517.
2. Roerig JL, Steffen KJ, Mitchell JE, Zunker C. Laxative abuse. *Drugs.* 2010;70(12):1487–1503.
3. Copeland PM. Renal failure associated with laxative abuse. *Psychother Psychosom.* 1994;62(3–4):200–202.
4. Logan MS, Logan JS. The treatment of myxoedema with raw sheep thyroid gland and its introduction into practice in County Londonderry in 1892. *Ulster Med J.* 1992;61(1):86–93.
5. Bray GA, Melvin KE, Chopra IJ. Effect of triiodothyronine on some metabolic responses of obese patients. *Am J Clin Nutr.* 1973;26(7):715–721.
6. Onigata K. Thyroid hormone and skeletal metabolism. *Clin Calcium.* 2014;24(6):821–827.
7. Mullur R, Liu Y-Y, Brent GA. Thyroid hormone regulation of metabolism. *Physiol Rev.* 2014;94(2):355–382.
8. Baxter JD, Webb P. Thyroid hormone mimetics: potential applications in atherosclerosis, obesity and type 2 diabetes. *Nat Rev Drug Discov.* 2009;8(4):308–320.
9. Villicev CM, Freitas FR, Aoki MS, et al. Thyroid hormone receptor beta-specific agonist GC-1 increases energy expenditure and prevents fat-mass accumulation in rats. *J Endocrinol.* 2007;193(1):21–29.
10. Elangbam CS. Review paper: current strategies in the development of anti-obesity drugs and their safety concerns. *Veterinary Pathol.* 2009;46(1):10–24.
11. Grundlingh J, Dargan PI, El-Zanfaly M, Wood DM. 2,4-Dinitrophenol (DNP): a weight loss agent with significant acute toxicity and risk of death. *J Med Toxicol.* 2011;7(3):205–212.

12. Harper JA, Dickinson K, Brand MD. Mitochondrial uncoupling as a target for drug development for the treatment of obesity. *Obes Rev*. 2001;2(4):255–265.

13. Cutting WC, Tainter ML. Metabolic actions of dinitrophenol. with the use of balanced and unbalanced diets. *J Am Med Assoc*. 1933;101(27):2099–2102.

14. Colman E. Dinitrophenol and obesity: an early twentieth-century regulatory dilemma. *Regul Toxicol Pharmacol*. 2007;48(2):115–117.

15. Agency FS. *Food Standards Agency Issues Urgent Advice on Consumption of 'fat Burner' Capsules Containing DNP*; 2011. http://www.food.gov.uk/news/pressreleases/2003/jun/fat burnpress.

16. Nelson DL, Gehlert DR. Central nervous system biogenic amine targets for control of appetite and energy expenditure. *Endocrine*. 2006;29(1):49–60.

17. Heal DJ, Smith SL, Gosden J, Nutt DJ. Amphetamine, past and present–a pharmacological and clinical perspective. *J Psychopharmacol Oxf Engl*. 2013;27(6):479–496.

18. Samuel PD, Burland W. Thyroid hormone. Paper presented at: obesity symposium: proceedings of a servier research Institute symposium held in December 1973 (1974).

19. Cohen PA, Goday A, Swann JP. The return of rainbow diet pills. *Am J Public Health*. 2012;102(9):1676–1686.

20. Fujioka K. Current and emerging medications for overweight or obesity in people with comorbidities. *Diabetes Obes Metab*. 2015;17(11):1021–1032.

21. Apovian CM, Aronne LJ, Bessesen DH, et al. Pharmacological management of obesity: an endocrine society clinical practice guideline. *J Clin Endocrinol Metab*. 2015;100(2):342–362.

22. Hendricks EJ, Srisurapanont M, Schmidt SL, et al. Addiction potential of phentermine prescribed during long-term treatment of obesity. *Int J Obes (2005)*. 2014;38(2):292–298.

23. Haddock CK, Poston WS, Dill PL, Foreyt JP, Ericsson M. Pharmacotherapy for obesity: a quantitative analysis of four decades of published randomized clinical trials. *Int J Obes Relat Metab Disord*. 2002;26(2):262–273.

24. Kernan WN, Viscoli CM, Brass LM, et al. Phenylpropanolamine and the risk of hemorrhagic stroke. *N Engl J Med*. 2000;343(25):1826–1832.

25. Kang JG, Park C-Y. Anti-obesity drugs: a review about their effects and safety. *Diabetes Metab J*. 2012;36(1):13–25.

26. Dietrich MO, Horvath TL. Limitations in anti-obesity drug development: the critical role of hunger-promoting neurons. *Nat Rev Drug Discov*. 2012;11(9):675–691.

27. Cercato C, Roizenblatt VA, Leanca CC, et al. A randomized double-blind placebo-controlled study of the long-term efficacy and safety of diethylpropion in the treatment of obese subjects. *Int J Obes (2005)*. 2009;33(8):857–865.

28. Byrne-Quinn E, Grover RF. Aminorex (Menocil) and amphetamine: acute and chronic effects on pulmonary and systemic haemodynamics in the calf. *Thorax*. 1972;27(1):127–131.

29. Barceloux DG. *Medical Toxicology of Drug Abuse: Synthesized Chemicals and Psychoactive Plants*. Wiley; 2012.

30. Lemke TL, Williams DA. *Foye's Principles of Medicinal Chemistry* Wolters Kluwer Health. ; 2012.

31. Nestler EJ, Hyman SE, Malenka RC. *Molecular Neuropharmacology: A Foundation for Clinical Neuroscience*. 2nd ed. McGraw-Hill Education; 2008.

32. Weintraub M. Long-term weight control: the National Heart, Lung, and Blood Institute funded multimodal intervention study. *Clin Pharmacol Ther*. 1992;51(5):581–585.

33. Khorassani FE, Misher A, Garris S. Past and present of antiobesity agents: focus on monoamine modulators. *Am J Health Syst Pharm*. 2015;72(9):697–706.

34. Szymanski C, Andrejak M, Peltier M, Marechaux S, Tribouilloy C. Adverse effects of benfluorex on heart valves and pulmonary circulation. *Pharmacoepidemiol Drug Saf*. 2014;23(7):679–686.

35. Tribouilloy C, Rusinaru D, Maréchaux S, et al. Increased risk of left heart valve regurgitation associated with benfluorex use in patients with diabetes mellitus. *Circulation*. 2012;126(24):2852.

36. Nisoli E, Carruba MO. An assessment of the safety and efficacy of sibutramine, an anti-obesity drug with a novel mechanism of action. *Obes Rev*. 2000;1(2):127–139.

37. James WPT, Caterson ID, Coutinho W, et al. Effect of sibutramine on cardiovascular outcomes in overweight and obese subjects. *N Engl J Med*. 2010;363(10):905–917.

38. Scheen AJ. Sibutramine on cardiovascular outcome. *Diabetes Care*. 2011;34(suppl 2):S114–S119.

39. Scheen AJ, Paquot N. Use of cannabinoid CB1 receptor antagonists for the treatment of metabolic disorders. *Best Pract Res Clin Endocrinol Metab*. 2009;23(1):103–116.

40. Topol EJ, Bousser M-G, Fox KAA, et al. Rimonabant for prevention of cardiovascular events (CRESCENDO): a randomised, multicentre, placebo-controlled trial. *Lancet*. 2010;376(9740):517–523.

CHAPTER 26

New Therapies in Obesity

CAROLINE DAY, PHD, FRSB

INTRODUCTION

Since 1980 the prevalence of obesity (BMI > 30 kg/m²) worldwide has more than doubled and now more than 1.9 billion adults (>18 years) and 41 million children <5 years of age have excess adiposity.[1] Being overweight or obese is considered a major driver in the development of insulin resistance, type 2 diabetes, cardiovascular diseases, and other comorbidities, which are associated with premature mortality. Increased ill health reduces the quality of life, burdens family finances, strains healthcare and social welfare provision, and impairs national economic productivity.

Despite conventional nonpharmacologic approaches such as health education, behavioral therapy, diet, exercise, and other lifestyle modifications, often supported by multimedia promotions, the obesity epidemic continues. This review will focus on newer therapies for obesity and consider agents with clinical antiobesity potential.

ANTIOBESITY DRUGS—SPECIAL CONSIDERATIONS

Caution surrounds the use of drug therapy for obesity. Is overweight or obesity wholly a "disease" or a state of disease risk? The United States has granted obesity an *International Classification of Diseases* (ICD) code (in *ICD-10-CM*, overweight and obesity codes are listed in category E66).[2] Recently an American Association of Clinical Endocrinologists (AACE) and the American College of Endocrinology (ACE) position statement recommended replacing the term obesity with "adiposity-based chronic disease (ABCD)" as a vehicle to refocus the conceptualization of obesity into a chronic disease with a defined pathophysiologic basis and adiposity-related complications.[3]

Obesity (or ABCD) is a relatively slowly generated chronic condition; generally it is not acutely life-threatening and is potentially treatable by nonpharmacologic measures (often termed lifestyle medicine), thus making drug safety paramount. Over the last 80 years a procession of licensed drug treatments for obesity have been withdrawn due to safety concerns (see Chapter 25).

Newer Approaches

Early in the 21st century there was optimism in Europe regarding the availability of treatments for obesity: in 1998 orlistat was introduced, followed by sibutramine in 2000 and rimonabant in 2006, but by the end of 2008 only orlistat remained (see Chapter 25). Although different in design, the orlistat and sibutramine registration trials provided the benchmarks for pharmacologic weight loss therapy, namely randomized placebo-controlled, parallel-group studies in overweight and obese patients noting placebo-subtracted weight loss at 12 months after randomization and number of patients achieving ≥5% and ≥10% decrease in body weight from baseline.[4] These criteria are now included in the regulatory requirements for registration of a weight management drug in the European Union and the United States.[5,6] Regulatory authorities also require (usually as a secondary end point) that a weight loss agent additionally benefits weight-related conditions, most notably type 2 diabetes, prediabetes, and other components of metabolic syndrome.

Orlistat

The intestinal lipase inhibitor orlistat has become the mainstay of weight management therapies and is available on prescription (*Xenical*, 120-mg capsule with meals, up to 3 times/day for up to 2 years) and also as a nonprescription medicine in some countries (*Alli*, 60-mg capsule, 3 times/day with meals for up to 6 months). Orlistat reduces the digestion of dietary fats and thereby cuts intestinal fat absorption by ~30%, but the resultant side effects (notably flatulence and loose stools) are often unacceptable to patients, although side effects can largely be remedied by reducing fat consumption—inadvertently supplying an add-on benefit of dietary modification. Orlistat treatment also reduces total cholesterol (~0.3 mmol/L) and low-density lipoprotein (~0.3 mmol/L) with smaller decreases in high-density lipoprotein (~0.06 mmol/L) and triglycerides (~0.08 mmol/L), as might be expected with lipid malabsorption, and decreases systolic (~1.8 mmHg) and diastolic (~1.6 mmHg) blood pressure.[7] Weight loss also improves glycemic control, and in the XENical in the Prevention of Diabetes in

Obese Subjects (XENDOS) study, 4 years of orlistat treatment reduced the cumulative incidence of type 2 diabetes to 6.3% (a 37.3% risk reduction, $P = .0032$). Weight loss was similar among patients with normal and impaired glucose tolerance at baseline (5.7 kg and 5.8 kg, respectively), but the difference in diabetes incidence was confined to the latter subgroup.[8] In studies that involve obese type 2 diabetes, orlistat reduced HbA1c by 0.5%.[9]

Safety

Safety is the most challenging issue in the licensing of all medicines, but for antiobesity agents the bar has been set even higher. This is partly due to a perception of weight loss as a cosmetic outcome, which increases the risk of drug abuse and adverse physiologic outcomes not associated with obesity (see Chapter 25). Indeed the worldwide withdrawal of fenfluramine and dexfenfluramine prompted the European regulators to also withdraw licenses for older products on the premise that they lacked proof of clinical benefits and explains the paucity of antiobesity agents in Europe compared with the United States. The potential for mental health and cardiovascular disease comorbidities are relatively high in the obese population and, on a practical level, this translates into a high risk for inappropriate prescribing.

Dietary interventions and other lifestyle measures are first-line strategies in obesity treatment, and pharmacologic agents supply adjunctive assistance. However, the extent of drug-induced weight loss is rarely sufficient to return an obese person to normal weight. Nevertheless, the obesity epidemic is increasing the demand for new agents from the public and health-related agencies and undoubtedly these pressures are being felt by regulatory bodies.

NEW AGENTS

In March 2015 liraglutide 3 mg (*Saxenda*) and a fixed-dose combination of naltrexone 8 mg + bupropion 90 mg (*Mysimba*) received EU marketing authorization as adjuncts to dietary and lifestyle management in the treatment of overweight (BMI ≥27) with ≥1 comorbid condition (e.g., dyslipidemia) and obesity (BMI ≥30).[11,12] It is anticipated that both preparations will be marketed in Europe in 2017. In the United States naltrexone 8 mg + bupropion 90 mg (*Contrave*) was launched in October 2014 and liraglutide 3 mg (*Saxenda*) entered the market in April 2015, and by mid-2015 they accounted for 27.9% and 4.3%, respectively, of antiobesity prescriptions.[10]

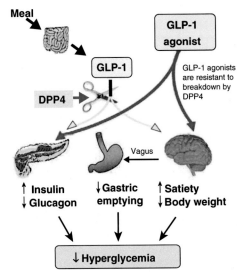

FIG. 26.1 Mode of action of glucagon-like peptide-1 (GLP-1) and GLP-1 receptor agonists, e.g., liraglutide. (From Bailey CJ, Feher MD. Diabetes Therapies: Treating Hyperglycaemia. Halesowen: Med Ed UK; 2009:150, with permission.)

Liraglutide 3 mg

Liraglutide is a glucagon-like peptide-1 (GLP-1) receptor agonist (RA). GLP-1RAs comprise a class of peptides that bind and activate receptors for the endogenous incretin hormone GLP-1. They potentiate insulin secretion and reduce glucagon secretion in a glucose-dependent manner to lower blood glucose, particularly after meals, and carry negligible risk of interprandial or fasting hypoglycemia. GLP-1RAs delay gastric emptying, which can cause temporary nausea in some patients. These agents also exert satiety effects that facilitate weight loss (Fig. 26.1).[13]

Liraglutide 0.6, 1.2, or 1.8 mg/day (*Victoza*) was licensed in Europe in 2009 and in the United States in 2010, to treat type 2 diabetes patients who are overweight (BMI ≥27) with ≥1 comorbid condition (e.g., hypertension) or obese (BMI ≥30)—i.e., they have diabesity.[14]

Unlike other antiobesity agents, liraglutide 3 mg (*Saxenda*) is delivered as a once-daily subcutaneous injection (supplied in a prefilled pen containing 18 mg of liraglutide in 3 mL) administered any time of day independently of food, but regularity of timing is recommended. Due to gastrointestinal tolerability issues (mainly nausea), dosing should commence at 0.6 mg daily and be increased weekly in 0.6 mg increments to the maintenance dose of 3 mg/day. Incretin therapy should be avoided in patients with a history of pancreatitis, gall bladder issues, and predisposing circumstances, such as alcoholism. In the liraglutide 3 mg Phase III trials, heart rate increased (2.5 beats/min), but this was reversed on treatment withdrawal. In the long-term clinical trials, there were 6 and 10 major adverse cardiovascular events (MACE) for patients treated with liraglutide 3 mg and placebo, respectively.[11]

SCALE was the study title given to the four randomized double-blind placebo-controlled trials with liraglutide 3 mg submitted for regulatory approval, and they are summarized in Table 26.1. All patients were overweight (BMI ≥27 with ≥1 comorbidity) or obese (BMI ≥30). In the SCALE studies all patients consumed a reduced calorie diet with increasing physical activity, and liraglutide was uptitrated to the "treatment dose" of 3 mg over a 4-week period.[14–18]

Liraglutide Effect and Action in Diabetes: Evaluation of Cardiovascular Outcome Results (LEADER) trial was a safety study in 9340 people with type 2 diabetes (HbA1c ≥7%) at high cardiovascular risk.[19] Over 60% of subjects had a BMI of ≥30, and treatment with liraglutide (median dose 1.78 mg/day) for a median of 3.8 years resulted in fewer deaths from any cause (8.2% vs. 9.6%, $P = .02$) and cardiovascular causes (4.7% vs. 6%, $P = .007$), and nonfatal myocardial infarction, nonfatal stroke, and hospitalization for heart failure were nonsignificantly lower in liraglutide versus placebo-treated patients. Liraglutide improved indices of increased cardiovascular risk (e.g., weight, HbA1c); however, heart rate was increased by 3 beats/minute; pancreatic cancer was higher than in placebo (13 vs. 5 patients) as was acute gallstone disease (145 vs. 90 patients), but acute pancreatitis only occurred in 18 patients in the liraglutide group compared with 23 in the placebo group. The main adverse events were gastrointestinal in nature.[19] Although the liraglutide dose for the treatment of obesity (3 mg/day) is higher than diabetes (0.6, 1.2, or 1.8 mg/day), it is hoped that the LEADER trial will allay concerns surrounding the use of liraglutide in obesity.

Naltrexone and Bupropion

In Europe the opioid receptor antagonist naltrexone (*Adepend*, a 50-mg tablet once daily) is licensed to reduce the craving for alcohol—the patient must be free of opioids when starting the treatment—and the noradrenaline and dopamine reuptake inhibitor bupropion (*Zyban*, a 150-mg prolonged release tablet uptitrated to a maximum of 300 mg daily) is used to assist smoking cessation.[20]

Naltrexone SR 8 mg + Bupropion SR 90 mg (NB)

NB (*Mysimba, Contrave*) is a slow-release fixed-dose combination of established agents with each NB tablet containing naltrexone 8 mg and bupropion 90 mg as slow release formulations. For regulatory purposes, pharmacodynamic studies were not undertaken using the fixed-dose combination tablet because it was presumed pharmacodynamics would be the same as for the agent as individual formulations. The exact mechanism of action of NB is still being elucidated. It has been suggested that these agents act synergistically on the central nervous system, with naltrexone blocking opioid-mediated proopiomelanocortin autoinhibition whilst bupropion stimulates proopiomelanocortin neurons in the hypothalamus. Theoretically these actions on the hypothalamus and mesolimbic dopamine circuit will promote satiety, additionally suppress appetite and increase metabolism.[21]

COR was the study title given to the four randomized double-blind placebo-controlled NB trials submitted for regulatory approval, and they are summarized in Table 26.2.

All patients were overweight (BMI ≥27 with ≥1 comorbidity) or obese (BMI ≥30). In the COR studies all patients consumed a reduced calorie diet and undertook lifestyle measures to aid weight loss. NB was uptitrated, one tablet in the morning for the first week adding in 1 tablet in the evening for the second week and so on until the treatment dose of naltrexone 32 mg-bupropion 360 mg was reached over a 4-week period.[22–25] The main adverse events reported with NB were gastrointestinal in nature, especially nausea that is about fivefold higher (32.5% vs. 6.7%) in patients taking NB.

Cautions and contraindications to treatment with NB also include those for each agent individually.[26] Increases in blood pressure and heart rate have been reported with NB and should be monitored, particularly at drug initiation and during the first 3 months of treatment.[27,28] The NB Phase IV cardiovascular outcome trials in obese people at cardiovascular risk have not completed: the LIGHT study (clinical trial. gov NCT01601704) was terminated in March 2015 due to the protocol breach of disclosure of interim results and the subsequent CONVENE trial (clinical trial. gov NCT02638129), which commenced recruiting in December 2015, had stopped by mid-2016, possibly due to financial constraints. However, NB does have a black box in its prescribing information in the United States, warning of suicidal thoughts and behaviors and risk for neuropsychiatric reactions.[26]

TABLE 26.1
Main Effects of Liraglutide 3 mg Once Daily Subcutaneous Injections in the Phase III SCALE Trials

	SCALE: Weight management (and prediabetes)[19] Randomized: n=3731; Completed: n=2590. BMI ≥30 or ≥27 with hypertension or dyslipidemia. No diabetes (61% prediabetes: HbA1c 5.7%–6.4%). Randomized 2:1 (liraglutide 3 mg, placebo) for 56 weeks (Followed by rerandomization 1:1 (i) if not had prediabetes at screening to continue liraglutide 3 mg or switch to placebo for 12 weeks; (ii) if had prediabetes at baseline enter 160-week extension trial. Data not shown below.)			SCALE: Diabetes[20] Randomized: n=846; Completed: n=628. BMI ≥27 with type 2 diabetes (HbA1c 7%–10%) on metformin, an SU or a TZD as mono or combination therapy. Randomized 2:1:1 (liraglutide 3 mg, 1.8 mg, placebo) for 56 weeks (Followed without treatment for further 12 weeks. Data not shown below.)			SCALE: Weight loss maintenance[21] Randomized: n=3731; Completed: n=2590. BMI ≥30 or ≥27 with comorbidities. No diabetes. If lost ≥5% body weight during 12-week diet and lifestyle run-in randomized 1:1 (liraglutide 3 mg, placebo) for 56 weeks (Followed without treatment for further 12 weeks. Data not shown below.)			SCALE: Sleep apnea[22] Randomized: n=359; Completed: n=276. BMI ≥3C. Sleep apnea (moderate: AHI 15–29.9 or severe: AHI ≥30) and not on continuous positive airway pressure. No diabetes. Randomized 1:1 (liraglutide 3 mg, placebo) for 32 weeks		
	Liraglutide 3 mg	Placebo	L vs P (95% CI)	Liraglutide 3 mg	Placebo	L vs P (95% CI)	Liraglutide 3 mg	Placebo	L vs P (95% CI)	Liraglutide 3 mg	Placebo	L vs P (95% CI)
Baseline weight	106.3 kg	106.3 kg		105.6 kg	106.7 kg		100.7 kg	98.9 kg		116.5 kg	118.7 kg	
Change in body weight	↓8.4 kg	↓2.8 kg	↓5.6 kg** (−6.0; −5.1)	↓6.2 kg (5.9%)	↓2.2 kg (2%)	↓4.1 kg** (−5.0; −3.1)	↓6.0 kg (6.3%)	↓0.2 kg (0.2%)	↓5.9 kg** (−7.3; −4.4)	↓6.8 kg (5.7%)	↓1.8 kg (1.8%)	↓4.9 kg** (−6.2; −3.7)
Lost ≥5% body weight	63.5%	26.6%	4.8%** (4.1; 5.6)	49.8%	13.5%	6.4%** (4.1; 10.0)	50.7%	21.3%	3.8%** (2.4; 6.0)	46.4%	18.1%	3.9%** (2.4; 6.4)
Lost >10% body weight	32.8%	10.1%	4.3** (3.5; 5.3)	22.9%	4.2%	6.8%** (3.4; 13.8)	27.4%	6.8%	5.1%** (2.7; 9.7)	22.4%	1.5%	19.0%** (5.7; 63.1)
Change HbA1c %	↓0.3	↓0.1	↓0.23** (−0.25; −0.21)	↓1.3	↓0.4	↓0.9** (−1.1; −0.8)				↓0.4	↓0.2	↓0.2 (−0.3; −0.1)**
AHI index events/hr										↓12.2	↓6.1	↓6.1* (−11.0; −1.2)

*P<.05; **P<.001 ↓=decrease. AHI, apnea-hypopnea index; vs, versus; CI, confidence interval.
Data from Marso SP, Daniels GH, Brown-Frandsen K, et al. Liraglutide and cardiovascular outcomes in type 2 diabetes. *N Engl J Med.* 2016;375:311–322, Summary of Product Characteristics. Electronic Medicines Compendium.www.medicines.org.uk/emc/, Sherman M, Ungureanu S, Rey JA. Naltrexone naltrexone/bupropion ER (Contrave). Newly approved treatment option for chronic weight management in obese adults. *Pharm Ther.* 2016;41:166–172, and Greenway FL, Fujioka K, Plodkowski RA, et al. Effect of naltrexone plus bupropion on weight loss in overweight and obese adults (COR-I): a multicentre, randomized, double-blind, placebo-controlled, phase 3 trial. *Lancet.* 2010;376:595–605.

TABLE 26.2

Main Effects of Fixed-Dose Naltrexone-Bupropion Combination Tablets (Daily Dosage Naltrexone 32 mg + Bupropion 360 mg) in the Phase III COR Trials

	COR-1[26]: Obesity. Randomized: n = 1742. Completed: n = 870. BMI 30–45 or BMI 27–45 + hypertension or dyslipidemia. No diabetes. Randomized 1:1:1 (NB 32–360 mg, 16–360 mg, placebo) for 56 weeks. Data for NB 16–360 mg not shown below			COR-Diabetes[27]: Randomized: n = 525. Completed: n = 275 (but data below for mITT population). Type 2 diabetes (HbA1c 7%–10%) on diet only, metformin, an SU or a TZD as mono or combination therapy. Randomized 2:1 (NB 32–360 mg) for 56 weeks			COR-II[28]: Obesity. Dosage Change if ≤5% weight loss weeks 28–44. Randomized: n = 1496. Completed: n = 701. BMI 30–47 or BMI 27–45 + hypertension and/or dyslipidemia. No diabetes. No opiates within previous 7 days. Randomized 2:1 (NB 32–360 mg, placebo). If in weeks 28–44 <5% weight loss, then rerandomized 1:1 (NB 32–360 mg, NB 48–360 mg) until 56 weeks			COR-BMOD[29]: Intense Behavior modification ± drug. Randomized: n = 793. Completed: n = 407. BMI 30–47 or BMI 27–45 + hypertension and/or dyslipidemia. No diabetes. No nicotine or tobacco within previous 6 months. Randomized 3:1 (NB 32–360 mg, placebo) for 56 weeks.		
	NB 32–360 mg	**Placebo**	**NB vs P (P)**	**NB 32–360 mg**	**Placebo**	**NB vs P (P)**	**NB 32–360 mg**	**Placebo**	**NB vs P (P)**	**NB 32–360 mg**	**Placebo**	**NB vs P (P)**
Baseline weight				104.2 kg	105.1 kg		100.3 kg	99.2 kg		100.2 kg	101.9 kg	
% weight change	↓6.1%	↓1.3%	<.001				↓8.2%	↓1.4%	<.001	↓7.3%	↓11.5%	<.001
X change							↓7.9 kg	↓1.5 kg	<.001			
Lost ≥5% body weight	48.0%	16.0%	<.0001	53.1%	24.0%	<.001	64.9%	21.7%	<.001	80.4%	60.4%	<.001
Lost >10% body weight	34%	11.0%	<.0001	26.3%	8.0%	<.001	39.4%	7.9%	<.001	55.2%	30.2%	<.001
Lost >15% body weight	17%	3.0%	<.0001				18.9%	3.4%	<.001	39.5%	17.9%	<.001
Change in HbA1c %				↓0.6	↓0.1	<.001						

↓ = decrease; vs, versus.

Data from Contrave Prescribing Information. Orexigen Therapeutics Inc: La Jolla, California, USA. https://contrave.com/content/pdf/Contrave_PI.pdf; September 2016, BELVIQ. Prescribing Information. http://www.accessdata.fda.gov/drugsatfda_docs/label/2014/022529s003lbl.pdf, Garber AJ. Anti-obesity pharmacotherapy and the potential for preventing progression from prediabetes to type 2 diabetes. *Endocr Pract.* 2015;21:634–644, and Scheen AJ, van Gaal LF. Comating the dual burden: therapeutic targeting of common pathways in obesity and type 2 diabetes. *Lancet Diabetes Endocrinol.* 2014;2:911–922.

NEW AGENTS NOT APPROVED IN EUROPE

Lorcaserin

Lorcaserin (*BELVIQ*) is a US-approved weight loss agent. Lorcaserin (10mg tablet twice daily) was approved in 2012 and a slow release preparation (*BELVIQ XR*, 20mg once daily) was approved in July and launched in October 2016.[27] Lorcaserin reduces food intake, possibly via suppressing appetite and increasing satiety, but the exact mechanism of action is unknown. It is a selective serotonin 2c(5-HT_{2c}) receptor agonist, and it is thought that this specificity will make serotonin-related valvulopathy unlikely. Nevertheless, caution is recommended in patients with valvular heart disease, as well as the risk of serotonin syndrome[28,29] A cardiovascular outcome study (NCT02019264), which is also investigating progression to type 2 diabetes (CAMELLIA-TIMI), is scheduled to complete by mid-2018.

The safety and efficacy of lorcaserin were evaluated in the Phase III trials: Behavioral modification and Lorcaserin for Overweight and Obesity Management (BLOOM), Behavioral modification and Lorcaserin Second Study for Obesity Management (BLOSSOM), and in patients with type 2 diabetes (BLOOM-DM). Over 1 year, patients treated with lorcaserin (20 mg per day) lost about 3–3.5kg more than those on placebo, and in patients with diabetes the enhanced weight loss was accompanied by a placebo-subtracted decrease in HbA1c of 0.5%[28,29] There are several side effects associated with the use of lorcaserin and the manufacturer withdrew its application to the European Medicines Agency (EMA) when it was informed that approval of lorcaserin was unlikely.[26]

Phentermine and Topiramate

Phentermine is an amphetamine analogue with anorectic activity, which was withdrawn in Europe due to safety issues and later reinstated (see Chapter 25), but is still not available in the United Kingdom.[4] However, phentermine (*Suprenza*; 15 mg, 30 mg tablets) has been a licensed antiobesity agent in the United States since 1959, where its use is restricted to a few weeks.[31]

Topiramate (*Topamax*) is licensed in Europe and the United States to treat epilepsy and migraine.[20,32] It should be uptitrated (weekly increase) until the minimal maintenance dose is attained and drug withdrawal should be gradual. It is speculated that topiramate aids weight loss by antagonizing α-amino-3-hydroxy-5-methyl-4-isoxazolepropionic acid and kainate receptors to reduce food cravings, decreasing lipogenesis and modifying taste via inhibition of carbonic anhydrase, as well as activating gamma-aminobutyric acid receptors to enhance energy expenditure.[28,29]

Phentermine + topiramate SR (PT)

PT (*Qysmia*, *Qnexa*) is a fixed-dose combination capsule of phentermine and extended release topiramate in the ratio of 3.75:23 mg; 7.5:46 mg; 11.25:69 mg, and 15:92 mg, respectively.[37] PT should be taken in the morning (to avoid insomnia) starting with the lowest PT dose and uptitrated to the maintenance dose. There is also a withdrawal schedule for termination of PT treatment. Increased heart rate (>5 to >20 beats/min) is an issue of concern with PT therapy.[30,33] Cautions and contraindications to treatment with PT also include those for each agent individually. To date a cardiovascular outcome trial has not been registered.

The safety and efficacy of PT was evaluated in Phase III clinical trials named EQUATE, EQUIP, CONQUER, and its 1-year extension termed SEQUEL. These studies showed improved weight loss with PT compared with placebo as well as with weight loss generally achieved with other weight loss agents.[28,29] However, PT (*Qsiva*) was refused marketing authorization in Europe in October 2012 and this was reaffirmed in February 2013. The EMA highlighted safety concerns, including effects on the cardiovascular system, psychiatric and cognitive effects, teratogenic risk, and off-label use.[30,34]

WEIGHT LOSS AS A SIDE EFFECT

Several drugs are known to effect body weight, and a recent metaanalysis has highlighted the weight loss associated with the antiepileptics zonisamide (7.7kg) and topiramate (3.8kg), the antidepressants fluoxetine (1.3kg) and bupropion (1.3kg), which is only licensed for smoking cessation in Europe, and several glucose lowering agents used in the treatment of type 2 diabetes.[35]

Antiepileptics and Antidepressants

Topiramate and bupropion as components of the fixed-dose combination therapies TP and NB are indicated in the treatment of obesity and overweight with ≥1 comorbidity in the United States; but only NB has received approval in Europe (see above).

Zonisamide

A 16-week study in obese adults recorded a placebo-subtracted weight loss of 5kg in subjects receiving zonisamide 400–600 mg per day, and weight loss continued during the 8-month study extension. However, fatigue and a rise in serum creatinine raise questions on the suitability of zonisamide as an antiobesity agent.[35]

Zonisamide + bupropion

Phase II studies using fixed-dose combinations of zonisamide + bupropion (*Empatic*), each as slow-release formulations, were said to have resulted in nearly 75% of obese patients losing ≥5% of initial body weight over 24 weeks, and by 52 weeks nearly half of them had lost ≥10% of their weight.[36] However, results have not been posted on ClinicalTrials.gov (NCT00339014, NCT00709371).

Fluoxetine

Despite the apparent weight loss efficacy of fluoxetine, its associated adverse events profile and its black box warning in the United States for suicidality undermine the potential of this drug as an antiobesity agent.[37]

Glucose-Lowering Agents

The weight loss utility of glucose-lowering agents has usually been demonstrated in patients with coexistent diabetes and excess adiposity—often referred to as diabesity. In the metaanalysis by Domecq et al. small, but statistically significant, decreases in body weight were associated with the biguanide metformin (1.1 kg) and the α-glucosidase inhibitors acarbose (0.4 kg) and miglitol (0.7 kg), which are all established antidiabetic agents.[35]

Metformin

Gastrointestinal incommode is a common side effect of metformin, which may help to reduce food intake. Splanchnic glucose cycling between the intestine and liver, such that glucose is converted to lactate and back to glucose consumes energy, and metformin's sensitizing actions to lower insulin levels reduces anabolic activity which may also assist weight loss in people with and without diabetes.[17]

α-Glucosidase inhibitors

The use of α-glucosidase inhibitors is associated with gastrointestinal discomfort and flatulence because they slow the digestion of complex carbohydrate and sucrose in the small intestine, thereby slowing the rate of glucose absorption and deferring the process to further along the intestine. Thus ingested calories may be lost in the feces in people with and without diabetes.[13]

Pramlintide

The amylin analogue pramlintide (*Symlin*) is an injectable agent approved in the United States in 2005 (but not in Europe) as an adjunct to insulin treatment in type 1 and type 2 diabetes. It acts mainly via central effects (area postrema) to decrease glucagon secretion, slow gastric emptying, and induce satiety.[38] The metaanalysis

by Domecq et al. noted a significant 2.3 kg weight loss with this agent and Dunican et al. have comprehensively reviewed trials with pramlintide in type 1 and type 2 diabetes where weight loss was monitored.[35,39] Three weight loss trials have been undertaken in obese (BMI >35) nondiabetic patients and treatment reduced caloric intake at each major meal. All treatment dosages and dosing strategies produced meaningful weight loss.[39] Nausea is the main side effect of pramlintide treatment.

Glucagon-like peptide-1 receptor agonists

Several GLP-1RAs are licensed for the treatment of type 2 diabetes in Europe and the United States and more are in development, including semaglutide, which has injectable and oral formulations. The GLP-1RAs are especially useful in the treatment of diabesity, having marginally different effects on basal and postprandial hyperglycemia as well as weight loss.[14,40] Liraglutide 3 mg (*Saxenda*) is the only member of the class licensed for use as an antiobesity agent (see above).

Sodium-glucose cotransporter 2 inhibitors

Sodium-glucose cotransporter (SGLT) 2 is located almost exclusively in the proximal renal tubule where it is responsible for reabsorption of filtered glucose from the nephron.[41] SGLT2 inhibition reduces the amount of glucose reabsorbed back into the circulation, resulting in excess glucose (and therefore calories) being eliminated in the urine—making these agents particularly helpful in the treatment of diabesity.[14] Since SGLT2 is not the only mechanism for renal glucose reabsorption, glycosuria only occurs in the presence of hyperglycemia. Thus SGLT2 inhibitors are unlikely to be of use as weight loss agents in people with normal glycemic control. In a metaanalysis in type 2 diabetes patients taking canagliflozin 300 mg (*Invokana*), dapagliflozin 10 mg (*Forxiga, Farxiga*), or empagliflozin 25 mg (*Jardiance*) achieved respectively a 2.66, 1.8, or 1.8 kg greater weight loss than placebo.[42]

NOVEL APPROACHES

Preclinical and clinical studies are in progress investigating novel approaches to antiobesity therapies (Fig. 26.2). Most of these approaches are aimed at controlling appetite, but from an evolutionary perspective it has been necessary to conserve fat and maintain body weight.[4,43] There are numerous mechanisms operating within the brain and the periphery which regulate feeding behavior and energy balance, providing a range of pathways to circumvent the actions of weight loss agents.

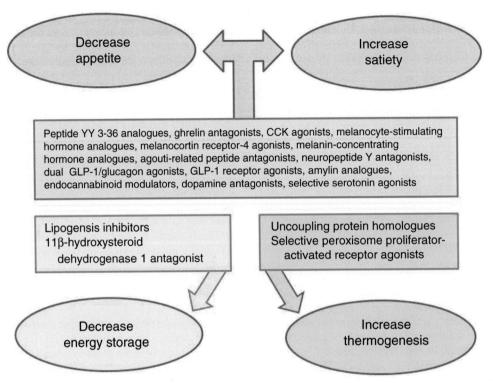

FIG. 26.2 Novel approaches to antiobesity therapy.

REFERENCES

1. World Health Organization. *Media Centre. Obesity and Overweight. Factsheet*; June 2016. http://www.who.int/mediacentre/factsheets/fs311/en/.
2. Gray L. *ICD-10 Corner: Overweight and Obesity Codes.* Code it Right online; December 2011. https://www.codeitright online.com/ciri/icd-10-corner-overweight-and-obesity-codes.html.
3. Mechanick JI, Hurley DL, Garvey T. Adiposity-based chronic disease as a new diagnositic term: American association of clinical Endocrinologists and the American College of Endocrinology position statement. *Endocr Pract.* 2017;23:372–378. http://dx.doi.org/10.4158/EP161688. PS. [Rapid Electronic Article in press].
4. Day C, Bailey CJ. Pharmacological approaches to adiposity. *Br J Diabetes Vasc Dis.* 2006;6:121–125.
5. European Medicines Agency, Committee for Medicinal Products for Human Use (CHMP). *Guideline on Clinical Evaluation of Medicinal Products Used in Weight Control*(Draft) ; June 2014. http://www.ema.europa.eu/docs/en_GB/document_library/Scientific_guideline/2014/07/WC500170278.pdf.
6. Food and Drug Administration (FDA), Center for Drug Evaluation and Research (CDER). Guidance for industry. *Developing Products for Weight Management*Draft Guidance, Revision 1 ; February 2007. http://www.fda.gov/downloads/Drugs/Guidances/ucm071612.pdf.
7. Drew BS, Dixon AF, Dixon JB. Obesity management: update on orlistat. *Vasc Health Risk Manag.* 2007;3:817–821.
8. Torgerson JS, Hauptman J, Boldrin MN, Sjöström L. XENical in the prevention of diabetes in obese subjects (XENDOS) Study. A randomized study of orlistat as an adjunct to lifestyle changes for the prevention of type 2 diabetes in obese patient. *Diabetes Care.* 2004;27:155–161.
9. Hollander PA, Elbein SC, Hirsch IB, et al. Role of orlistat in the treatment of obese patients with type 2 diabetes: a 1-year randomized double-blind study. *Diabetes Care.* 1998;21:1288–1294.
10. Weight Loss Industry Analysis 2016 – Cost and Trends. https://www.franchisehelp.com/industry-reports/weight-loss-industry-report/.
11. *Saxenda (Liraglutide 3 mg) Summary of Product Characteristics.* March 2015. http://www.ema.europa.eu/docs/en_GB/document_library/EPAR_-_Product_Information/human/003780/WC500185786.pdf.
12. *Mysimba (Nalrexone+bupropion) Summary of Product Characteristics.* March 2015. http://www.ema.europa.eu/docs/en_GB/document_library/EPAR_-_Product_Information/human/003687/WC500185580.pdf.
13. Bailey CJ, Feher MD. *Diabetes Therapies: Treating Hyperglycaemia.* Halesowen: Med Ed UK; 2009:pp 150.
14. Day C, Bailey CJ. Pharmacotherapies to manage diabesity: an up-date. *Diabesity Pract.* 2015;4:14–22.

15. Pi-Sunyer X, Astrup A, Fujioka K, et al. For the SCALE Obesity and Prediabetes NN8022-1839 Study Group. A randomized, controlled trial of 3.0 mg of liraglutide in weight management. *N Engl J Med*. 2015;373:11–22.

16. Davies MJ, Bergenstal R, Bode B, et al. Efficacy of liraglutide for weight loss among patients with type 2 diabetes: the SCALE diabetes randomized clinical trial. *JAMA*. 2015;314:687–699.

17. Blackman A, Foster GD, Zammit G, et al. Effect of liraglutide 3.0 mg in individuals with obesity and moderate or severe obstructive sleep apnea: the SCALE sleep apnea randomized clinical trial. *Int J Obes*. 2016;40:1310–1319.

18. Wadden TA, Hollander P, Klein S, Niswender K, et al. Weight maintenance and additional weight loss with liraglutide after low-calorie-diet-induced weight loss: the SCALE Maintenance randomized study. *Int J Obes*. 2013;37:1443–1451.

19. Marso SP, Daniels GH, Kirstine Brown-Frandsen K, et al. Liraglutide and cardiovascular outcomes in type 2 diabetes. *N Engl J Med*. 2016;375:311–322.

20. Summary of Product Characteristics. Electronic Medicines Compendium. www.medicines.org.uk/emc/.

21. Sherman M, Ungureanu S, Rey JA. Naltrexone naltrexone/bupropion ER (Contrave). Newly approved treatment option for chronic weight management in obese adults. *Pharm Ther*. 2016;41:166–172.

22. Greenway FL, Fujioka K, Plodkowski RA, et al. Effect of naltrexone plus bupropion on weight loss in overweight and obese adults (COR-I): a multicentre, randomised, double-blind, placebo-controlled, phase 3 trial. *Lancet*. 2010;376:595–605.

23. Hollander P, Gupta AK, Plodkowski R, et al. Effects of naltrexone sustained release/bupropion sustained-release combination therapy on body weight and glycemic parameters in overweight and obese patients with type 2 diabetes. *Diabetes Care*. 2013;36(12):4022–4029.

24. Apovian CM, Aronne L, Rubino D, et al. A randomized, phase 3 trial of naltrexone SR/bupropion SR on weight and obesity-related risk factors (COR-II). *Obesity*. 2013;21:935–943.

25. Wadden TA, Foreyt JP, Foster GD, et al. Weight loss with naltrexone SR/bupropion SR combination therapy as an adjunct to behavior modification: the COR-BMOD trial. *Obesity*. 2011;19:110–120.

26. *Contrave Prescribing Information*. La Jolla, California, USA: Orexigen Therapeutics Inc; September 2016. https://contrave.com/content/pdf/Contrave_PI.pdf.

27. BELVIQ. *Prescribing Information*. http://www.accessdata.fda.gov/drugsatfda_docs/label/2014/022529s003lbl.pdf.

28. Garber AJ. Anti-obesity pharmacotherapy and the potential for preventing progression from prediabetes to type 2 diabetes. *Endocr Pract*. 2015;21:634–644.

29. Scheen AJ, van Gaal LF. Comating the dual burden: therapeutic targeting of common pathways in obesity and type 2 diabetes. *Lancet Diabetes Endocrinol*. 2014;2:911–922.

30. Woloshin S, Schwartz LM. The new weight-loss drugs, lorcaserin and phentermine topiramate. Slim Pickings? *JAMA Intern Med*. 2014;17:615–619.

31. Suprenza. *Prescribing Information*. http://www.accessdata.fda.gov/drugsatfda_docs/label/2011/202088s001lbl.pdf.

32. *Topamax Prescribing Information*. Titusville, New Jersey, USA: Janssen Pharmaceuticals Inc. http://www.topamaxepilepsy.com/prescribing-info.html.

33. *Qsymia Prescribing Information*. Moutain View, California: Vivus Inc; 2014. https://qsymia.com/patient/include/media/pdf/prescribing-information.pdf.

34. European Medicines Agency. *Refusal of the Marketing Authorisation for Qsiva (Phentermine/Topiramate)*. Outcome of re-examination; February 2013. http://www.ema.europa.eu/docs/en_GB/document_library/Summary_of_opinion_-_Initial_authorisation/human/002350/WC500139215.pdf.

35. Domecq JP, Prutsky G, Leppin A, et al. Drugs commonly associated with weight change: a systematic review and meta-analysis. *J Clin Endocrinol Metab*. 2015;100:363–370.

36. Empatic. http://www.tesofensine-information.com/empatic.html.

37. Prozac. *Prescribing Information*. https://www.accessdata.fda.gov/drugsatfda_docs/label/2011/018936s091lbl.pdf.

38. Day C. Amylin analogue as an antidiabetic agent. *Br J Diabetes Vasc Dis*. 2005;5:151–154.

39. Dunican KC, Adams NM, Desilets AR. The role of pramlintide for weight loss. *Ann Pharmacother*. 2010;44:538–545.

40. Trujillo JM, Nuffer W, Ellis SL. GLP-1 receptor agonists: a review of head-to-head clinical studies. *Ther Adv Endocrinol Metab*. 2015;6:19–28.

41. Bailey CJ. The challenge of managing coexistent type 2 diabetes and obesity. *BMJ*. 2011;342. http://dx.doi.org/10.1136/bmj.d1996. 8 pp.

42. Pinto LC, Rados DV, Remont LR, et al. Efficacy of SGLT2 inhibitors in glycemic control, weight loss and blood pressure reduction: a systematic review and meta-analysis. *Diabetol Metab Syndr*. 2015;7(suppl 1). A58.

43. Chen Y. Regulation of food intake and the development of anti-obesity drugs. *Drug Disc Ther*. 2016;10:62–73.

CHAPTER 27

Medical Management of Patients Before and After Bariatric Surgery

ARUTCHELVAM VIJAYARAMAN, MD, FRCP

INTRODUCTION

Obesity is recognized as a major health problem internationally. In 2014, more than 1.9 billion adults were overweight and more than 600 million of them were obese.[1] Only recently, the medical fraternity is developing structured ways of managing weight-related disorders. The success of medical interventions in terms of weight reductions remains very low at 5%–10% of body weight.[2] Additionally, most of these patients regain the weight. Hence, currently, bariatric surgery is the only intervention resulting in a sustained, life-changing weight reduction in a significant number of patients. However, it remains extremely important to identify the suitable patients for bariatric surgery and prepare them both physically and mentally along with providing them with the help and support they need to achieve the required lifestyle changes before they undergo bariatric surgery. In the United Kingdom, it has been made mandatory for the patients planning to undertake bariatric surgery to work with the multidisciplinary specialized nonsurgical weight management services for a minimum period of 6 months and up to 1 year.[3,4]

STRUCTURE OF NONSURGICAL WEIGHT MANAGEMENT SERVICE

Ideally, a nonsurgical weight management service should be designed as a multidisciplinary service including bariatric physicians, dieticians, psychologists, physiotherapists, and health trainers.[5] There is no separate training program yet for bariatric medicine, but in most places the diabetes specialists train themselves with expertise to manage patients with weight-related problems.

There are different models of this service, but most will provide at least 1 year of support for the patients,

with the chance to meet all the professionals with regular input throughout the year.

An educational seminar as a group program is a good starting point, explaining about the service, providing the motivation, and creating faith in the patients' mind that the team will aim to maximize their effort to help them. This is particularly important because most patients are already frustrated with the failure of any medical treatment they received so far.

INITIAL ASSESSMENT

At the first visit, it will be effective, if it is used as a listening exercise. The patient meets up with all the members of the multidisciplinary team (MDT) and explains the story of their life with obesity. This opens up significant aspects of psychologic problems, including the complex relationship with food, which will be picked by the psychologists and will form the basis for further regular counseling. The dietitian will identify the areas to work on in the subsequent dietary counseling. The physiotherapists shall address the factors causing limitations with mobility and will provide future support on increasing physical activity levels including exercise on prescription.

The physician will make a full assessment on various aspects of obesity. From the history and physical examination, the physician will identify any evidence for secondary causes of obesity such as Cushing's syndrome as in Box 27.1. If there is any suspicion in the history such as periods of accelerated weight gain, physical signs suggestive of hormonal conditions, or laboratory results such as hypokalemia, further investigations shall be planned.

We commonly use BMI to assess obesity and there is evidence with observational data showing consistently

---

BOX 27.1
Secondary Causes of Obesity

ENDOCRINE CAUSES
Hypothyroidism
  Cushing's disease
  Polycystic ovaries
  Growth hormone deficiency
  Hypothalamic obesity
  Hypogonadism
  Insulinoma
  Pseudohypoparathyroidism

DRUG INDUCED
Atypical antipsychotics
  Tricyclic antidepressants
  Lithium
  Steroids

EATING DISORDERS
Binge eating disorder
  Bulimia nervosa

GENETIC CAUSES
Monogenic Obesity
Leptin and leptin receptor deficiency
  Proopiomelanocortin (POMC) deficiency
  Melanocortin receptor 4 deficiency
  Brain-derived neurotrophic factor (BDNF) and tropo-myosin-related kinase B (TrkB) deficiency
  Single-minded homologue 1 (SIM1) insufficiency

Syndromic Obesity
Prader-Willi syndrome
  Bardet-Biedl syndromes
  Beckwith-Wiedemann syndrome
  Alstrom-Hallgren syndrome
  Carpenter syndrome
  Cohen syndrome

BOX 27.2
Who Should Be Offered Bariatric Surgery

Body mass index (BMI) >40 kg/m^2 without comorbidities
or
  BMI 35 kg/m^2 with significant obesity-related comorbidities
  All secondary causes of obesity excluded
  Adequate engagement with all nonsurgical weight loss programs (6 months to 1 year)
  Required lifestyle changes achieved
  10% of "excess body weight" reduction by lifestyle changes demonstrated
  Treatment for comorbidities optimized
  Satisfactory psychologic assessment
  Well-informed and motivated patient
  Supportive family/social environment
  Suitable for general anesthesia
  Nonsmoker or stopped smoking

---

diabetes, economic complications, functional limitations, gonadal axis, perceived health status, and body image.

The pharmacologic agents available for weight reduction are limited with drugs such as orlistat. Recently, liraglutide 3 mg is licensed to be used in obese patients for weight reduction purposes.[10] Although some evidence is available, we need to wait for long-term studies to fully assess the efficacy and the cost-effectiveness of this treatment.[11]

The patients continue to work with the MDT to achieve all the prerequirements for bariatric surgery as in Box 27.2.

BARIATRIC SURGERY AND MANAGEMENT OF DIABETES

Bariatric surgery is increasingly included in the treatment algorithm of the management of type 2 diabetes. It is well known that type 2 diabetes may undergo remission following bariatric surgery. Hence, it is important to address management of diabetes with the bariatric surgery perspective. The type of diabetes is reconfirmed with investigations as it is important to differentiate between type 1 and type 2 diabetes before bariatric surgery. While type 2 diabetes may achieve remission, type 1 diabetes will still require insulin but in lesser amount following bariatric surgery. The treatment of type 2 diabetes is revisited, and medications that help with weight reduction such as GLP-1 analogues and SGLT 2 inhibitors are preferred over sulfonylurea and insulins in the treatment algorithm. The treatment is escalated to achieve an optimal HbA1c of less than 64 mmol/mol before surgery.

deleterious associations between elevated BMI and morbidity and mortality.[6] It is increasingly identified that body weight and BMI alone are not enough to assess and stratify the severity of obesity and its effects. Many other tools like Edmonton Obesity Staging System (EOSS)[7] and King's obesity staging criteria[8] are being used.

EOSS is a 5-point ordinal classification system that is quite practical. It makes assessments on mental health, medical conditions, and functional status in all patients with obesity and groups into stage 0 to stage 5. Studies have been performed and confirmed that these stages correlate well with the mortality and morbidity related to obesity.[9] The King's obesity staging criteria includes nine health domains including airways, BMI, cardiovascular disease,

All patients are assessed with the duration of diabetes, recent HbA1c, and their current medications. During bariatric surgery, to achieve access to the stomach the left lobe of the liver needs to be moved by retractors. Patients with morbid obesity invariably suffer from a certain degree of fatty liver, technically complicating the procedure. Hence, before bariatric surgery, a very-low-calorie and low-carbohydrate diet with 100 g of carbohydrate a day and 600 calories a day is prescribed to the patients to reduce the size of the liver. This will dramatically increase the insulin sensitivity and may cause hypoglycemia in patients on various hypoglycemic agents. Hence during this period of liver-reducing diet, the diabetes medications should be appropriately altered. Usually the GLP-1 analogues, DPP-4 inhibitors, and SGLT-2 inhibitors are stopped during this period. If the patients are on insulin, the basal insulin dose is reduced by 50% with a plan to appropriately titrate.

Perioperatively, patients are managed with a glucose insulin infusion.

In the immediate postoperative period, as the type 2 diabetes improves dramatically, the medications are carefully optimized. The GLP-1, DPP-4 inhibitor, and SGLT-2 inhibitors are stopped. Metformin can be restarted as a suspension when the patient is able to eat. If the patient was on insulin preoperatively, it will be restarted at a much lower dose and titrated slowly with a close monitoring of capillary blood glucose. The patient will be discharged with optimum dose with an advice to closely self-monitor the blood glucose and a plan to review in the clinic within 6 weeks. Usually, metformin is continued long term.

ASSESSMENT FOR SLEEP APNEA

Preoperatively, all patients are clinically screened for obstructive sleep apnea with Epworth sleepiness scale, which has its limitations. Hence the 8-point STOP BANG tool is used, which includes Snoring, Tiredness (Epworth score >12), Obstruction signs with apneic episodes, blood Pressure, BMI >35, Age >50, Neck circumference >40 cm, and Gender: Male.[12] A score of >3 needs further sleep studies with overnight pulse oximetry or Embletta studies. All patients who are confirmed to have sleep apnea are treated with home CPAP, which reduces anesthetic risk. Appropriate identification and management of obstructive sleep apnea is important to reduce anesthetic complications.[13]

ASSESSMENT OF OTHER MEDICAL PROBLEMS PREOPERATIVELY

Hypertension is quite commonly associated with obesity because of multiple mechanisms including increased sympathetic activity and alterations in renal tubular reabsorption of sodium.[14,15] When an obese patient presents with hypertension and diabetes mellitus, it always triggers investigations for secondary causes for obesity. Long-standing hypertension may be associated with other complications such as left ventricular hypertrophy, congestive heart failure, and atrial fibrillation, which will have an effect on the outcome of bariatric surgery. Hence it is important to optimize antihypertensive treatment before preanesthetic assessment. A plan is made to reduce the antihypertensive drugs after bariatric surgery because the blood pressure improves following bariatric surgery and patients need less number of medications.[16]

There is a well-established association between low vitamin D levels and obesity.[17] Vitamin D deficiency in obesity is multifactorial including altered behavior causing reduced exposure to sun, high sequestration of vitamin D in adipose tissue, and altered metabolism of vitamin D.[18] Because low vitamin D is associated with symptoms leading to reduced physical activity, it will have an impact on increasing weight. Because vitamin D deficiency is a modifiable factor, it helps to measure and replace vitamin D in all obese patients. Bariatric surgery, particularly Roux-en-Y gastric bypass (RYGB) could cause malabsorption; hence routinely vitamin D is replaced postoperatively.[19] If patients are found to be severely vitamin D deficient (with serum 25 hydroxy vitamin D levels <25 nmol/L), it is advisable to use high-dose vitamin D of up to 60,000 IU every week for 3 months followed by around 1000–2000 IU per day for maintenance.[18] There is evidence that weight loss increases the serum vitamin D levels.[19]

Hypogonadotropic hypogonadism is found to be very prevalent in men with obesity.[20,21] This male obesity–associated secondary hypogonadism still remains incompletely understood and underdiagnosed, leading to poor health outcome in obese men. Low levels of testosterone were found in obese men with or without type 2 diabetes with an inverse relationship with BMI. The prevalence is reported to be up to 40%.[22] Obesity in men is known to cause increased aromatase activity within adipocytes. This results in increased peripheral conversion of testosterone into estradiol leading to increased levels of serum estradiol. This estradiol has a negative feedback effect on LH secretion, resulting in suppression of hypothalamic–pituitary–gonadal axis, eventually resulting in low testosterone levels.[21] Presence of hypogonadism causes increased fat mass, which in turn causes further hypogonadism leading to the vicious cycle of worsening obesity. This interplay of testosterone levels and adipose tissue is known to make the management of obesity more difficult.[23] Hence it is beneficial to investigate all men with obesity for hypogonadism at the earliest stage and treat with testosterone replacement appropriately, well before patients are prepared for bariatric surgery. However, because most obese patients have obstructive sleep apnea and testosterone replacement could make OSA worse, appropriate investigations to rule out OSA should be undertaken. Although there is no evidence to show testosterone replacement will result in significant weight reduction by itself, it is known to improve mood, and energy, might reduce fatigue, and will result in higher motivation for men to adhere to diet and exercise regimens designed to combat obesity.[24]

Women undergoing bariatric surgery would be advised not to get pregnant for up to 2 years following surgery.[25] Around 83% of weight loss surgeries were done for women in reproductive age group as shown in one review.[26] Hence it is important to counsel these patients about contraception during the preparation period for surgery. This is particularly relevant, because immediately after bariatric surgery, the women will start ovulating regularly and the fertility chances increase. The chances of maternal and fetal malnutrition and the risks of "small for age babies" are high if women get pregnant, particularly during the rapid weight loss phase. Because pregnant patients need extra calories, immediate post–bariatric surgery period will make it difficult for women to meet with the nutritional requirements. However, there remain some differing views in this domain. The studies and reviews have not shown significant difference in maternal and perinatal complications in women who got pregnant within the 12 months postsurgery period.[27,28] Considering the possible risks associated with pregnancy during the accelerated weight loss period, the current guidelines recommend to avoid pregnancy for 12 months up to 24 months.[25,29,30]

The importance of psychologic counseling is very important during the preparatory period. Issues around body image should actively be counseled. Many patients worry about the development of loose skin and abdominal apron following weight loss with bariatric surgery.[31] Patients should be given appropriate advice and guidance and provided with help from the physician and psychologists.

POST–BARIATRIC SURGERY MANAGEMENT OF MEDICAL PROBLEMS

All patients with diabetes mellitus are revisited with the diabetes treatment. Becasue many patients achieve remission of type 2 diabetes, generally all medications are stopped with regular monitoring of blood glucoses and HbA1c. Many patients with type 2 diabetes who were on insulin are able to stop insulin post–bariatric surgery and keep a good glycemic control.[32] Most physicians continue to use a small dose of metformin even in patients who have achieved remission. This ensures that patients remember about their diabetes and have regular review for complications of diabetes in addition to weight loss related to metformin itself.

Patients, who have not achieved remission of type 2 diabetes, will need complete adjustment of their antidiabetes treatment. The patients who commonly do not achieve remission are the people who had type 2 diabetes for a long time of more than 10 years, who already are on insulin and who had a poor control despite maximal medical treatment.[33] These patients should be regularly reviewed in specialist clinics to optimize the treatment. A probability score, namely DIArem score has been found useful for preoperative prediction of remission of type 2 diabetes following RYGB based on four variables including the use of insulin, age, HbA1c, and type of antidiabetic medication.[34]

The other medical problems such as hypertension should be revisited by reducing the number of antihypertensive medications with blood pressure monitoring. Patients diagnosed with obstructive sleep apnea will be able to return their home CPAP if their symptoms improve.

Most patients develop nutritional deficiencies including vitamins A, D, E, K, B12, zinc; iron; ferritin; selenium; folate; and thiamine. This is more common following malabsorptive procedures such as RYGB. Patients who lost more than 10% of their body weight in the first month, those with anastomotic stenosis, those who had revision surgeries, and those having persistent vomiting are at a higher risk of developing nutritional deficiencies. A clear strategy for replacing all these nutrients is developed following the bariatric surgery with a plan to monitor the levels every 6 months. Occasionally, patients develop protein–energy malnutrition following RYGB. To prevent this, patients should be provided with dietary advice on taking appropriate amount of proteins in the daily intake.[35]

POST–BARIATRIC SURGERY HYPOGLYCEMIA

Symptoms of hypoglycemia have been encountered by a significant number of patients following RYGB.[36,37] Many patients develop neuroglycopenic symptoms of hypoglycemia following RYGB. Although it was reported that the incidence of post–bariatric surgery hyperinsulinemic hypoglycemia is only 0.2%,[38] in practice it is reported to be significantly higher than this. Patients who had diabetes, as well as patients who never had diabetes preoperatively, develop this complication. In many patients these symptoms are recurrent, severe, and intractable. It is considered to be due to inappropriately high levels of secretion of insulin as a response to food, which is mediated through the incretin pathway.[36]

It is increasingly recognized that adequate education should be provided to the patients preoperatively, to recognize the symptoms of hypoglycemia. If patients report hypoglycemic symptoms, they should be provided with glucose monitoring devices. In patients with proven hypoglycemia with the capillary blood glucose monitoring, further testing with either prolonged oral glucose tolerance test or a mixed meal test should be administered to establish the presence of hyperinsulinemic hypoglycemia. In severe cases CT or MRI imaging of pancreas may be needed to rule out the presence of nesidioblastosis and insulin-secreting tumors.

Most patients with hypoglycemia are treated with dietary advice to have small frequent meals with low glycemic index diet. There are reports with variable success of using acarbose, verapamil, nifedipine, diazoxide, and octreotide.[39–41] All patients receive adequate dietary advice followed by a trial period of acarbose 50 g tds. If the hypoglycemia persists, a trial with Octreotide injections, 50 mcg two to three times a day for 3–6 months would be appropriate. Rarely, patients needed surgical procedures such as pancreatectomy to resolve the symptoms in severe cases.[42]

CONCLUSION

Because the number of patients undergoing bariatric surgery is in the increase globally, the surgical resources and expertise have expanded. However, there is an increasing need for structured nonsurgical management of these patients both before and after surgery. Detailed assessment of all obese patients by a nonsurgical team providing a multiprofessional support for a period of 6 months to 1 year before surgery is extremely important to achieve excellent postoperative results with the physical, mental, and social well-being of all patients.

REFERENCES

1. World Health Organization. *Obesity and Overweight, Fact Sheet N 311;* 2015. Available at: http://www.who.int/mediacentre/factsheets/fs311/en/.
2. Bray GA. Lifestyle and pharmacological approaches to weight loss: efficacy and safety. *J Clin Endocrinol Metab.* 2008;93(11 suppl 1):S81–S88. http://dx.doi.org/10.1210/jc.2008-1294.
3. NICE Guidelines for Identification, Assessment and Management of Obesity. https://www.nice.org.uk/guidance/cg189/chapter/1-recommendations; November 2014.
4. Clinical Commissioning Policy: Complex and Specialised Obesity Surgery. https://www.engage.england.nhs.uk/consultation/ssc-area-a/supporting_documents/a5policy.pdf:8.
5. Commissioning Gude: Weight Assessment and Management Clinics. http://www.bomss.org.uk/wp-content/uploads/2014/04/Commissioning-guide-weight-assessment-and-management-clinics-published.pdf:6.
6. Whitlock G, Lewington S, Sherliker P, et al. Body-mass index and cause-specific mortality in 900 000 adults: collaborative analyses of 57 prospective studies. *Lancet.* 2009;373:1083–1096.
7. Sharma AM, Kushner RF. A proposed clinical staging system for obesity. *Int J Obes (Lond).* March 2009;33(3):289–295.
8. Asheim ET, Aylwin SJB, Radhakrishnan ST, et al. Assessment of obesity beyond body mass index to determine benefit of treatment. *Clin Obes.* 2011;1:77–84. http://dx.doi.org/10.1111/j.1758-8111.2011.00017.
9. Padwal RS, Pajewski NM, Allison DB, Sharma AM. Using the Edmonton obesity staging system to predict mortality in a population-representative cohort of people with overweight and obesity. *CMAJ.* 2011;183(14):e1059–e1066.
10. FDA: Liraglutide Approved by FDA for Obesity. Available at: https://www.fda.gov/NewsEvents/Newsroom/PressAnnouncements/ucm427913.htm.
11. Pi-Sunyer X, Astrup A, Fujioka K, et al. A randomized controlled trial of 3 mg of Liraglutide in weight management. *N Engl J Med.* July 2, 2015;373:11–22.
12. STOP BANG Sleep Apnoea Screening Questionnaire. Available at: https://www.sleepassociation.org/sleep-apnea-screening-questionnaire-stop-bang/.
13. Kaw R, Gali B, Collop NA. Perioperative care of patients with obstructive sleep apnea. *Curr Treat Options Neurol.* 2011;13(5):496–507. http://dx.doi.org/10.1007/s11940-011-0138-5.
14. Re RN. Obesity-related hypertension. *Ochsner J.* 2009;9(3):133–136.

15. Wenzel UO, Krebs C. Management of arterial hypertension in obese patients. *Curr Hypertens Rep*. 2007;9(6):491–497.
16. Wilhelm SM, Young J, Kale-Pradhan PB. Effect of bariatric surgery on hypertension. *Ann Pharmacother*. 2014vol 48(6):674–682.
17. Parikh SJ, Edelman M, Uwaifo GI, et al. The relationship between obesity and serum 1,25-dihydroxy vitamin D concentrations in healthy adults. *J Clin Endocrinol Metab*. March 2004;89(3):1196–1199.
18. Vanlint S. Vitamin D and obesity. *Nutrients*. 2013;5(3):949–956.
19. Hewitt S, Søvik TT, Aasheim ET, et al. Secondary hyperparathyroidism, vitamin D sufficiency, and serum calcium 5 years after gastric bypass and duodenal switch. *Obes Surg*. March 2013;23(3):384–389.
20. Hofstra J, Loves S, van Wageningen B, et al. High prevalence of hypogonadotropic hypogonadism in men referred for obesity treatment. *Neth J Med*. 2008;66:103–109.
21. Dandona P, Dhindsa S. Update: hypogonadotropic hypogonadism in type 2 diabetes and obesity. *J Clin Endocrinol Metab*. 2011;96:2643–2651.
22. Hindsa S, Miller MG, McWhirter CL, et al. Testosterone concentrations in diabetic and nondiabetic obese men. *Diabetes Care*. 2010;33:1186–1192.
23. Mammi C, Calanchini M, Antelmi A, et al. Androgens and adipose tissue in males: a complex and reciprocal interplay. *Int J Endocrinol*. 2012;2012:789653.
24. Saad F, Aversa A, Isidori AM, Gooren LJ. Testosterone as potential effective therapy in treatment of obesity in men with testosterone deficiency: a review. *Curr Diabetes Rev*. 2012;8(2):131–143. http://dx.doi.org/10.2174/15733991 2799424573.
25. Armstrong C. ACOG guidelines on pregnancy after bariatric surgery. *Am Fam Physician*. April 1, 2010;81(7):905–906.
26. Maggard MA, Yermilov I, Li Z, et al. Pregnancy and fertility following bariatric surgery: a systematic review. *JAMA*. November 19, 2008;300(19):2286–2296.
27. Sheiner E, Edri A, Balaban E, Levi I, Aricha-Tamir B. Pregnancy outcome of patients who conceive during or after the first year following bariatric surgery. *Am J Obstet Gynecol*. January 2011;204(1):50. e1–e6.
28. Dao T, Kuhn J, Ehmer D, et al. Pregnancy outcomes after gastric-bypass surgery. *Am J Surg*. 2006;192:762–766.
29. *Role of Bariatric Surgery in Improving Reproductive Health: Royal College of Obstetrics and Gynaecology*. October 2015. Available at: https://www.rcog.org.uk/globalassets/documents/guidelines/scientific-impact-papers/sip_17.pdf.
30. Khan R, Bashir D, Chappatte O. Pregnancy outcome following bariatric surgery. *Obstet Gynaecol*. 2013;15:37–43.
31. Pecori L, Giacomo G, Cervetti S, Marinari GM, Miglior F, Adami GF. Attitudes of morbidly obese patients to weight loss and body image following bariatric surgery and body contouring. *Obes. Surg*. 2007;17:68–73.
32. Ardestani A, Rhoads D, Tavakkoli A. Insulin cessation and diabetes remission after bariatric surgery in adults with insulin-treated type 2 diabetes. *Diabetes Care*. April 2015;38(4):659–664.
33. Hamza N, Abbas MH, Darwish A, Shafeek Z, New J, Ammori BJ. Predictors of remission of type 2 diabetes mellitus after laparoscopic gastric banding and bypass. *Surg Obes Relat Dis*. 2011;7:691–696.
34. Still CD, Wood GC, Benotti P, et al. A probability score for preoperative prediction of type 2 diabetes remission following RYGB surgery. *Lancet Diabetes Endocrinol*. 2014;2(1):38–45. http://dx.doi.org/10.1016/S2213-8587 (13)70070-6.
35. Davies DJ, Baxter JM, Baxter JN. Nutritional deficiencies after bariatric surgery. *Obes Surg*. September 2007;17(9):1150–1158.
36. Goldfine AB, Mun EC, Devine E, et al. Patients with neuroglycopenia after gastric bypass surgery have exaggerated incretin and insulin secretory responses to a mixed meal. *J Clin Endocrinol Metab*. 2007;92:4678–4685.
37. Service GJ, Thompson GB, Service FJ, Andrews JC, Collazo-Clavell ML, Lloyd RV. Hyperinsulinemic hypoglycemia with nesidioblastosis after gastric-bypass surgery. *N Engl J Med*. 2005;353:249–254.
38. Marsk R, Jonas E, Rasmussen F, Näslund E. Nationwide cohort study of post-gastric bypass hypoglycaemia including 5,040 patients undergoing surgery for obesity in 1986–2006 in Sweden. *Diabetologia*. November 2010;53(11):2307–2311.
39. Mordes JP, Alonso LC. Evaluation, medical therapy, and course of adult persistent hyperinsulinemic hypoglycemia after roux-en-y gastric bypass surgery: a case series. *Endocr Pract*. 2015;21(3):237–246.
40. Moreira RO, Moreira RB, Machado NA, Gonçalves TB, Coutinho WF. Post-prandial hypoglycemia after bariatric surgery: pharmacological treatment with verapamil and acarbose. *Obes Surg*. December 2008;18(12):1618–1621.
41. Bernard B, Kline GA, Service FJ. Hypoglycaemia following upper gastrointestinal surgery: case report and review of the literature. *BMC Gastroenterol*. 2010;10:77.
42. Patti ME, McMahon G, Mun EC, et al. Severe hypoglycaemia post-gastric bypass requiring partial pancreatectomy: evidence for inappropriate insulin secretion and pancreatic islet hyperplasia. *Diabetologia*. 2005;48:2236–2240.

FURTHER READING

1. Pearce SHS, Cheetham TD. Diagnosis and management of vitamin D deficiency. *BMJ*. 2010;340:b5664.
2. Rock CL, Emond JA, Flatt SW, et al. Weight loss is associated with increased serum 25-hydroxyvitamin D in overweight or obese women. *Obes (Silver Spring)*. November 2012;20(11):2296–2301.

CHAPTER 28

Surgical Management of Obesity

ARUTCHELVAM VIJAYARAMAN, MD, FRCP

INTRODUCTION

There is increasing awareness of obesity as a medical disorder amenable to surgical treatment. The debate is still ongoing about, if obesity should be coded as disease, albeit few countries, such as the United States and Canada, have already done so.[1,2] There has been significant development in understanding the pathophysiology of obesity and associated comorbidities. However, the treatment modalities available are still very limited. The various nonsurgical treatments for obesity are based on motivational consultations, behavior modification sessions, behavioral contracting, reinforcement, goal setting, psychologic interventions, dietary modifications, and very few pharmacologic agents. The current evidences from various studies suggest that nonsurgical interventions result in around 1%–5% of total body weight loss.[3,4] Unfortunately, these measures are not found to produce a sustained weight reduction and improvement with weight-related comorbidities in majority of patients with morbid obesity. Bariatric surgery, on the other hand, has shown significant weight reduction in multiple studies. A systematic review by Gloy et al.,[5] with a metaanalysis of 11 randomized controlled trials (RCTs), concluded that bariatric surgery resulted in significantly higher body weight loss and greater remission rates of type 2 diabetes, although the results were limited to 2-year follow-up and were based on small numbers of studies and individuals.[5] A review of the Swedish obesity subjects trial showed that mean changes in body weight after 2, 10, 15, and 20 years were 23%, 17%, 16%, and 18% in the surgery group and 0%, 1%, –1%, and –1% in the control group, respectively.[6] Hence, currently, bariatric surgery appears to be the only definitive way of achieving a sustained weight reduction, resulting in remission of type 2 diabetes and improvement in other comorbidities in a significant number of patients.

ELIGIBILITY FOR BARIATRIC SURGERY

Most centers offer surgery for patients with a body mass index (BMI) of ≥35 without comorbidities or ≥40 with weight-related comorbidities. In the United Kingdom, the National Institute of Clinical Excellence (NICE) guidelines CG 189, which was amended and published in November 2014, in addition suggested that bariatric surgery should be offered as the first line of management for adult patients with BMI more than 50.[7] It also recommended that people with type 2 diabetes of recent onset, and a BMI of ≥35, should be offered bariatric surgery as treatment for the type 2 diabetes. The NICE guidelines also suggested that people with a BMI of 30–34.9 with recent onset of type 2 diabetes mellitus should be considered for an assessment for bariatric surgery. The recent onset is defined as diabetes of less than 10-year duration.[7] Both the International Diabetes Federation (IDF) and American Diabetes Association (ADA) have advised that bariatric surgery should be considered for people with type 2 diabetes at a BMI of 30, although it is highlighted that the evidence in this group is limited.

Patients are expected to work with a multidisciplinary specialist weight management team for a period of 6–12 months and exhaust all nonsurgical treatment. The NICE guidelines in the United Kingdom mandates that all patients considered for bariatric surgery should be treated with a tier 3 specialist weight management or equivalent service with a multidisciplinary team. Patients are expected to stop smoking before they are considered for surgery and provided support with smoking cessation. Management of all comorbidities is optimized and plans are made for the perioperative period. Patients with sleep apnea are known to have higher anesthetic risk. Hence, all patients are assessed clinically and, if needed, assessed with sleep studies and treated with home Continuous Positive Airway Pressure (CPAP), if diagnosed to have obstructive sleep apnea (OSA) at least for 6 weeks preoperatively.

CHOICE OF BARIATRIC SURGERY

Various types of bariatric procedures are considered (Fig. 28.1). The three major types of bariatric surgery are restrictive, malabsorptive, or combined as shown in

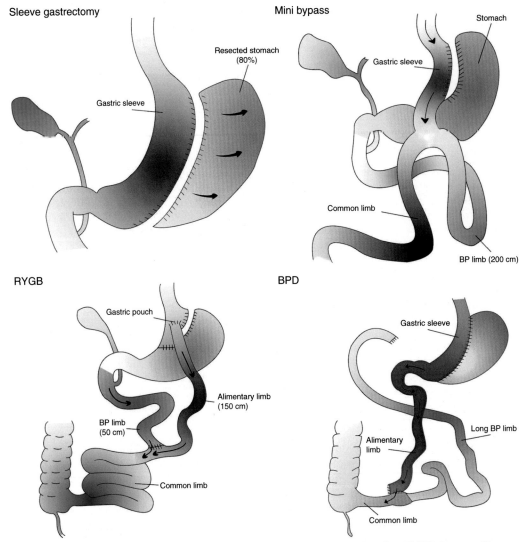

FIG. 28.1 Various types of bariatric procedures. *BPD*, biliary pancreatic diversion; *RYGB*, Roux-en-Y gastric bypass.

Box 28.1. Restrictive procedures include laparoscopic adjustable gastric banding (LAGB), sleeve gastrectomy (SG), and vertical banded gastroplasty (VBG). The biliary pancreatic diversion (BPD), with or without a duodenal switch, is a malabsorptive procedure. The more commonly used laparoscopic Roux-en-Y gastric bypass (RYGB) is a procedure that combines both the restrictive and malabsorptive elements. Single anastomosis gastric bypass is a variant of RYGB. This procedure is also known as "mini gastric bypass" (MGBP), and it simplifies the surgical technique slightly by advocating a single anastomosis, instead of the double anastomosis required in RYGB (Fig. 28.1). This, in turn, results in lesser chances of anastomotic leaks and lesser sites for internal hernias.[8,9] Hence, many centers increasingly use this procedure. The main disadvantage of MGBP appears to be increased chances of bile reflux.[10]

The type of surgery is chosen based on the individual patient characteristics and suitability for the procedure after having a multidisciplinary discussion, which also considers patient choice.

BOX 28.1
Types of Bariatric Procedures

RESTRICTIVE

Laparoscopic adjustable gastric banding (less frequently used in the United Kingdom)

    Sleeve gastrectomy (commonly used in the United Kingdom)

        Vertical banded gastroplasty

        Intragastric balloon (temporary)

MALABSORPTIVE

Biliary pancreatic diversion—with or without duodenal switch

COMBINED

Roux-en-Y gastric bypass (most commonly used in the United Kingdom)

    Minigastric bypass (single anastomosis gastric bypass)

EXPERIMENTAL (NOT WIDELY AVAILABLE)

Laparoscopic implantable gastric pacing device

        Endoscopic duodenal-jejunal bypass sleeve

        Endoluminal restriction procedures

The characteristics of the procedures are listed in Table 28.1, which helps in choosing the right procedure for the individual patient depending on patient factors and surgical choices.

Gastric banding is a reversible procedure with low complication rates. Hence, many patients will prefer this procedure because they perceive it to be less invasive. However, it needs regular adjusting by the surgeon and many patients become noncompliant. The weight loss is slow and many patients regain the weight.[11] As filling the band involves a needle, many patients who have needle phobia will not choose this. In the United Kingdom, in the last few years, the use of gastric band has declined steadily and it is the least commonly used procedure now.

Intragastric balloon placement is a temporary procedure used in patients with morbid obesity to reduce the weight to make them suitable for a definitive procedure such as RYGB. A balloon can be kept for 6 months and, if necessary, repeated until the patient is fit for RYGB.

Both SG and RYGB are permanent procedures, resulting in significant weight reduction. However, RYGB produces a quicker weight reduction, slightly higher percentage of total body weight reduction

TABLE 28.1
Characteristics of Common Bariatric Procedures

Factors to Consider for the Choice of Bariatric Surgery	Sleeve Gastrectomy (SG)	Laparoscopic Adjustable Gastric Band	Roux-en-Y Gastric Bypass (RYGB)
Hormonal	Eliminates ghrelin	None	Higher GLP effect
Type of diet before surgery	Large volume eater		Grazer
Conversion	Convertible to RYGB	Straight forward	Not reversible
Dumping	No dumping	None	Dumping more common
Hypoglycemia	Less common	No hypoglycemia	More common
GERD	Aggravates GERD		Less chances of GERD
Technical difficulty	Straight forward	Straight forward	Complex
Rate of weight loss	Immediate	Slow	Immediate
Remission of T2DM/metabolic	Less than RYGB	None	More than SG
Surgical risk	Lower than RYGB	Very low	Higher than SG
Bridging procedure	Part of two-step procedure in superobese patients		One-step procedure
Complications	Heart burn, weight regain	Erosion, slippage	Dumping, anastomotic leak, marginal ulcers, bowel obstruction, vitamin deficiency

GERD, gastroesophageal reflux disease; *GLP*, glucagon-like peptide; *T2DM*, type 2 diabetes mellitus.

and higher rate of remission for type 2 diabetes.[12,13] The long-term sustainability of the weight reduction depends on the permanent changes in the lifestyle and behavior than the type of procedure. Recent evidence has suggested that SG also produces remission of type 2 diabetes in significant percentage of patients. It has the advantage of being a bridging procedure, which could be converted to gastric bypass later if desired weight reduction is not achieved. Nutrient deficiencies are less common in SG because it does not involve malabsorption. Hunger is significantly reduced as SG reduces the ghrelin levels. Recently, it was found that SG was done more frequently than RYGB in many centers.[14]

In patients with family history of gastric carcinoma, it will be difficult to perform surveillance endoscopy after RYGB, and this will be taken into consideration when a choice is made. SG does not cause dumping syndrome and, hence, hyperinsulinemic hypoglycemia is less common. It was postulated that in some patients with morbid obesity with a BMI of more than 50, development of dumping syndrome is considered to be helpful in achieving a sustained weight reduction. The morbidly obese patients usually have an eating disorder and have an adverse relationship with food. As gastric bypass procedure results in dumping syndrome, the patient gets a negative reinforcement with nausea and sweating and a general ill feeling after they eat large amount of carbohydrates. However, studies did not confirm this and showed that there was no correlation between weight reduction and the presence of dumping syndrome, post-RYGB, but the eating behavior of the patient mainly seems to influence the weight loss.[15]

The BPD surgery is very effective in terms of weight reduction and remission of type 2 diabetes but has significantly high rates of complications. Hence, it is advocated only in few centers with the availability of expertise. It is rarely performed in the United Kingdom.

Generally, people with a BMI of more than 50, who have type 2 diabetes with poor diabetes control; people at high risk of gastroesophageal reflux disease; or/ and people who need to achieve the weight reduction quicker will be chosen for RYGB, and it remains the gold standard surgery currently.

People who would like to achieve the weight reduction slowly, who could stick to healthy diet and regular exercise, and patients who will have higher surgical and anesthetic risks with whom it is better to leave the option of converting into the bypass at a later date are chosen for SG.

However, it is fair to say that these factors are quite subjective and usually decided after having a good discussion with the patient and the multidisciplinary team of professionals.

Different types of endoscopic endobarrier procedures have been advocated for obesity for weight reduction purposes and to improve comorbidities, such as type 2 diabetes, although the availability of these procedures is still limited. A recent metaanalysis showed a mean weight reduction of 4–19 kg along with variable levels of improvement in glycemic control in people with obesity.[16] Currently, these procedures are used as a noninvasive alternative to gastric bypass surgery.

BARIATRIC SURGERY AND WEIGHT REDUCTION

The success of bariatric surgery in causing a sustained weight reduction is well established now. Many systematic reviews have shown that both malabsorptive and restrictive procedures result in a significant, life-changing weight reduction with malabsorptive procedures achieving relatively more weight reduction than the restrictive procedures.

A recent Cochrane review studied 22 RCTs with 1798 participants with follow-up for 12, 24, or 36 months.[17] Seven RCTs, comparing surgery with intensive medical measures, showed significantly higher weight reduction with surgery along with improvement in health-related quality of life. Three RCTs found that laparoscopic RYGB surgery resulted in significantly greater reduction in the BMI up to 5 years after surgery compared with LAGB. Seven other RCTs compared RYGB with SG and did not find a consistent difference between these two procedures, in terms of weight loss with a mean difference of 0.2 kg/m² in BMI (95% confidence interval [CI] 1.8–1.3). No significant difference in the quality of life was found between these two procedures. Additionally, the effects on comorbidities, such as type 2 diabetes and surgical and other complications, were found to be neutral, except that gastroesophageal reflux disease was found to be improved following RYGB in one RCT. These results showing relatively comparable weight reduction with SG explains the increasing use of SG for bariatric purposes worldwide.

A systematic review of bariatric surgery was reported in 2004, extracting 136 studies, with a total of 22,094 patients and a mean age of 39 years (range, 16–64 years) with 19% as men.[18] The baseline mean BMI was 46.9 (range, 32.3–68.8). The mean percentage of excess body weight loss was 61.2% (58.1%–64.4%) for all patients, 47.5% (40.7%–54.2%) for patients who underwent gastric banding, 61.6% (56.7%–66.5%) for gastric bypass, 68.2% (61.5%–74.8%) for gastroplasty, and 70.1% (66.3%–73.9%) for biliopancreatic diversion/duodenal switch (BPD-DS). The operative mortality for purely restrictive procedures was reported to be 0.1%, for gastric bypass 0.5%, and for BPD 1.1%. This review gave insight into the effect of different bariatric procedures with RYGB being the procedure producing relatively higher weight reduction than SG and with relatively fewer side effects than BPD.

An updated systematic review published in 2014 included 164 RCTs and 127 observational studies analyzing 161,756 patients with a mean BMI of 46 kg/m^2.[19] The analysis of RCTs reporting percentage of excess body weight reduction showed the first year reduction to be 60% (range 50%–70%), second year 71% (61%–79%), and third year 57% (52%–62%). Eleven studies within the review reported BMI change over a 5-year period with a mean reduction of 12–17 kg/m^2. The study concluded that RYGB and SG produced comparable weight loss and LAGB had lower mortality and complication rates; yet, the reoperation rate was higher and weight loss was less substantial than RYGB and SG.

Another systematic review assessed 147 studies, 89 of which were contributing to the weight loss analysis and 134 contributing to the mortality analysis.[20] Surgery resulted in a weight loss of 20–30 kg, which was maintained for up to 10 years. The overall mortality for all the procedures was found to be less than 1%. As reported in other studies, this review also showed that gastric bypass procedures resulted in relatively more weight loss than gastric band and SG.

A recently published review used the bariatric outcomes longitudinal database (BOLD) in the United States from 2007 to 2012 and compared 50,987 patients with BMI more than 50, who underwent either RYGB (n = 42,119) or SG (n = 8868).[21] The percentage reduction of total body weight was higher for patients who underwent RYGB compared with those who underwent SG at 3 months (14.1 vs. 13.1%, P < .001), 6 months (25.2 vs. 22.4%, P < .001), and 12 months (34.5 vs. 29.7%, P < .001). The overall 30-day complication rates showed no difference.

The Swedish obesity study, although limited by the fact it is not a randomized study, is an important study because it has provided significant insight into the long-term results up to 20 years after bariatric surgery.[22] Although the follow-up data available at 15 years and 20 years are low (at 15 years, 150 patients underwent banding, 487 patients underwent VBG, and 37 patients underwent RYGB and, at 20 years, 50, 82, and 13, respectively), the trend in weight reduction gives convincing information. The mean (±SD) percentage weight reduction in the surgical groups was maximal after 1–2 years followed by some weight regain in the

following years. This increase in weight seems to level off at around 8–10 years. At 10 years, the percentage weight reductions were 25 ± 11% for RYGB, 16 ± 11% for VBG, and 14 + 14% for banding. At 15 years, the weight reductions were 27 ± 12%, 18 ± 11%, and 13 ± 14%, respectively. The numbers are too small to interpret the 20-year data, but the trend seems to continue. The primary outcome of the effect on overall mortality was reported at 16 years of follow-up. The risk reduction with any-cause mortality was reported to be close to 30% (HR = 0.71, 95% CI 0.54–0.92). This long-term data has shown convincing results that bariatric surgery has caused sustained weight reduction and was associated with significant reduction in all-cause mortality.

Bariatric surgery was found to produce equally good weight reduction with comparable rate of complications in people with BMI more than 60. A single-center, retrospective study reviewed 135 patients who underwent RYGB (n = 93) or SG (n = 42).[23] The study looked at the percentage of patients who achieved more than 30% of their excess weight loss. 72% of the patients who underwent RYGB achieved more than 30% excess body weight loss at 6 months and 94.5% at 12 months. SG showed comparable results with 59% achieving more than 30% excess body weight reduction by 6 months and 100% at 12 months. However, preoperative comorbidities, conversion to open surgery from laparoscopic surgery, and the average length of hospital stay are all reported to be higher in this group of patients.

A case-matched 5-year follow-up study matched 30 patients with BMI more than 60 (mean BMI of 64.1) with 60 patients with BMI less than 60 (mean BMI of 46).[24] The percentage of initial weight loss was found to be comparable between the two groups (27.4 ± 11.8 vs. 29.7 ± 9.2; P = .35). However, the percentage of excess weight loss was found to be higher for the group with the lesser initial BMI (44.9 ± 19.9 vs. 66.5 ± 21.2; P < .0001). No difference was noted in the rate of remission or improvement of comorbidities, such as type 2 diabetes or hypertension, in both the groups. It should be noted, in most countries, surgery for this group of patients with a BMI of more than 60 is performed only in centers with adequate experience. Sometimes, these patients are encouraged to lose weight to a BMI of less than 60, by advocating intragastric balloon insertion temporarily.

There is enough evidence to show the cost-effectiveness of bariatric procedures by way of not only improving the comorbidities but also causing simple weight reduction. A metaanalysis has shown the cost effectiveness of bariatric surgery in people with obesity of BMI more than 35, without any comorbidity, just by way of causing weight reduction. It was particularly found to be cost saving for patients with BMI more than 50.[25]

Although most of these structured systematic reviews included a heterogeneous group of studies and included both RCTs and observational studies, there is enough evidence to conclude the following with regards to bariatric surgery and weight reduction.

- Bariatric surgery produces a life-changing weight reduction, resulting in a percentage excess weight reduction of 50%–65%.
- RYGB and SG are commonly used procedures.
- RYGB produces relatively more weight reduction than SG.
- SG is being increasingly advocated because of relatively less operative time, simpler surgical technique, and slightly less complications. However, the procedure is chosen based on the patient's characteristics.
- Bariatric procedures are found to be effective to cause weight reduction in patients with a BMI of more than 60, but the procedures are usually conducted in centers with experience.

BARIATRIC SURGERY AND DIABETES

It has been recognized for 15 years that bariatric surgery could result in remission of type 2 diabetes as an additional beneficial effect. Since then, there has been mounting evidence to confirm this phenomenon. Moreover, it has been shown that the complications of type 2 diabetes also improves following bariatric surgery with reduction in diabetes-related mortality and morbidity. Studies have shown that blood glucoses return to normal with no treatment within days following surgery, and this appears to be independent of weight loss. Various mechanisms are postulated, including reduced calorie intake, malabsorption of nutrients, alterations in the structure of the gastrointestinal anatomy leading onto modification of incretin system, and hormonal changes such as reduction of ghrelin, to name a few. However, as more patients with type 2 diabetes are offered bariatric surgery as a treatment for poor glycemic control, it is important to make appropriate perioperative adjustment in medications for these patients.

The most important first step is to confirm the type of diabetes preoperatively. There are reports about diabetic ketoacidosis developing up to 30 days after bariatric surgery.[26] This is attributed to a combination of underinsulinization and surgical stress. Additionally, if a patient with type 1 diabetes is wrongly diagnosed as type 2, it has led on to DKA. It is mandatory to revisit the diagnosis of the type of diabetes with appropriate investigations, including diabetes antibody profile and C-peptide estimation to correctly label the type preoperatively. This will also help, when the patients are on a low-carbohydrate, liver reducing diet, just before surgery, careful insulin dose titrations with more frequent blood glucose tests are advocated. New medications, such as SGLT-2 inhibitors, are known to be associated with DKA in patients with dehydration following surgery, which might need to be considered stopping before starting the liver reducing diet along with close monitoring of blood glucoses.[26]

DEFINITION FOR REMISSION OF TYPE 2 DIABETES:

Different studies used a variety of criteria to define remission of type 2 diabetes following bariatric surgery. The ADA position statement listed stringent criteria to confirm remission of type 2 diabetes following bariatric surgery.[27] This defined complete remission as normal glycemic measures for more than 1-year duration. Partial remission is clarified as hyperglycemia below diagnostic thresholds for diabetes for at least 1-year duration with no active pharmacologic therapy or ongoing procedures.

The ADA criteria, based on the diagnostic criteria for diagnosis of diabetes, defined complete remission as HbA1c of less than 42 mmol/mol (6%) and fasting blood glucose of less than 100 mg/dL (5.6 mmol/L) for more than 1 year. The IDF defines optimization of the metabolic state following bariatric surgery as HbA1c less than 42 mmol/mol (6%) with no hypoglycemia.[28]

There are many mechanisms postulated for the improvement of type 2 diabetes following bariatric surgery.

Rubino et al. suggested three mechanisms, including the effect of weight loss, degree of malabsorption, and hormonal changes.[29] The hormonal effects, such as increased levels of glucagon-like peptide-1 following bariatric surgery, explain the improvement in blood glucose levels within days after the surgery, independent of weight reduction. Other gut hormones, such as PPY and ghrelin, play a role.

There are many nonrandomized, observational studies published with reliable evidence, suggesting remission of type 2 diabetes in a significant number of patients.

In an earlier systematic review,[18] type 2 diabetes was reported to be completely resolved in 76.8% of bariatric surgery patients. A metaanalysis of 621 studies, involving 135,246 patients undergoing bariatric surgery, reported a 78.2% of patients with type 2 diabetes undergoing remission.[30] However, the studies included in these metaanalyses were heterogeneous and observed different, less stringent criteria for defining remission.

Another metaanalysis, which included both observational studies and RCTs till 2013, compared bariatric surgery with intensive medical therapy for remission of type 2 diabetes.[31] The overall type 2 diabetes remission rates were reported to be 63.5% (range, 38.2–100.0) compared with the control group with 15.6% (0.0–46.7) (*P*<.001). Another cross-sectional, nonrandomized, controlled study analyzed improvement of type 2 diabetes after RYGB, 1 week and 3 months after surgery, and found fasting blood glucose to fall to a level as in lean control subjects within that short period.[32]

The Swedish obese subjects (SOS) study, which is a prospective matched cohort study, demonstrated type 2 diabetes remission rates 2 years after surgery as 72.3% (95% CI, 66.9%–77.2%; 219/303) for bariatric surgery patients (odds ratio, 13.3; 95% CI, 8.5–20.7; *P*<0.001) compared with 16.4% (95% CI, 11.7%–22.2%; 34/207) for control patients.[33] At 15 years, although the diabetes remission rates decreased to 30.4%, it is still considered significant. This study also observed marked reduction in the microvascular and macrovascular complications of type 2 diabetes.

A retrospective cohort study of adults with uncontrolled or medication-controlled type 2 diabetes, who underwent gastric bypass from 1995 to 2008 in three integrated healthcare delivery systems in the United States, observed an overall remission rate of 68.2% in 5 years. 35% of these patients were found to redevelop diabetes in this study.[34]

Another interesting observational study enrolled 2458 patients undergoing bariatric surgery, with 627 patients with diabetes.[35] After 3 years, it was reported that 68.7% of RYGB and 30.2% of LAGB participants were in diabetes remission.

Another study assessed changes in insulin-treated type 2 diabetes patients after bariatric surgery. 10% of the 113,638 adult surgical patients in the BOLD were insulin-treated type 2 diabetes patients. Of the 3318 patients who underwent RYGB, 62% were off insulin at 12 months compared with 34% (n=1907) after gastric band (*P*<.001).[36]

Although there is an abundance of data available from observational studies and retrospective reviews, the data from RCT were limited. This is partly due to the difficulty in recruiting patients to be randomized to surgery or medical therapy because patients prepared for bariatric surgery will be highly motivated and disappointed if they are randomized to the medical therapy arm. However, there are quite a few, high-quality RCTs recently published comparing bariatric surgery with intensive medical therapy in achieving remission with type 2 diabetes.

A RCT compared conventional diabetes therapy with LAGB in achieving diabetes remission with a criteria of HbA1c <6.2% and fasting blood glucose of 126 mg/dL (7 mmol/L), over a 2-year period.[37] 73% were reported to have achieved remission in the surgical group and 13% in the medical treatment group.

A 1-year RCT compared RYGB, gastric band, and medical therapy and randomized 69 participants with a BMI of 30–40 and type 2 diabetes.[38] Although the study was limited by the small numbers, it did show 12 of 24 (50%) undergoing RYGB being classified with partial type 2 diabetes mellitus remission at 12 months and 4 (16.7%) with complete remission, compared with 6 of 22 (27.3%) and 5 (22.7%) of those undergoing LAGB, respectively. No patient on medical therapy achieved remission.

An RCT, STAMPEDE, published the initial results in 2012 comparing the effect of intensive medical therapy with RYGB and SG in patients with uncontrolled type 2 diabetes.[39] 150 patients were randomized to the three arms of intensive medical treatment as per ADA guidelines, SG, or RYGB. The 1-year results showed that the target HbA1c of 6% (42 mmol/mol) was achieved in 12% patients in the medical therapy group compared with 42% in the RYGB group and 37% in the SG group. Although this study showed a significant number of patients achieved target HbA1c in the SG group, 28% of those patients needed one or more antiglycemic drugs, whereas the RYGB group sustained the target without any medications. This trend was shown to continue at 3 years because 38% of the participants in the RYGB

group and 24% in the SG group sustained the target HbA1c at 3 years, whereas only 5% achieved that in the medical treatment group.[40]

The 5-year data from STAMPEDE, presented in the American College of Cardiology meeting in 2016, showed that the glycemic benefits of bariatric surgery are sustained in a significant number of patients. At 5 years, more than 88% of patients in both surgery groups had maintained healthy HbA1c levels without the use of insulin. In addition, 29% of patients in the gastric bypass group and 23% in the SG group had achieved and maintained healthy HbA1c levels versus the 5% in the medical therapy group.[41]

Another RCT by Mingrone et al. was published in 2012 comparing RYGB, BPD, and medical therapy in patients with type 2 diabetes and obesity.[42] This study presented an initial 2-year data with 75% of patients in the RYGB group, 95% in the BPD group, and 0% in the medical therapy group, achieving remission of type 2 diabetes. Although the study was limited with the sample size, it gave good insight into the efficacy of bariatric procedures for glycemic management.

Another multicenter RCT analyzed RYGB compared with intensive medical therapy.[43] With a criterion of achieving HbA1c <7% (53 mmol/mol), 120 randomized patients were studied with a mean BMI of 34.6 kg/m² (30–39.9). The glycemic goal with HbA1c 7.0% was achieved with 75% patients who underwent RYGB with a mean of 6.3% with 65% fewer medications. The triple end point as the primary outcome, which included HbA1c <7%, low-density lipoprotein cholesterol <100 mg/dL, and systolic BP <130, was achieved by 49% in the RYGB group and 19% in the intensive medical therapy group. Interestingly, this study included patients with a lower BMI of 30–34.9, showing similar results.

A probability scoring system has been developed, namely "DiaRem" score, to predict remission of type 2 diabetes following bariatric surgery. Using four variables, including the use of insulin, age, HbA1c, and type of antidiabetic medication, with a probable score range of 0–22, could identify patients preoperatively into 5 probability range.[44] This might help in predicting which patients have a higher chance of remission of type 2 diabetes and assist in counseling the patients.

Bariatric surgery also has some evidence that it can prevent the development of type 2 diabetes in obese patients. A nonrandomized, matched control study assessed 1658 patients who underwent bariatric surgery with 1771 obese matched controls.[45] The results showed an incidence rate of 28.4 cases per 1000 person-years in the control group as opposed to 6.8 cases per 1000 person-years in the bariatric surgery group with an adjusted hazard ratio with bariatric surgery of 0.17 (95% CI, 0.13–0.21; $P<.001$).

The cost-effectiveness of bariatric surgery in patients with type 2 diabetes is difficult to establish with evidence base. The savings in the cost of medications in the patients who achieve remission of type 2 diabetes will be high, but it is difficult to quantify the benefits of preventing diabetes-related microvascular and macrovascular complications. A two-group RCT conducted in China, showed that SG and laparoscopic RYGB appear to be relatively cost-effective treatments for people with diabetes, with cost-effectiveness ratios ranging from $1028.97 to $1197.44/quality-adjusted life year (QALY) compared with $1589.02/QALY for medical treatment.[46]

NICE UK has made the cost-effectiveness analysis and has recommended that bariatric surgery should be offered as a treatment for people with recent onset of type 2 diabetes with poor glycemic control.[7]

Analyzing all the evidence with these observational studies and available RCTs, the key messages are as follows:

- Bariatric surgery has convincing evidence for remission of type 2 diabetes.
- Although long-term data are needed, a significant number of patients seem to have sustained the glycemic improvement.
- Although RYGB is superior to SG in achieving remission of type 2 diabetes, SG also achieves remission in a significant number of patients with relatively less complications.
- There is enough evidence that bariatric procedures are cost-effective in patients with a BMI of more than 35 and type 2 diabetes. Hence, many agencies, such as ADA, IDF, and NICE UK, have recommended that these procedures should be offered in the treatment algorithm of type 2 diabetes.
- Although it could be effective in the cohort of patients with BMI 30–34.9 kg/m² (and lesser in some ethnic groups such as South Asians at 27.5), there still is not enough evidence to recommend bariatric surgery to this group as treatment for type 2 diabetes. However, it is reasonable to discuss this as an option with the patients if they have poor glycemic control despite maximizing medical treatment.

BARIATRIC SURGERY AND DEPRESSION

It is well known that obesity is associated with significant mental health problems, influenced by behavioral, social, psychologic, and biologic factors with a clear bidirectional association between depression and obesity.[47,48] 43% of patients with obesity were found to be obese, and across all age groups, women with depression were more likely to be obese than women without depression.[49] When we prepare patients for bariatric surgery, it is extremely important to assess their mental health status and take every step to improve depression. Psychologists play a major role in the multidisciplinary team involved with bariatric surgery.

A metaanalysis on mental health conditions was performed among patients seeking and undergoing bariatric surgery.[50] 68 publications were identified with 59 reporting prebariatric surgery prevalence of mental health problems. 27 studies reported an association between preoperative problems and the postoperative outcome. The most common illness was depression (19%) and binge eating (17%). However, the evidence on the association of mental health problems with postoperative weight loss was found to be conflicting.

Rapid weight reduction was known to be associated with increased suicide risk. In a retrospective cohort study, the long-term mortality was determined among 9949 patients who had undergone gastric bypass surgery and 9628 severely obese persons who applied for driver's licenses.[51] This showed, during a mean follow-up period of 7.1 years, any-cause mortality was reduced by 40% in the surgery group and cause-specific mortality reduced by 56% for coronary artery diseases, by 60% for cancer, and by 92% for diabetes. However, death caused by accidents and suicide were found to be 58% higher in the surgery group. The hazard ratio for suicide was reported to be 2.03 (95% CI 0.66–6.27), compared with matched control subjects. Similar to our experience with weight loss medications, such as sibutramine and rimonabant, there seem to be an association between bariatric surgery–induced weight loss and increased incidence of suicide. A variety of mechanisms are reported to cause the increased incidence of suicide, including psychosocial, weight, eating factors and changes in a multitude of peptidergic systems following bariatric surgery.[52] Recently, studies also showed that there is an increased risk of substance abuse, including drugs and alcohol, in patients who underwent bariatric surgery.[53] Although further evidence need to be gathered, it is safe to say careful preoperative counseling is absolutely needed, which could help to reduce this.

A population-based, self-matched, longitudinal cohort analysis, studied 8815 adults from Canada, reported that self-harm emergencies significantly increased after bariatric surgery (3.63 per 1000 patient-years) compared with that before surgery (2.33 per 1000 patient-years).[54] This was found to be particularly high in patients aged more than 35 with high risk ratio of 1.76. An important finding was that 93% of these self-harm emergency events happened in patients having mental health disorder during the 5-year period before surgery. This illustrates the importance of astute and detailed preoperative psychologic assessment.

BARIATRIC SURGERY AND OBSTRUCTIVE SLEEP APNEA

The association of obesity and OSA is well established. It is very important to assess for OSA and treat before bariatric surgery. The incidence of OSA in obese population is reported to be as high as 45%.[55,56] Obesity may worsen OSA because of fat deposition at specific tissues surrounding the upper airway, resulting in a smaller lumen and increased collapsibility of the upper airway, predisposing to apnea.

Patients with OSA are at a higher anesthetic risk, including difficulties with intubation. The perioperative complications are significantly increased in patients with OSA.[57] Hence, all patients are assessed preoperatively for OSA with clinical tools, such as STOP BANG and Epworth sleepiness scale, followed by studies like overnight oximetry and Embletta studies as appropriately. In patients with diagnosed OSA, a period of treatment with domiciliary CPAP is advocated before planning for bariatric surgery.

In Buchwald's metaanalysis, 94.5% of patients showed either resolution or improvement in OSA following RYGB.[18] A systematic review on the effect of bariatric surgery on OSA analyzed 69 studies with 13,900 patients with data on OSA. In patients undergoing RYGB, 34.9% of patients were found to have varying grades of sleep apnea and by average 79% patients showed either resolution or improvement of OSA. Similar results were observed in the gastric band (73%), SG (86%), and BPD (99%) groups.[58]

The improvement in OSA seems to be related to the weight reduction, and the improvement after bariatric surgery was observed to be sustained, resulting in the improved quality of life.

BARIATRIC SURGERY AND HYPERTENSION, DYSLIPIDEMIA, AND CARDIOVASCULAR RISK

Apart from type 2 diabetes, most weight-associated comorbidities were found to improve following bariatric surgery. All the observational studies and some RCTs have demonstrated improvement of other comorbidities, such as hypertension.

The Buchwald metaanalysis showed that hyperlipidemia improved in 70% or more of patients.[18] Hypertension was resolved in 61.7% of patients and resolved or improved in 78.5%. A metaanalysis on the effect of bariatric surgery on hypertension analyzed 31 prospective and 26 retrospective studies with a variety of bariatric procedures performed.[59] A total of 96,460 patients were evaluated; 52,151 had hypertension prior to surgery. Resolution of hypertension was reported in around 50% of patients after bariatric surgery, with 63.7% reporting improvement in blood pressure.

In another study, longer duration and severity of hypertension were reported to predict nonresolution of hypertension following bariatric surgery.[60]

The SOS study observed, with 10-year data, a clear improvement in cardiovascular risk factors, including hypertension, hypercholesterolemia, hypertriglyceridemia, and hyperuricemia, along with type 2 diabetes, in the surgical group compared with the control group. Interestingly, the rate with which the hypercholesterolemia recovered did not differ much between the surgery and control groups after either 2 or 10 years.[61]

Vogel et al. reported a prediction that, during an average follow-up of 17 months, using the Framingham risk score, the coronary heart disease (CHD) risks reduced by 39% in men and 25% in women.[62] Another study reported that the overall CHD risk represented an absolute risk reduction of 3.3% or a relative risk reduction of 52%.[63]

The overall quality of life is shown to improve after bariatric surgery. In a study on 65 patients who underwent bariatric surgery, the quality of life was assessed using SF-36 and MA-QOL-QII (Moorehead-Ardelt Quality of Life Questionnaire II) 1 year after bariatric surgery. There was a significant improvement found in all the domains of SF-36 in both the RYGB and SG groups without any difference between the groups.[64] 70.6% of all patients showed a significant improvement in the MA-QOL-QII scale as well. De Zwann et al. published a study on patients undergoing RYGB, with a mean follow-up period of 13.8 years, in which all aspects of quality of life were found to improve except for certain aspects of mental health.[65] A systematic review, reported in 2015, reviewed the data available on 9433 patients undergoing surgery and found that bariatric surgery had a significant positive impact on the quality of life.[66]

CONCLUSION

Obesity has developed into a major international health problem. There has been a massive level of health investment on the preventative aspects of obesity. Also, there is an increased realization that the condition of morbid obesity is causing a huge burden on the healthcare delivery and hence needs development of models of active therapeutic intervention. The evidence for intensive lifestyle modification shows only a moderate reduction in the weight, and there are not many pharmacologic agents available currently. Hence, currently, bariatric surgery remains the only definitive way of achieving a life-changing weight reduction for patients with obesity.

The initial evidence for the effects of bariatric surgery on weight reduction and improvement of weight-related comorbidities were largely based on retrospective, observational data and systematic reviews. However, there is an increasing number of RCT results being published, largely confirming the findings on the observational data.

It is well known that patients do well following bariatric surgery if they are well prepared by working with a multidisciplinary team of professionals. This has increased the need for specialist professionals, including bariatric physicians, surgeons, dieticians, psychologists, physiotherapists, sleep specialists, and health trainers to work collaboratively as a team.

More research and trials are being developed to understand the mechanisms of bariatric surgery, resulting in metabolic improvement of weight-related comorbidities. This, in the near future, might lead onto the development of newer nonsurgical techniques, such as novel drugs and simplified endoscopic endo-barrier techniques.

As recently as 40 years ago, the gold standard treatment for peptic ulcer was surgical with partial gastrectomy and truncal vagotomy. The development of H2 receptor blockers and proton pump inhibitors transformed that. A similar development may be in the horizon for obesity management. However, until then, we are in need of developing expertise in bariatric procedures and making it available more widely.

REFERENCES

1. CMA Recognises Obesity as Disease. Available at: https://www.cma.ca/En/Pages/cma-recognizes-obesity-as-a-disease.aspx:10.9.2015.
2. Fitzgerald K. *Obesity Is Now a Disease*; August 17, 2013. Available at: http://www.medicalnewstoday.com/articles/262226.php.
3. Bray GA. Lifestyle and pharmacological approaches to weight loss: efficacy and safety. *J Clin Endocrinol Metab.* 2008;93(11 suppl 1):S81–S88.
4. Norris SL, Zhang X, Avenell A, et al. Long-term effectiveness of lifestyle and behavioural weight loss interventions in adults with type 2 diabetes: a meta-analysis. *Am J Med.* November 15, 2004;117(10):762–774.
5. Gloy VL, Briel M, Bhatt DL, et al. Bariatric surgery versus non-surgical treatment for obesity: a systematic review and meta-analysis of randomised controlled trials. *Database Abstr Rev Eff (DARE).* 2013. Quality-assessed Reviews.
6. Sjostrom L. Review of the key results from the Swedish obese subjects (SOS) trial – a prospective controlled intervention study of bariatric surgery. *J Intern Med.* 2013;273:219–234.
7. *NICE Guidelines for Identification, Assessment and Management of Obesity.* November 2014. Available at: https://www.nice.org.uk/guidance/cg189/chapter/1-recommendations.
8. Mini Gastric Bypass : BOMSS Position Statement. Available at: http://www.bomss.org.uk/wp-content/uploads/2014/09/BOMSS-MGB-position-statement-September-20141.pdf.
9. Rutledge R. The mini-gastric bypass: experience with the first 1274 cases. *Obes Surg.* 2001;11(3):276–280.
10. Johnson WH, Fernanadez AZ, Farrell TM, et al. Surgical revision of loop ("mini") gastric bypass procedure: multicenter review of complications and conversions to Roux-en-Y gastric bypass. *Surg Obes Relat Dis.* 2007 Jan-Feb;3(1):37–41.

11. *Deleat : Gastric Banding Summary Statement.* 2011. Available at: http://bestpractice.bmj.com/best-practice/evidence/intervention/0604/0/sr-0604-i1254832461700.html#summary-statement.

12. Zak Y, Petrusa E, Gee DW. Laparoscopic Roux-en-Y gastric bypass patients have an increased lifetime risk of repeat operations when compared to laparoscopic sleeve gastrectomy patients. *Surg Endosc.* 2015;30:1833–1838.

13. Young MT, Gebhart A, Phelan MJ, Nguyen NT. Use and outcomes of laparoscopic sleeve gastrectomy vs laparoscopic gastric bypass: analysis of the American College of Surgeons NSQIP. *J Am Coll Surg.* 2015;220(5):880–885.

14. Spaniolas K, Kasten KR, Brinkley J, et al. The changing bariatric surgery landscape in the USA. *Obes Surg.* 2015;25:1544–1546.

15. Banerjee A, Ding Y, Mikami DJ, et al. The role of dumping syndrome in weight loss after gastric bypass surgery. *Surg Endosc.* 2013;27:1573.

16. Jain D. Endoscopic bypass using endobarrier devices: efficacy in treating obesity and metabolic syndrome. *J Clin Gastroenterol.* 2015;49(10):799–803.

17. Colquitt JL, Pickett K, Loveman E, Frampton GK. Surgery for weight loss in adults. *Cochrane Database Syst Rev.* 2014;(8):CD003641.

18. Buchwald H, Avidor Yoav, Braunwald Eugene, et al. Bariatric surgery, a systematic review and meta-analysis. *JAMA.* 2004;292(14):1724–1737.

19. Su-Hsin C, Stoll CRT, Song J, Esteban Varela J, Eagon CJ, Colditz GA. Bariatric surgery: an updated systematic review and meta-analysis, 2003–2012. *JAMA Surg.* March 1, 2014;149(3):275–287.

20. Maggard MA, Shugarman LR, Suttorp M, et al. Meta-analysis: surgical treatment of obesity. *Ann Intern Med.* April 5, 2005;142(7):547–559.

21. Celio AC, Wu Q, Kasten KR, et al. Comparative effectiveness of Roux-en-Y gastric bypass and sleeve gastrectomy in super obese patients. *Surg Endosc.* 2017;31:317.

22. Sjöström L, The Sahlgrenska Academy, The University of Gothenburg, Gothenburg, Sweden. Review of the key results from the Swedish Obese Subjects (SOS) trial – a prospective controlled intervention study of bariatric surgery (Review). *J Intern Med.* 2013;273:219–234.

23. Serrano OK, Tannebaum JE, Cumella L, et al. Weight loss outcomes and complications from bariatric surgery in the super super obese. *Surg Endosc.* 2016;30:2505.

24. Jérémie T, et al. Five-year outcomes of gastric bypass for super-super-obesity (BMI ≥60 kg/m²): a case matched study. *Surg Obes Relat Dis.* 2015;11(1):p32–p37.

25. Chang SH, Stoll CR, Colditz GA. Cost-effectiveness of bariatric surgery: should it be universally available? *Maturitas.* July 2011;69(3):230–238.

26. Andalib A, Elbahrawy A, Alshlwi S, et al. Diabetic ketoacidosis following bariatric surgery in patients with type 2 diabetes. *Diabetes Care.* August 2016;39(8):e121–e122.

27. Buse JB, Caprio S, Cefalu WT, et al. How do we define cure of diabetes? *Diabetes Care.* 2009;32(11):2133–2135. http://dx.doi.org/10.2337/dc09-9036.

28. Mas-Lorenzo A, Benaiges D, Flores-Le-Roux JA, et al. Impact of different criteria on type 2 diabetes remission rate after bariatric surgery. *Obes Surg.* 2014;24:1881. http://dx.doi.org/10.1007/s11695-014-1282-2.

29. Rubino F. Bariatric surgery: effects on glucose homeostasis. *Curr Opin Clin Nutr Metab Care.* July 2006;9(4):497–507.

30. Buchwald, Henry, et al. Weight and type 2 diabetes after bariatric surgery: systematic review and meta-analysis. *Am J Med.* March 2009;122(3):248–256. e5.

31. Ribaric G, Buchwald JN, McGlennon TW. Diabetes and weight in comparative studies of bariatric surgery vs conventional medical therapy: a systematic review and meta-analysis. *Obes Surg.* 2014;24(3):437–455. http://dx.doi.org/10.1007/s11695-013-1160-3.

32. Reed MA, Pories WJ, Chapman W, et al. Roux-en-Y gastric bypass corrects hyperinsulinemia implications for the remission of type 2 diabetes. *J Clin Endocrinol Metab.* August 2011;96(8):2525–2531.

33. Sjöström L, Peltonen M, Jacobson P, et al. Association of bariatric surgery with long-term remission of type 2 diabetes and with microvascular and macrovascular complications. *JAMA.* 2014;311:2297–2304.

34. Arterburn DE, Bogart A, Sherwood NE, et al. A multisite study of long-term remission and relapse of type 2 diabetes mellitus following gastric bypass. *Obes Surg.* 2013;23:93–102.

35. Purnell JQ, et al. Type 2 diabetes remission rates after laparoscopic gastric bypass and gastric banding: results of the longitudinal assessment of bariatric surgery study. *Diabetes Care.* June 2016. http://dx.doi.org/10.2337/dc15-2138. dc152138.

36. Ali A, Rhoads D, Tavakkoli A. Insulin cessation, diabetes remission after bariatric surgery in adults with insulin-treated type 2 diabetes. *Diabetes Care.* April 2015;38(4):659–664. http://dx.doi.org/10.2337/dc14-1751.

37. Dixon JB, O'Brien PE, Playfair J, et al. Adjustable gastric banding and conventional therapy for type 2 diabetes; a randomized controlled trial. *JAMA.* 2008;299(3):316–323. http://dx.doi.org/10.1001/jama.299.3.316.

38. Courcoulas AP, Goodpaster BH, Eagleton JK, et al. A randomized trial to compare surgical and medical treatments for type 2 diabetes: the triabetes study. *JAMA Surg.* 2014;149(7):707–715. http://dx.doi.org/10.1001/jamasurg.2014.467.

39. Schauer PR, Kashyap SR, Wolski K, et al. Bariatric surgery versus intensive medical therapy in obese patients with diabetes. *N Engl J Med.* April 26, 2012;2012(366):1567–1576. http://dx.doi.org/10.1056/NEJMoa1200225.

40. Schauer PR, Bhatt DL, Kirwan JP, et al. For STAMPEDE Investigators. *N Engl J Med 2014.* May 22, 2014;(370):2002–2013.

41. *STAMPEDE 5 Year Data.* April 5, 2016. Available at: http://www.ajmc.com/focus-of-the-week/0416/cleveland-clinic-5-year-data-show-glycemic-benefits-last-after-bariatric-surgery.

42. Geltrude M, Panunzi S, De Gaetano A, et al. Bariatric surgery versus conventional medical therapy for type 2 diabetes. *N Engl J Med 2012*. April 26, 2012;366:1577–1585.

43. Ikramuddin S, Korner J, Lee W, et al. Roux-en-Y gastric bypass vs intensive medical management for the control of type 2 diabetes, hypertension, and hyperlipidemia the diabetes surgery study randomized clinical trial. *JAMA*. 2013;309(21):2240–2249. http://dx.doi.org/10.1001/jama.2013.5835.

44. Still CD, Wood GC, Benotti P, et al. A probability score for preoperative prediction of type 2 diabetes remission following RYGB surgery. *Lancet Diabetes Endocrinol*. 2014;2(1):38–45. http://dx.doi.org/10.1016/S2213-8587(13)70070-6.

45. Carlsson LMS, Peltonen M, Ahlin S, et al. Bariatric surgery and prevention of type 2 diabetes in Swedish obese subjects. *N Engl J Med*. 2012;367:695–704. PMID:22913680.

46. Tang Q, Sun Z, Zhang N, et al. Cost-effectiveness of bariatric surgery for type 2 diabetes mellitus: a randomized controlled trial in China. *Med Baltim*. 2016;95(20):e3522.

47. Napolitano MA, Foster GD. Depression and obesity: implications for assessment, treatment, and research. *Clin Psychol Sci Pract*. 2008;15(1):21–27.

48. Obesity and Mental Health. Available at: http://www.noo.org.uk/uploads/doc/vid_10266_Obesity%20and%20mental%20health_FINAL_070311_MG.pdf.

49. Pratt LA. *Depression and Obesity in US*; October 2014. Available at: https://www.cdc.gov/nchs/products/databriefs/db167.htm NCHS.

50. Dawes AJ, Maggard-Gibbons M, Maher AR, et al. Mental health conditions among patients seeking and undergoing bariatric SurgeryA meta-analysis. *JAMA*. 2016;315(2):150–163.

51. Adams TD, Gress RE, Smith SC, et al. Long-term mortality after gastric bypass surgery. *N Engl J Med*. 2007;357:753–761.

52. Mitchell JE, Crosby R, de Zwaan M, et al. Possible risk factors for increased suicide following bariatric surgery. *Obes (Silver Spring, Md)*. 2013;21(4):665–672.

53. Conason A, Teixeira J, Hsu C-H, Puma L, Knafo D, Geliebter A. Substance use following bariatric weight loss surgery. *JAMA Surg*. 2013;148:145–150.

54. Bhatti JA, Nathens AB, Thiruchelvam D, Grantcharov T, Goldstein BI, Redelmeier DA. Self-harm emergencies after bariatric Surgery a population-based cohort study. *JAMA Surg*. 2016;151(3):226–232. http://dx.doi.org/10.1001/jamasurg.2015.3414.

55. Sharma SK, Kumpawat S, Banga A, Goel A. Prevalence and risk factors of obstructive sleep apnea syndrome in a population of Delhi. *India Chest*. July 2006;130(1):149–156.

56. Resta O, Foschino-Barbaro MP, Legari G, et al. Sleep-related breathing disorders, loud snoring and excessive daytime sleepiness in obese subjects. *Int J Obes Relat Metab Disord*. May 2001;25(5):669–675.

57. Shin CH, Zaremba S, Devine S. Effects of obstructive sleep apnoea risk on postoperative respiratory complications: protocol for a hospital-based registry study. *BMJ Open*. 2016;6:e008436. http://dx.doi.org/10.1136/bmjopen-2015-008436.

58. Sarkhosh K, Switzer NJ, El-Hadi M, et al. Effect of Bariatric surgery on sleep apnoea: a systematic review. *Obes Surg*. 2013;23:414. http://dx.doi.org/10.1007/s11695-012-0862-2.

59. Wilhelm SM, Young J, Kale-Pradhan PB. Effect of bariatric surgery on hypertension. *Ann Pharmacother*. 2014;48(6):674–682.

60. Flores L, Vidal J, Canivell S, Delgado S, Lacy A, Esmatjes E. *Surg Obes Relat Dis*. August 2014;10(4):661–666.

61. Sjöström L, Anna-Karin L, Peltonen M, et al. Lifestyle, diabetes, and cardiovascular risk factors 10 years after bariatric surgery. *N Engl J Med*. December 23, 2004;2004(351):2683–2693.

62. Vogel JA, Franklin BA, Zalesin KC, et al. Reduction in predicted coronary heart disease risk after substantial weight reduction after bariatric surgery. *Am J Cardiol*. January 15, 2007;99(2):222–226.

63. Kligman MD, Dexter DJ, Omer S, Park AE. Shrinking cardiovascular risk through bariatric surgery: application of Framingham risk score in gastric bypass. *Surgery*. April 2008;143(4):533–538.

64. Major P, Matłok M, Pędziwiatr M, et al. Quality of life after bariatric surgery. *Obes Surg*. 2015;25(9):1703–1710. http://dx.doi.org/10.1007/s11695-015-1601-2.

65. De Zwaan M, Lancaster KL, Mitchell JE, et al. Health-related quality of life in morbidly obese patients: effect of gastric bypass surgery. *Obes Surg*. December 2002;12(6):773–780.

66. Lindekilde N, Gladstone BP, Lübeck M, et al. The impact of bariatric surgery on quality of life: a systematic review and meta-analysis. *Obes Rev*. 2015;16:639–651. http://dx.doi.org/10.1ss111/obr.12294.

CHAPTER 29

Psychological Management Before and After Weight Loss Surgery

LYNNE JOHNSTON, BA, MSC, PHD, CBT DIPLOMA, DCLIN PSYCH, AFBPSS •
CHARLOTTE HILTON, BSC, PHD •
CLAIRE LANE, BA, PHD, DIPPSYCH, DCLIN PSYCH

In this chapter, we offer a psychological perspective on obesity. We begin with a discussion of the need to understand obesity in terms of an individualized conceptualization. We then offer a brief review of the literature examining psychological factors and weight loss surgery (WLS). Specifically, we explore the psychological predictors of outcomes following WLS, next we examine the psychological status in severely obese patients seeking weight loss surgery, and then we discuss what psychological factors are contraindications for WLS. Our chapter then introduces a discussion of the role of practitioner psychologists within obesity services, and demonstrates how psychologists contribute to patient care via a worked case conceptualization (formulation). Specifically, we discuss how psychologically informed treatments can be integrated from a case formulation and how this can help improve outcomes for WLS patients. This chapter ends with an overview and discussion of a suggested treatment plan that addresses co-maintaining cycles of behavioral avoidance and lifestyle dysregulation, internal rumination (overthinking), and binge eating behaviors.

DECONSTRUCTING OBESITY

In the United Kingdom, the current National Institute for Health and Care Excellence (NICE) guidance for obesity[1] states that WLS is a suitable treatment option for patients with a body mass index (BMI) of >40 (or >35 with significant comorbidities). In line with a medical model approach, treatment is suggested in terms of a solution to the obesity itself, rather than addressing the factors that have resulted in obesity. The "solution" is highly variable in terms of available provision in the United Kingdom.[2,3] The down side to a medical model approach is that simply classifying an individual as obese, and providing generic treatments based on diet and activity alone, fails to address the underlying cause(s) of an individual's obesity. If we view all obese patients as one homogenous group, then we risk adopting a "one-size-fits-all" approach to treatment. It makes more conceptual and pragmatic sense to understand the causes (and associated comorbidities) as a multifaceted biopsychosocial construct.[4,5] For patients who find themselves at the end point of tiered weight management services (e.g., WLS patients), generic, prescribed, lifestyle interventions are (usually) insufficient. The causes of obesity may be better understood by adopting a nonmedicalized, formulation-based approach to treatment.[6]

In practice, a common pervasive problem for WLS patients is that the length of their weight management journey may have exacerbated their underlying difficulties. As an individual's level of obesity rises, their chance of developing comorbid long-term psychiatric conditions (e.g., major depressive disorder [MDD], social anxiety) also increases (see Chapters 16–18). For patients who have struggled to manage their weight for many years without success, previous maladaptive attempts at managing weight may have inadvertently reinforced the development, and maintenance, of disordered eating patterns, as well as ongoing mood difficulties. Clinically, we have observed, time and again, the negative reinforcing and *maintaining* impact of many *nonsurgical measures* (e.g., failed commercial diets, fad diets, diet pills). Sadly, this has a deep and very damaging impact on patients' negative self-beliefs, underlying self-judgments of worthlessness, and a dispositional sense of failure and shame. Tragically, for those exposed to *weight cycling*[7] from a very young age (5–11 years) via inappropriate diet regimes, this developed a sense of hopelessness (learned helplessness) and has consistently been shown to be associated with depression and low self-worth.[8–11]

As clinical psychologists working with WLS patients, we believe it is essential to work *with* a person to conceptualize their obesity within a broader framework of distal and proximal causal mechanisms, as well as factors that maintain their obesity. Importantly, we aim to identify protective or resilience factors (e.g., social support networks, employment) to maximize a strength-based approach. An inherent focus on a deficit-based (medical model) approach runs the risk of becoming a *self-fulfilling prophecy*. Rather than something that is "done to" a patient, a client-centered, strength-based approach to treatment considers that the quality of the patient-practitioner interpersonal processes, and the clinician's ability to build hope and optimism with the patient impacts directly on treatment outcomes.[12] Further information regarding *how* to engage patients in a client-centered, strength-based approach is discussed in Chapter 19.

LITERATURE REVIEW OF PSYCHOLOGICAL FACTORS AND WEIGHT LOSS SURGERY

Although WLS can be successful,[13] the surgery itself is not a panacea. Patients undertaking WLS still need to make, and crucially *maintain*, changes to their lifestyle behaviors (e.g., eating, drinking, activity, sleep).[14] Clinically, the patients who appear to find this *most* problematic are those with more severe underlying psychological difficulties that remain unidentified, untreated, or poorly managed (e.g., people who use food, alcohol, or other substances to regulate their emotions; those who have more severe mental health difficulties and emotional disturbances; those who are fixated on body image or evaluate their self-worth on their body size/weight; and those with chronic low self-worth). We now consider what the emerging literature tells us about those who may require additional psychological screening and support prior to WLS, as well as those for whom WLS may be a contraindication or a serious risk.

Psychological Predictors of Outcomes Following Weight Loss Surgery

Kewin and Boyle[15] reviewed the psychological predictors of outcomes following WLS and report that the academic literature is contradictory and nonconclusive. They explained this in terms of a self-selecting bias (i.e., the exclusion of people with more severe psychological difficulties leads to psychologically homogenous and healthier samples). Nevertheless, disordered eating *was* highlighted as a "negative predictor of weight loss".[15(p42)] Those who used food to "emotionally regulate" prior to surgery experienced "suboptimal" weight loss postoperatively. Sheets[16] identified empirical support for postoperative binge eating, uncontrolled eating/grazing, and the presence of a depressive disorder as negative predictors of weight loss outcomes. Unresolved emotional eating may also impact poorly on surgery outcomes.[17] Fourteen of fifteen studies examining

the association of binge eating disorder (BED) and loss of control eating on weight outcomes after surgery identified that both are associated with less weight loss and/or more weight regain post-WLS.[18] The authors have urged clinicians to identify patients who may have BED so that appropriate pre- and postoperative tailored interventions can be provided.

Formal "diagnosis" of BED as an eating disorder per se did not emerge until the most recent version of the *Diagnostic and Statistical Manual of Mental Disorders*.[19] Consequently, until 2013, BED is likely to have been underdiagnosed. Evidence is emerging to support this. One study[20] that retrospectively reassessed WLS candidates (using *DSM-V* criteria) for BED has found significantly ($P < 0.001$) more met the diagnostic threshold. This is still likely to be an underestimate because we know that clinically we are often the first person that a patient discloses their binge eating to. Typically, this follows many lonely years of silent self-berating—a ruminative process that has perpetuated their sense of shame, guilt, and internalized anger. Underreporting is likely to be exacerbated further if patients are told that WLS is their "last chance" and that WLS may not be available if an eating disorder is disclosed.

Psychological Status in Severely Obese Patients Seeking Weight Loss Surgery

The inclusion criteria for consideration of WLS[1] dictate that patients are at the higher end of the BMI spectrum (e.g., we routinely work with patients with a BMI between 40 and 80). People with a higher BMI are significantly *more* likely to present with psychiatric comorbidities,[21–25] with prevalence rates of BED (although not *usually* formally diagnosed at referral), as a common comorbidity of obesity, reported from 2% to 50%.[23,24,26–31] A key issue to unpack is the extent to which prior psychiatric condition(s) have had a *causal* impact/influence on the development and maintenance of an individual's obesity versus the extent to which an individual's obesity has *caused* and maintained their psychiatric comorbidities, and as such how this might be treated[32] (e.g., see Clinical Case Study section).

Common comorbid mental health difficulties tend to be depression, anxiety, and substance misuse difficulties.[15,23,24] The relationship between obesity and MDD is well documented. For example, one metaanalysis[33] found a significant association between both conditions (particularly in women). A second metaanalysis demonstrated a bidirectional association: "obese persons had a 55% increased risk of developing depression [and] depressed persons had a 58% increased risk of becoming obese".[34(p225)] Key moderators were *levels of obesity* (higher BMI, higher levels of obesity) and *gender* (stronger link in females). A summary of factors that impact on the bidirectional relationship between obesity and MDD is discussed in more depth elsewhere.[35] Chapter 16 of this book provides an updated review of this literature.

Clinically, it is essential to extricate this complex relationship. For some people treating their obesity via WLS *may* have a positive impact on their low mood *if* their low mood was being maintained by their obesity. However, for those with a preexisting MDD, or other associated psychiatric diagnosis (e.g., Post Traumatic Stress Disorder (PTSD)), it would be extremely important to treat the underlying reasons for their psychological disorder first, or instead of the WLS. The risk of *not* treating the psychological disorder first is that the WLS may simply be removing one coping strategy (food/drinks), which then leaves the person seeking an alternative coping strategy (e.g., other substances), or without a coping strategy, for the underlying issues that remain untreated (e.g., trauma, abuse, loss issues). Emerging evidence, from interviews with patients who have undergone WLS, suggests that, for some, it was perceived as the "wrong journey."[36] Interviews with people 5 years post-WLS have revealed that experiencing weight gain is associated with emotional stress, shame, and self-contempt.[37] A recent assessment of the use of therapeutic patient education for WLS candidates identified that a short duration of obesity, a limited number of past diets, and low levels of anxiety/depression were factors that predicted surgery success.[38] Yet, the clinical reality is that patients referred for presurgery assessment often present with quite the opposite characteristics (e.g., adjustment disorders, depression, and/or personality disorders[39]; emotional eating; history of abuse).[40] These factors have all been associated with less successful post-surgery outcomes. Higher preoperative depression and binge eating also predict poorer improvement in physical, psychosocial, and sexual quality of life (QoL) and comfort with food.[41] These presentations often reflect the complexity of obesity that builds a convincing argument of the necessity to fully assess and treat underlying psychological issues before (or instead of) WLS.

For some patients treating a mood disorder with initial behavioral activation (BA), work[42] can impact positively on mood and lifestyle patterns (e.g., sleep, activity, diet) and can have a beneficial impact on weight. For others (e.g., loss or trauma history) it is important to address the underlying issues that are often *the* causal factor(s) in their MDD (and indirectly obesity via behavioral avoidance or use of food to emotionally regulate). This is not simply a *chicken and egg* logic argument. Clinically, the psychological driver for *both* the mood disorder and obesity is the untreated trauma/

loss. For example, greater levels of sudden weight gain have been observed in patients seeking bariatric surgery who have experienced childhood parental death or separation.[43] The importance of addressing these underlying psychological mechanisms, such that programs that specifically target the prevention of obesity for individuals who have experienced multiple losses, has been recommended.[44] This is where the use of a formulation-based approach is absolutely essential because it helps both the practitioner and client to disentangle the complex array of factors that have caused and maintained the person's comorbid difficulties. The formulation can then be used to outline the plan for treatment within a team (see Clinical Case Study below).

What Psychological Factors Are Contraindications for Weight Loss Surgery?

Psychological factors that have been highlighted as potential contraindications for WLS include active or recent substance misuse, addictive behaviors (including "food addiction"), past or current eating disorder (particularly BED), active or recent depression, and a history of trauma/abuse.[45,46] However, published studies suffer from small sample sizes, high attrition rates, and follow-up periods of 12 months or less (i.e., before the end of the "honeymoon period" following WLS).[47] Consequently, this makes it difficult to draw concrete conclusions regarding accepted contraindications. Kerwin and Boyle[15] also concluded that there was a lack of consensus and pointed to limited evidence regarding those *diagnosed* with a personality disorder and a history of trauma (e.g., weight being "used" as a "protective buffer" to avoid intimacy). They suggest that the most common contraindications identified include "active substance abuse; uncontrolled major mental illness; severe learning difficulties; or having a clear history of non-compliance with medical advice".[15(p44)] Arguably, it makes sense to examine the severity and existing management of a psychological problem, to assess if the extent to which any psychological difficulty is likely to impact the individual's ability to make and adhere to behavioral changes postsurgery, rather than simply looking for the presence or absence of particular diagnostic labels.

Stevens et al.[48] note that there are no agreed recommendations to guide clinicians when considering WLS for patients with diagnosed mental health disorders. They emphasize that using surgery to "treat" an underlying psychiatric disorder poses risk and that any patients receiving treatment within a secondary care mental health service within the previous 12 months should be offered a full assessment by a mental health professional prior to *any* decision-making regarding

WLS (not to exclude patients, but rather to optimize mental health management and assist with preparation for WLS). They suggest that the following areas should be included in the assessment:

- Lifetime history of weight gain, including precipitating events
- History of weight loss attempts
- Expectations from surgery
- Current eating habits and patterns
- Drug and alcohol use
- Past physical activity
- Past psychiatric history
- Current social circumstances
- Screening for current mental disorder, including depression and eating disorders
- Assessment of capacity.[48(p421)]

Clinically, it is essential that these assessments are conducted in a patient-centered way. Patients want to *feel* understood and to be helped to understand their difficulties via a collaborative formulation process. We would refer the reader to Chapter 19, which describes how best to engage with, and involve, patients in the formulation process and in their own treatment planning. When patients feel judged and blamed, they are much less likely to provide an accurate, authentic account to those that they view as authoritarian figures. An individual must understand the relative risks and benefits of surgery, have capacity to fully understand the processes involved, and be realistic about WLS outcome expectations.[48] For example, patients may be told to expect a 60%–70% loss of their *excess* weight initially but then to expect an approximate percentage of weight regain within 2 years. Clinically, it is not unusual for patients to hold on to beliefs that they will lose and maintain 60/70% of their *total* body weight. Patients may hear what they want to hear rather than the clinical reality. This highlights the importance of the way in which the information is exchanged with clients (see Chapter 19).

A traffic light framework has been suggested as a useful way to highlight psychological risks for WLS and to aid multidisciplinary team (MDT) discussions regarding suitability.[48] Unstable psychosis, active substance misuse, severe learning difficulty, dementia, severe personality disorder, self-harm within the last 12 months, active bulimia nervosa, and current nonadherence to treatment may suggest unsuitability for WLS.[48] Furthermore, the following may warrant more detailed MDT team discussions: severe (but stable in the last 12 months) mental illnesses, history of substance misuse (including an eating disorder), mild learning difficulties, poor motivation/nonadherence or poor adherence/inadequate insight into eating behaviors, and unrealistic expectations.[48]

Clearly, some patients do regain all of their weight lost.[49,50] Yet, published evidence is still somewhat limited regarding the psychological characteristics of these patients and further research is urgently required to fully explicate who these patients are and, crucially, why they are regaining all the weight lost. Initial studies have suggested that approximately 20%–30% of patients undergoing bariatric surgery did not achieve successful weight outcomes.[50,51] Systematic psychological investigation is extremely challenging because these patients are likely to feel disenfranchised ("I've failed again") and lacking in hope, leading to increased risk of depression.

Clinically, on the occasions when these patients have been referred to psychology services (postsurgery), we have found them to be suffering from *severe* levels of depression. If these patients have not been referred for a full psychological assessment and formulation *before* surgery, it may be difficult to establish the extent to which their postsurgery levels of depression were present and/or if their depression has been triggered by factors associated with the surgery or adjustment difficulties postsurgery. Arguably, these patients are likely to be the patients who we know least about because they are less likely to attend follow-up appointments postsurgery (and to respond to research requests) if they have not succeeded in their anticipated weight loss targets. For example, in a study exploring post–bariatric surgery weight regain, all 59 participants reported that they stopped treatment with the MDT in the first year after the operation.[49] Ironically it is these individuals that researchers need to be speaking with via future in-depth qualitative research to more fully understand the patient experience of a "failed WLS journey."

In sum, "checklist" approaches[48] tend to be driven by a medical approach (i.e., psychiatric diagnoses), rather than a psychological[15] formulation-based approach. The disadvantage of a diagnostic approach is that we do not fully understand *how* and *why* the patients are eating in the way that they do, what kinds of changes may be needed to ensure surgery works for the patient, how to help them get to the point where they are ready to make these changes, and which factors help mitigate some of the potentially problematic factors. Without this information, it is difficult to determine how surgery might be helpful and how best to work *with* the patient to ensure that surgery is successful *in the long term*. There is often much confusion among health professionals regarding what psychologists do; where they fit in to the process of patient care before, during, and after WLS; and how the psychologist's input differs to that of a psychiatrist. We hope to further clarify these issues in the following section.

THE ROLE OF PSYCHOLOGISTS IN MULTIDISCIPLINARY TEAMS

Psychologists are trained in understanding *how* and *why* individual people act in particular ways at particular times. If things were genuinely as simple as "calories in-calories out," then few people would struggle with obesity. Typically, health professionals understand the role of psychologists in teams to be delivering treatments for psychological problems or assessments to establish suitability for WLS. Although this forms part of the psychologists' role, their remit is far wider than this. Psychologists can foster and support psychological thinking and ways of working within teams. This includes consulting on cases, providing input to care and treatment plans, and supporting nonpsychologist colleagues to integrate psychological aspects of care into patients' treatment plans via indirect working. Many patients do not need direct psychological therapy for a particular issue (or may struggle to engage with this). Understanding a patient's needs from a psychological perspective enables treatment planning to be tailored in such a way that it directly targets the complex interaction of specific variables that have led the individual to gain weight over time and, as such, increases the likelihood of a successful treatment outcome.

Patients treated in WLS settings usually present with a whole host of comorbid "symptoms," which may include observable medical diagnoses (e.g., hypothyroidism, Cushing's syndrome, polycystic ovary syndrome, depression, diabetes, sleep apnea, metabolic syndrome, stroke, gallbladder disease, respiratory problems, osteoarthritis, cancers, cardiovascular disease, chronic pain).[52] Yet, there are also the less observable psychological "symptoms," such as the dysregulation of various lifestyle behaviors (e.g., eating, activity, sleep), beliefs about low self-worth, reduced ability to plan, avoidant coping styles, lack of emotional processing, intolerance of uncertainty, and all-or-nothing thinking/behaviors. These observable and nonobservable "symptoms" are linked because they are the result of multiple, deeper, underlying causes that involve a complex mix of biologic, psychological and social factors. If these factors are not identified (assessed), understood (formulated), and addressed (treatment), then they are likely to persist beyond the surgical procedure and may negatively impact the outcome of WLS over the longer term.

Psychologists help teams to make sense of this via the process of formulation,[53,54] rather than diagnosis. Clearly the factors outlined above are complex, and they can feel overwhelming. Formulation seeks to highlight the interaction between the biological, psychological and social factors in a clear, digestible way, providing a map for treatment planning that addresses the different aspects of the patient's presentation. Formulations can be created with the patient directly or within a team. It is essential that formulations are conducted in a patient-centered, collaborative manner to help the patient and practitioner(s) to work within a strong/safe alliance. Both parties need to "own" the formulation process. When both parties see *how* and *why* the patient's complex comorbid "symptoms" are linked, this helps them to see things as less overwhelming and usually identifies a clear *path through the fog*. Having a shared, working formulation in a team guides individual team members to address issues underlying the physical presentation(s) in a consistent way, as well as with a clear rationale. Diagnosis is a process that results in a "yes/no" answer, whereas formulation is more about exploring the "how" and "why" to find a workable plan.

There are a number of different formulation frameworks that a psychologist may use. One that we have found helpful within a physical healthcare context is known as the "five P's" formulation.[55-57] This involves understanding the patient's Presenting difficulty in relation to their Past life history (i.e., Pre-disposing factors), the biopsychosocial factors that Precipitated the difficulty (triggering events), the factors that Perpetuate (or maintain) it, as well as the factors that Protect the patient from further deterioration. In the following section, we use a case example to demonstrate how such a formulation might be used to develop the treatment Plan (sometimes referred to as a sixth P). We have provided other examples of formulations within a weight management context elsewhere.[56-58]

CASE STUDY: JANET
Presenting Difficulty

We receive a referral from Janet's primary care physician. Janet is a 47-year-old female with a BMI of 56.7. Her physician is concerned about the impact of her weight on her diabetes and chronic lower back pain. She is currently taking medication for insulin resistance, high cholesterol, high blood pressure, and pain. Janet states that she cannot lose weight. Her weight has stayed within a 3-kg range for over 12 months. She has lost weight previously through various diet and exercise regimes but has never maintained these losses; she is now at her heaviest. Diet pills worked in the past, but she regained all her weight (and more) when she could no longer access them (they were likely to have been amphetamine based; explaining her reported lack of appetite and boundless energy). Janet is now seeking WLS as she feels it is her only hope. She believes that if her stomach is physically smaller, it will be impossible for her to overeat. She longs to be a size 12, but even a size 16 is "normal enough not to stand out and much better than being a size 32."

So What?

Janet has a history of weight cycling[7] and may have a tendency toward "all-or-nothing" patterns in relation to diet and activity.[59,60] Her self-efficacy (a person's belief in his/her ability to succeed)[61] is likely to be low, and she may have an external locus of control (a belief that weight is influenced by factors beyond her own personal control)[62] in relation to making sustainable changes. In essence, her levels of self-determination are likely to be low.[63]

Past History

Janet's mother passed away from breast cancer when she was five. Thereafter, her primary caregiver was her father. He never really talked about feelings: "he couldn't handle seeing me upset and he'd fall to pieces." Janet described herself as "broken" following her mother's death. Nobody seemed to want to talk about it, leading her to believe that she was "making too big a deal out of it." When her father saw her upset, he tried to soothe Janet's grief by "taking her mind off it"; she was usually given something "nice to eat" to make her feel better (e.g., chocolate, ice cream, crisps, or cake), and sometimes they would "watch something good on TV together." Janet learned that her dad became distressed when she was upset, which made her feel guilty. She learned to keep her emotions private and would hide her distress with humor. She learned to absorb herself in the TV to take her mind off feeling sad. She ate biscuits, chocolate, and crisps rapidly (in her bedroom) to give her *mood a boost* and hide her sadness.

So What?

Janet has learned that it is unacceptable to express sadness. Her ability to regulate her emotions was dependent on distraction from her feelings, rather than working through them. Responding to a child's emotional needs helps them to process the trauma of grief and loss,[64] as well as creating an opportunity to build emotional self-regulation skills.[65] Dopamine will

likely have been released by overeating, giving Janet a mood boost by activating the brain functions associated with reward and pleasure. Over the long term, this may have led to Janet being reliant on food to regulate her emotions.[66] Sedentary, mentally absorbing activity and overeating certain foods are now associated with a calming, soothing feeling. If Janet is given advice to drastically reduce her food intake, sedentary behavior, and certain food choices, this will leave her with no capacity to be able to manage difficult emotions. Janet associates sadness with shame: something that must not be seen by others. Similarly, her overeating appears to be associated with shame as it is an indicator of sadness. As such, certain food choices and eating need to be hidden, and not talked about, potentially presenting challenges in conversations about managing weight.

Precipitating Factors

Some key life events seem to have triggered habits that contribute to her weight management difficulties.

Bullying

Janet started school just after her mother died. At first, she enjoyed it. However, by age 7, she hated it. Janet had started to gain weight, and some children would tease her and exclude her from games. She pretended she did not care and would absorb herself in her school work to block them out (she cried in private most days). She kept a "stash" of sweet, salty, and stodgy foods under her bed and ate large quantities of these foods in front of the TV in her room, hiding them when she heard dad come home. She did not tell dad about the bullying; she did not want to upset him. She believed that the feelings of others were more important than her own; she felt guilty for feeling so upset.

Food Shaming

Aged 8, Janet was put on her first diet by the school nurse, who advised the dinner ladies not to allow her to eat puddings because she was "too fat." Janet felt deprived and singled out. People would berate her for eating, saying this was why she was so fat. She became increasingly ashamed of her eating and body size. She ate little of her school dinner and then ate as much as she wanted in the privacy of her bedroom. At secondary school, Janet chose to go home at lunchtimes. If others did not see her eat, maybe they would not think she was such a bad person.

Body Shaming and Weight Cycling

Aged 13, Janet began to read teenage magazines and found out ways to lose weight. She desperately wanted (and still does) to look like those beautiful women in the magazines. She was successful with the diets, but struggled to maintain any loss. She often felt hungry and saw this as her fault. Janet's weight began fluctuating. No matter how much weight she lost, her peers still bullied her. She believed she just needed to be slimmer. Every New Year she would promise herself that she would starve to get that perfect body, but was unsuccessful. During physical education (PE) at school, Janet was always the last to be picked; she was "too fat to be fit." When showering afterward, her peers would make fun of her size and would hide her towel and/or her clothes on a regular basis. Janet would try to avoid PE lessons if she could.

Loss

Janet saw the most significant weight gain (30 kg) in the 12 months after her father died from cancer when she was in her mid-20s. She tried to "carry on as usual" despite feeling devastated. She did not want to "infect" others with her sadness. She would binge (privately) on comfort foods, away from "their judging eyes" and "whispered ridicule." She would watch endless TV Box Sets (in bed) to block her pain until she was exhausted enough to fall asleep.

So What?

Here are the building blocks that develop the beliefs and habits that set the course for Janet's weight management difficulties. She has made an association between abuse and rejection (e.g., peers, health professionals, media) and her body/weight.[67] Her self-worth is based strongly on her food choices, weight, and shape. She has developed a sense of "good foods," "bad foods," and strict dietary rules, reinforced by weight loss following dieting. As such, she has developed "all-or-nothing" patterns in relation to food and eating. Her inability to maintain weight loss has reduced her self-efficacy, making it hard to believe she can achieve successes; let alone have *any* self-worth. Self-determination theory,[68] one model of motivation, suggests that three basic psychological needs must be satisfied to foster positive heath behaviors: competence (ability to master the task and have control over it); autonomy (to have freedom to make choices based on the person's own needs); and relatedness (a desire to have connection with others). Janet's description suggests that she does not feel competent, struggles to recognize and prioritize her own needs, and has had difficult experiences with others that make her want to avoid rather than connect. This impacts on her ability to make/sustain changes. Finally, Janet seems to regulate her emotions

by avoidance. She copes by escaping from her emotions (e.g., absorbing herself in the TV; soothing herself with food), rather than working through her difficulties. As a consequence, many issues will go unresolved. She gradually starts to avoid others, fearful of the judgments they make, creating further isolation and increasing her anxiety regarding social contact. This lowers her confidence, self-worth, and self-efficacy, which in turn contributes to an inability to resist emotional cues to eating.[69]

Perpetuating Factors

Several factors maintain Janet's weight management difficulties.

Weight Cycling

Janet's weight fluctuated from the age of 13. She is aspiring to a potentially unrealistic body type and associates this ideal with being confident, popular, likeable, and loveable. She feels unable to adopt these traits until she has achieved an ideal body. This has reinforced a sense of failure in relation to maintaining changes and a belief that she has to resort to extremes to achieve her goal. She adopts an *all-or-nothing* approach to diet and exercise—she is either "on it" and "succeeding" or "off it" and "worthless." Over the long term, her weight cycling may have increased her risk for cardiovascular disease and long-term weight gain.[70]

Body Image

Janet has developed a hatred for her body (maintained by verbal abuse, media images of "perfect" bodies, and messages about the burden on society of being overweight). Janet believes she is not worthy of being liked by others until she achieves her ideal body. This impacts her mood. Janet has learned to avoid social contact and building relationships with others for fear of judgment and rejection. She desperately craves closeness, yet fears it greatly. This leaves her feeling lonely and depressed.

Avoidant Emotional Coping

When low in mood/lonely, Janet attempts to soothe herself by overeating foods that boost her mood and block her distress. This helps her manage daily stressors. She will often go to bed with large quantities of food, watching films, or surfing the net until she falls asleep (the TV is on in the background).

Low Self-worth

Janet does not believe that she is truly likeable/lovable due to her weight/shape. She derives gratification from helping and pleasing others. She does not view her own physical and emotional needs as a priority. Her job, as a carer for people with learning disabilities, enables her to have social contact in a safe way, protected by her "professional role." However, this is likely to be detrimental to her weight, as she is likely to rely on external appraisals. She is likely to prioritize what others need from her, rather than caring for herself (leading her to abandon any plans or behavior changes). Her busy job often leads to irregular eating and grabbing food "on the go." She arrives home exhausted and has a tendency to go straight to bed with a takeaway in front of the TV. She follows this with her favorite comfort foods (chocolate, crisps, and ice cream) to help her relax.

Low Self-efficacy

Janet feels she has failed. Her beliefs about body image and low self-worth have been further reinforced by health professionals repeatedly providing vouchers to attend slimming clubs to "solve the problem," leading to further experiences of failure. Janet has had the experience of short-term success via medical means (diet pills), reinforcing the belief that she is unable to manage her weight. She dreads going to the primary care physician because she fears she will be "spoken down to" and be "blamed" for her weight/health problems: "Even if I went in with a broken eyelash they would tell me it's due to my weight." Her strategy for coping is to "switch off" when she is being "told off," often missing valuable information that medical staff are trying to provide. She rarely asks any questions because "it will just prolong the lecture." She "rewards" herself with a treat when she "escapes" from the consultation.

Physical Health Problems

Janet has a number of physical health conditions that leave her feeling depressed and hopeless. These include lower back pain, hypertension, hyperlipidemia, and type 2 diabetes. She is fearful for her future. It is not so much the early death but rather the poor QoL with long-term conditions that she may have to endure. She hates the thought of a carer having to take care of her personal hygiene as she has witnessed some poor practice firsthand. Janet's back problem also impacts the amount of physical activity she can engage in. Just walking from the car is becoming increasingly difficult, and she is starting to worry that she may eventually lose her job because of her own physical decline.

Sleep Problems

Janet struggles to sleep at night due to her back pain and having to get up to pass urine frequently. She is undergoing tests for sleep apnea. Janet has made her bed her place of comfort, where she engages in activities (eating, playing on her phone, watching TV) to distract herself away from her mood. Having the TV on all night helps her to distract herself from her loneliness. These activities are not conducive to a good night's sleep, but Janet is unaware of the link between sleep problems and weight gain/diabetes. She heard the nurse say "weight" and then "switched off." She has therefore not "heard" any of the information regarding the role of leptin and ghrelin in those who are experiencing less than 6 h of quality sleep per night.[71,72]

So What?

Janet's experience with dieting has led to a pathologic relationship with food and has led her to deal with this in an "all-or-nothing way." She continues to engage in dieting behaviors, despite these clearly not working for her in the long term. She relies on the scales and perception of her body as an indication of progress. She does not see progress; all she notices is failure. Not prioritizing her needs impacts on the regularity of her eating, her food choices, and her tiredness. Many of her hunger/satiety cues are driven by her need to soothe herself rather than by physical cues. With such low self-efficacy in relation to managing weight, it is hard for Janet to begin to initiate changes or take onboard help (particularly if she feels she is being judged). Her physical problems and mood also present barriers to change.

Protective Factors

Janet is currently maintaining her job, despite her health threatening this. Caring for others really boosts Janet's sense of self-worth and helps her to be a little active every day. It helps her mood as she is engaged in focused, purposeful activity. Janet has lived through traumatic life events and has managed to carry on despite the early loss of her parents and the bullying at school. This shows a lot of personal resolve. She is dedicated and does not give up easily when something is important to her, as demonstrated by her repeated attempts to lose weight. She is a kind person, who is keen to help others, which enables her to connect and value herself to some extent (albeit through pleasing or helping others).

The initial descriptive formulation is summarized in Fig. 29.1. This is typically what a formulation would look like when produced either with a patient or within a team. It summarizes the relevant information in one schematic and starts to help the patient/team to understand the key factors that have caused, and are maintaining, the patient's weight management difficulties. The next step is to work with the patient/team to clarify

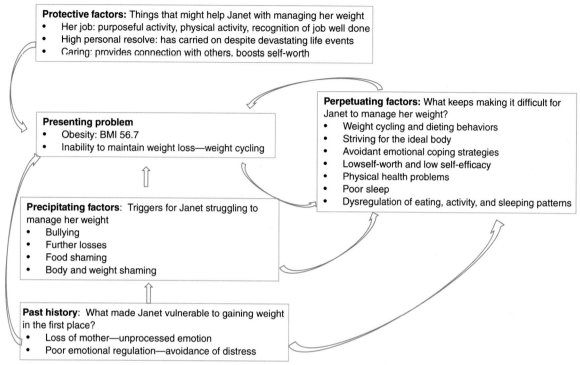

FIG. 29.1 Initial five P's formulation for Janet.

how the formulation can lead to the specific treatment plan. When patients understand their difficulties in this way, they tend to feel less overwhelmed and are more likely to engage with the treatment plan *because* they have been actively engaged in the development process (see Chapter 19 for more discussion of ways in which patient engagement can be maximized).

TREATMENT PLANNING

Fig. 29.2 provides an overview of our example treatment plan for Janet. The first layer of our pyramid, and as such the first phase of treatment, involves conducting psychological work to help Janet process her underlying trauma/loss. This factor is underlying all the others as it is driving the strategies and behaviors that are leading Janet to struggle with managing her weight. Failing to address the emotional processing work before helping her to make changes, or indeed Janet having WLS, means that she is vulnerable to further failure, even after surgery. Failure to process the grief and trauma and continued avoidance of emotional distress will likely make any new emotional management strategies difficult to engage with, as well as any lifestyle management changes (i.e., sleep, activity, dietary patterns).

This first phase of treatment is akin to the foundations of a building, failing to get this right prior to building a (therapeutic) structure on it is likely to lead to eventual collapse. Therapeutic emotional processing work is a *fundamental* component of Janet's journey toward managing her weight and having WLS.

Following the foundational work, in Phase II, we would introduce a more specific treatment model (see Fig. 29.3) to focus on the comaintaining cycles that are perpetuating Janet's comorbid symptoms. This model was developed to specifically treat patients (like Janet) with comorbid depression, social anxiety, and disordered eating (either binge eating and/or bulimia). Fig. 29.3 addresses the comaintaining factors by combining key elements of cognitive and behavioral treatment models for depression,[73] social anxiety,[74] and BED.[59,*] In cases, such as Janet, the limitation with these existing treatment models is that they address each "diagnosis" in isolation. The clinical reality is that we rarely (if ever) receive a referral for a patient with a single diagnosis. This makes it difficult to apply one standard Cognitive

---

* The reader is referred to the original treatment models and associated self-help workbooks for a full discussion and explanation of each treatment.

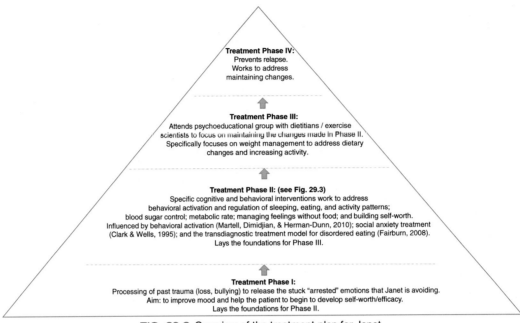

FIG. 29.2 Overview of the treatment plan for Janet.

Behavioral Therapy (CBT) treatment model. We have found that the treatment model outlined in Fig. 29.3 works extremely well with patients like Janet. The process of talking through this model to help patients formulate (understand) the clear links between their emotions, physical symptoms, behaviors, and cognitions is highly therapeutic. Essentially, Fig. 29.3 helps patients/team members to understand the comaintaining negative impact of three cycles—Behavioral Avoidance; Overthinking (Rumination); and Binge Eating; and crucially why all three cycles have a reinforcing impact on an individual's long standing beliefs about their worth.

Fig. 29.3 shows that behavioral avoidance and associated dysregulation (sleep, eating, and activity) typically acts as a vicious cycle leading to lower mood and confidence, as well as increased levels of social anxiety. There has been an increased interest in BA approaches over the last 20 years, including complex and comorbid physical health conditions.[42] Given the high levels of comorbidity between obesity and depression,[22] evidence for the use of BA, to treat both conditions, is emerging.[22,75] The thinking behind this is that in depressed patients, obesity could be a consequence of the use of food to emotionally regulate, as well as behavioral avoidance (i.e., decreased physical activity and increased sedentary behavioral patterns).[76] The advantages of using a BA intervention with patients such as Janet are that it is a relatively simple, parsimonious intervention for

severely depressed patients, and there is an increasing evidence base for its use generally and with comorbid obese and depressed women specifically.

Working through Fig. 29.3 with patients who can help them to conceptualize how they use avoidance strategies (e.g., staying in bed; lack of social interaction; use of substances such as food, alcohol, or drugs) as a "coping strategy" for their low mood/anxiety is a short-term palliative response that *maintains* and/or exacerbates their difficulties in the longer term. The vicious cycle can be represented as *digging to get out of a hole*.[77] Continuing to dig (i.e., making the problem worse) is actually acting as a trigger for their BED, usually because of dysregulation of eating (usually long gaps) and/or associated emotional changes (low mood/heightened anxiety). In some instances the trigger may simply be due to a context or situation. Clinically, we have found physiological (hunger) triggers, due to long gaps, to be the main cause. This is consistent with Fairburn[59,60] who points out that triggers for BED are particularly likely to happen to people (like Janet) who already have an overevaluation of their weight/shape, which has been reinforced by continued (and often extreme) diets, an all-or-nothing approach to dieting/exercise behaviors, and a long history of weight cycling. These behaviors activate the diet-binge cycle, and Fairburn[59,60] explains that this is why developing a collaborative formulation to help patients fully understand why they binge is such

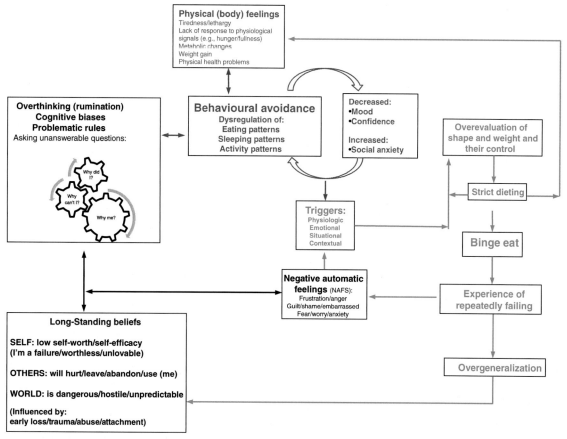

FIG. 29.3 Enhanced Cognitive Behavioral Therapy (CBT-E) treatment model for comorbid depression and binge eating disorder. (Data from references Fairburn C. Cognitive Behaviour Therapy and Eating Disorders. Chichester: Guilford Press; 2008, Martell CR, Dimidjian S, Herman-Dunn R. Behavioral Activation for Depression: A Clinician's Guide. New York: Guilford Press; 2010, and Clark DM, Wells AA. Cognitive model of social phobia. *Soc Phobia Diag Ass Treat*. 1995;41:00022–00023.)

an essential part of the first phase of treatment. Thus, for the vast majority of patients, it is the dysregulation of eating and sleeping behaviors, together with a lack of activity scheduling linked to their core values, that maintains the cycle outlined in Fig. 29.3. We have written elsewhere about the importance of value-matched activities in long-term activity change.[78]

Within a weight management context specifically, it is arguably essential that the "intervention" begins by breaking the dysregulation and avoidance cycle. There is a significant danger in prematurely focusing on dietary change (for weight management purposes) *before* the individuals disordered eating and dysregulated sleeping/activity patterns have been fully addressed because patients' experiences of traditional (often extreme)

commercial diets can reinforce their beliefs regarding an overevaluation of weight/shape and ridged rules around what they can/cannot eat (reinforcing all-or-nothing thinking/behaviors). There is therefore a risk that if patients perceive themselves to be "dieting," rather than adopting a permanent lifestyle change (in the form of health eating, sleeping, exercise patterns), then their prior "dieting beliefs" and sense of failure, from extreme weight loss products and commercial diets, will be reactivated. This then becomes a reinforcing (maintaining) factor in their disordered eating via overgeneralization. Fig. 29.3 highlights that a patient's response to a binge episode is highly likely to cycle back to reinforce various maintaining cycles. First, the emotional response to the experience of repeatedly failing (postbinge) may act as a direct (emotional) trigger to a further binge. Second, it may reactivate the rumination (overthinking) cycle associated with the guilt/anger/shame, whereby patients further self-berate by asking themselves (unanswerable) questions such as "why did I do that," "here I go again," "why do I continue to fail," "why am I so useless," etc. Third, the binge can have a reinforcing impact on the patients' underlying beliefs about their worth in addition to reinforcing their sense of failure and efficacy belief that change may not actually be possible for them.

Returning to our case study, we can see how regulating appetite and eating patterns is so important given the erratic nature of Janet's eating (before looking to make any changes to the content of her diet). She currently has no sense of physical hunger and satiety cues, and these would need to be identified and learned. Similarly, Janet's sleep and diabetes control are likely to impact on her physical hunger and satiety cues and need to be stabilized. This would also be a good point for Janet to begin to learn some new strategies for managing emotional distress with the team psychologist. Failure to undertake these steps prior to WLS could potentially lead to poor outcomes. Phase II would also provide an excellent opportunity for the health professionals involved to help Janet to begin to build her self-worth in line with Fairburn's BED treatment model.[59,60] A fundamental key to Janet succeeding with WLS would be an internal sense that she can achieve weight loss through maintaining changes that are driven by her. Given that Janet's sense of this is currently low, helping her to recognize her own progress will help increase her confidence that she can succeed. When patients, such as Janet, focus on increased levels of regulation in their behaviors (eating, sleeping, and activity), this typically results in a steady reduction in both the number of binge episodes and their volume. These reductions are associated with a reduced likelihood of the activation of the secondary maintaining cycle of overthinking (rumination) because of the reduced level of negative automatic feelings associated with binge eating (e.g., guilt/anger/frustration); improved physical symptoms (e.g., energy levels, blood sugar regulation); and weight loss. Thus, although weight loss is not a specific focus of the intervention at this stage (this comes in Phase III of Fig. 29.2), many of our patients report weight loss due to the reduction in binge frequency and content (i.e., less fat/sugar), as well as increased levels of valued, purposeful physical activities linked to life goals.

An important aspect of Fig. 29.3 is that when patients implement behavioral changes, these impact directly on their long-standing beliefs (self-worth, self-efficacy). These beliefs are now being challenged because they are no longer being reinforced via uncontrolled binges and self-berating internal dialogue. Patients report feeling more in control over their eating behaviors. At this stage, they are ready to move into Phase III of treatment (see Fig. 29.2). In Phase III, the focus is more directly on psychoeducational work with dietitians and exercise professionals to maintain the progress made in Phase II and in making specific, realistic, long-term changes to eating and activity patterns in a way that is both regulated and consistent with their life goals and values. We would strongly recommend that health professionals who work with patients to implement these changes are first aware of the work that has been completed in Phases I and II and that they are well trained in client-centered treatment approaches that maximize patient activation and increase their levels of self-determination. In our own practice we have specifically worked with allied health professionals to ensure they are trained in motivational interviewing (MI) as an approach that is inherently linked to increasing levels of self-determination.[63] The reader is referred to Chapter 19 for more information on how to implement MI consistent practitioner behaviors.

Finally, Phase IV of our treatment model (Fig. 29.2) highlights the importance of a relapse prevention phase, prior to any WLS. We would suggest that a period of consolidation of up to 12 months is built into this intervention. Clearly the level of contact with patients lessens during this time, and we would suggest that face-to-face visits would reduce in quantity (and duration) perhaps to monthly and then quarterly contacts. Some of our current patients have set up their own virtual support groups using social media as part of their own relapse prevention plan, and we have encouraged them to take ownership of this process to increase their levels of self-determination (i.e., control, responsibility, relatedness).

It is interesting that for many weight management interventions what we suggest as Phase IV is considered to be the first line of treatment. However, we would argue that, in Janet's case, this would be akin to *putting a roof on a building* before the rest of the building is there to support it. Once the other layers are in place, this will provide a solid foundation and structure for Janet to succeed at making changes, boost her self-efficacy, and have a successful outcome with or without WLS (we say with or without, because it is not uncommon for patients to reach this point and no longer feel the need for WLS). Ideally, we would advocate that this work is carried out within an MDT, with a consistency of approach between team members. Realistically, there is likely to be around 2 years of quite intensive work to be completed to prepare Janet for WLS. We are mindful that for Janet, and the many patients like her, it has not been easy for them to open up and tell the complexity of their story. It is important, therefore, that Janet feels safe and understood and that she has built a good rapport. One good predictor of outcome for patients generally is the strength of the relationship between the health professional and the patient;[79] therefore, we would be keen not to disrupt this. Unfortunately, in the United Kingdom, national commissioning arrangements do not necessarily support this way of working. Many specialist weight management services have to refer to mental health and third-sector services for underlying trauma/loss work (although there is the expertise within their teams to deliver this). This is due to the constraints of their own treatment pathways and/or commissioning arrangements locally viewing factors, such as mood disorders and related health conditions, as separate entities from weight issues (although we can see clearly from the above case example, that they are not). In the case that Janet would need to be referred out to other services for Phase I of her treatment, we would recommend liaising closely with those services regarding Janet, to ensure continuity of care in line with the treatment models outlined in this chapter.

REFERENCES

1. NICE. *Obesity*. London: National Institute for Health and Clinical Excellence; 2014. Available from: https://www.nice.org.uk/guidance/cg189.
2. BOMSS. *Commissioning Guide: Weight Assessment and Management Clinics (Tier 3)*. London: British Obesity & Metabolic Surgery Society; 2014. Available from: http://www.bomss.org.uk/commissioning-guide-weight-assessment-and-management-clinics-tier-3/.
3. Hughes CA. The rewards and challenges of setting up a Tier 3 adult weight management service in primary care. *Brit J Obes*. 2015;1:25–31.
4. Andrasik F, Goodie J, Peterson A. Biopsychosocial assessment. In: *Clinical Health Psychology*. 1st ed. London: Guilford Press; 2015.
5. Suls J, Rothman A. Evolution of the biopsychosocial model: prospects and challenges for health psychology. *Health Psychol*. 2004;23(2):119–125. http://dx.doi.org/10.1037/0278-6133.23.2.119.
6. British Psychological Society. *Good Practice Guidelines on the Use of Psychological Formulation*. Leicester: The British Psychological Society; 2011.
7. Glovsky E. *Wellness, Not Weight: Health at Every Size and Motivational Interviewing*. San Diego, CA: Cognella; 2013.
8. Klein D, Fencil-Morse E, Seligman M. Learned helplessness, depression, and the attribution of failure. *J Pers Soc Psychol*. 1976;33(5):508–516. http://dx.doi.org/10.1037//0022-3514.33.5.508.
9. Ozment J, Lester D. Helplessness and depression. *Psychol Rep*. 1998;82(2):434–438. http://dx.doi.org/10.2466/pr0.1998.82.2.434.
10. Rotenberg K, Costa P, Trueman M, Lattimore P. An interactional test of the reformulated helplessness theory of depression in women receiving clinical treatment for eating disorders. *Eat Behav*. 2012;13(3):264–266. http://dx.doi.org/10.1016/j.eatbeh.2012.03.001.
11. Taylor J, Neitzke D, Khouri G, et al. A pilot study to investigate the induction and manipulation of learned helplessness in healthy adults. *Psychiatry Res*. 2014;219(3):631–637. http://dx.doi.org/10.1016/j.psychres.2014.05.045.
12. Miller W, Rollnick S. *Motivational Interviewing*. 1st ed. New York, NY: Guilford Press; 2013.
13. Buchwald H, Estok R, Fahrbach K, et al. Weight and type 2 diabetes after bariatric surgery: systematic review and meta-analysis. *Am J Med*. 2009;122(3):248–256. http://dx.doi.org/10.1016/j.amjmed.2008.09.041.
14. Mundi M, Lorentz P, Swain J, Grothe K, Collazo-Clavell M. Moderate physical activity as predictor of weight loss after bariatric surgery. *Obes Surg*. 2013;23(10):1645–1649. http://dx.doi.org/10.1007/s11695-013-0979-y.
15. Kewin E, Boyle S. Weight loss surgery. In: BPS Working Group, ed. *Obesity in the UK: A Psychological Perspective*. Leicester: British Psychological Society; 2011:39–50.
16. Sheets C, Peat C, Berg K, et al. Post-operative psychosocial predictors of outcome in bariatric surgery. *Obes Surg*. 2014;25:330–345. http://dx.doi.org/10.1007/s11695-014-1490-9.
17. Canetti L, Berry E, Elizur Y. Psychosocial predictors of weight loss and psychological adjustment following bariatric surgery and a weight-loss program: the mediating role of emotional eating. *Int J Eat Disord*. 2009;42(2):109–117. http://dx.doi.org/10.1002/eat.20592.
18. Meany G, Conceição E, Mitchell J. Binge eating, binge eating disorder and loss of control eating: effects on weight outcomes after bariatric surgery. *Eur Eat Disord Rev*. 2013;22(2):87–91. http://dx.doi.org/10.1002/erv.2273.
19. *Diagnostic and statistical manual of mental disorders*. 5th ed. Washington, DC: American Psychiatric Association; 2013.
20. Marek R, Ben-Porath Y, Ashton K, Heinberg L. Impact of using DSM-5 criteria for diagnosing binge eating disorder in bariatric surgery candidates: change in prevalence rate, demographic characteristics, and scores on the Minnesota multiphasic personality inventory – 2 restructured form (MMPI-2-RF). *Int J Eat Disord*. 2014;47(5):553–557. http://dx.doi.org/10.1002/eat.22268.
21. Onyike CU, Crum RM, Lee HB, Lyketsos CG, Eaton WW. Is obesity associated with major depression? Results from the third National Health and Nutrition Survey. *Am J Epid*. 2003;58:1136–1147.
22. Pagoto S, Schneider K, Whited M, et al. Randomized controlled trial of behavioral treatment for comorbid obesity and depression in women: the Be Active Trial. *Int J Obes (Lond)*. 2013;37(11):1427–1434. http://dx.doi.org/10.1038/ijo.2013.25.

23. Rish JR, Heinberg LJ. Psychosocial morbidity and the effect of weight loss. In: *The Clinician's Guide to the Treatment of Obesity*. New York, NY: Springer; 2015.

24. Sogg S, Lauretti J, West-Smith L. Recommendations for the presurgical psychosocial evaluation of bariatric surgery patients. *Surg Obes Relat Dis*. 2016;12:731–749.

25. Vaidya V. Psychosocial aspects of obesity. *Adv Psychosom Med*. 2006;27:73–85.

26. Adami G, Gandolfo P, Bauer B, Scopinaro N. Binge eating in massively obese patients undergoing bariatric surgery. *Int J Eat Disord*. 1995;17(1):45–50. http://dx.doi.org/10.1002/1098-108x(199501)17:1<45::aid-eat2260170106>3.0.co;2-s.

27. Allison K, Wadden T, Sarwer D, et al. Night eating syndrome and binge eating disorder among persons seeking bariatric surgery: prevalence and related features. *Surg Obes Relat Dis*. 2006;2(2):153–158. http://dx.doi.org/10.1016/j.soard.2006.03.014.

28. Dymek-Valentine M, Rienecke-Hoste R, Alverdy J. Assessment of binge eating disorder in morbidly obese patients evaluated for gastric bypass: SCID versus QEWP-R. *Eat Weight Disord*. 2004;9(3):211–216. http://dx.doi.org/10.1007/bf03325069.

29. Kalarchian M, Wilson G, Brolin R, Bradley L. Binge eating in bariatric surgery patients. *Int J Eat Disord*. 1998;23(1):89–92. http://dx.doi.org/10.1002/(sici)1098-108x(199801)23:1<89::aid-eat11>3.3.co;2-r.

30. Hsu L, Sullivan S, Benotti P. Eating disturbances and outcome of gastric bypass surgery: a pilot study. *Int J Eat Disord*. 1997;21(4):385–390. http://dx.doi.org/10.1002/(sici)1098-108x(1997)21:4<385::aid-eat12>3.3.co;2-z.

31. Zimmerman M, Francione-Witt C. Presurgical psychiatric evaluations of candidates for bariatric surgery, Part 1. *J Clin Psychiatry*. 2007;68(10):1557–1562. http://dx.doi.org/10.4088/jcp.v68n1014.

32. Bean M, Stewart K, Olbrisch M. Obesity in America: implications for clinical and health psychologists. *J Clin Psychol Med Settings*. 2008;15(3):214–224. http://dx.doi.org/10.1007/s10880-008-9124-9.

33. de Wit L, Luppino F, van Straten A, Penninx B, Zitman F, Cuijpers P. Depression and obesity: a meta-analysis of community-based studies. *Psychiat Res*. 2010:230–235.

34. Luppino FS, de Wit LM, Bouvy PF, Stijnen T, Cuijpers P, Penninx BWJH Overweight, obesity, and depression: a systematic review and meta-analysis of longitudinal studies. *Arch Gen Psychiat*. 2010;67:220–229.

35. National Obesity Observatory (N.O.O.). *Treating Adult Obesity through Lifestyle Change Interventions. A Briefing Paper for Commissioners*. LONDON: National Obesity Observatory; 2010. Available at: http://www.noo.org.uk/uploads/doc/vid_5189_Adult_weight_management_Final_220210.pdfMarch.

36. Ogden J, Birch A, Wood K. 'The wrong journey': patients' experience of plastic surgery post weight loss surgery. *Qual Res Sport Ex Health*. 2014;7(2):294–308. http://dx.doi.org/10.1080/2159676x.2014.926967.

37. Natvik E, Gjengedal E, Råheim M. Totally changed, yet still the same: patients' lived experiences 5 years beyond bariatric surgery. *Qual Health Res*. 2013;23:1202–1214. http://dx.doi.org/10.1177/1049732313501888.

38. Piacentino D, Prosperi E, Guidi G, et al. Effectiveness and factors predicting success of therapeutic patient education in obese patients candidates for bariatric surgery. *Eur Psychiatry*. 2016;33:S235–S236. http://dx.doi.org/10.1016/j.eurpsy.2016.01.590.

39. Kinzl J, Schrattenecker M, Traweger C, Mattesich M, Fiala M, Biebl W. Psychosocial predictors of weight loss after bariatric surgery. *Obes Surg*. 2006;16(12):1609–1614. http://dx.doi.org/10.1381/096089206779319301.

40. Wedin S, Madan A, Correll J, et al. Emotional eating, marital status and history of physical abuse predict 2-year weight loss in weight loss surgery patients. *Eat Behav*. 2014;15(4):619–624. http://dx.doi.org/10.1016/j.eatbeh.2014.08.019.

41. Brunault P, Frammery J, Couet C, et al. Predictors of changes in physical, psychosocial, sexual quality of life, and comfort with food after obesity surgery: a 12-month follow-up study. *Qual Life Res*. 2014;24(2):493–501. http://dx.doi.org/10.1007/s11136-014-0775-8.

42. Dimidjian S, Barrera M, Martell C, Muñoz R, Lewinsohn P. The origins and current status of behavioral activation treatments for depression. *Annu Rev Clin Psychol*. 2011;7(1):1–38. http://dx.doi.org/10.1146/annurev-clinpsy-032210-104535.

43. Alciati A, Caldirola D, Foschi D, Perna G. Psychiatric disorders and childhood parental loss in obesity: relationship with the mode of weight gain. *J Loss Trauma*. 2015;21(3):213–224. http://dx.doi.org/10.1080/15325024.2015.1075796.

44. Alciati A, Caldirola D, Grassi M, Foschi D, Perna G. Mediation effect of recent loss events on weight gain in obese people who experienced childhood parental death or separation. *J Health Psychol*. 2017;22(1):101–110. http://dx.doi.org/10.1177/1359105315595451.

45. Fabricatore AN, Wadden TA, Sarwer DB, et al. Self-reported eating behaviors of extremely obese persons seeking bariatric surgery: a factor analytic approach. *Obes*. 2006;14:83S–89S. http://dx.doi.org/10.1038/oby.2006.287.

46. Bauchowitz AU, Gonder-Frederick LA, Olbrisch ME, et al. Psychosocial evaluation of bariatric surgery candidates: a survey of present practices. *Psychosom Med*. 2005;67:825–832.

47. Parkes C. *After the Honeymoon Period; an Interpretative Phenomenological Analysis of the Experiences of Bariatric Surgery Patients 12 Months to Three Years Post Operatively*. University of Wolverhampton, UK: Doctoral Thesis in Counselling Psychology; 2014. http://hdl.handle.net/2436/561196.

48. Stevens T, Spavin S, Scholtz S, McClelland L. Your patient and weight-loss surgery. *Adv Psychiat Treat*. 2012;18:418–425. http://dx.doi.org/10.1192/apt.bp.111.008938.

49. Cambi M, Marchesini S, Baretta G. Post-bariatric surgery weight regain: evaluation of nutritional profile of candidate patients for endoscopic argon plasma coagulation. *ABCD Arq Bras Cir Dig*. 2015;28(1):40–43. http://dx.doi.org/10.1590/s0102-67202015000100011.

50. Magro D, Geloneze B, Delfini R, Pareja B, Callejas F, Pareja J. Long-term weight regain after gastric bypass: a 5-year prospective study. *Obes Surg*. 2008;18(6):648–651. http://dx.doi.org/10.1007/s11695-007-9265-1.

51. Sjöström L, Narbro K, Sjöström C, et al. Effects of bariatric surgery on mortality in Swedish obese subjects. *N Engl J Med.* 2007;357(8):741–752. http://dx.doi.org/10.1056/nejmoa066254.

52. Apovian CM. Obesity: definition, comorbidities, causes and burden. *Am J Manag Care.* 2016;22:S176–S185.

53. British Psychological Society. *Clinical psychology forum special issue: team formulation.* Leicester: British Psychological Society; 2015.

54. Johnstone L, Dallos R. *Formulation in Psychology and Psychotherapy : Making Sense of People's Problems.* 2nd ed. London: Guilford Press; 2014.

55. Dudley R, Kuyken W. Cognitive-behavioural case formulation. In: Johnstone L, Dallos R, eds. *Formulation in Psychology and Psychotherapy: Making Sense of People's Problems.* London: Routledge; 2006:17–46.

56. Johnston LH, Hutchison AJ. Influencing health behaviour: applying theory to practice. In: Scott A, Gidlow C, eds. *Clinical Exercise Science.* London: Routledge; 2016:224–246.

57. Johnston LH, Hutchison AJ, Ingham B. The utility of biopsychosocial models of clinical formulation within stress and coping and applied practice. In: Devonport T, ed. *Managing Stress from Theory to Application.* NY: Nova Science Publishers; 2011:259–290.

58. Hutchison A, Johnston L. Exploring the potential of case formulation within exercise psychology. *J Clin Sport Psychol.* 2013;7(1):60–76. http://dx.doi.org/10.1123/jcsp.7.1.60.

59. Fairburn C. *Cognitive Behaviour Therapy and Eating Disorders.* Chichester: Guilford Press; 2008.

60. Fairburn C. *Overcoming Binge Eating: The Proven Program to Learn Why You Binge and How You Can Stop.* London: Guildford Press; 2013.

61. Bandura, A. *Social Learning Theory.* Englewood Cliffs, NJ: Prentice-Hall.

62. Rotter JB. Generalized expectancies for internal versus external control of reinforcement. *Psych Mono.* 1966:80–81.

63. Markland D, Ryan R, Tobin V, Rollnick S. Motivational interviewing and self–determination theory. *J Soc Clin Psychol.* 2005;24(6):811–831. http://dx.doi.org/10.1521/jscp.2005.24.6.811.

64. Crenshaw D, Van Ornum W. *Bereavement.* 1st ed. New York: Continuum; 2002.

65. Morris A, Silk J, Steinberg L, Myers S, Robinson L. The role of the family context in the development of emotion regulation. *Soc Dev.* 2007;16(2):361–388. http://dx.doi.org/10.1111/j.1467-9507.2007.00389.x.

66. Bello N, Hajnal A. Dopamine and binge eating behaviors. *Pharmacol Biochem Behav.* 2010;97(1):25–33. http://dx.doi.org/10.1016/j.pbb.2010.04.016.

67. McClure Brenchley K, Quinn D. Weight-based rejection sensitivity: scale development and implications for well-being. *Body Image.* 2016;16:79–92. http://dx.doi.org/10.1016/j.bodyim.2015.11.005.

68. Deci EL, Ryan RM. *Intrinsic Motivation and Self-determination in Human Behavior.* New York, NY: Plenum; 1985.

69. Annesi J, Mareno N. Improvement in emotional eating associated with an enhanced body image in obese women: mediation by weight-management treatments' effects on self-efficacy to resist emotional cues to eating. *J Adv Nurs.* 2015;71(12):2923–2935. http://dx.doi.org/10.1111/jan.12766.

70. Montani J, Viecelli A, Prévot A, Dulloo A. Weight cycling during growth and beyond as a risk factor for later cardiovascular diseases: the 'repeated overshoot' theory. *Int J Obes (Lond).* 2006;30:S58–S66. http://dx.doi.org/10.1038/sj.ijo.0803520.

71. Chaput J, Després J, Bouchard C, Tremblay A. Association of sleep duration with type 2 diabetes and impaired glucose tolerance. *Diabetologia.* 2007;50(11):2298–2304. http://dx.doi.org/10.1007/s00125-007-0786-x.

72. Chaput J, Després J, Bouchard C, Tremblay A. The association between sleep duration and weight gain in adults: a 6-year prospective study from the quebec family study. *Sleep.* 2008;31(4):517–523. http://dx.doi.org/10.1093/sleep/31.4.517.

73. Martell CR, Dimidjian S, Herman-Dunn R. *Behavioral Activation for Depression: A Clinician's Guide.* New York: Guilford Press; 2010.

74. Clark DM, Wells AA. Cognitive model of social phobia. *Soc Phobia Diag Ass Treat.* 1995;41:00022–00023.

75. Pagoto SL, Bodenlos JS, Schneider KL, Olendzki B, Spates RC, Ma Y. Initial investigation of behavioral activation therapy for co-morbid major depressive disorder and obesity. *Psychotherapy.* 2008;45:410–415.

76. Pagoto SL, Spring B, Cook JW, McChargue D, Schneider K. High BMI and reduced frequency and enjoyment of pleasant events. *Per Ind Diff.* 2006;40:1421–1431.

77. Stott R, Mansell W, Salkovskis P, Lavender A, Cartwright-Hatton S. *Oxford Guide to Metaphors in CBT: Building Cognitive Bridges (Oxford Guides in Cognitive Behavioural Therapy).* 1st ed. Oxford University Press; 2010.

78. Hutchison A, Johnston L, Breckon J. A grounded theory of successful long-term physical activity behaviour change. *Qual Res Sport Ex Health.* 2013;5(1):109–126. http://dx.doi.org/10.1080/2159676x.2012.693529.

79. Kelley J, Kraft-Todd G, Schapira L, Kossowsky J, Riess H. The influence of the patient-clinician relationship on healthcare outcomes: a systematic review and meta-analysis of randomized controlled trials. *PLoS One.* 2014;9(4):e94207. http://dx.doi.org/10.1371/journal.pone.0094207.

CHAPTER 30

Dietary Interventions for Weight Loss and Essential Aspects of Nutrition Post–Bariatric Surgery

JORDAN BARNARD, BSC (HONS) • DEBORAH SNOWDON, BSC (HONS) • LUCY HEWITSON, BMEDSCI, MA, PGDIP

INTRODUCTION TO THE ROLE OF DIETARY INTERVENTIONS IN WEIGHT MANAGEMENT

Obesity is a very complex condition that can be caused by numerous external and internal factors, which may be medical, psychologic, physiologic, social, and economical, as well as lifestyle behaviors. With this in mind, it is important to understand that obesity is not always managed by addressing diet and energy input and output in isolation. Dietary intervention in the management of obesity is of upmost importance, and it is clear that there is a relationship between diet and body weight. However, dietary interventions are only useful when a client is ready and willing to change and when his/her other needs are being addressed, e.g., psychologic, medical, and physical activity. Therefore a multidisciplinary team (MDT) is essential for effective weight management. A clinician specializing in dietary interventions for weight management is an essential part of a weight management MDT and plays a very important role in promoting behavior change in these clients.

Diet may not always be the sole cause of someone's obesity, but it is usually a contributing factor and needs to be carefully managed for effective weight loss and improvement of health. Clinicians working in the dietary management of obesity will routinely offer clients dietary assessment, dietary counseling, and/or other dietary interventions and lifestyle advice. The main role of a clinician working in the dietary management of obesity is to offer evidence-based dietary advice that will help overweight or obese clients to lose weight. Within this remit, one of the main tasks of a weight management clinician is to help people achieve dietary changes that will establish weight loss (often restricting the diet) while ensuring the nutritional adequacy of the diet. Research shows that reduction

in dietary energy intake usually corresponds with a reduction in micronutrient intake.[1,2] It is often highly impractical to monitor the macronutrient and micronutrient content of every weight management client. However, by making sure that healthy dietary proportions and portion sizes are being adhered to, the risk of nutritional inadequacy is minimalized. It may also help to keep in mind the higher-risk nutrients, which are more likely to be inadequate in people who restrict their diet, such as protein; vitamins B1, C, and E; calcium; magnesium; and iron.[2]

Clinicians working in the dietary management of obesity will help clients to make evidence-based dietary changes within their personal preferences that will enable them to lose weight. There is evidence to suggest that a client's personal choice of dietary intervention may be one of the main factors influencing successful weight loss. The more acceptable the dietary changes are to the client, the more likely they are to adhere to them and achieve weight loss.[3,4] It is certainly beneficial to understand and use this knowledge when working in the dietary management of obesity.

STANDARD DIETARY COUNSELING

Standard dietary counseling is the process of helping people to apply evidence-based nutritional advice and healthy eating guidelines in their own lifestyle. Many clinicians know the basic nutritional advice for weight management and general healthy eating principles, such as reducing calorie and fat intake and healthy portion sizes, at least 400 g fruit and vegetables per day (5-a-day). However, it is clear to see in the developed world that although this knowledge seems to be present with many clinicians, this has not been effective at reducing the rising levels of obesity. It can be difficult for most clinicians

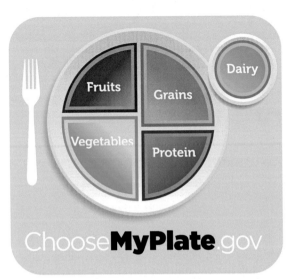

FIG. 30.1 MyPlate image. (From https://choosemyplate-prod.azureedge.net/sites/default/files/printablematerials/myplate_green.jpg.)

to express this knowledge to people in a way that they understand and can use, especially in time-limited consultations. The following tools offer practical ways to help express dietary advice for weight loss.

Dietary Proportion Models

Dietary proportion models display the recommended daily dietary proportions for each defined food group (Figs. 30.1 and 30.2). Many clinicians would think that dietary proportion models are the most useful tool in weight management nutrition education. Dietary proportion models are, of course, useful and should be used to help people understand the proportions of a healthy diet, and they are an excellent basis for education and discussion around healthy eating. However, in practice, if dietary proportion models are used in isolation, clients may find it hard to translate the information in dietary proportion models into everyday food and meal choices. This is mainly because dietary proportion models display healthy proportions of daily food intake and are not necessarily representative of healthy proportions of

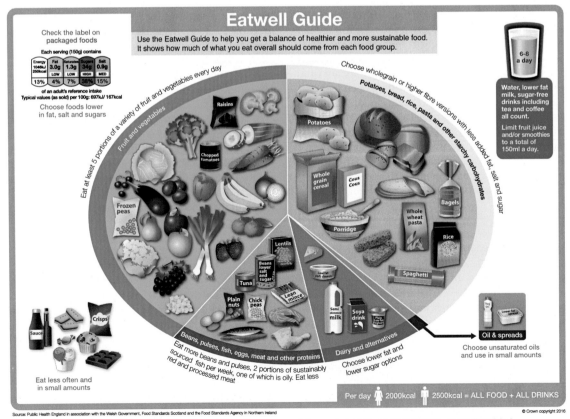

FIG. 30.2 Eatwell Guide. (From https://www.gov.uk/government/publications/the-eatwell-guide.)

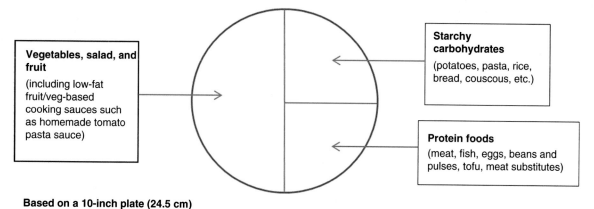

Based on a 10-inch plate (24.5 cm)

FIG. 30.3 Example of a weight loss plate model.

individual meals. Knowing the daily proportion of food groups is useful when analyzing the diet as a whole, but it is unlikely to offer clients quick help to decide what to prepare for the next meal. To address this, it is often best to use dietary proportion models alongside other tools such as plate models and portion size information. Dietary proportion models are based on guidance for the general population and may not be appropriate for more obese clients trying to achieve weight loss. It is also necessary to understand that dietary proportion models on their own do not effectively educate about portion sizes. That is why dietary proportion models are best used along with plate models.

Weight Loss Plate Model

Plate models are useful tools that can help to educate people about healthy dietary proportions and portion sizes for individual meals. In nutrition, proportions and portions are practically very different. Someone can have excellent dietary proportions but have poor portion sizes (too big or too small). Therefore there is a need to educate about both dietary proportions and portion sizes simultaneously. Practically, most clients trying to lose weight prefer to think in terms of healthy meals and snack choices instead of daily dietary proportions. Plate models help to achieve this while also educating about healthy meal choices. See Fig. 30.3 for an example of a weight loss plate model that can be used for most obese clients trying to achieve dietary changes for weight loss.

Food and Drink Record

A food and drink record is a useful tool in which a person records all of the food and drink that he/she consumes each day. Information is best recorded

throughout the day as a person is eating or soon after eating to avoid memory bias. A food and drink diary can be recorded in many different forms, including notepads, Internet sites, and smartphone applications. Clients should be encouraged to use the format that is most acceptable to them to improve adherence. Food and drink diaries can obviously be used by clinicians to analyze a client's diet. However, it could be argued that a food and drink diary is most valuable to clients themselves. When someone records what they eat and drink, it is highly likely to make them more aware of what they are eating and drinking. It is also likely to lead people to make healthier food choices because they are monitoring their own dietary intake. Obviously, there is the potential for people to underreport or overreport, but generally food and drink diaries are very useful tools. Self-analysis of food and drink diaries should be encouraged under the supervision of a weight management clinician.

24-h Dietary Recall and Typical Day Diet History

A 24-h dietary recall is a method of dietary assessment where a client is asked to report what he/she has eaten over a very recent 24-h period (usually the last 24 h or the previous day). A typical day diet history differs from a 24-h dietary recall in that a client is asked to talk through his/her typical daily diet. During a typical day diet history a clinician would use simple open-ended questions to guide a client through this process such as, "what is the first thing that you would normally eat or drink in a normal day?" Or, "What is the next thing you would normally have to eat and drink?"

Both the 24-h dietary recall and the typical day diet history are a means of helping a clinician analyze a client's diet and both carry a low respondent burden. However, they are likely to lead to a degree of inaccuracy. For example a 24-h dietary recall relies on memory, and most people will have some difficulty in reporting their recent dietary intake accurately. Even if someone can report accurately, the last 24-h period may not be representative of his/her diet.[5] Multiple 24-h dietary recalls can be used to help alleviate some of these problems, but this can be time-consuming and is likely to be impractical in a clinical environment although it may be useful in clinical research or large-scale surveys such as the Low Income Nutrition and Diet Survey in the United Kingdom.[6] A typical day diet history may help to overcome some of the inaccuracies of a 24-h dietary recall, but it is still prone to its own inaccuracies. For example, clients may not bring up negative dietary behaviors that happen less often but still significantly contribute to their weight. Despite the inherent inaccuracies, both a 24-h dietary recall and a typical day diet history are useful tools for weight management clinicians to use during a consultation. However, it is widely considered by weight management clinicians that a typical day diet history is a more useful dietary analysis tool than a 24-h dietary recall for use in a clinic appointment because it allows for a more broad analysis of someone's diet. It is important to state that both of these methods should be viewed as tools that give an indication of a person's diet and dietary habits. They should not be relied on for in-depth dietary analysis because of the inherent inaccuracies.

Food Frequency Questionnaires

A food frequency questionnaire (FFQ) is a document that clients or clinicians use to categorize the frequency of consumption of certain foods. Estimated nutritional intakes can then be derived from this.[7] FFQs are most often presented as a "checklist" style document where a category is ticked that is most appropriate to the client. In the previous research, FFQs have been shown to give similar results to multiple 2-day food records.[8] However, the main advantage is that shorter FFQs can take less time to conduct than a food and drink record or diet history. It is important to understand that there are many different types of FFQs and that each FFQ is often developed for a specific use. Therefore careful consideration should be given before deciding on which FFQ to use with clients. FFQs can be used in individual consultations to assess diet, but they are more commonly used in research studies, especially large-scale studies or surveys such as the Health Survey for England.[5] In practice, FFQs can identify aspects of a client's diet that may not have been raised in a 24-h dietary recall or a typical

day diet history. However, if an FFQ is used as the only means of dietary assessment during a consultation, it may not collect sufficient evidence to allow for specific dietary goals to be set with a client.

Portion Size Information

Information about portion sizes of specific foods is very helpful to clients who are trying to change their diet to lose weight. Clients will be given much information about healthy eating, but sometimes this can be difficult to interpret when actually preparing a meal. Portion size information will give a client advice about the amount of a specific food that can be enjoyed as part of a healthy meal or as a snack. Written and pictorial information of specific portion sizes are tools that should be considered as necessary for all weight management clinicians.

Portion size information is best given in conjunction with dietary proportion models and plate models to ensure that it is understood in the correct context.

Motivational Interviewing and Behaviural Change Techniques

Having evidence-based advice and the right tools is important for clinicians working in weight management. However, in practice, knowledge and advice alone is often not enough to elicit change in a client. In addition to understanding the correct advice, clients need to be motivated and prepared to make changes; they need to understand the benefit that this will give them and take responsibility for making the change happen. Motivational interviewing is a counseling approach, which aims to help patients change their behavior. It is client centered and elicits change from the client and not from outside forces. Motivational interviewing was developed by Miller and Rollnick[9] originally for use in clients with alcohol addiction. However, motivational interviewing skills are useful in almost all clinical settings, especially in weight management. It may be beneficial to use motivational interviewing skills to help clients to apply dietary advice. It can also help those clients who have lower motivation and may not otherwise make necessary changes.

SPECIFIC DIETARY INTERVENTIONS FOR WEIGHT LOSS

Partial Meal Replacement Diets

A partial meal replacement diet (PMRD) is a diet that involves replacing one to two meals per day with a meal replacement product. Meal replacement products normally take the form of shakes but can also come in the form of other drinks, meal bars, and soups. Meal replacement products are specially formulated products that provide the nutrition of a balanced meal (e.g., protein, carbohydrate, vitamins, and minerals) but with a relatively small amount of calories (usually 200–230 calories per meal replacement product).

PMRDs are usually low-calorie diets that commonly provide a daily calorie intake of 1000–1600 depending on the need of client and the advice given.

PMRDs are a convenient way to help people achieve a calorie-controlled diet. Calorie-controlled diets can be very difficult for weight management clients to achieve with free food choice partly because it is difficult to know the nutritional content of the foods and drinks that are present in different situations. There is much scientific evidence to show that PMRDs are effective at helping people to lose weight in the shorter and longer term.[10-13] There is some evidence to suggest that liquid meal replacements may help to control appetite and reduce feelings of hunger better than an isocaloric solid food diet. This is possibly due to a change in appetite-regulating hormones (such as ghrelin and leptin) and a reduction in insulin levels, which can occur while on a PMRD.[14,12]

The standard advice for starting a PMRD is to replace two meals per day with a meal replacement product and have a balanced third meal in the day. Appropriate snacks are also recommended if needed. In practice, most clients find the following structure the easiest to follow when on a PMRD although this is just an example and will depend on the client's lifestyle:
Breakfast: meal replacement product ~200–230 kcal
Midmorning: snack ~100 kcal
Lunch: meal replacement product ~200–230 kcal
Midafternoon: snack ~100 kcal
Evening meal: balanced meal as stated above ~400–800 kcal

It is usually advised that clients on a PMRD are allowed up to three 100-kcal snacks per day. These can be used to increase satiety, keep energy levels up, and improve compliance. These snacks may also help clients to control their blood glucose levels. Clients should be advised to have appropriate snacks if they feel that they need them. Having three snacks per day is not compulsory on a PMRD; however, most clients will require one to two snacks per day. Examples of appropriate snacks while on a PMRD are one portion of fruit, one pot of low-fat yoghurt, or a cereal bar that is approximately 100 kcal. Many PMRD product ranges produce their own snacks that are approximately 100 kcal for people on PMRDs. These may be useful, but care must be taken before recommending these snacks because these products can be expensive and are not necessary to a PMRD.

It should also be advised that clients drink at least 2 L of water or other low-calorie fluids every day (such as tea and coffee with no or a little milk and no sugar or no added sugar cordial) while on a PMRD to increase satiety and prevent dehydration. In practice, clients find it relatively easy to establish a PMRD and it can also be quite an efficient intervention. When this is combined with the evidence base, it makes PMRDs a valuable tool in the management of obesity.

Very-Low-Calorie Diets

A very-low-calorie diet (VLCD) is any diet that is 800 kcal/day or less. It is commonly stated that these diets should not be used routinely in the management of obesity, and there is great caution about their use in some weight management services.[15] Although it is true that VLCDs should not be used in the majority of weight management cases because of their restrictive nature, they do have a place in the management of obesity. Some people require quick weight loss under medical supervision. For example, someone who has very limited mobility due to osteoarthritis in hips or knees can be stuck in a difficult cycle. They have limited mobility due to pain and this restricts their energy output, which makes it difficult to lose weight. People in this situation are often waiting for joint replacement surgery, but their body mass index (BMI) may be too high to be considered, even though such surgery will likely improve their health and quality of life. Someone in situation such as this may benefit from a VLCD if other dietary interventions have not been successful in providing the desired weight loss. There has been increased interest in VLCDs recently due to recent research that demonstrates that they may have a role in putting type 2 diabetes into remission.[16-18] It is advised by some health organizations that people do not follow a VLCD for more than 12 weeks if using it every day.[15] This advice is useful to know, especially if a VLCD is being used without sufficient prior experience. However, there is no robust evidence with which to base the 12-week restriction.

It is always important in weight management to ensure that dietary interventions are likely to meet a client's nutritional requirements while still providing an energy deficit. This is no different when using a VLCD. In practice liquid VLCDs are an attractive option. This is because making food choices within an 800 kcal/day restriction is very difficult to do and it is highly likely that such a diet would be nutritionally deficient. Using a liquid-based VLCD may be more satiating than using solid food. This may be because liquids or meal replacements used in VLCDs may also affect hormones

TABLE 30.1
Example of a Cost-effective Liquid-Based Very-Low-Calorie Diet

Food/Fluid	Amount	Energy (kcal)	Protein (g)	Fluid (mL)
Semiskimmed milk	1500 mL	700–750	52–54	1500
Low/no calorie fluids	1000 mL	–	0	1000
Nonstarchy vegetables	240 g	0–75	–	–
A-Z multivitamin and mineral (daily)	–	–	–	–
Total	–	**700–825**	**52–54**	**2500**

involved in appetite regulation.[14,12] However, there are VLCD plans developed by weight management clinicians available using relatively normal food choices.

Some commercial VLCDs can be quite expensive, usually $65–90 or £50–70 per week, and consequently may not be appropriate for some clients. However, a simple and cost-effective liquid-based VLCD can be developed and adjusted to a client's specific needs using cow's milk, A-Z vitamin and mineral supplements, and additional low-calorie fluids such as water or no added sugar cordial. Some low-calorie solid foods such as nonstarchy vegetables may also be added to this depending on the need of the client and include some fiber into the diet (see Table 30.1).

People with diabetes who are on hypoglycemic medication, such as sulfonylureas (i.e. gliclazide, glimepiride), insulins, or any combinations with those, will find it difficult and potentially dangerous to use a VLCD without medical supervision because of the increased risk of hypoglycemia. However, if the right supervision is provided, then a VLCD may be used despite this if there is a clinically justifiable need. A recent systematic review of 17 studies looking at the use of VLCDs in people with type 2 diabetes concluded that they are safe and effective at reducing weight and improving other metabolic risk factors.[19] Intermittent use of VLCDs for 2 days per week has also been shown to have a similar effect on weight and health biomarkers than consecutive use of VLCDs.[20] This presents a distinct advantage due to the regularly advised restricted use of continuous VLCDs.

As with everyone following a dietary intervention for weight loss, clients will benefit from having regular support and a means of contacting medical and healthcare professionals for advice while following a VLCD.

Higher-Protein Diets

There is evidence to show that higher-protein diets are an effective way of helping people to lose weight.[21] Greater loss of weight and fat mass has been observed

when using higher-protein diets when compared with standard low-fat diets in some studies.[22] However, most of this evidence is in reference to the short-term use of these diets. Higher-protein diets are often accompanied with a carbohydrate restriction, but this varies greatly from diet to diet. Diets moderately increased in protein and modestly restricted in carbohydrate and fat, particularly saturated fat, may have beneficial effects on body weight, body composition, and associated metabolic parameters.[21] If these diets are being considered for use, it may therefore be beneficial to use a modest increase in protein to ~25% of total energy intake (approximately 100–150 g per day) and a modest reduction in starchy carbohydrates and fat by means of portion control and healthier food choices.[23] One of the main benefits of a higher-protein diet is that they are more satiating and therefore may be useful to people who report regularly feeling hungry throughout the day.[21,22] In practice, clients often find it relatively simple to establish a higher-protein diet with portion-controlled starchy carbohydrates. It is because of this that these diets present an attractive option to many clients and clinicians.

Intermittent Fasting

Intermittent fasting refers to any diet where there is one or more "fast day" per week. On a fast day, a person may consume between 0 and 800 kcal/day. Most commonly these diets take the "5:2" form whereby a person eats a healthy balanced diet for 5 days/week and consumes 500–600 kcal/day for 2 days/week. Currently, there is less evidence to support the use of these diets in practice compared with the dietary interventions already mentioned. However, despite this, intermittent fasting diets are gaining popularity. There is some evidence to show that resting energy expenditure can be increased after short-term fasting.[24,25] Some studies have also shown that intermittent fasting can be as effective as calorie-restricted diets for weight loss and cardioprotection.[26,27] As previously stated, intermittent use of VLCDs has been shown to have a similar effect on weight and health biomarkers when compared with consecutive use of a VLCD.[20] In practice, anecdotal evidence also suggests that intermittent fasting helps people to lose a moderate amount of weight. However, there is currently limited evidence to suggest that these diets can help people to lose weight over the long term.

An intermittent fasting diet is likely to be safe for most people except for those on hypoglycemic medications (i.e., gliclazide, glimepiride, or insulins) and other medications that require a regular food intake, such as allopurinol. In most cases, such medications can be adjusted under medical supervision to allow trialing an intermittent fasting diet. Clients who want to try an intermittent fasting diet and for whom it is safe to do so should not be discouraged from trying them. However, it should be recommended that they follow a nutritionally complete plan developed by a qualified medical and/or healthcare professional.

Weight Maintenance

It has been suggested that people who have successfully lost weight may need specific diets to maintain their body weight. For example, if two people both have the same body weight but one used to be 50 kg heavier than the other, it may be that the person who has lost 50 kg will need a different diet to maintain his/her weight than the other person who has not lost weight. A large-scale international randomized control trial of people who had lost 8% of their body weight using a VLCD showed that a higher-protein diet with lower glycemic index (GI) carbohydrates helped to prevent weight regain more than the other diets studied.[23] In this study participants were randomly assigned to one of five diets:

1. a low-protein (13% of total energy consumed) with low-GI diet;
2. a low-protein with high-GI diet;
3. a higher-protein diet (25% of total energy consumed, ~100–150 g per day) with low-GI diet;
4. a high-protein and high-GI diet; or
5. a control diet.

The group following the high-protein with low-GI diet was the only one to maintain the weight lost with the VLCD. It is therefore possible that this type of diet may be protective against weight regain after a weight loss.

Specific dietary intervention to improve weight maintenance and prevent weight regain is a relatively new area of study. More research is required into this area before more solid conclusions can be made.

PREPARATION FOR BARIATRIC SURGERY

The previous sections have discussed the potential ways of losing weight with or without the plan to progress to bariatric surgery. At this point, bariatric surgery or weight loss surgery would depend on a client's BMI and the amount of weight loss they have achieved with dietary and lifestyle intervention. Guidance from National Institute for Health and Clinical Excellence (NICE) in United Kingdom states that for anyone with a BMI >35 with comorbidities or a BMI >40, weight loss surgery should be considered as an option after diet and exercise have been promoted and medical management has been provided by a specialist obesity service. However, for clients presenting with a BMI >50, bariatric surgery is to be considered as the first-line option for treatment.[15]

It is essential that clients are well educated and aware of the nutritional requirements before weight loss surgery. Research suggests that preoperative dietary intervention will improve postoperative outcomes after gastric bypass surgery.[28] Some of the dietary aspects and healthy eating principles discussed previously are excellent preparation; however, the following dietary aspects are more specific to a client who is planning toward weight loss surgery.

Firstly, a comprehensive assessment of the client's dietary intake either by a dietary recall or preferably by a food diary would be advantageous. Clinicians should look for a routine or frequent eating pattern and check if standard healthy eating principles, such as "5-a-day," are being followed, as well as decreased portion sizes and healthier snacking options replacing high-fat and high-sugar options. Key factors should be discussed, such as reducing the pace of eating, chewing 15–20 times, and using smaller plates: it is essential for the client to understand all these and put into practice because after surgery the diet needs to be nutritionally complete and meals cannot be rushed. Hydration is paramount before and after bariatric surgery; therefore assessing a client's fluid intake is essential. However, clients should be advised to avoid carbonated drinks, high sugar drinks and drinking with a meal. Post bariatric surgery the stomach capacity is greatly reduced and fluid is often not tolerated when eating.

Assessing micronutrient intake and ensuring that the client is aware of the importance of foods rich in calcium, vitamin D, protein, and iron in the diet is more important. It is well documented that morbidly obese clients can be nutrient deficient before bariatric surgery.[29,30] This is due to their poor dietary choices that can be predominantly energy dense with very little nutrient content. The micronutrients that are more commonly seen to be deficient in obese clients are iron (low levels of ferritin) and vitamins such as B12 and D. Inadequate vitamin D status has been observed in nearly 90% of individuals considering bariatric surgery.[31] Therefore a thorough assessment of the client's dietary intake and biochemistry should be completed to ensure there are no nutrient deficiencies before bariatric surgery.

During the time with the MDT, an evaluation would be made assessing individual eating behaviors and identifying any possible eating disorders. Identifying eating behaviors and disordered eating, such as comfort eating, grazing, or binge eating, is essential. It is also important to look for eating behaviors that are habitual or hedonistic. Habitual eating is where the client has adopted an unhealthy eating routine that has become a habit and hedonistic eating is where they eat for pleasure or self-gratification. These behaviors or disordered eating can easily result in indulging in excessive food intake and therefore is a main contributing factor to the development of obesity. Appropriate treatment and support is given before bariatric surgery by a trained member of the team depending on the outcome of the MDT assessment. Some clients will have input from the clinical psychologist to explore the reasons for their eating behavior and support will be given around coping mechanisms and strategies to manage these behaviors. Before the bariatric referral is made, the clinical psychologist will make a final report and recommendations. However, other clients may not require psychologic input and it would be more appropriate for them to see the dietitian with behavior change skills training or the health trainer to cover mindful eating and distraction techniques.

Bariatric assessment may highlight the need to place an intragastric balloon depending on BMI and risk factors. This is a nonsurgical procedure where the balloon is placed in the stomach and expanded usually for 6 months. The intragastric balloon helps a client feel full, eat less, and lose weight. Approximately 60% of clients lose a third of their excess body weight in 6 months.[32] The main reason for using an intragastric balloon is to achieve further weight loss preoperatively in the severely obese to reduce the surgical risk for the client.[33]

PRE–BARIATRIC SURGERY

Preoperatively, a restrictive diet low in fat, sugar, and carbohydrates is commonly recommended by many bariatric services. This restriction is used short term usually for 1–2 weeks before bariatric surgery. The purpose of the dietary restriction is to reduce glycogen stores in the liver thus shrinking the liver.[34] The liver is a large organ that

is positioned over the stomach; therefore gastric surgery is made easier laparoscopically if the liver-reducing diet is followed. The liver-reducing diet is low in calories and ranges from 800–1000 calories per day. Because of the restrictive nature of such a diet, a multivitamin/mineral supplement would generally be recommended.

ESSENTIAL ASPECTS OF NUTRITION POST–BARIATRIC SURGERY

Bariatric surgery is the most effective medical treatment for morbid obesity.[35] However, bariatric surgery is not a simple intervention and there is much that should be considered before this treatment is offered to clients.

Bariatric surgery can affect appetite, food tolerance, taste, intake, and absorption of a client, which can compromise nutritional status. It is essential that clients are monitored following bariatric surgery to prevent nutritional deficiencies and to provide additional support and advice to help them maximize their weight loss and continue with their improved lifestyle behaviors. NICE guidance in the United Kingdom advises that clients who undergo a bariatric procedure should be monitored by their bariatric service for a minimum of 2 years postprocedure.[15] Recommendations and guidelines following a bariatric procedure vary widely depending on the bariatric service and the type of bariatric intervention. However, there is general consensus among most of the bariatric surgery community about the following topics.

Consistency

Following bariatric surgery, clients are advised to monitor not only the volume that they eat but also the consistency. As with most surgery involving the gastrointestinal tract, a gradual buildup back to a normal consistency diet is advised immediately following the procedure. It is advised that clients start with a liquid diet, then advance to a puree diet, then to a soft diet, finally building up to solid food. This texture progression should take place over a period of 6–8 weeks. Specific advice varies between bariatric services. Typical foods that clients can struggle to tolerate following a bariatric procedure are bread, meat, and fibrous vegetables. In some cases, these foods will be best avoided, but this should be approached in an individual client-centered way.

Eating Technique

Clients who have had a bariatric procedure have described a process of "learning to eat all over again" immediately after the procedure. To prevent symptoms such as vomiting, discomfort, loose stools, or dumping syndrome, it is important for clients to adapt to their eating technique. Eating slowly is advantageous and behaviors such as allowing 20 seconds between each mouthful and putting cutlery down between each mouthful are advised. This also helps prevent overeating. Clients should be encouraged to allow themselves 20–30 min to have a meal, to prevent eating quickly. Additionally, it is recommended that distractions are avoided at meal times, e.g., eating in front of the television or while reading, again to prevent eating too quickly or overeating (mindless eating).

Clients are encouraged to chew their food well: up to 20 times per mouthful has been suggested. This helps clients to tolerate their food; it also slows down their consumption. Smaller portion sizes, eating off a small plate (approximately 17-20 cm in diameter), and stopping as soon as one feels full should be advised to prevent overeating. Portion size information is essential for clients post–bariatric surgery because of the reduced volume of food that one can tolerate; however, in practice the amount of food that a client may tolerate post–bariatric surgical procedure varies greatly. Therefore portion size information should be tailored to the individual client.

Dumping Syndrome

Dumping syndrome occurs when food moves from the stomach to the intestines too quickly. The body reacts to this by moving a large amount of fluid into the small intestine.[36] Dumping syndrome is common in clients following a malabsorptive bariatric procedure. Dumping syndrome is generally caused by eating foods high in sugar or fat, eating too quickly, and/or drinking and eating at the same time. Symptoms can vary but commonly include vomiting, loose stools, abdominal cramps, nausea, hot sweats and flushes, light headedness, and heart palpitations.[36] There is no medical treatment for Dumping syndrome; therefore clients are simply advised to avoid foods high in sugar and fat, to eat slowly, and not to eat and drink at the same time. Some clinicians may refer to this as "early dumping syndrome."

Late Dumping Syndrome

Late Dumping syndrome occurs when there is a rapid movement of sugar into the intestine and bloodstream. This causes a quick increase in blood glucose levels, which in turn triggers the pancreas to produce insulin. In late Dumping syndrome, too much insulin is produced to deal with the blood glucose and consequently hypoglycemia occurs.[36] Late Dumping syndrome may be referred to as "reactive hypoglycemia" by some clinicians because it can occur 2–3 h after eating. The main symptoms of late Dumping syndrome are hypoglycemia, sweating, weakness, rapid or irregular heartbeat, flushing, and dizziness.[36] Dietary modification is the main treatment for late Dumping syndrome. It is advised that clients consume lower-GI carbohydrates (sometimes referred to as complex carbohydrates), such as whole grains and wholemeal alternatives, sweet potato, pasta, instead of higher-GI carbohydrates (sometimes called refined carbohydrates), e.g., potatoes, white bread, high-sugar breakfast cereals. The dietary advice for those with early dumping syndrome may also benefit those with late dumping syndrome.

Fluid

Clients are encouraged to drink 2 L of fluid per day following a bariatric procedure. In practice, it is often difficult for people to meet fluid requirements after surgery. This is likely to be due to the reduced stomach capacity; therefore clients are unable to drink large volumes at one time. Patients are often encouraged to drink from a sports bottle or a straw to prevent "gulping." Clients should not drink 30 min before or after a meal to prevent malnutrition and dumping syndrome. Carbonated drinks should be avoided because they can create discomfort.

Protein

Education should be provided on dietary sources of protein because clients are encouraged to eat 60–80 g of protein per day.[37] To prevent inadequate protein intake, clients are encouraged to first eat the protein component of their meal. It is common for clients to have difficulty swallowing and digesting red meat and poultry post–bariatric surgery. Education should be provided on alternate sources of protein, such as fish, eggs, beans, and pulses, or different cooking methods, such as slow-cooked casseroles to soften the texture. Clients also tend to find the addition of sauces and condiments, such as gravy and tomato, make foods easier to swallow.

Vitamins and Minerals Supplementation

It is recommended that clients take two A-Z multivitamin and mineral supplements per day lifelong post–bariatric procedure.[38] Two supplements are recommended because the content of A-Z multivitamins and minerals vary and, additionally, to compensate for the reduced intake and malabsorptive effect of some bariatric procedures. Compliance with nutritional supplements is usually sufficient to keep trace elements (such as iron, zinc, copper, and selenium) within healthy parameters; however, adherence may wane over time. It is therefore important that clients who have had procedures such as a duodenal switch, a Roux-en-Y gastric bypass (RYGB), or a single anastomosis loop gastric bypass have their blood checked regularly: this is most commonly completed annually.

Calcium and Vitamin D

Calcium, vitamin D, and parathyroid hormone should be monitored annually following a bariatric procedure because of being at a greater risk of metabolic bone disease. Clients who have a malabsorptive bariatric procedure are more likely to suffer from vitamin D and calcium deficiency because calcium is absorbed in the duodenum and proximal jejunum and vitamin D in the jejunum and ileum (see Fig. 30.4). Parathyroid hormone should be monitored annually for hyperparathyroidism because blood calcium levels may be within normal parameters because of calcium mobilization from bone rather than from adequate nutrition.[39]

Education should be provided on dietary sources of calcium and vitamin D, and clients should be informed that our main source of vitamin D is from exposure to sunlight. A daily vitamin D and calcium supplement should be prescribed to prevent deficiencies in addition to the A-Z multivitamin and mineral supplements.

B12 Injection

Clients who have had a surgical bariatric procedure receive an intramuscular 1 mg B12 injection every 3 months.[38] There are limited high doses of oral vitamin B12 available on prescription.[38] Some bariatric teams only recommend B12 injections following malabsorptive surgical procedures.

Vitamin B12 deficiency occurs for two main reasons. Firstly, a reduced contact with stomach acid due to a smaller stomach and prescription of a proton pump inhibitor reduces the production of stomach acid, consequently reducing the release of B12 from protein food sources.

Secondly, vitamin B12 would normally bind with intrinsic factor in the stomach to aid its absorption in the intestines. The area of the stomach that produces intrinsic factor is bypassed in bariatric surgery; therefore less B12 is absorbed in the intestines.

Iron

Clients who have had a surgical bariatric procedure are at risk of iron deficiency, particularly following an RYGB, because iron is mostly absorbed in the duodenum and proximal jejunum. For clients who have had a surgical bariatric procedure, it is recommended that an iron supplement is taken in addition to the A-Z multivitamin and mineral supplement. Iron tablets should be taken alongside citrus fruits or drinks as vitamin C aids absorption. Iron supplements and a calcium supplements should not be taken at the same time, optimum at least 2 h apart.[38]

It is advised that menstruating women have 100 mg additional requirement of iron.[38]

A good diet and oral nutritional supplements are sometimes insufficient to meet a client's nutritional requirements. In addition, compliance with a diet rich in iron and supplement consumption may also be poor. In these circumstances an iron infusion would need to be considered.

Pregnancy

Clients are encouraged not to become pregnant for at least 18 months following bariatric surgery. Clients are encouraged to follow standard pre- and postconception advice and to change their A-Z multivitamin and mineral supplement to a pregnancy-based multivitamin and mineral supplement to prevent intake of too much vitamin A. They are encouraged to continue to follow a healthy balanced diet to ensure adequate nutrition.

Weight Loss

Most weight loss occurs in the first 12 months following surgery, with maximum weight loss being reached 18–24 months following the bariatric procedure.[41] Weight loss from bariatric procedures is expressed as percentage loss of excess body weight. Excess body weight is defined as weight in excess of body weight that is equivalent to a BMI of 25 kg/m^2 for a specific client.

$$\text{Height } (m)^2 \times 25 = \text{healthy body weight (kg)}$$

$$\text{Body weight pre–bariatric surgery} - \text{healthy body weight} = \text{excess body weight}$$

$$\frac{\text{Weight lost following bariatric surgery}}{\text{Excess body weight}} \times 100 = \% \text{ loss of excess body weight}$$

Depending on the bariatric procedure performed, an excess body weight loss of between 10% and >70% can be expected. It should be emphasized to clients that bariatric procedures are a tool to aid weight loss and without continued appropriate lifestyle behaviors weight regain can occur.

Follow-up

Following a bariatric procedure, many bariatric teams offer a 2 year follow-up as standard. General practitioners will often be requested to continue annual follow-up and monitor following discharge.

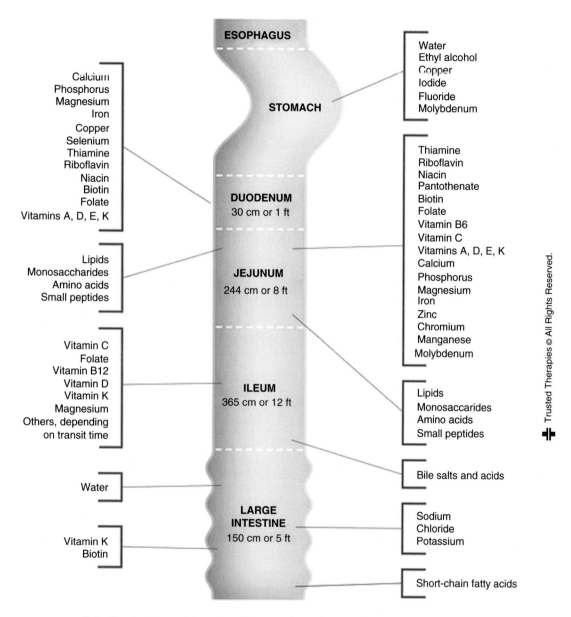

Note: The duodenum, jejunum, and ileum make up the small intestine.

FIG. 30.4 Illustration of the site of absorption of nutrients in the gastrointestinal tract. (From Bressler B, Charlebois A. Meeting Energy and Nutrient Needs With Crohn's Disease. https://www.trustedtherapies.com /articles/14-meeting-energy-and-nutrient-needs-with-crohn-s-disease.)

SUMMARY AND CONCLUSIONS

It is clear that diet is an important factor in the cause and management of obesity; therefore it must be addressed for effective weight management. However, because of the complex nature of obesity, dietary intervention should not be the sole form of treatment. An MDT is highly beneficial when helping a client to address the issue of obesity and make long-term changes. A weight management clinician specializing in dietary interventions for weight loss will often be more effective in helping clients to lose weight when working in conjunction with medical, psychologic, and physiotherapy input.

As can be seen in this chapter, there are many evidence-based dietary interventions available to help people to achieve healthy weight loss and weight loss maintenance. Adherence to an evidence-based dietary intervention is the most important predictor of weight loss. Therefore the best evidence-based dietary intervention is the one that a client makes an educated choice to adhere to.[3,4] Dietary changes are also necessary pre–bariatric surgery and post–bariatric surgery to ensure the long-term weight loss and maintenance of clients choosing this line of treatment.

REFERENCES

1. Webber KH, Lee E. The diet quality of adult women participating in a behavioural weight-loss programme. *J Hum Nutr Diet.* 2011;24:360–369.
2. Gardner CD, Kim S, Bersamin A, et al. Micronutrient quality of weight-loss diets that focus on macronutrients: results from the A TO Z study. *Am J Clin Nutr.* 2010;92:304–312.
3. Bray GA. Lifestyle and pharmacological approaches to weight loss: efficacy and safety. *J Clin Endocrinol Metab.* 2008;93(11 suppl 1):S81–S88.
4. Drummond S. Obesity: a diet that is acceptable is more likely to succeed. *J Fam Health Care.* 2007;17(6):219–221.
5. National Obesity Observatory. *Dietary Surveillance and Nutritional Assessment in England: What Is Measured and Where Are the Gaps?* 2010.
6. Nelson M, Erens B, Bates B, Church S, Boshier T. *Low Income Diet and Nutrition Survey – Summary of Key Findings.* Norwich: TSO; 2007.
7. Thompson FE, Subur AF. Dietary assessment methodology. In: Coulston AM, Bouchey CJ, eds. *Nutrition in the Prevention of Treatment and Disease.* London: Elsevier; 2008:3–22.
8. Mares-Perlman JA, Klein BE, Klein R, et al. A diet history questionnaire ranks nutrient intakes in middle-aged and older men and women similarly to multiple food records. *J Nutr.* 1993;123(3):489–501.
9. Miller W, Rollnick S. *Motivational Interviewing: Preparing People to Change Addictive Behaviour.* London: Guildford Press; 1991.
10. Flechtner-Mors M, Ditschuneit HH, Johnson TD, et al. Metabolic and weight loss effects of long-term dietary intervention in obese patients: four-year results. *Obes Res.* 2000;8(5):399–402.
11. Li Z, Saltman P, DeShields S, Bellman M, et al. Long-term efficacy of soy-based meal replacements vs. an individual diet plan in obese type 2 diabetes mellitus patients: relative effects on weight loss, metabolic parameters, and C-reactive protein. *Eur J Clin Nutr.* 2005;59:411–418.
12. König D, Deibert P, Frey I, et al. Effect of meal replacement on metabolic risk factors in overweight and obese subjects. *Ann Nutr Metab.* 2008;52(1):74–78.
13. Wadden TA, West DS, Neiberg RH, et al. One-year weight losses in the Look AHEAD study: factors associated with success. *Obes.* 2009;17:713–722.
14. Konig D, Muser K, Berg A, et al. Fuel selection and appetite-regulating hormones after intake of a soy protein-based meal replacement. *Nutr.* 2012;28(1):35–39.
15. National Institute for Health and Care Excellence. *Obesity: Identification, Assessment and Management CG189.* Available at: https://www.nice.org.uk/guidance/cg189/chapter/1-Recommendations; 2014. Accessed October 27, 2016.
16. Steven S, Hollingsworth KG, Al-Mrabeh A, et al. Very low-calorie diet and 6 months of weight stability in type 2 diabetes: pathophysiological changes in responders and nonresponders. *Diabetes Care.* 2016;39(5):808–815.
17. Lim EL, Hollingsworth KG, Aribisala BS, et al. Reversal of type 2 diabetes: normalisation of beta cell function in association with decreased pancreas and liver triacylglycerol. *Diabetologia.* 2011;54(10):2506–2514.
18. Steven S, Lim EL, Taylor R. Population response to information on reversibility of type 2 diabetes. *Diabet Med.* 2013;30(4):e135–e138.
19. Sellahewa L, Khan C, Lakkunarajah S, et al. A systematic review of evidence on the use of very low calorie diets in people with diabetes. *Curr Diabetes Rev.* 2015.
20. Harvie MN, Pegington M, Mattson MP, et al. The effects of intermittent or continuous energy restriction on weight loss and metabolic disease risk markers: a randomised trial in young overweight women. *Int J Obes Lond.* 2011;35(5):714–727.
21. Brehm BJ, D'Alessio DA, et al. Benefits of high-protein weight loss diets: enough evidence for practice? *Cur Opin Endocrinol Diabetes Obes.* 2008;15(5):416–421.
22. Wycherley TP, Moran LJ, Clifton PM, et al. Effects of energy-restricted high-protein, low-fat compared with standard-protein, low-fat diets: a meta-analysis of randomized controlled trials 1–3. *Am J Clin Nutr.* 2012;96(6):1281–1298.
23. Larsen TM, Dalskov SM, van Baak M, et al. Diets with high or low protein content and glycemic index for weight-loss maintenance. *N Engl J Med.* November 25, 2010;363(22):2102–2113.
24. Zauner C, Schneeweiss B, Kranz A, et al. Resting energy expenditure in short-term starvation is increased as a result of an increase in serum norepinephrine. *Am J Clin Nutr.* 2000;71(6):1511–1515.
25. Mansell PI, Fellows IW, Macdonald IA. Enhanced thermogenic response to epinephrine after 48-h starvation in humans. *Am J Physiol.* 1990;258(1 pt 2):R87–R93.
26. Barnosky AR, Hoddy KK, Unterman TG, et al. Intermittent fasting vs daily calorie restriction for type 2 diabetes prevention: a review of human findings. *Transl Res.* 2014;164(4):302–311.
27. Varady KA. Intermittent versus daily calorie restriction: which diet regimen is more effective for weight loss? *Obes Rev.* 2011;12(7):e593–e601.
28. Sarwer DB, Wadden TA, Moore RH, et al. Preoperative eating behaviour, postoperative dietary adherence, and weight loss after gastric bypass surgery. *Surg Obes Relat Dis.* 2008;4(5):640–646.

29. Lefebvre P, Letois F, Sultan A, et al. Nutrient deficiencies in patients with obesity considering bariatric surgery: a cross-sectional study. *Surg Obes Relat Dis.* 2014;10(3):540–546.

30. De Luis DA, Pacheco D, Izaola O, et al. Micronutrient status in morbidly obese women before bariatric surgery. *Surg Obes Relat Dis.* 2013;9(2):323–328.

31. Grace C, Vincent R, Aylwin SJ. High prevalence of vitamin D insufficiency in a United Kingdom urban morbidly obese population: implications for testing and treatment. *Surg Obes Relat Dis.* 2014;10:355–360.

32. Gottig S, Weiner RA, Daskalakis M. Preoperative weight reduction using the intragastric balloon. *Obes Facts.* 2009;2(suppl 1):20–23.

33. British Obesity Surgery Patient Association. *Intragastric Balloon.* Available at: http://www.bospa.org/Information _Page_8.html; 2014. Accessed November 7th, 2016..

34. Colles SL, Dixon JB, Marks P, et al. Preoperative weight loss with a very-low-energy diet: quantitation of changes in liver and abdominal fat by serial imaging. *Am J Clin Nutr.* 2006;84:304–311.

35. Kissler HJ, Settmacher U. Bariatric surgery to treat obesity. *Semin Nephrol.* 2013;33(1):75–89.

36. National Institute of Diabetes and Digestive and Kidney Diseases. *Dumping Syndrome.* https://www.niddk.nih.gov/ health-information/digestive-diseases/dumping-syndrome; 2013. Accessed January 6th, 2017.

37. Aills L, Blankenship J, Buffington C, et al. ASMBS allied health nutritional guidelines for the surgical weight loss patient. *Surg Obes Relat Dis.* 2008;4:S73–S108.

38. BOMSS British Obesity and Metabolic Surgery Society. BOMSS Guidelines on Peri-Operative and Postoperative Biochemical Monitoring and Micronutrient Replacement for Patients Undergoing Bariatric Surgery. http://www. bomss.org.uk/wp-content/uploads/2014/09/BOMSS-guide-lines-Final-version1Oct14.pdf. Accessed January 13th, 2017.

39. Slater GH, Ren CJ, Seigel N, et al. Serum fat soluble vitamin deficiency and abnormal calcium metabolism after malabsorptive bariatric surgery. *J Gastrointest Surg.* 2004;8:48–55.

40. Bressler B, Charlebois A. Meeting Energy and Nutrient Needs With Crohn's Disease. https://www.trustedtherapies .com/articles/14-meeting-energy-and-nutrient-needs-with-crohn-s-disease. Accessed January 13th, 2017.

41. Pinnock G, O'Kane M. Bariatric surgery. In: Gandy J, ed. *Manual of Dietetic Practice.* 5th ed. Wiley-Blackwell; 2014.

CHAPTER 31

The Future of Obesity Medicine

JOLANTA U. WEAVER, MRCS, MRCP, FRCP, PHD, CTLHE

The heterogeneity of the physical appearance in obesity and its association with various endocrine disorders has led some clinicians and almost every patient with obesity to believe that there was an underlying hormonal imbalance to account for their problem. It is for this reason that endocrinologists are frequently consulted to advice on the possible underlying diagnosis for a secondary obesity. The term "secondary" means that the obesity accompanies another illness that is considered to be the primary disease state.

DISEASE STATES ASSOCIATED WITH OBESITY

Secondary morbid obesity (body mass index [BMI] ≥40) due to endocrine causes is quite rare and is usually associated with hypothalamic disorders. Lesser degrees of a weight problem (BMI 26–39) may be associated with thyroid disorders, polycystic ovarian syndrome (PCOS), or Cushing's syndrome/disease.

An appropriate assessment is the first step in developing a treatment plan for overweight patients. A medical history is paramount to evaluate the history of the development of obesity and the etiological factors involved. The physical examination and laboratory testing should extend this evaluation to exclude treatable endocrine causes. The results of this evaluation then provide a guide to selecting an appropriate treatment plan if required.

HYPOTHYROIDISM

Although one of the symptoms of hypothyroidism is weight gain, most patients with obesity have normal thyroid function tests. Dr. Angelos has clearly explained in Chapter 5 that although weight gain occurs in hypothyroidism, the reverse relation between obesity and thyroid hormones does not apply. Excessive thyroid hormone therapy is associated with loss of lean body mass; thus it is

detrimental to future weight maintenance. Lean mass is required for maintaining a sufficient metabolic rate responsible for calorie loss. Thus therapy with excessive thyroid hormones will be counterproductive and have a detrimental effect because it will cause loss of lean body mass and promote obesity in addition to increasing the risk of atrial fibrillation and osteoporosis.

Care should be taken not to mistake central hypothyroidism (low T4, low T3, inappropriately normal or slightly raised TSH) for primary hypothyroidism (low T4, low T3, and significantly raised TSH).[1] The treatment of central hypothyroidism with thyroxine before excluding hypothalamic-pituitary-adrenal axis axis deficiency may lead to an Addisonian crisis (acute cortisol deficiency).

An interpretation of thyroid function test results is provided in Table 31.1.

POLYCYSTIC OVARIAN SYNDROME

PCOS is a very common endocrine problem occurring in up to 10% of premenopausal women.[2] It is by far the most complex endocrine disorder associated with obesity. The diagnosis of PCOS is made by excluding nonclassic adrenal hyperplasia, androgen-secreting tumors, Cushing's syndrome or Cushings disease, and hyperprolactinemia. PCOS is viewed as a heterogeneous disorder of multifactorial etiology.

Both simple obesity and PCOS-associated obesity are characterized by the endogenous mechanisms of limiting exposure to cortisol by reducing cortisol generation from cortisone.

Two key enzymes are involved in the metabolism of cortisol: 11β-hydroxysteroid dehydrogenase type 1 (11β-HSD1), which converts cortisone to cortisol, and 5α-reductase, which catabolizes cortisol in addition to converting testosterone to dihydrotestosterone.[3,4] The more central obesity an individual has, the less cortisone is converted to cortisol, thus providing a

TABLE 31.1
Laboratory Investigations for Suspected Hypothyroidism

TSH, Free T4	TPO Antibodies	Diagnosis
TSH <0.4 mU/L FT4 low/low normal	–/+	Posthyperthyroid hypothyroidism
TSH 0.4–4.0 mU/L FT4 low	–	Central hypothyroidism
TSH >4 and <10 mU/L FT4 normal/low	–/+	Subclinical hypothyroidism Early primary autoimmune hypothyroidism Central hypothyroidism
TSH >10 mU/L FT4 low	+	Primary hypothyroidism due to autoimmune thyroid disease
TSH >10 mU/L FT4 low/low-normal	–	Intercurrent illness, drug-induced external radiation, iodine deficiency
TSH >10 nmol/L FT4 normal/elevated	–/+	Thyroid hormone resistance, drugs Assay artifact

FT4, free thyroxine; *TPO*, thyroid peroxidase antibodies; *TSH*, thyrotropin stimulating hormone.

negative feedback loop for the generation of cortisol and adipogenesis.

Two Chapters (Chapters 6 and 12) of this book provide a detailed outline of the management of PCOS. It suffices to say that PCOS continues to be a challenge to patients (need for exercise and weight loss to improve insulin resistance), clinicians, and researchers.

CUSHING'S DISEASE OR SYNDROME

Obese patients may present an opportunity for the early diagnosis of Cushing's disease or syndrome. This requires a high level of clinical suspicion because the patient may not display all the typical symptoms or signs. Awaiting a textbook presentation of Cushing's as first described by Harvey Cushing in 1932 consisting of the constellation of symptoms of obesity, hirsutism, and amenorrhea and attributed to a primary pituitary abnormality associated with

adrenal hyperplasia, is likely to lead to a delayed diagnosis. The most discriminating symptoms and signs of Cushing's disease/syndrome are bruising, muscle weakness, skin thinning, plethora, and truncal obesity. The symptoms and signs of *Cushing's syndrome* arise as a result of prolonged exposure to excessive levels of free cortisol levels, either endogenous cortisol or exogenous cortisol (iatrogenic Cushing's syndrome), due to prednisolone, dexamethasone, or various types of topical and inhaled steroids. A summary of investigations for excluding endogenous cortisol excess and the differential diagnosis is provided in Table 31.2.

Because very few investigations for Cushing's syndrome have 100% sensitivity and specificity, endocrine expertise combined with clinical experience is essential for the correct diagnosis of Cushing's disease/syndrome.

HYPOTHALAMIC OBESITY

Acquired obesity not present from infancy, coupled with headache, a growth disorder, or other growth dysfunction, requires investigations for hypothalamic/pituitary disease. It is associated with severe hyperphagia and is described in further detail in Chapter 15.

One can conclude that obesity due to endocrine causes is not as common as perceived by patients and some physicians. However, because the effective treatment of less common underlying endocrine causes is available, the clinical management of patients with obesity should include appropriate screening for endocrine conditions, which may be amenable to pharmacological treatment.

Having excluded endocrine causes of obesity, one is invariably challenged how to proceed further.

NEXT STEP

Many of us regulate our own weight by various methods; therefore we never get to the stage of having an abnormal BMI. The triggers for our behavior are very individual and frequently personal, and the methods we use to achieve our normal weight vary. However, only those who fail to regulate their weight end up being referred to health care professionals (HCPs) for advice regarding their BMI. When advice is being sought from an HCP the patient usually presents late and have obesity (BMI >30). Assistance from an HCP is very useful for identifying the potential triggers to initiate a change in behavior. This may include a variety of reasons identified during the consultation, but the

TABLE 31.2
Diagnostic Tests for the Investigations of Cushing's Disease

Screening for Glucocorticoid Excess	Application	Sensitivity/Specificity %[a]
Spot urine cortisol/creatinine ratio	Ambulatory	85–92/95
24-h urinary free cortisol (2–3×)	Ambulatory	85–92/95
Overnight 1 mg dex suppression test (F < 50 nmol/L)	Ambulatory	100/82
Low-dose dexamethasone suppression test	Ambulatory	95/99
Midnight cortisol >200 nm/L	In-patient	90/100
DIFFERENTIAL DIAGNOSIS		
9 a.m. plasma ACTH (Cushing's disease)	Ambulatory	50/70
ACTH >5 pmol/L at midnight (ACTH dependent)	In-patient	100/99
Plasma potassium, bicarbonate (ectopic ACTH)	Ambulatory	95/90
High-dose dex suppression test (Cushing's disease)	Ambulatory	90/100[b]
High-dose dex suppression test (ectopic ACTH)	Ambulatory	50/95
CRH test (Cushing's disease)	Ambulatory	90/90
CRH test (exclude ectopic ACTH)	Ambulatory	100/100[c]
Imaging pituitary and adrenal (MRI)	Ambulatory	80/78
Imaging pituitary and adrenal (CT)	Ambulatory	20–60/78
Inferior petrosal sinus sampling	In-patient	97/100

[a]Sensitivity and specificity values calculated from data provided in Ref. 5.
[b]90% suppression of urinary basal cortisol.
[c]100% rise in ACTH and 50% rise in cortisol excludes ectopic ACTH.
ACTH, adrenocorticotropic hormone; *CT*, computed tomography; *dex*, dexamethasone; *F*, cortisol; *MRI*, magnetic resonance imagining.

common ones are infertility, hirsutism, arthritis, cholesterol, diabetes, asthma, sleep apnea, hypertension, heart attack, cancer, and liver disease. This list is not exclusive.

New research discussed in this book (Chapter 17) highlights the reasons why many individuals gravitate to abnormal BMI without noticing. In the Western world, particularly in countries with a high prevalence of obesity individuals no longer recognize their own weight problem because the majority of people around are overweight or obese. Consequently, the individual feels this is normal and underestimates his/her weight. This misconception is not just unique to overweight/obese patients but also to parents of obese children and healthcare professionals, who fail to recognize a weight problem in their patients as discussed in the Chapter 17 on Visual Biases in Estimating Body Size. Equally, it is common that patients frequently report that they lost some weight and then they must have regained it without realizing it. Simple solutions can be promoted and include a regular recording of weight and/or a physical solution as suggested by John Garrow (personal communication). He provided patients with nylon waist cord that did not stretch and was difficult to cut. When the patient started regaining weight, the discomfort from the cord signaled to the patient that his/her weight had changed. Homemade obesity solutions may include wearing a tight belt or tight trousers (without Lycra). Such physical solutions, however, require a change in behavior: it is all too easy to wear loose clothes or buy the next size up.

Society has turned to constantly ruminating behavior. The food industry is promoting their products under an umbrella of "individual choice." This includes exporting pop drinks to developing countries and promoting unhealthy lifestyles in these countries as they are in the Western world.

Consumption of ready-made meals with high fat and salt content and high-energy foods rich in sugar are on the increase, and they are frequently more expensive than the alternative, healthier options.

We frequently see in supermarkets, money-saving offers, "buy two pizzas for the price of one" but rarely see such initiatives for healthy foods such "buy two lettuces for the price of one."

New initiatives such as the sugar tax in the United Kingdom may change sugar consumption for some. It remains to be seen for the majority. Some good news is that food labeling has improved, but many obese individuals lack the basic literacy and numeracy skills to read and understand these labels and are unable to use a recipe to cook healthy food for themselves; therefore they resort to convenience and fast foods, high in fat and salt.

Promoting healthy behavior in schools, work canteens, and universities is likely to have a lifelong effect and bridge the perceived knowledge gap from a home upbringing.

There is an unmet need for more education on healthy eating from an early age and education of the whole family. Celebrity chefs such as Jamie Oliver, in the United Kingdom, have influenced the healthy food content of school meals and promoted healthy eating. However, there is still an imbalance in the media between cookery programs and "get fit" programs.

There is also frantic media interest in magic weight loss cures; therefore the public is constantly bombarded with conflicting misinformation about the causes, consequences, and cures for their weight problem. Press releases on the research findings of these "cures" are frequently exaggerated to increase the sales of newspapers, thus misguiding readers. In our book we provide evidence-based advice on diets, in addition to various weight-reducing programs.

In accordance with the first law of thermodynamics, obesity results from a state of positive energy balance in which energy intake exceeds energy expenditure over a prolonged period of time. Long-standing advice exists that by eating breakfast one can prevent obesity.

Dr. Gonzalez, in his eloquent Chapter 22, provides evidence that the calorie intake associated with breakfast although will induce postprandial thermogenesis may not provide calorie deficit when compared with missed breakfast calorie intake (Chapter 22). There is clearly more research to come.

In the past 50 years, it was noted that the obesity epidemic has been paralleled by a concomitant shortening of sleep duration with an increase in the prevalence of obstructive sleep apnea (OSA). More recently, a cross-sectional study identified an inverse relationship between length of sleep and calorie intake. A deficit in sleep duration of 30-min per day was translated to approximately 83 kcal/day increase in energy intake. In addition, OSA was associated with a shift from carbohydrate to fat intake. Furthermore, alcohol intake was equally inversely related to sleep duration.[6] Although sleep is our most sedentary behavior, it, paradoxically, may protect us from obesity. A metaanalysis of 18 studies in 604,509 adults demonstrated a pooled obesity odds ratio of 1.55 (1.43–1.68; $P < .0001$) for less than 5 h of sleep and a dose effect of sleep duration such that for each additional hour of sleep, the BMI decreased by 0.35 kg/m².[7] The results of sleep extension interventional studies are still awaited.

One of the problems in society is that our general socializing activities involve food. This has always been a case, but the issue now lies in the calorie-dense food, which lands on our plate and not always by choice. Because the obesogenic environment includes modalities to improve our lives (cars, shopping trolleys, shopping online, escalators, suitcases on wheels, automatic doors, electric mowers, to name a few), the current calorie intake is no longer used for daily activities. Some individuals still think, "Why should I walk if I can afford a car."

Society has started investing in gym facilities, providing cycle paths, etc., thus taking a step back to the lifestyle of the past. The challenge of energy-dense food to be remedied by exercise is provided in this book, with clear help in conceptualizing energy excess and how to battle it. "Those individuals seeking to lose weight or prevent weight regain over the long-term are advised to increase their exercise duration to 200-300 min per week.... For most individuals, this equates to expending over 2000 kcal/week (or over 400 kcal/session). To put this into perspective, most individuals would need to walk or jog 1 mile to expend 100 calories which is the same as consuming one slice of bread or 4 heaped tablespoons of sugar," say Dr. Campbell and Dr. Rutherford in this book (Chapter 20). Therefore the challenge is *on* for everyone aiming for a normal body weight. Exercise benefits are not just calorie loss but also socializing in a different way. Such an approach may not to be that daunting; however, it is very important to realize the penalty we may encounter for indulging in calorie-dense food on regular basis.

A multifaceted approach to obesity management is summarized in a graphic representation (Trigger wheel: Fig. 31.1) of the patient's obesity journey. The wheel can be redesigned according to the different facilities available to the individuals worldwide, but the principle is the same. Patients are likely to stick to the intervention they choose for themselves. Their choice of action for accessing help will vary during their journey with their weight problem. They may try different ways to regulate their weight.

In the United Kingdom alone, new healthy lifestyle initiatives are commissioned regularly to cope with chronic ill health, depression, diabetes, obesity, etc.

One of them is "social prescribing," defined as a service for advising patients on non-NHS matters in deprived communities such as Gateshead (where I practice medicine). The service educates disadvantaged patients on basic money matters, consumer laws, basic nutrition, practical cooking skills, shopping, etc., which are crucial for a healthy lifestyle.

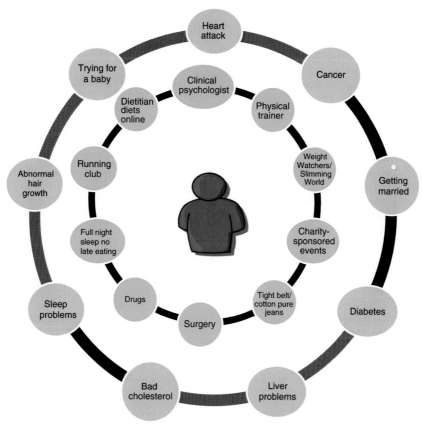

FIG. 31.1 A trigger wheel. The outer ring contains triggering factors for invoking behavioral change. The inner circle contains the methods for achieving the behavior change to cause weight loss.

Most obese people decline referrals to the dietitian or an exercise program: despite their familiarity with this health education advice they still struggle to achieve weight loss because they are using food to deal with personal stress, low mood, tiredness, inappropriate reward, and to solve other "nonhunger" problems.

The "Foresight Report" (UK Government Office of Science, 2007 https://www.gov.uk/government/publications/reducing-obesity-future-choices) indicates that two-thirds of individuals regain the weight they have lost on traditional weight management plans within 1–5 years. Psychologically based approaches to weight management, including mindfulness, cognitive behavioral therapy, dialectical, compassionate, and solution-focused approaches, are necessary for long-term avoidance of weight gain as discussed in this book by Dr. Johnston and coauthors.

A psychologic assessment is likely to identify the multifactorial etiology of obesity. To encourage this line of management, it is vitally important to engage patients in agreeing to seek this help. In this book, examples of "change talk" are provided to overcome the barrier of seeking help from a clinical psychologist. This year's workshop at Diabetes UK National Conference on "nonhunger eating" introduced an Internet-based support for individuals with weight problems available at www.EatingBlueprint.com, which is part of www.successfuldiabetes.com. Motivational interviewing is likely to help patients to take this very step toward unpacking the complex behavior that underlines their problem because their weight gain is not necessarily about food. Human behavior is very complex. The triggers for change vary between different individuals. Our preference for an adopted lifestyle also varies between a stricter diet to doing more exercise, things we will give up, and things that we will not. Our health beliefs and expectations vary. The presence of a family history of premature heart disease for some may be a *faint accompli*, whereas for others it is the reason to undertake exercise and a healthy diet. Many obese patients are constantly looking somewhere else and not within themselves for easier weight loss solution: better drugs or better surgery. However, the most exciting part of being a practicing clinician is that each patient is a mystery until we get to know them better through unpacking their complex behavior, establishing what motivates them and what they are afraid of? Sowing the seeds of self-management can reap lasting benefits for the individual and society. Let us appreciate more the clinical psychologist's skills by practicing *change talk* with patients so that they will be more likely to accept their referrals to behavioral scientists to make life-long lifestyle changes. Behavioral experts with knowhow and experience in motivational techniques can successfully nudge people to initiate and maintain healthy lifestyles. They should be the new professionals providing the lead on obesity management. The future of Obesity Medicine belongs to behavioral scientists.

REFERENCES

1. Khatami Z, Handley G, Brandon H, Weaver J. Borderline thyroid function tests: so easy to look at, so hard to define. *Ann Clin Biochem*. 2006;43(Pt 1):77–79.
2. Asuncion M, Calvo RM, San Millan JL, Sancho J, Avila S, Escobar-Morreale HF. A prospective study of the prevalence of the polycystic ovary syndrome in unselected Caucasian women from Spain. *J Clin Endocrinol Metab*. 2000;85(7):2434–2438.
3. Andrew R, Phillips DI, Walker BR. Obesity and gender influence cortisol secretion and metabolism in man. *J Clin Endocrinol Metab*. 1998;83(5):1806–1809.
4. Weaver JU, Taylor NF, Monson JP, Wood PJ, Kelly WF. Sexual dimorphism in 11 beta hydroxysteroid dehydrogenase activity and its relation to fat distribution and insulin sensitivity; a study in hypopituitary subjects. *Clin Endocrinol (Oxf)*. 1998;49(1):13–20.
5. Stewart PM. The adrenal cortex. In: Wilson JD, Foster DW, eds. *William's Textbook of Endocrinology*. 10th ed. Philadelphia: WB Saunders Co; 2003:357–487.
6. Galli G, Piaggi P, Mattingly MS, et al. Inverse relationship of food and alcohol intake to sleep measures in obesity. *Nutr Diabetes*. 2013;3. e58.
7. Cappuccio FP, D'Elia L, Strazzullo P, Miller MA. Sleep duration and all-cause mortality: a systematic review and meta-analysis of prospective studies. *Sleep*. 2010;33(5):585–592.

Index

'*Note*: Page numbers followed by "f" indicate figures, "t" indicate tables, and "b" indicate boxes.'

335